Essential Haematology

FIFTH EDITION

Essential Haematology

A.V. Hoffbrand

MA DM FRCP FRCPath FRCP(Edin) DSc FMED Sci
Emeritus Professor of Haematology, Royal Free
and University College Medical School, London

P.A.H. Moss

PhD FRCP FRCPath
Professor of Haematology,
University of Birmingham

J.E. Pettit

MD FRCPA FRCPath
Haematologist, Medlab South,
Christchurch, New Zealand

Blackwell
Publishing

Published by Blackwell Publishing Ltd
Blackwell Publishing, Inc., 350 Main Street, Malden, Massachusetts 02148-5020, USA
Blackwell Publishing Ltd, 9600 Garsington Road, Oxford OX4 2DQ, UK
Blackwell Publishing Asia Pty Ltd, 550 Swanston Street, Carlton, Victoria 3053, Australia

First published 1980
Reprinted 1981, 1982, 1983 (twice)
Second edition 1984
Reprinted 1985
Reprinted with corrections 1985, 1988 (twice), 1989
German edition 1986 (reprinted 1996)
Japanese edition 1986
Spanish edition 1987 (reprinted twice)
Indonesian edition 1987
Third edition 1993
Hungarian edition 1997
Chinese edition 1998
Reprinted with corrections 1993, 1994, 1995, 1996, 1997, 1998, 1999, 2000
Fourth edition 2001
Fifth edition 2006

3 2008

Library of Congress Cataloging-in-Publication Data

Hoffbrand, A.V.
Essential haematology / A.V. Hoffbrand, P.A.H. Moss, and J.E. Pettit. — 5th ed.
p. ; cm.
Includes bibliographical references.
ISBN 978-1-4051-3649-5 (alk. paper)

1. Blood—Diseases. 2. Hematology. I. Moss, P.A.H. II. Pettit, J.E. III. Title.
[DNLM: 1. Hematologic Diseases. WH 120 H698e 2006]

RC633.H627 2006
616.1′5—dc22

2006016791

A catalogue record for this title is available from the British Library

Set in 9/12pt Palatino by Graphicraft Limited, Hong Kong
Printed and bound by Fabulous Printers Pte Ltd, Singapore

Commissioning Editor: Martin Sugden
Development Editor: Rebecca Huxley
Production Controller: Kate Charman

For further information on Blackwell Publishing, visit our website:
http://www.blackwellpublishing.com

The publisher's policy is to use permanent paper from mills that operate a sustainable forestry policy, and which has been manufactured from pulp processed using acid-free and elementary chlorine-free practices. Furthermore, the publisher ensures that the text paper and cover board used have met acceptable environmental accreditation standards.

Contents

Preface to the fifth edition

Major advances in the understanding at a molecular level of the genetic changes underlying many inherited and acquired haematological disorders have necessitated revisions in many chapters for this new edition. The introduction of new diagnostic laboratory tests and imaging techniques for diagnosis and monitoring of malignant blood disorders and the major changes in their therapy has required expansion of these sections with many new figures. Chapters on principles of treatment and support care and on the spleen have been added while Hodgkin's disease and the non-Hodgkin's lymphomas are now given separate chapters. The greatly increased knowledge of iron absorption, metabolism and iron loading diseases is recognized by allocating increased space to these topics. In order to keep the book as concise as possible, topics that are now no longer in routine practice have been omitted (e.g. radioactive chromium red cell survival studies and immunofluorescent microscopy).

Essential Haematology is intended for medical students but we realize there is more information than most medical students can be expected to know, given the new knowledge in all areas of medicine. We have therefore indicated by means of vertical blue lines in the margins, material that we consider more suitable for honours candidates and for postgraduates, leaving unmarked core material appropriate for medical students taking final examinations. We hope, therefore, that this new edition provides 'two books', one more basic, the other more advanced. We hope the book will be used as previously, by science graduates, medical laboratory technicians and general physicians, indeed all those wishing to learn about the exciting topic of the blood and its diseases.

As previously, we are grateful to Rebecca Huxley for her expert help during the publishing process and to Jane Fallows for the beautiful clear scientific diagrams which illustrate the text throughout. We are also grateful to Dr Clare Taylor for advice in Chapters 27 and 28, and Dr Pratima Chowdary for advice on Chapters 22–25. We also wish to thank Blackwell Publishing for their continuing support for this book since it was first published in 1980.

Sir John Dacie, FRS was mentor to AVH and JEP, and Per Saugman, Chairman of Blackwell Scientific Publications commissioned the First Edition of *Essential Haematology*. Both sadly died during the last year. We wish to dedicate this fifth edition of *Essential Haematology* to their memory.

A.V. Hoffbrand, P.A.H. Moss and J.E. Pettit
September 2006

Preface to the first edition

The major changes that have occurred in all fields of medicine over the last decade have been accompanied by an increased understanding of the biochemical, physiological and immunological processes involved in normal blood cell formation and function and the disturbances that may occur in different diseases. At the same time, the range of treatment available for patients with diseases of the blood and blood-forming organs has widened and improved substantially as understanding of the disease processes has increased and new drugs and means of support care have been introduced.

We hope the present book will enable the medical student of the 1980s to grasp the essential features of modern clinical and laboratory haematology and to achieve an understanding of how many of the manifestations of blood diseases can be explained with this new knowledge of the disease processes.

We would like to thank many colleagues and assistants who have helped with the preparation of the book. In particular, Dr H.G. Prentice cared for the patients whose haematological responses are illustrated in Figs 5.3 and 7.8 and Dr J. McLaughlin supplied Fig. 8.6. Dr S. Knowles reviewed critically the final manuscript and made many helpful suggestions. Any remaining errors are, however, our own. We also thank Mr J.B. Irwin and R.W. McPhee who drew many excellent diagrams, Mr Cedric Gilson for expert photomicrography, Mrs T. Charalambos, Mrs B. Elliot, Mrs M. Evans and Miss J. Allaway for typing the manuscript, and Mr Tony Russell of Blackwell Scientific Publications for his invaluable help and patience.

AVH, JEP

Bibliography

Arceci R.J., Hann I.M., Smith O.P. (eds) (2006) *Pediatric Hematology*, 3rd edn. Blackwell Publishing Ltd, Oxford.

Bain B.J. (2005) *A Beginner's Guide to Blood Cells*, 2nd edn. Blackwell Publishing, Oxford.

Bain B.J., Clark D.M., Lampert I.A., Wilkins B.S. (2001) *Bone Marrow Pathology*, 2nd edn. Blackwell Science, Oxford.

Beutler E., Kipps T.J., Lichtman M.A. *et al.* (eds) (2000) *William's Hematology*, 6th edn. McGraw-Hill, New York.

Degos L., Linch D.C., Lowenberg B. (eds) (2005) *Textbook of Malignant Hematology*, 2nd edn. Taylor & Francis, London & New York.

Hoffbrand A.V. and Pettit J.E. (2000) *Color Atlas of Clinical Hematology*, 3rd edn. Mosby, London.

Hoffbrand A.V., Tuddenham E.G. and Catovsky D. (eds) (2005) *Postgraduate Hematology*, 5th edn. Blackwell Publishing, Oxford.

Hoffman R., Benz E.J., Shatill S.J. *et al.* (2005) *Hematology: Basic Principles and Practice*, 4th edn. Elsevier, New York.

Klein H.G. and Anstee D.J. (2005) *Mollison's Blood Transfusion in Clinical Medicine*, 11th edn. Blackwell Publishing, Oxford.

Provan D. and Gribben J. (eds) (2005) *Molecular Haematology*, 2nd edn. Blackwell Publishing, Oxford.

Stamatoyannopous G., Perlmutter R.M., Majerus P.W., Varmus H. (eds) (2000) *The Molecular Basis of Blood Diseases*, 3rd edn. W.B. Saunders, Philadelphia.

CHAPTER 1

1 Haemopoiesis

This first chapter is concerned with the general aspects of blood cell formation (haemopoiesis). The processes that regulate haemopoiesis and the early stages of formation of red cells (erythropoiesis), granulocytes and monocytes (myelopoiesis) and platelets (thrombopoiesis) are also discussed.

Site of haemopoiesis

In the first few weeks of gestation the yolk sac is the main site of haemopoiesis. However, definitive haemopoiesis derives from a population of stem cells first observed on the dorsal aorta termed the AGM (aorta-gonads-mesonephros) region. These common precursors of endothelial and haemopoietic cells (haemangioblasts) are believed to seed the liver, spleen and bone marrow and from 6 weeks until 6–7 months of fetal life the liver and spleen are the major haemopoietic organs and continue to produce blood cells until about 2 weeks after birth (Table 1.1) (see Fig. 6.1b). The bone marrow is the most important site from 6 to 7 months of fetal life. During normal childhood and adult life the marrow is the only source of new blood cells. The developing cells are situated outside the bone marrow sinuses and mature cells are released into the sinus spaces, the marrow microcirculation and so into the general circulation.

Table 1.1 Sites of haemopoiesis.

Fetus	0–2 months (yolk sac) 2–7 months (liver, spleen) 5–9 months (bone marrow)
Infants	Bone marrow (practically all bones)
Adults	Vertebrae, ribs, sternum, skull, sacrum and pelvis, proximal ends of femur

In infancy all the bone marrow is haemopoietic but during childhood there is progressive fatty replacement of marrow throughout the long bones so that in adult life haemopoietic marrow is confined to the central skeleton and proximal ends of the femurs and humeri (Table 1.1). Even in these haemopoietic areas, approximately 50% of the marrow consists of fat (Fig. 1.1). The remaining fatty marrow is capable of reversion to haemopoiesis and in many diseases there is also expansion of haemopoiesis down the long bones. Moreover, the liver and spleen can resume their fetal haemopoietic role ('extramedullary haemopoiesis').

Haemopoietic stem and progenitor cells

Haemopoiesis starts with a pluripotential stem cell that can give rise to the separate cell lineages.

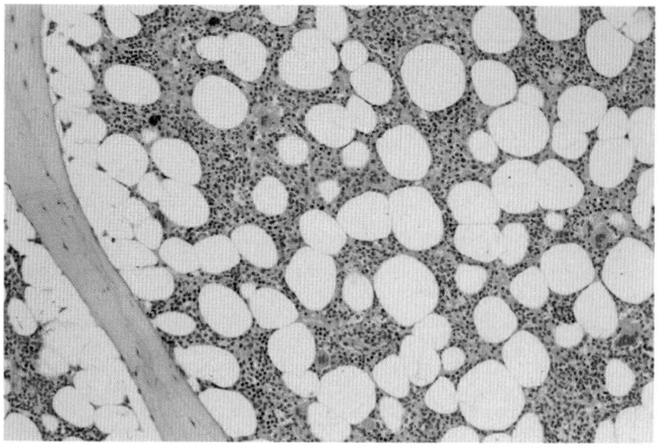

Fig. 1.1 A normal bone marrow trephine biopsy (posterior iliac crest). Haematoxylin and eosin stain; approximately 50% of the intertrabecular tissue is haemopoietic tissue and 50% is fat.

This ***haemopoietic stem cell*** is rare, perhaps 1 in every 20 million nucleated cells in bone marrow. Although its exact phenotype is unknown, on immunological testing it is $CD34^+$ $CD38^-$ and has the appearance of a small or medium-sized lymphocyte (Fig. 21.3). Cell differentiation occurs from the stem cell via the committed ***haemopoietic progenitors*** which are restricted in their developmental potential (Fig. 1.2). The existence of the separate progenitor cells can be demonstrated by *in vitro* culture techniques. Very early progenitors are assayed by culture on bone marrow stroma as long-term culture initiating cells whereas late progenitors are generally assayed in semi-solid media. An example is the earliest detectable mixed myeloid precursor which gives rise to granulocytes, erythrocytes, monocytes and megakaryocytes and is termed

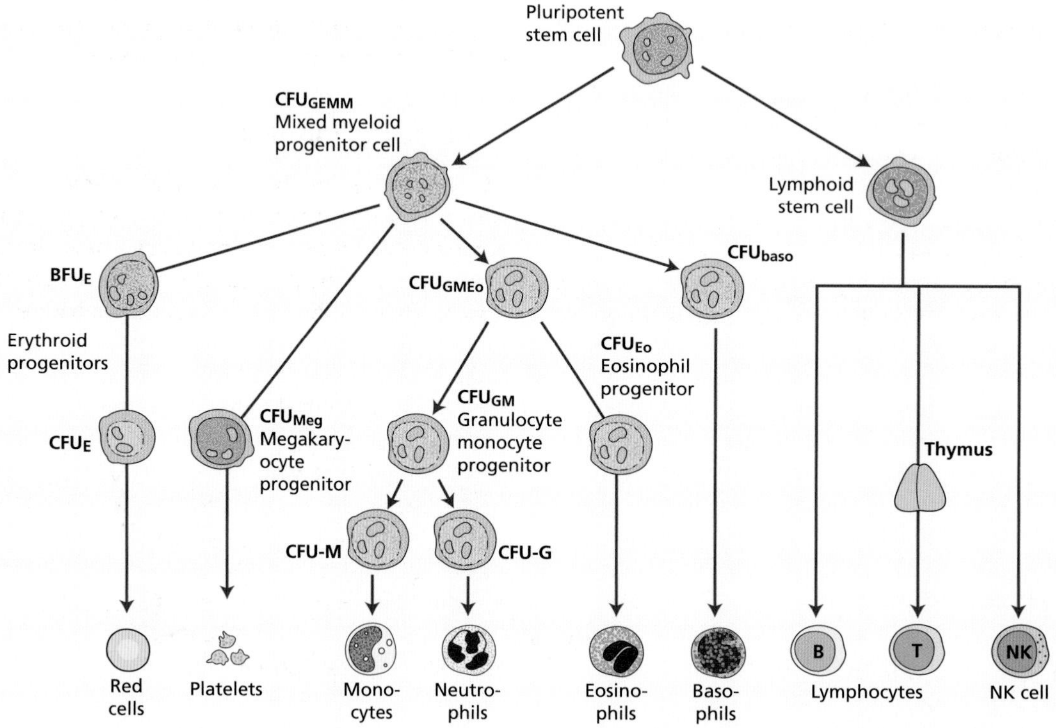

Fig. 1.2 Diagrammatic representation of the bone marrow pluripotent stem cell and the cell lines that arise from it. Various progenitor cells can be identified by culture in semi-solid medium by the type of colony they form. Baso, basophil; BFU, burst-forming unit; CFU, colony-forming unit; E, erythroid; Eo, eosinophil; GEMM, granulocyte, erythroid, monocyte and megakaryocyte; GM, granulocyte, monocyte; Meg, megakaryocyte; NK, natural killer.

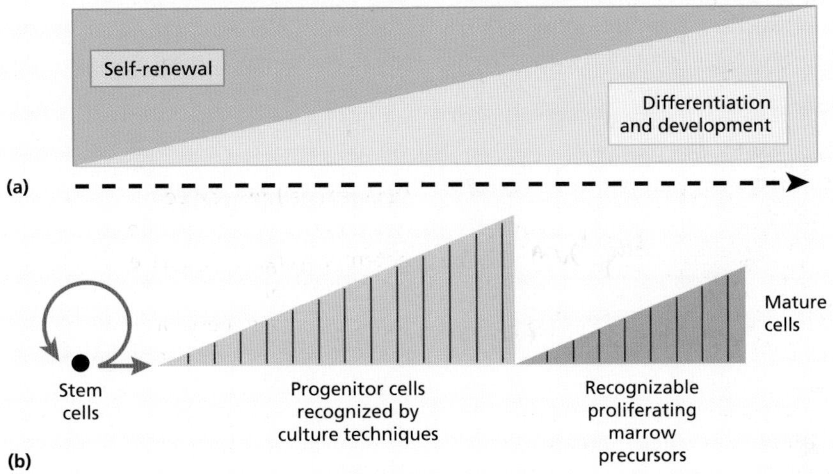

Fig. 1.3 **(a)** Bone marrow cells are increasingly differentiated and lose the capacity for self-renewal as they mature. **(b)** A single stem cell gives rise, after multiple cell divisions (shown by vertical lines), to >10^6 mature cells.

CFU (colony-forming unit)-GEMM (Fig. 1.2). The bone marrow is also the primary site of origin of lymphocytes (Chapter 8) which differentiate from a common lymphoid precursor.

The stem cell has the capability for ***self-renewal*** (Fig. 1.3) so that marrow cellularity remains constant in a normal healthy steady state. There is considerable amplification in the system: one stem cell is capable of producing about 10^6 mature blood cells after 20 cell divisions (Fig. 1.3). The precursor cells are, however, capable of responding to haemopoietic growth factors with increased production of one or other cell line when the need arises. The development of the ***mature cells*** (red cells, granulocytes, monocytes, megakaryocytes and lymphocytes) is considered further in other sections of this book.

Bone marrow stroma

The bone marrow forms a suitable environment for stem cell survival, growth and development. It is composed of stromal cells and a microvascular network (Fig. 1.4). The stromal cells include adipocytes, fibroblasts, endothelial cells and macrophages and

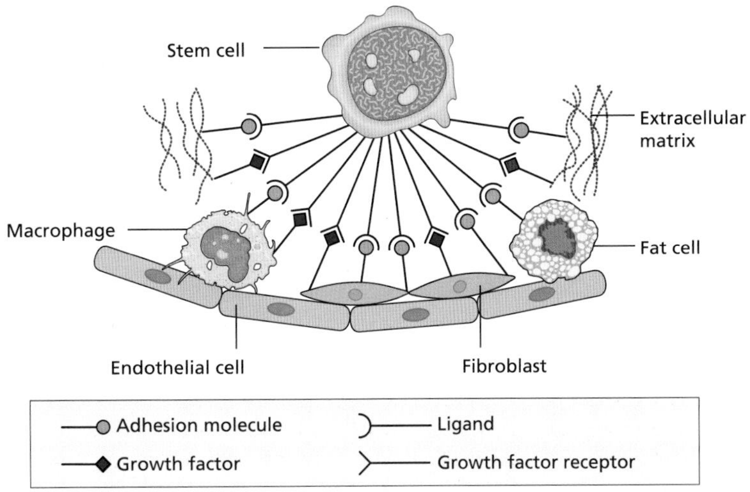

Fig. 1.4 Haemopoiesis occurs in a suitable microenvironment provided by a stromal matrix on which stem cells grow and divide. There are probably specific recognition and adhesion sites (p. 11); extracellular glycoproteins and other compounds are involved in the binding.

they secrete extracellular molecules such as collagen, glycoproteins (fibronectin and thrombospondin) and glycosaminoglycans (hyaluronic acid and chondroitin derivatives) to form an extracellular matrix. In addition, stromal cells secrete several growth factors necessary for stem cell survival. ***Mesenchymal stem cells*** are thought to be critical in stromal cell formation.

Stem cells are able to traffic around the body and are found in peripheral blood in low numbers. In order to exit the bone marrow, cells must cross the blood vessel endothelium and this process of ***mobilization*** is enhanced by administration of cytokines such as granulocyte colony-stimulating factor (G-CSF) or granulocyte–macrophage colony-stimulating factor (GM-CSF) (p. 97). The reverse process of stem cell ***homing*** appears to depend on a chemokine gradient in which the stromal-derived factor (SDF-1) is critical. Several critical interactions maintain stem cell viability and production in the stroma including stem cell factor (SCF) and Jagged proteins expressed on stroma and their respective receptors c-Kit and Notch expressed on stem cell.

Stem cell plasticity

There is some evidence that adult stem cells in different organs are ***pluripotent*** and can generate various types of tissue (Fig. 1.5). Studies in patients and animals who have received haemopoietic stem cell transplants (Chapter 21) have suggested that donor cells may contribute to tissues such as neurons, liver and muscle. The contribution of adult donor bone marrow cells to non-haemopoietic tissues is at most small. The persistence of pluripotential stem cells in postnatal life, organ-specific stem cells and fusion of transplanted cells with host cells

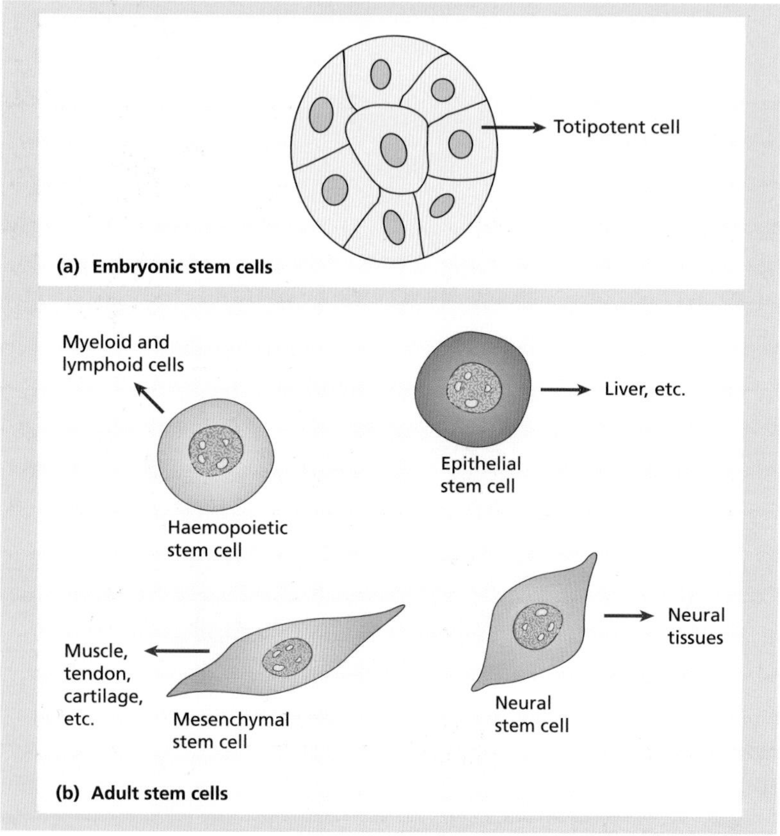

Fig. 1.5 **(a)** Cells in the early embryo are able to generate all the tissues of the body and are known as totipotent. **(b)** Specialized adult stem cells of the bone marrow, nervous tissue, epithelial and other tissues give rise to differentiated cells of the same tissue and possibly to other tissues (see text).

have all been proposed, however, to explain many of the findings suggesting stem cell plasticity.

The regulation of haemopoiesis

Haemopoiesis starts with stem cell division in which one cell replaces the stem cell (***self-renewal***) and the other is committed to differentiation. These early committed progenitors express low levels of transcription factors that may commit them to discrete cell lineages. Which cell lineage is selected for differentiation may depend both on chance and on the external signals received by progenitor cells. Several transcription factors have been isolated that regulate differentiation along the major cell lineages. For instance, PU.1 commits cells to the myeloid lineage whereas GATA-1 has an essential role in erythropoietic and megakaryocytic differentiation.

Haemopoietic growth factors

The haemopoietic growth factors are glycoprotein hormones that regulate the proliferation and differentiation of haemopoietic progenitor cells and the function of mature blood cells. They may act locally at the site where they are produced by cell–cell contact or circulate in plasma. They also bind to the extracellular matrix to form niches to which stem and progenitor cells adhere. The growth factors may cause cell proliferation but can also stimulate differentiation, maturation, prevent apoptosis and affect the function of mature cells (Fig. 1.6).

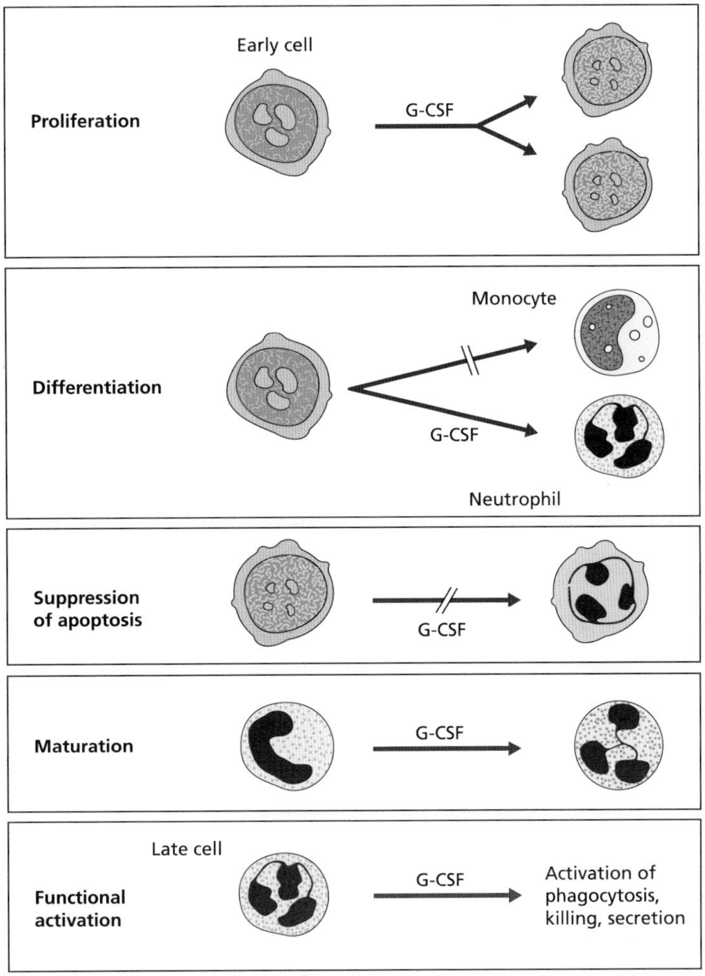

Fig. 1.6 Growth factors may stimulate proliferation of early bone marrow cells, direct differentiation to one or other cell type, stimulate cell maturation, suppress apoptosis or affect the function of mature non-dividing cells, as illustrated here for granulocyte colony-stimulating factor (G-CSF) for an early myeloid progenitor and a neutrophil.

Table 1.2 General characteristics of myeloid and lymphoid growth factors.

Glycoproteins that act at very low concentrations
Act hierarchically
Usually produced by many cell types
Usually affect more than one lineage
Usually active on stem/progenitor cells and on functional end cells
Usually show synergistic or additive interactions with other growth factors
Often act on the neoplastic equivalent of a normal cell
Multiple actions: proliferation, differentiation, maturation, functional activation, prevention of apoptosis of progenitor cells

Table 1.3 Haemopoietic growth factors.

Act on stromal cells
IL-1
TNF
Act on pluripotential stem cells
SCF
Flt-L
Act on multipotential progenitor cells
IL-3
GM-CSF
IL-6
G-CSF
Thrombopoietin
Act on committed progenitor cells
G-CSF*
M-CSF
IL-5 (eosinophil-CSF)
Erythropoietin
Thrombopoietin*

Flt-L, Flt ligand; G- and GM-CSF, granulocyte and granulocyte–macrophage colony-stimulating factor; IL, interleukin; M-CSF, macrophage colony-stimulating factor; SCF, stem cell factor; TNF, tumour necrosis factor.
* These also act synergistically with early acting factors on pluripotential progenitors.

They share a number of common properties (Table 1.2) and act at different stages of haemopoiesis (Table 1.3; Fig. 1.7). Stromal cells are the major source of growth factors except for erythropoietin, 90% of which is synthesized in the kidney, and thrombopoietin, made largely in the liver. An important feature of growth factor action is that two or more factors may synergize in stimulating a particular cell to proliferate or differentiate. Moreover, the action of one growth factor on a cell may stimulate production of another growth factor or growth factor receptor. SCF and Flt ligand (Flt-L) act locally on the pluripotential stem cells and on early myeloid and lymphoid progenitors (Fig. 1.7). Interleukin 3 (IL-3) and GM-CSF are multipotential growth factors with overlapping activities. G-CSF and thrombopoietin enhance the effects of SCF, Flt-L, IL-3 and GM-CSF on survival and differentiation of the early haemopoietic cells.

These factors maintain a pool of haemopoietic stem and progenitor cells on which later acting factors erythropoietin, G-CSF, M-CSF, IL-5 and thrombopoietin act to increase production of one or other cell lineage in response to the body's need. Granulocyte and monocyte formation, for example, can be stimulated by infection or inflammation through release of IL-1 and tumour necrosis factor (TNF) which then stimulate stromal cells to produce growth factors in an interacting network (Fig. 7.4). In contrast, cytokines such as transforming growth factor-β (TGF-β) and γ-interferon (IFN-γ) can exert a negative effect on haemopoiesis and may have a role in the development of aplastic anaemia (p. 244).

Growth factor receptors and signal transduction

The biological effects of growth factors are mediated through specific receptors on target cells. Many receptors (e.g. erythropoietin (epo) receptor (R), GM-CSF-R) are from the ***haematopoietin receptor superfamily*** which dimerize after binding their ligand.

Dimerization of the receptor leads to activation of a complex series of intracellular signal transduction pathways of which the three major ones are the JAK/STAT, the mitogen activated protein (MAP) kinase and the phosphatidylinositol 3 (PI3) kinase pathways (Figs 1.8, 19.2). The Janus associated kinase (JAK) proteins are a family of four tyrosine-specific protein kinases that associate with the intracellular domains of the growth factor receptors (Fig. 1.8). A growth factor molecule binds simultaneously to the extracellular domains of two or three receptor

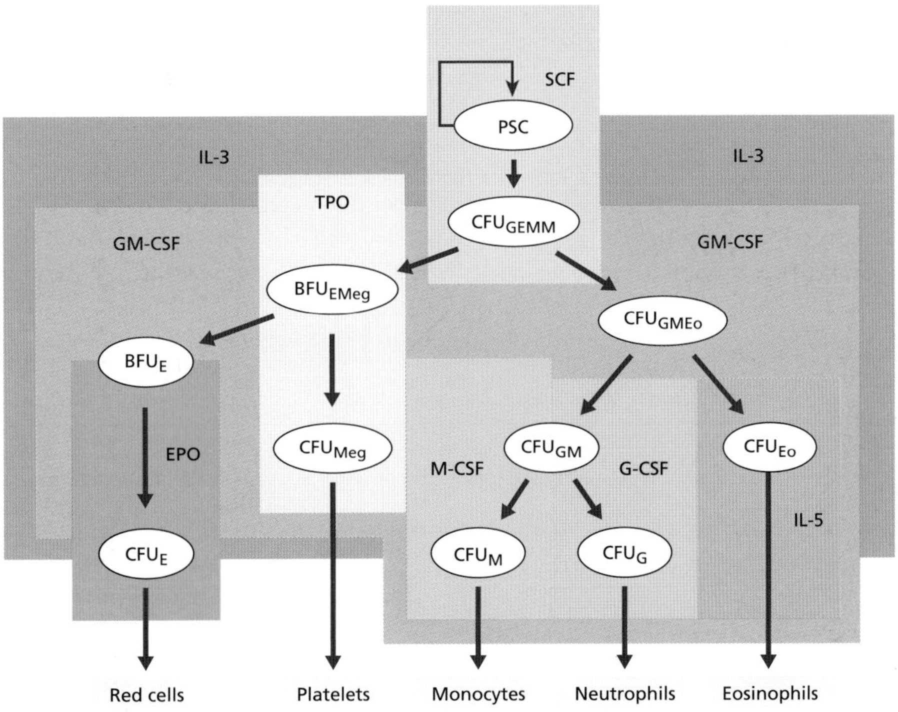

Fig. 1.7 A diagram of the role of growth factors in normal haemopoiesis. Multiple growth factors act on the earlier marrow stem and progenitor cells. EPO, erythropoietin; PSC, pluripotential stem cell; SCF, stem cell factor; TPO, thrombopoietin. For other abbreviations see Fig. 1.2.

molecules, resulting in their aggregation. Receptor aggregation induces activation of the JAKs which now phosphorylate members of the signal transducer and activator of transcription (STAT) family of transcription factors. This results in their dimerization and translocation from the cell cytoplasm across the nuclear membrane to the cell nucleus. Within the nucleus STAT dimers activate transcription of specific genes. A model for control of gene expression by a transcription factor is shown in Fig. 1.9. The clinical importance of this pathway is revealed by the finding of an activating mutation of the *JAK2* gene as the cause of polycythaemia rubra vera (p. 230).

JAK can also activate the MAPK pathway which is regulated by Ras and controls proliferation. PI3 kinases phophorylate inositol lipids which have a wide range of downstream effects including activation of AKT (protein kinase B) leading to block of apoptosis and other actions (Fig. 1.8, 19.2). Different domains of the intracellular receptor protein may signal for the different processes (e.g. proliferation or suppression of apoptosis) mediated by growth factors.

A second smaller group of growth factors, including SCF, Flt-3L and macrophage colony-stimulating factor (M-CSF) (Table 1.3), bind to receptors that have an extracellular immunoglobulin-like domain linked via a transmembrane bridge to a cytoplasmic tyrosine kinase domain. Growth factor binding results in dimerization of these receptors and consequent activation of the tyrosine kinase domain. Phosphorylation of tyrosine residues in the receptor itself generates binding sites for signalling proteins which initiate complex cascades of biochemical events resulting in changes in gene expression, cell proliferation and prevention of apoptosis.

The cell cycle

The cell division cycle, generally known simply as the ***cell cycle***, is a complex process that lies at

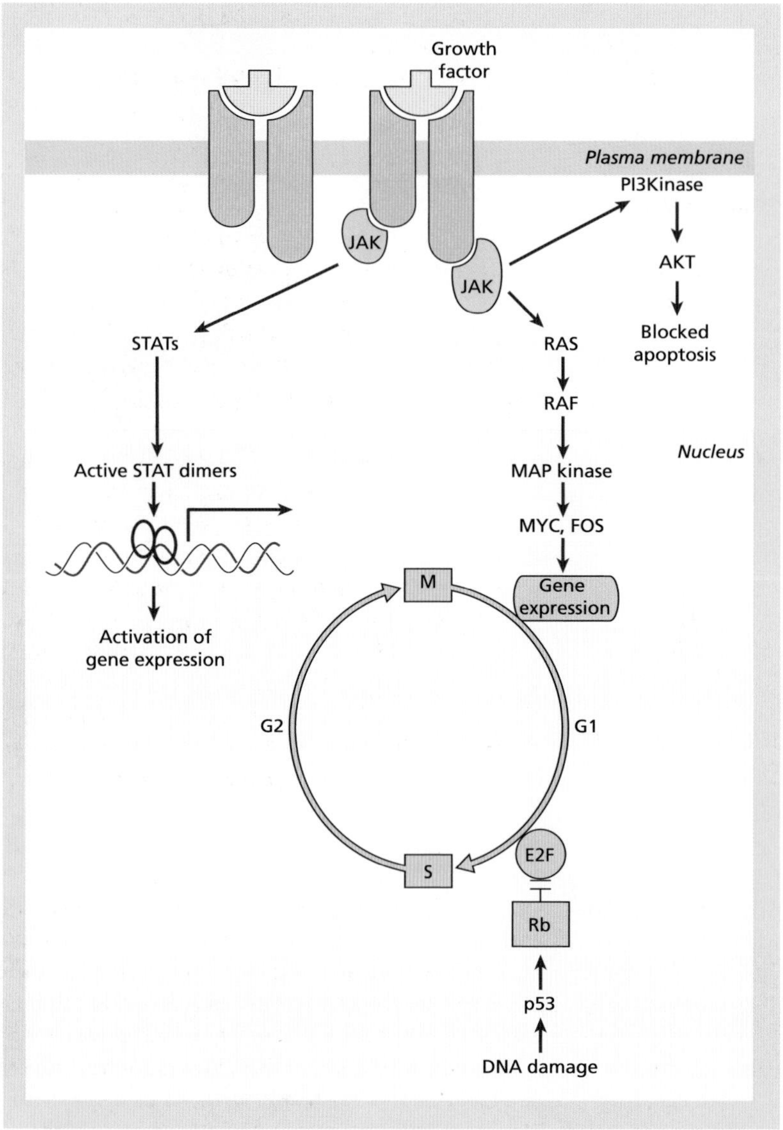

Fig. 1.8 Control of haemopoiesis by growth factors. The factors act on cells expressing the corresponding receptors. Binding of a growth factor to its receptor activates the JAK/STAT, MAPK and phosphatidyl-inositol3-kinase (PI3K) pathways (Fig. 19.2) which leads to transcriptional activation of specific genes. E2F is a transcription factor needed for cell transition from G1 to S phase. E2F is inhibited by the tumour suppressor gene *Rb* (retinoblastoma) which can be indirectly activated by p53. The synthesis and degradation of different cyclins (Fig. 1.10) stimulates the cell to pass through the different phases of the cell cycle. The growth factors may also suppress apoptosis by activating AKT (protein kinase B).

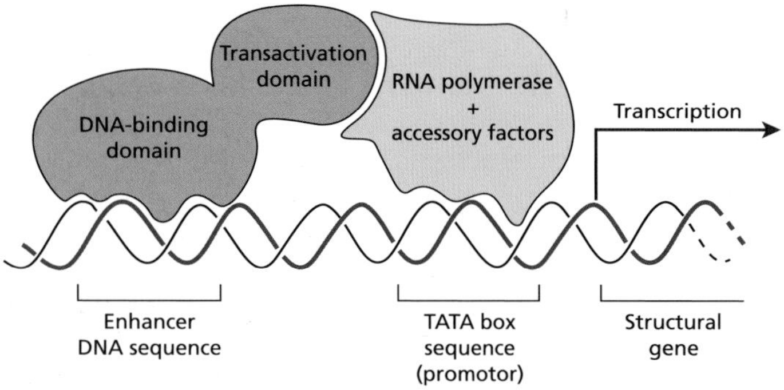

Fig. 1.9 Model for control of gene expression by a transcription factor. The DNA-binding domain of a transcription factor binds a specific enhancer sequence adjacent to a structural gene. The transactivation domain then binds a molecule of RNA polymerase, thus augmenting its binding to the TATA box. The RNA polymerase now initiates transcription of the structural gene to form mRNA. Translation of the mRNA by the ribosomes generates the protein encoded by the gene.

the heart of haemopoiesis. Dysregulation of cell proliferation is also the key to the development of malignant disease. The duration of the cell cycle is variable between different tissues but the basic principles remain constant. The cycle is divided in to the mitotic phase (***M phase***), during which the cell physically divides, and ***interphase*** during which the chromosomes are duplicated and cell growth occurs prior to division (Fig. 1.10). The M phase is further partitioned into classical ***mitosis*** in which nuclear division is accomplished, and ***cytokinesis*** in which cell fission occurs.

Interphase is divided into three main stages: a ***G_1 phase*** in which the cell begins to commit to replication, an ***S phase*** during which DNA content doubles (Fig. 1.10b) and the chromosomes replicate and the ***G_2 phase*** in which the cell organelles are copied and cytoplasmic volume is increased. If cells rest prior to division they enter a G_0 state where they can remain for long periods of time. The number of cells at each stage of the cell cycle can be assessed by exposing cells to a chemical or radiolabel that gets incorporated into newly generated DNA or by flow cytometry.

The cell cycle is controlled by two ***checkpoints*** which act as brakes to coordinate the division process at the end of the G_1 and G_2 phases. Two major classes of molecules control these checkpoints, ***cyclin dependent protein kinases*** (Cdk) which phosophorylate downstream protein targets and ***cyclins*** which bind to Cdks and regulate their activity. An example of the importance of these systems is demonstrated by mantle cell lymphoma which results from the constitutive activation of cyclin D1 as a result of a chromosomal translocation (p. 212).

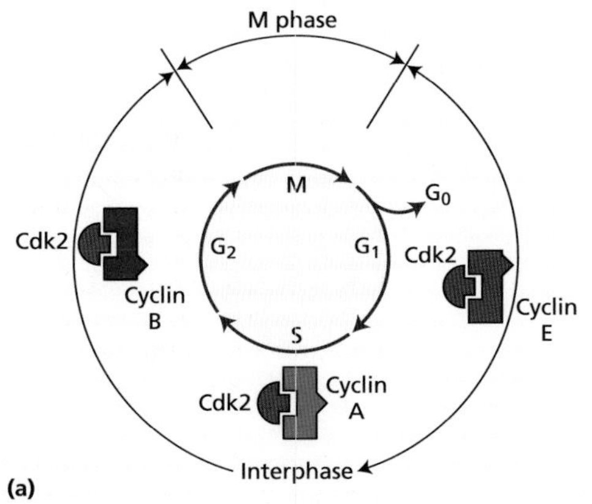

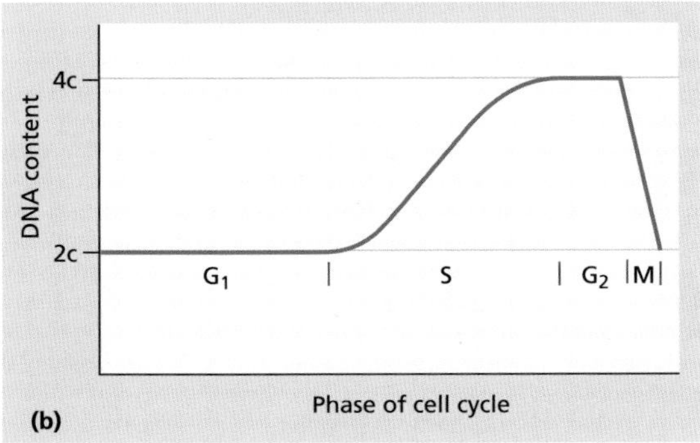

Fig. 1.10 **(a)** The stages of the cell cycle. Progression through cell cycle is regulated by specific combinations of cyclin dependent protein kinases (Cdk) and cyclin proteins. The synthesis and degradation of different cyclins stimulates the cell to pass through the different phases of the cell cycle although the exact role of each heterodimer is currently uncertain. **(b)** Relationship between the DNA content of a cell expressed in arbitrary units as 2c increasing to 4c and its position in the cell cycle. (Adapted from Wickramasinghe S.N. (1975) *Human Bone Marrow*, Blackwell Scientific, Oxford, p. 13.)

Apoptosis

Apoptosis is a regulated process of physiological cell death in which cells are triggered to activate intracellular proteins that lead to the death of the cell. Morphologically it is characterized by cell shrinkage, condensation of the nuclear chromatin, fragmentation of the nucleus and cleavage of DNA at internucleosomal sites. It is an important process for maintaining tissue homoeostasis in haemopoiesis and lymphocyte development.

Apoptosis results from the action of intracellular cysteine proteases called ***caspases*** which are activated following cleavage and lead to endonuclease digestion of DNA and disintegration of the cell skeleton (Fig. 1.11). There are two major pathways by which caspases can be activated. The first is by signalling through membrane proteins such as Fas or TNF receptor via their intracellular death domain. An example of this mechanism is shown by activated cytotoxic T cells expressing Fas ligand which induce apoptosis in target cells. The second

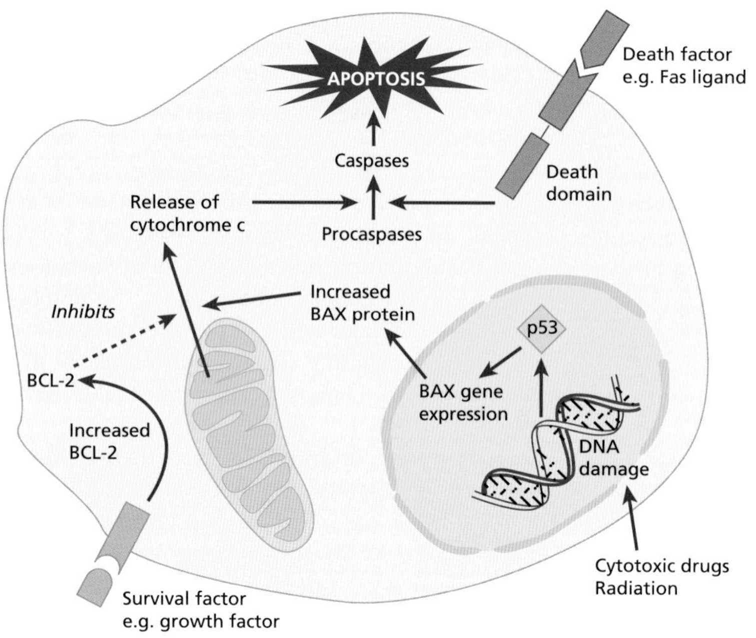

Fig. 1.11 Representation of apoptosis. Apoptosis is initiated via two main stimuli: (i) signalling through cell membrane receptors such as FAS or tumour necrosis factor (TNF) receptor; or (ii) release of cytochrome c from mitochondria. Membrane receptors signal apoptosis through an intracellular death domain leading to activation of caspases which digest DNA. Cytochrome c binds to the cytoplasmic protein Apaf-1 leading to activation of caspases. The intracellular ratio of pro- (e.g. BAX) or anti-apoptotic (e.g. BCL-2) members of the BCL-2 family may influence mitochondrial cytochrome c release. Growth factors raise the level of BCL-2 inhibiting cytochrome c release whereas DNA damage, by activating p53, raises the level of BAX which enhances cytochrome c release.

pathway is via the release of cytochrome c from mitochondria. Cytochrome c binds to Apaf-1 which then activates caspases. DNA damage induced by irradiation or chemotherapy may act through this pathway. The protein p53 has an important role in sensing DNA damage. It activates apoptosis by raising the cell level of BAX which then increases cytochrome c release (Fig. 1.11). P53 also shuts down the cell cycle to stop the damaged cell from dividing (Fig. 1.8). The cellular level of p53 is rigidly controlled by a second protein MDM2. Following death, apoptotic cells display molecules that lead to their ingestion by macrophages.

As well as molecules that mediate apoptosis there are several intracellular proteins that protect cells from apoptosis. The best characterized example is BCL-2. BCL-2 is the prototype of a family of related proteins, some of which are anti-apoptotic and some, like BAX, pro-apoptotic. The intracellular ratio of BAX and BCL-2 determines the relative susceptibility of cells to apoptosis and may act through regulation of cytochrome c release from mitochondria.

Many of the genetic changes associated with malignant disease lead to a reduced rate of apoptosis and hence prolonged cell survival. The clearest example is the translocation of the *BCL-2* gene to the immunoglobulin heavy chain locus in the t(14; 18) translocation in follicle centre lymphoma. Overexpression of the BCL-2 protein makes the malignant B cells less susceptible to apoptosis. Apoptosis is the normal fate for most B cells undergoing selection in the lymphoid germinal centres.

Several translocations leading to the generation of fusion proteins such as t(9; 22), t(1; 14) and t(15; 17) also result in inhibition of apoptosis (Chapter 10). In addition, genes encoding proteins that are involved in mediating apoptosis following DNA damage, such as p53 and ATM, are also frequently mutated and therefore inactivated in haemopoietic malignancies.

Transcription factors

Transcription factors regulate gene expression by controlling the transcription of specific genes or gene families. Typically, they contain at least two domains: a ***DNA-binding domain*** such as a leucine zipper or helix-loop-helix motif which binds to a specific DNA sequence, and an ***activation domain*** which contributes to assembly of the transcription complex at a gene promoter.

Adhesion molecules

A large family of glycoprotein molecules termed adhesion molecules mediate the attachment of marrow precursors, leucocytes and platelets to various components of the extracellular matrix, to endothelium, to other surfaces and to each other. The adhesion molecules on the surface of leucocytes are termed receptors and these interact with molecules (termed ligands) on the surface of potential target cells. Three main families exist:

1 ***Immunoglobulin superfamily*** This includes receptors that react with antigens (the T-cell receptors and the immunoglobulins) and antigen-independent surface adhesion molecules.

2 ***Selectins*** These are mainly involved in leucocyte and platelet adhesion to endothelium during inflammation and coagulation.

3 ***Integrins*** These are involved in cell adhesion to extracellular matrix (e.g. to collagen in wound healing and in leucocyte and platelet adhesion).

The adhesion molecules are thus important in the development and maintenance of inflammatory and immune responses, and in platelet–vessel wall and leucocyte–vessel wall interactions. Expression of adhesion molecules can be modifed by extracellular and intracellular factors and this alteration of expression may be quantitative or functional. IL-1, TNF, IFN-γ, T-cell activation, adhesion to extracellular proteins and viral infection may all up-regulate expression of these molecules.

The pattern of expression of adhesion molecules on tumour cells may determine their mode of spread and tissue localization (e.g. the pattern of metastasis of carcinoma cells or non-Hodgkin's lymphoma cells into a follicular or diffuse pattern). The adhesion molecules may also determine whether or not cells circulate in the bloodstream or remain fixed in tissues. They may also partly determine whether or not tumour cells are susceptible to the body's immune defences.

Bibliography

Adolfsson J., Mansson R., Buza-Vidas N. *et al.* (2005) Identification of Flt3+ lympho-myeloid stem cells lacking erythro-megakaryocytic potential: a revised road map for adult blood lineage commitment. *Cell* **121**,295–306.

Cantor A.B. and Orkin S.H. (2002) Transcriptional regulation of erythropoiesis: an affair involving multiple partners. *Oncogene* **21**,3368–76.

Hochedlinger K. and Jaenisch R. (2003) Nuclear transplantation, embryonic stem cells and potential for cell therapy. *N Engl J Med* **349**,275–86.

Kaushansky K. (2006) Lineage-specific hematopoietic growth factors. *N Engl J Med* **354**,2034–45.

Lanza R., Gearhart J., Hogan B. *et al.* (eds) (2006) *Essentials of Stem Cell Biology*. Elsevier Academic Press, San Diego, California.

Lapidot T., Dar A., Kollet O. (2005) How do stem cells find their way home? *Blood* **106**,1901–10.

Lensch M.W. and Daley G.Q. (2006) Scientific and clinical opportunities for modeling blood disorders with embryonic stem cells. *Blood* **107**,2605–12.

Lemoli R.M., Bertolini F., Cancedda R. *et al.* (2005) Stem cell plasticity: time for a reappraisal. *Haematologica* **90**,360–81.

Martin-Rendon E. and Watt S.M. (2003) Skin cell plasticity. *Br J Haematol* **122**,877–91.

Orkin S.H. and Zon L.I. (2002) Hematopoiesis and stem cells: plasticity versus developmental heterogeneity. *Nat Immunol* **4**,323–8.

Taichman R.S. (2005) Blood and bone: two tissues whose fates are intertwined to create the hematopoietic stem-cell niche. *Blood* **105**,2631–9.

Vats A., Bielby R.C., Tolley N.S., Nerem R., Polak J.M. (2005) Stem cells. *Lancet* **366**,592–602.

CHAPTER 2

2 Erythropoiesis and general aspects of anaemia

We each make approximately 10^{12} new erythrocytes (red cells) each day by the complex and finely regulated process of erythropoiesis. Erythropoiesis passes from the stem cell through the progenitor cells colony-forming unit granulocyte, erythroid, monocyte and megakaryocyte (CFU_{GEMM}), burst-forming unit erythroid (BFU_E) and erythroid CFU (CFU_E) (see Figs 1.2 and 2.2) to the first recognizable erythrocyte precursor in the bone marrow, the pronormoblast. This is a large cell with dark blue cytoplasm, a central nucleus with nucleoli and slightly clumped chromatin (Fig. 2.1). The pronormoblast gives rise to a series of progressively smaller normoblasts by a number of cell divisions. They also contain progressively more haemoglobin (which stains pink) in the cytoplasm; the cytoplasm stains paler blue as it loses its RNA and protein synthetic apparatus while nuclear chromatin becomes more condensed (Figs 2.1 and 2.2). The nucleus is finally extruded from the late normoblast within the marrow and a reticulocyte stage results which still contains some ribosomal RNA and is still able to synthesize haemoglobin (Fig. 2.3). This cell is slightly larger than a mature red cell, spends 1–2 days in the marrow and also circulates in the peripheral blood for 1–2 days before maturing, mainly in the spleen, when RNA is completely lost. A completely pink-staining mature erythrocyte results which is a non-nucleated biconcave disc. A single pronormoblast usually gives rise to 16 mature red cells (Fig. 2.2). Nucleated red cells (normoblasts) are not present in normal human peripheral blood. They appear in the blood if erythropoiesis is occurring outside the marrow (extramedullary erythropoiesis) and also with some marrow diseases. Normoblasts.

Erythropoietin

Erythropoiesis is regulated by the hormone erythropoietin. The erythropoietin gene contains a hypoxia-response element at its 3′ end. Erythropoietin is a heavily glycosylated polypeptide of 165 amino acids with a molecular weight of 34 kDa. Normally, 90% of the hormone is produced in the peritubular interstitial cells of the kidney and 10% in the liver and elsewhere. There are no preformed stores and the stimulus to erythropoietin production is the oxygen (O_2) tension in the tissues of the kidney (Fig. 2.4). Erythropoietin production therefore increases in anaemia, when haemoglobin for some metabolic or structural reason is unable to give up O_2 normally, when atmospheric O_2 is low or when defective cardiac or pulmonary function or damage to the renal circulation affects O_2 delivery to the kidney.

Erythropoietin stimulates erythropoiesis by increasing the number of progenitor cells committed to erythropoiesis. The transcription factors GATA-1 and FOG-1 are activated by erythropoietin receptor stimulation and are important in enhancing expression of erythroid-specific genes (e.g. haem

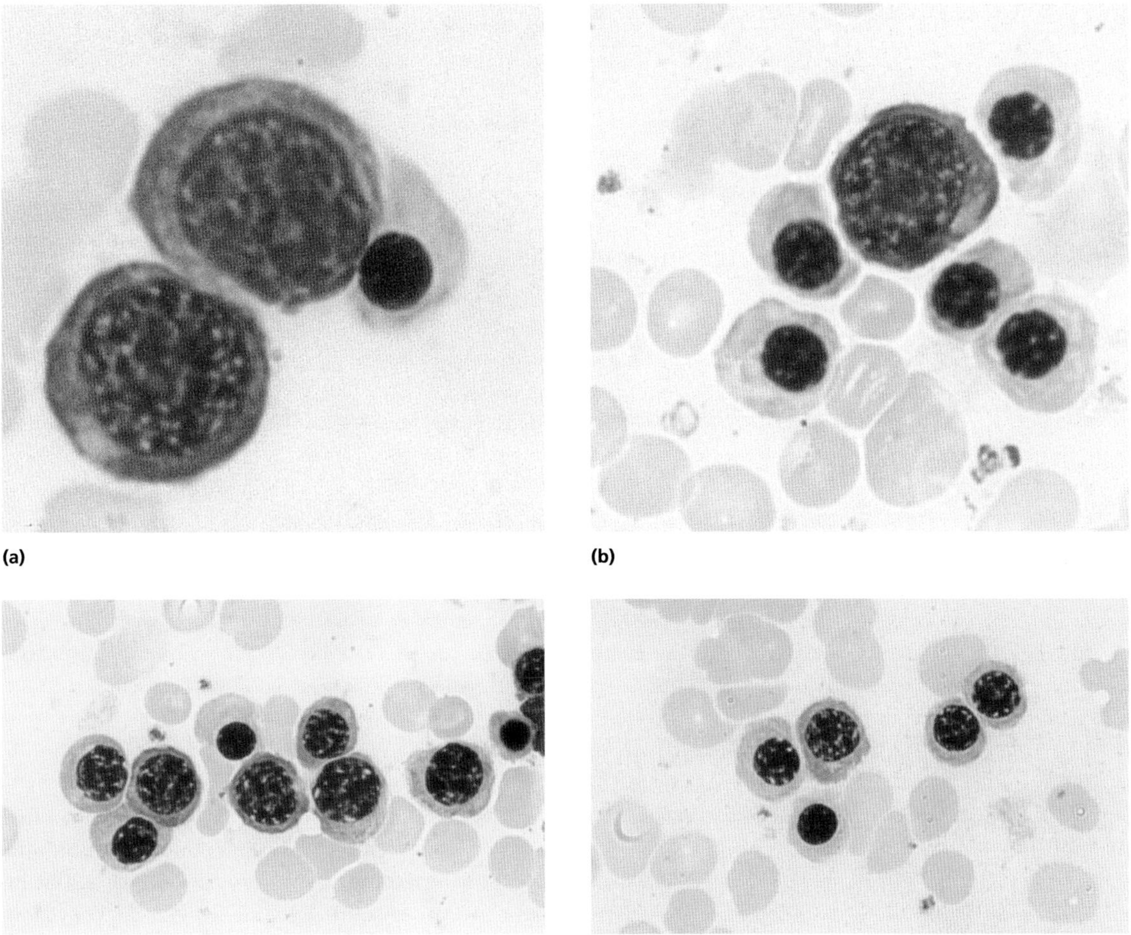

(a) (b) (c) (d)

Fig. 2.1 Erythroblasts (normoblasts) at varying stages of development. The earlier cells are larger, with more basophilic cytoplasm and a more open nuclear chromatin pattern. The cytoplasm of the later cells is more eosinophilic as a result of haemoglobin formation.

biosynthetic and red cell membrane proteins) and also enhancing expression of anti-apoptotic genes and of the transferrin receptor (CD71). Late BFU_E and CFU_E which have erythropoietin receptors are stimulated to proliferate, differentiate and produce haemoglobin. The proportion of erythroid cells in the marrow increases and, in the chronic state, there is anatomical expansion of erythropoiesis into fatty marrow and sometimes into extramedullary sites. In infants, the marrow cavity may expand into cortical bone resulting in bone deformities with frontal bossing and protrusion of the maxilla (p. 78).

Conversely, increased O_2 supply to the tissues (because of an increased red cell mass or because haemoglobin is able to release its O_2 more readily than normal) reduces the erythropoietin drive. Tissue hypoxia also stimulates new blood vessel formation by vascular endothelial growth factor (VEGF).

Plasma erythropoietin levels can be valuable in clinical diagnosis. They are high if a tumour-secreting erythropoietin is causing polycythaemia but low in severe renal disease or polycythaemia rubra vera (Fig. 2.5).

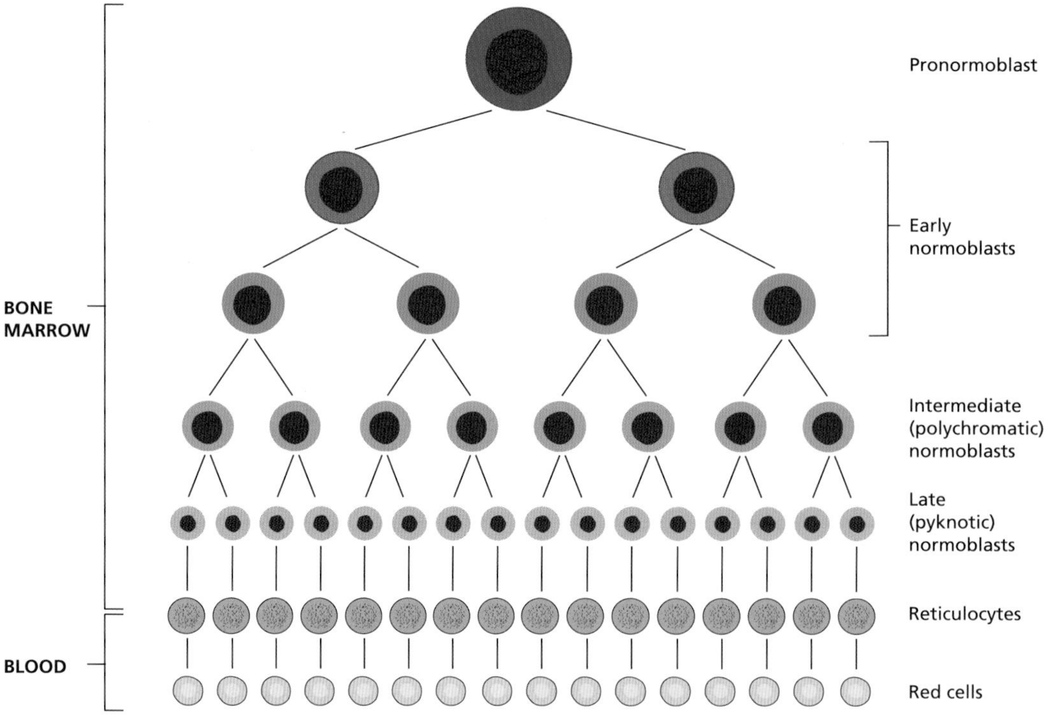

Fig. 2.2 The amplification and maturation sequence in the development of mature red cells from the pronormoblast.

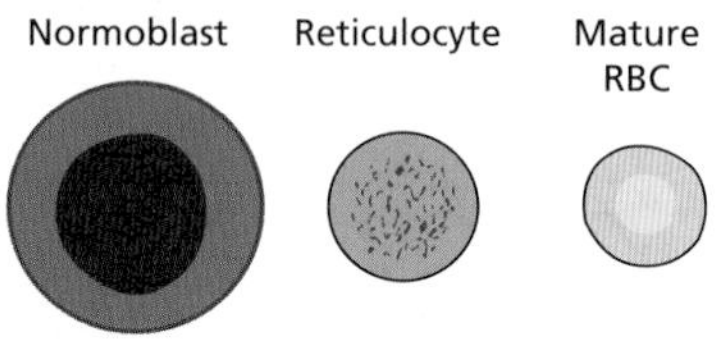

	Normoblast	Reticulocyte	Mature RBC
Nuclear DNA	Yes	No	No
RNA in cytoplasm	Yes	Yes	No
In marrow	Yes	Yes	Yes
In blood	No	Yes	Yes

Fig. 2.3 Comparison of the DNA and RNA content, and marrow and peripheral blood distribution, of the erythroblast (normoblast), reticulocyte and mature red blood cell (RBC).

Indications for erythropoietin therapy

Recombinant erythropoietin is of great value in treating anaemia resulting from renal disease or from various other causes. It is given intravenously or subcutaneously either 3–7 times weekly or once every 1–2 weeks depending on the indication and on the preparation used (erythropoietin alpha or beta or darbepoetin alpha, a heavily glycosylated longer acting form). The main indication is end-stage renal disease (with or without dialysis). Other uses include pre-autologous blood transfusions, the anaemia of chronic disorders (e.g. in rheumatoid arthritis or cancer) and some cases of myelodysplasia or myeloma. In these conditions, often higher doses are used (Table 2.1) and the quality of life is improved (Chapter 11). A low serum erythropoietin

Table 2.1 Clinical uses of erythropoietin.

Anaemia of chronic renal disease
Myelodysplastic syndrome
Anaemia associated with malignancy and chemotherapy
Anaemia of chronic diseases
AIDS
Anaemia of prematurity
Perioperative uses

AIDS, acquired immunodeficiency syndrome.

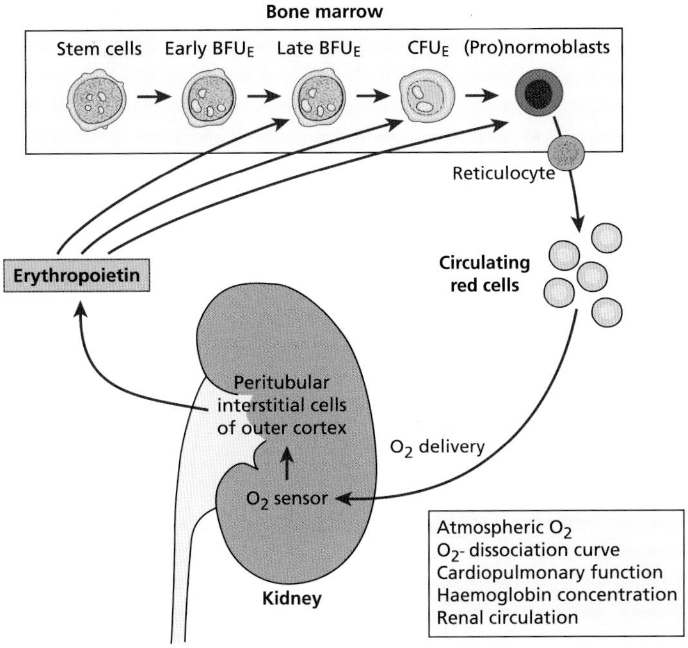

Fig. 2.4 The production of erythropoietin by the kidney in response to its oxygen (O_2) supply. Erythropoietin stimulates erythropoiesis and so increases O_2 delivery. BFU$_E$, erythroid burst-forming unit; CFU$_E$, erythroid colony-forming unit.

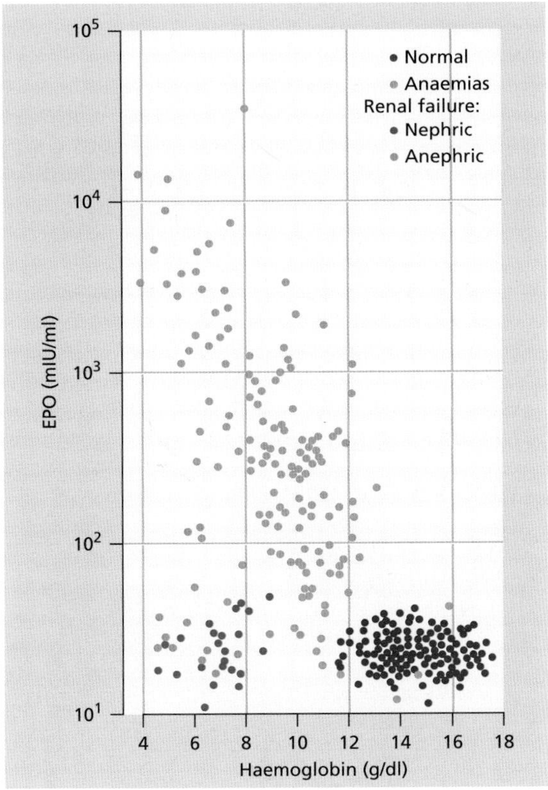

Fig. 2.5 The relation between radioimmunoassay estimates of erythropoietin (EPO) in plasma and haemoglobin concentration. Anaemias exclude conditions shown to be associated with impaired production of EPO. (From M. Pippard *et al.* 1992 with permission)

level prior to treatment is valuable in predicting an effective response. Oral or parenteral iron is often needed to maximize the response to erythropoietin therapy. Side-effects include a rise in blood pressure and platelet count and local injection site reactions.

The marrow requires many other precursors for effective erythropoiesis. These include metals such as iron or cobalt, vitamins (especially vitamin B_{12}, folate, vitamin C, vitamin E, vitamin B_6, thiamine and riboflavin) and hormones such as androgens and thyroxine. Deficiency in any of these may be associated with anaemia.

Haemoglobin

Haemoglobin synthesis

The main function of red cells is to carry O_2 to the tissues and to return carbon dioxide (CO_2) from the

Table 2.2 Normal haemoglobins in adult blood.

	Hb A	Hb F	Hb A_2
Structure	$\alpha_2\beta_2$	$\alpha_2\gamma_2$	$\alpha_2\delta_2$
Normal (%)	96–98	0.5–0.8	1.5–3.2

tissues to the lungs. In order to achieve this gaseous exchange they contain the specialized protein haemoglobin. Each red cell contains approximately 640 million haemoglobin molecules. Each molecule of normal adult haemoglobin (Hb) A (the dominant haemoglobin in blood after the age of 3–6 months) consists of four polypeptide chains, $\alpha_2\beta_2$, each with its own haem group. The molecular weight of Hb A is 68 000. Normal adult blood also contains small quantities of two other haemoglobins: Hb F and Hb A_2. These also contain α chains, but with γ and δ chains, respectively, instead of β (Table 2.2). The synthesis of the various globin chains in the fetus and adult is discussed in more detail in Chapter 6.

Table 2.3 Normal adult red cell values.

	Male	Female
Haemoglobin (g/dL)	13.5–17.5	11.5–15.5
Haematocrit (PCV) (%)	40–52	36–48
Red cell count ($\times10^{12}$/L)	4.5–6.5	3.9–5.6
Mean cell haemoglobin (MCH) (pg)	27–34	
Mean cell volume (MCV) (fL)	80–95	
Mean cell haemoglobin concentration (g/dL)	30–35	
Reticulocyte count ($\times10^9$/L)	25–125	

PCV, packed cell volume.

The major switch from fetal to adult haemoglobin occurs 3–6 months after birth (Table 2.2; see Fig. 6.1b).

Haem synthesis occurs largely in the mitochondria by a series of biochemical reactions commencing with the condensation of glycine and succinyl coenzyme A under the action of the key rate-limiting enzyme δ-aminolaevulinic acid (ALA) synthase (Fig. 2.6). Pyridoxal phosphate (vitamin B_6)

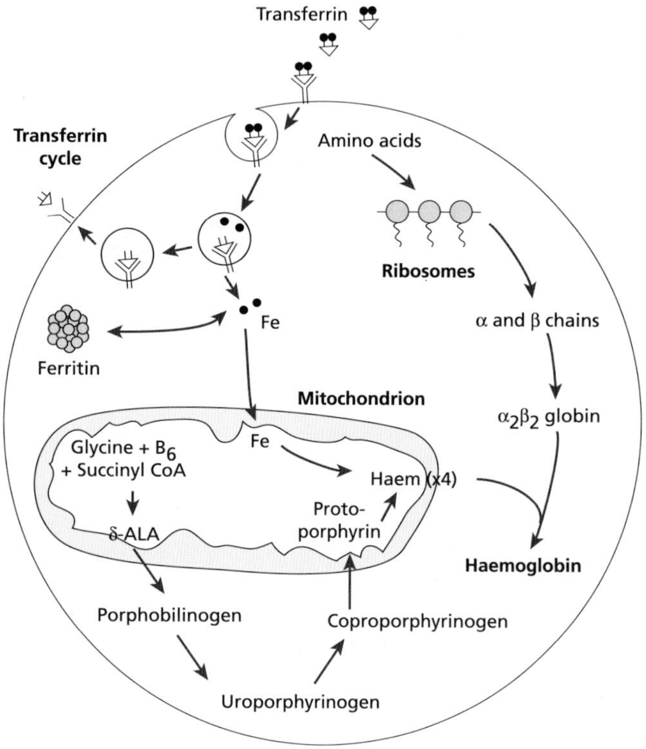

Fig. 2.6 Haemoglobin synthesis in the developing red cell. The mitochondria are the main sites of protoporphyrin synthesis, iron (Fe) is supplied from circulating transferrin; globin chains are synthesized on ribosomes. δ-ALA, δ-aminolaevulinic acid; CoA, coenzyme A.

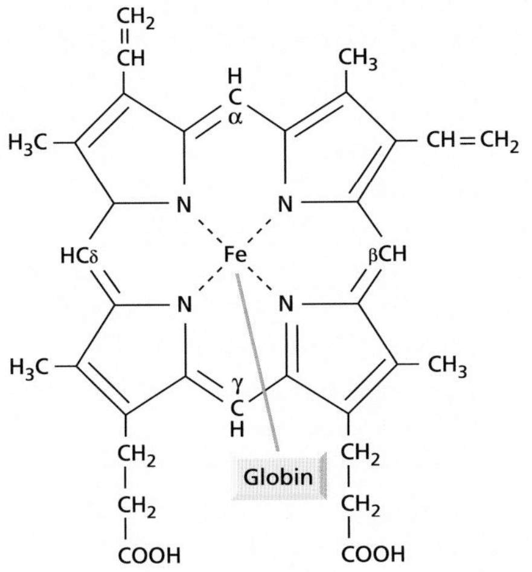

Fig. 2.7 The structure of haem.

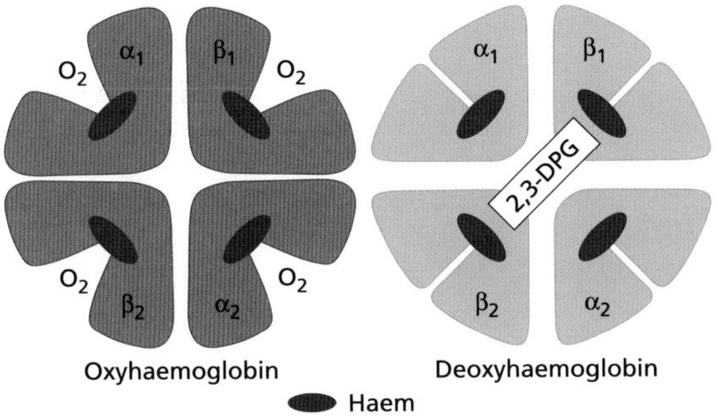

Fig. 2.8 The oxygenated and deoxygenated haemoglobin molecule. α, β, globin chains of normal adult haemoglobin (Hb A). 2,3-DPG, 2,3-diphosphoglycerate.

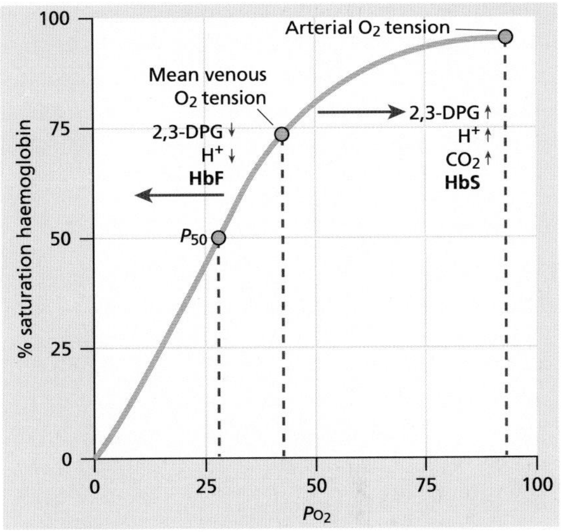

Fig. 2.9 The haemoglobin oxygen (O_2) dissociation curve. 2,3-DPG, 2,3-diphosphoglycerate.

is a coenzyme for this reaction which is stimulated by erythropoietin. Ultimately, protoporphyrin combines with iron in the ferrous (Fe^{2+}) state to form haem (Fig. 2.7), each molecule of which combines with a globin chain made on the polyribosomes (Fig. 2.6). A tetramer of four globin chains each with its own haem group in a 'pocket' is then formed to make up a haemoglobin molecule (Fig. 2.8).

Haemoglobin function

The red cells in systemic arterial blood carry O_2 from the lungs to the tissues and return in venous blood with CO_2 to the lungs. As the haemoglobin molecule loads and unloads O_2 the individual globin chains in the haemoglobin molecule move on each other (Fig. 2.8). The $\alpha_1\beta_1$ and $\alpha_2\beta_2$ contacts stabilize the molecule. The β chains slide on the $\alpha_1\beta_2$ and $\alpha_2\beta_1$ contacts during oxygenation and deoxygenation. When O_2 is unloaded the β chains are pulled apart, permitting entry of the metabolite 2,3-diphosphoglycerate (2,3-DPG) resulting in a lower affinity of the molecule for O_2. This movement is responsible for the sigmoid form of the haemoglobin O_2 dissociation curve (Fig. 2.9). The P_{50} (i.e. the partial pressure of O_2 at which haemoglobin is half saturated with O_2) of normal blood is 26.6 mmHg. With increased affinity for O_2, the curve shifts to the left (i.e. the P_{50} falls) while with decreased affinity for O_2 the curve shifts to the right (i.e. the P_{50} rises).

Normally *in vivo*, O_2 exchange operates between 95% saturation (arterial blood) with a mean arterial O_2 tension of 95 mmHg and 70% saturation (venous blood) with a mean venous O_2 tension of 40 mmHg.

The normal position of the curve depends on the concentration of 2,3-DPG, H^+ ions and CO_2 in the red cell and on the structure of the haemoglobin molecule. High concentrations of 2,3-DPG, H^+ or CO_2, and the presence of certain haemoglobins (e.g. sickle haemoglobin, Hb S), shift the curve to the right (oxygen is given up more easily) whereas fetal haemoglobin (Hb F)—which is unable to bind 2,3-DPG—and certain rare abnormal haemoglobins associated with polycythaemia shift the curve to the left because they give up O_2 less readily than normal.

Methaemoglobinaemia

This is a clinical state in which circulating haemoglobin is present with iron in the oxidized (Fe^{3+}) instead of the usual Fe^{2+} state. It may arise because of a hereditary deficiency of reduced nicotinamide adenine dinucleotide (NADH), diaphorase or inheritance of a structurally abnormal haemoglobin (Hb M). These contain an amino acid substitution affecting the haem pocket of the globin chain. Toxic methaemoglobinaemia (and/or sulphaemoglobinaemia) occurs when a drug or other toxic substance oxidizes haemoglobin. In all these states, the patient is likely to show cyanosis.

The red cell

In order to carry haemoglobin into close contact with the tissues and for successful gaseous exchange, the red cell, 8 μm in diameter, must be able: to pass repeatedly through the microcirculation whose minimum diameter is 3.5 μm, to maintain haemoglobin in a reduced (ferrous) state and to maintain osmotic equilibrium despite the high concentration of protein (haemoglobin) in the cell. Its total journey throughout its 120-day lifespan has been estimated to be 480 km (300 miles). To fulfil these functions, the cell is a flexible biconcave disc with an ability to generate energy as adenosine triphosphate (ATP) by the anaerobic glycolytic (Embden–Meyerhof) pathway (Fig. 2.10) and to generate reducing power as NADH by this pathway and as reduced nicotinamide adenine dinucleotide phosphate (NADPH) by the hexose monophosphate shunt (Fig. 2.11).

Red cell metabolism

Embden–Meyerhof pathway

In this series of biochemical reactions, glucose that enters the red cell from plasma by facilitated transfer is metabolized to lactate (Fig. 2.10). For each molecule of glucose used, two molecules of ATP and thus two high-energy phosphate bonds are generated. This ATP provides energy for maintenance of red cell volume, shape and flexibility. The red cell has an osmotic pressure five times that of plasma and an inherent weakness of the membrane results in continual Na^+ and K^+ movement. A membrane ATPase sodium pump is needed, and this uses one molecule of ATP to move three sodium ions out and two potassium ions into the cell.

The Embden–Meyerhof pathway also generates NADH which is needed by the enzyme methaemoglobin reductase to reduce functionally dead methaemoglobin (oxidized haemoglobin) containing ferric iron (produced by oxidation of approximately 3% of haemoglobin each day) to functionally active, reduced haemoglobin. The Luebering–Rapoport shunt, or side arm, of this pathway (Fig. 2.10b) generates 2,3-DPG which forms a 1 : 1 complex with haemoglobin and, as mentioned above, is important in the regulation of haemoglobin's oxygen affinity.

Hexose monophosphate (pentose phosphate) pathway

Approximately 10% of glycolysis occurs by this oxidative pathway in which glucose-6-phosphate is converted to 6-phosphogluconate and so to ribulose-5-phosphate (Fig. 2.11). NADPH is generated and is linked with glutathione which maintains sulphydril (SH) groups intact in the cell including those in haemoglobin and the red cell membrane. NADPH is also used by another methaemoglobin reductase to maintain haemoglobin iron in the functionally active Fe^{2+} state. In one of the most common inherited abnormalities of red cells, glucose-6-phosphate dehydrogenase (G6PD) deficiency, the red cells are extremely susceptible to oxidant stress (p. 63).

Red cell membrane

The red cell membrane comprises a lipid bilayer, integral membrane proteins and a membrane skeleton (Fig. 2.12). Approximately 50% of the membrane is protein, 20% phospholipids, 20% cholesterol molecules and up to 10% is carbohydrate. Carbohydrates occur only on the external surface while

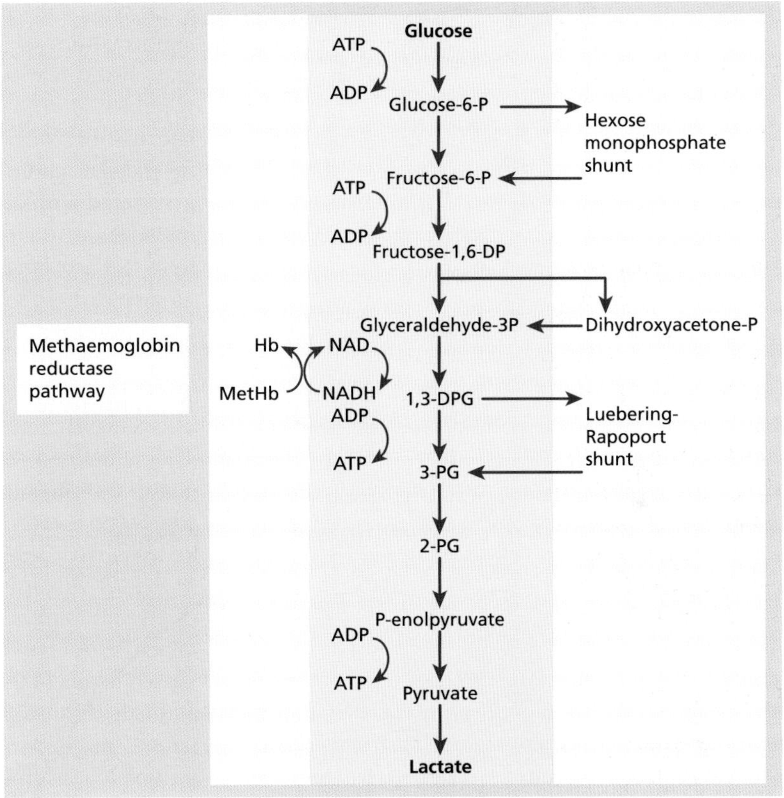

(a)

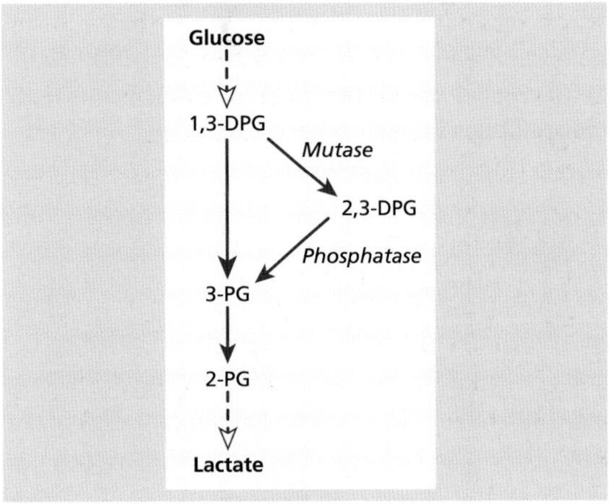

(b)

Fig. 2.10 (a) The Embden–Meyerhof glycolytic pathway. **(b)** The Luebering–Rapoport shunt which regulates the concentration of 2,3-diphosphoglycerate (2,3-DPG) in the red cell. ADP, adenosine diphosphate; ATP, adenosine triphosphate; Hb, haemoglobin; NAD, NADH, nicotinamide adenine dinucleotide; PG, phosphoglycerate.

proteins are either peripheral or integral, penetrating the lipid bilayer. Several red cell proteins have been numbered accordingly to their mobility on polyacrylamide gel electrophoresis (PAGE), e.g. Band 3, proteins 4.1, 4.2 (Fig. 2.12).

The membrane skeleton is formed by structural proteins that include α and β spectrin, ankyrin, protein 4.1 and actin. These proteins form an horizontal lattice on the internal side of the red cell membrane and are important in maintaining the biconcave

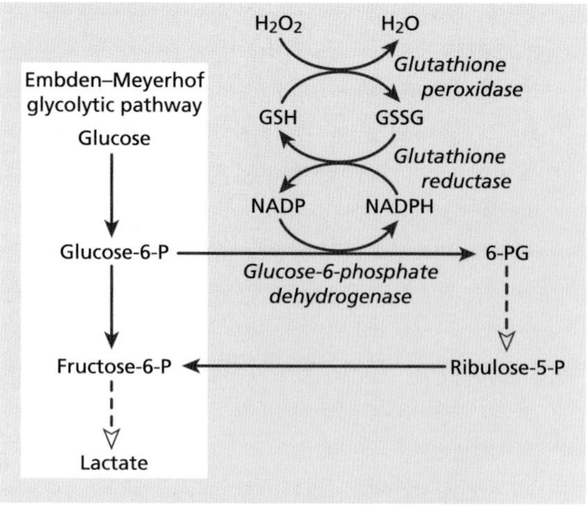

Fig. 2.11 The hexose monophosphate shunt pathway. GSH, GSSG, glutathione; NADP, NADPH, nicotinamide adenine dinucleotide phosphate; P, phosphate; PG, phosphoglycerate.

shape. Spectrin is the most abundant and consists of two chains, α and β, wound around each other to form heterodimers which then self-associate head-to-head to form tetramers. These tetramers are linked at the tail end to actin and are attached to protein band 4.1. At the head end, the β spectrin chains attach to ankyrin which connects to band 3, the transmembrane protein that acts as an anion channel ('vertical connections') (Fig. 2.12). Protein 4.2 enhances this interaction.

Defects of the proteins may explain some of the abnormalities of shape of the red cell membrane (e.g. hereditary spherocytosis and elliptocytosis) (Chapter 5) while alterations in lipid composition because of congenital or acquired abnormalities in plasma cholesterol or phospholipid may be associated with other membrane abnormalities. For instance, an increase in cholesterol and phospholipid has been suggested as one cause of target cells whereas a large selective increase in cholesterol may cause acanthocyte formation (see Fig. 2.16).

Anaemia

This is defined as a reduction in the haemoglobin concentration of the blood. Although normal values can vary between laboratories, typical values would be less than 13.5 g/dL in adult males and less than 11.5 g/dL in adult females (Fig. 2.13). From the age of 2 years to puberty, less than 11.0 g/dL indicates anaemia. As newborn infants have a high haemoglobin level, 14.0 g/dL is taken as the lower limit at birth (Fig. 2.13). Reduction of haemoglobin is usually accompanied by a fall in red cell count and packed cell volume (PCV) but these may be normal in some patients with subnormal haemoglobin levels (and therefore by definition anaemic). Alterations in total circulating plasma volume as well as of total circulating haemoglobin mass determine the haemoglobin concentration. Reduction in plasma volume (as in dehydration) may mask anaemia or even

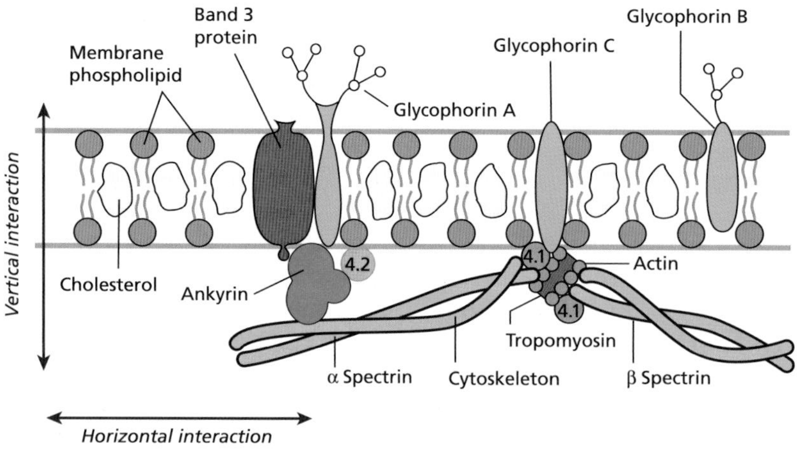

Fig. 2.12 The structure of the red cell membrane. Some of the penetrating and integral proteins carry carbohydrate antigens; other antigens are attached directly to the lipid layer.

Table 2.4 Classification of anaemia.

Microcytic, hypochromic	Normocytic, normochromic	Macrocytic
MCV <80 fL MCH <27 pg Iron deficiency Thalassaemia Anaemia of chronic disease (some cases) Lead poisoning Sideroblastic anaemia (some cases)	MCV 80–95 fL MCH ≥27 pg Many haemolytic anaemias Anaemia of chronic disease (some cases) After acute blood loss Renal disease Mixed deficiencies Bone marrow failure (e.g. post-chemotherapy, infiltration by carcinoma, etc.)	MCV >95 fL Megaloblastic: vitamin B_{12} or folate deficiency Non-megaloblastic: alcohol, liver disease, myelodysplasia, aplastic anaemia, etc. (Table 4.11)

MCH, mean corpuscular haemoglobin; MCV, mean corpuscular volume.

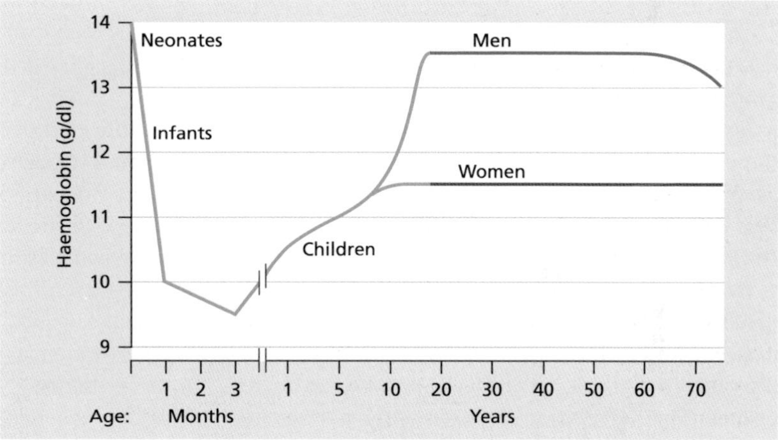

Fig. 2.13 The lower limit of normal blood haemoglobin concentration in men, women and children of various ages.

cause (pseudo) polycythaemia (p. 236); conversely, an increase in plasma volume (as with splenomegaly or pregnancy) may cause anaemia even with a normal total circulating red cell and haemoglobin mass.

After acute major blood loss, anaemia is not immediately apparent because the total blood volume is reduced. It takes up to a day for the plasma volume to be replaced and so for the degree of anaemia to become apparent (p. 350). Regeneration of the haemoglobin mass takes substantially longer. The initial clinical features of major blood loss are therefore a result of reduction in blood volume rather than anaemia.

Clinical features of anaemia

The major adaptations to anaemia are in the cardiovascular system (with increased stroke volume and tachycardia) and in the haemoglobin O_2 dissociation curve. In some patients with quite severe anaemia there may be no symptoms or signs, whereas others with mild anaemia may be severely incapacitated. The presence or absence of clinical features can be considered under four major headings.

1 ***Speed of onset*** Rapidly progressive anaemia causes more symptoms than anaemia of slow onset because there is less time for adaptation in the cardiovascular system and in the O_2 dissociation curve of haemoglobin.

2 ***Severity*** Mild anaemia often produces no symptoms or signs but these are usually present when the haemoglobin is less than 9–10 g/dL. Even severe anaemia (haemoglobin concentration as low as 6.0 g/dL) may produce remarkably few symptoms,

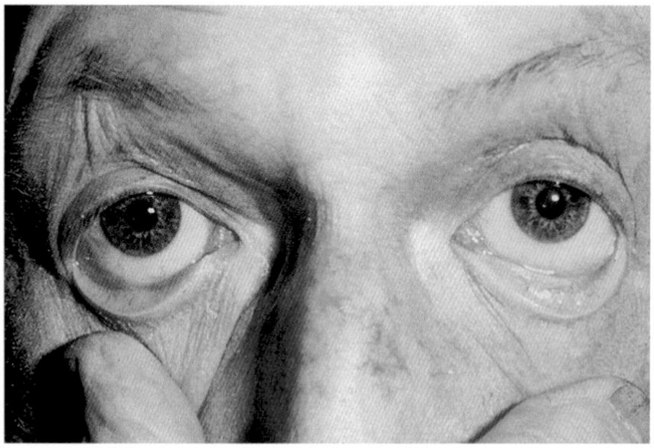

(a)

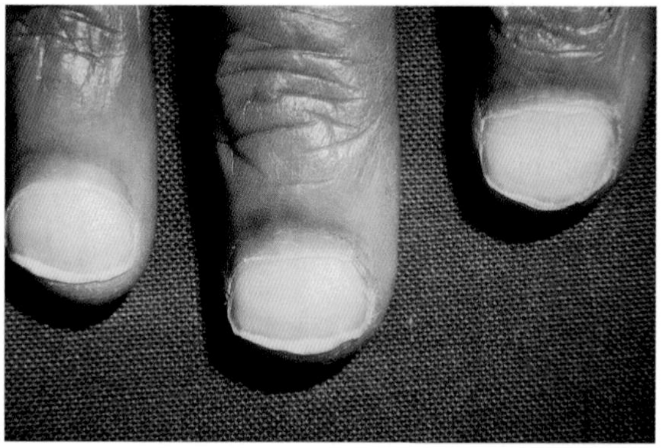

(b)

Fig. 2.14 Pallor of the conjunctival mucosa **(a)** and of the nail bed **(b)** in two patients with severe anaemia (haemoglobin 6.0 g/dL).

however, when there is very gradual onset in a young subject who is otherwise healthy.

3 *Age* The elderly tolerate anaemia less well than the young because of the effect of lack of oxygen on organs when normal cardiovascular compensation (increased cardiac output caused by increased stroke volume and tachycardia) is impaired.

4 ***Haemoglobin*** O_2 ***dissociation curve*** Anaemia, in general, is associated with a rise in 2,3-DPG in the red cells and a shift in the O_2 dissociation curve to the right so that oxygen is given up more readily to tissues. This adaptation is particularly marked in some anaemias which either affect red cell metaboism directly (e.g. the anaemia of pyruvate kinase deficiency which causes a rise in 2,3-DPG concentration in the red cells) or which are associated with a low affinity haemoglobin (e.g. Hb S) (Fig. 2.9).

Symptoms

If the patient does have symptoms these are usually shortness of breath particularly on exercise, weakness, lethargy, palpitation and headaches. In older subjects, symptoms of cardiac failure, angina pectoris or intermittent claudication or confusion may be present. Visual disturbances because of retinal haemorrhages may complicate very severe anaemia, particularly of rapid onset.

Signs

These may be divided into *general* and *specific*. General signs include pallor of mucous membranes which occurs if the haemoglobin level is less than 9–10 g/dL (Fig. 2.14). Conversely, skin colour is not a reliable sign. A hyperdynamic circulation may be present with tachycardia, a bounding pulse, cardiomegaly and a systolic flow murmur especially at the apex. Particularly in the elderly, features of congestive heart failure may be present. Retinal haemorrhages are unusual (Fig. 2.15).

Specific signs are associated with particular types of anaemia (e.g. koilonychia 'spoon nails' with iron deficiency, jaundice with haemolytic or megaloblastic anaemias, leg ulcers with sickle cell and other haemolytic anaemias, bone deformities with

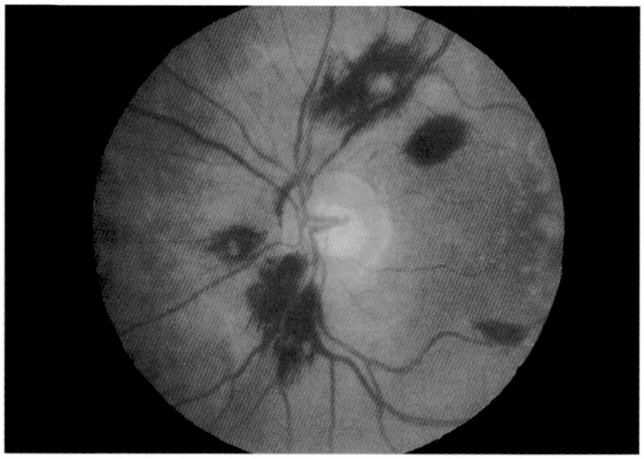

Fig. 2.15 Retinal haemorrhages in a patient with severe anaemia (haemoglobin 2.5 g/dL) caused by severe chronic haemorrhage.

thalassaemia major and other severe congenital haemolytic anaemias).

The association of features of anaemia with excess infections or spontaneous bruising suggest that neutropenia or thrombocytopenia may be present, possibly as a result of bone marrow failure.

Classification and laboratory findings in anaemia

Red cell indices

The most useful classification is that based on red cell indices (Table 2.4) and divides the anaemia into microcytic, normocytic and macrocytic. As well as suggesting the nature of the primary defect, this approach may also indicate an underlying abnormality before overt anaemia has developed.

In two common physiological situations the mean corpuscular volume (MCV) may be outside the normal adult range. In the newborn for a few weeks the MCV is high but in infancy it is low (e.g. 70 fL at 1 year of age) and rises slowly throughout childhood to the normal adult range. In normal pregnancy there is a slight rise in MCV, even in the absence of other causes of macrocytosis (e.g. folate deficiency).

Other laboratory findings

Although the red cell indices will indicate the type of anaemia, further useful information can be obtained from the initial blood sample.

Leucocyte and platelet counts

Measurement of these helps to distinguish 'pure' anaemia from 'pancytopenia' (a drop in red cells, granulocytes and platelets) which suggests a more general marrow defect (e.g. caused by marrow hypoplasia or infiltration) or general destruction of cells (e.g. hypersplenism). In anaemias caused by haemolysis or haemorrhage, the neutrophil and platelet counts are often raised; in infections and leukaemias the leucocyte count is also often raised and there may be abnormal leucocytes or neutrophil precursors present.

Reticulocyte count

The normal percentage is 0.5–2.5%, and the absolute count $25–125 \times 10^9/L$. This should rise in anaemia because of erythropoietin increase and be higher the more severe the anaemia. This is particularly so when there has been time for erythroid hyperplasia to develop in the marrow as in chronic haemolysis. After an acute major haemorrhage there is an erythropoietin response in 6 h, the reticulocyte count rises within 2–3 days, reaches a maximum in 6–10 days and remains raised until the haemoglobin returns to the normal level. If the reticulocyte count is not raised in an anaemic patient this suggests impaired marrow function or lack of erythropoietin stimulus (Table 2.5).

Blood film

It is essential to examine the blood film in all cases of anaemia. Abnormal red cell morphology (Fig. 2.16) or red cell inclusions (Fig. 2.17) may suggest a particular diagnosis. When causes of both microcytosis and macrocytosis are present (e.g. mixed iron and folate or B_{12} deficiency) the indices may be normal but the blood film reveals a 'dimorphic' appearance (a dual population of large well-haemoglobinized cells and small hypochromic cells). During the blood film examination the white cell differential count is performed, platelet number and morphology are assessed and the presence or absence of abnormal cells (e.g. normoblasts, granulocyte precursors or blast cells) is noted.

Table 2.5 Factors impairing the normal reticulocyte response to anaemia.

Marrow diseases (e.g. hypoplasia, infiltration by carcinoma, lymphoma, myeloma, acute leukaemia, tuberculosis)
Deficiency of iron, vitamin B_{12} or folate
Lack of erythropoietin (e.g. renal disease)
Reduced tissue O_2 consumption (e.g. myxoedema, protein deficiency)
Ineffective erythropoiesis (e.g. thalassaemia major, megaloblastic anaemia, myelodysplasia, myelofibrosis, congenital dyserythropoietic anaemia)
Chronic inflammatory or malignant disease

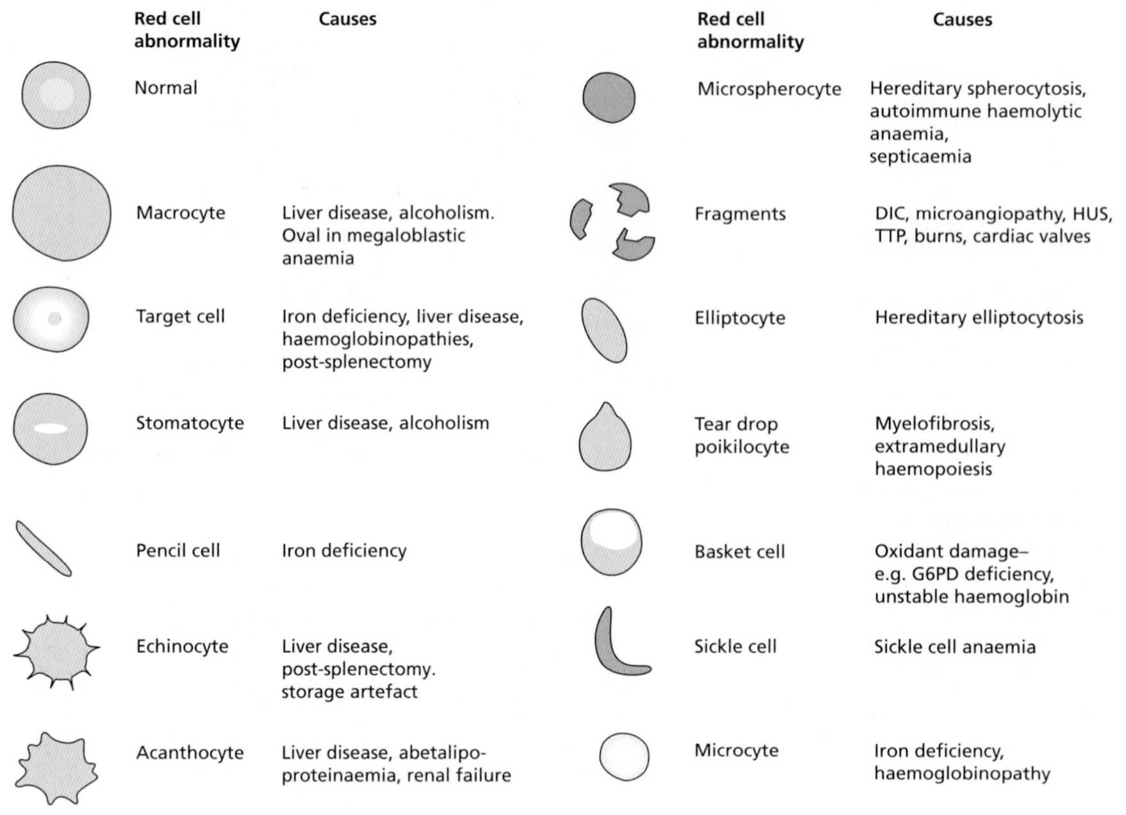

Fig. 2.16 Some of the more frequent variations in size (anisocytosis) and shape (poikilocytosis) that may be found in different anaemias. DIC, disseminated intravascular coagulopathy; G6PD, glucose-6-phosphate dehydrogenase; HUS, haemolytic uraemic syndrome; TTP, thrombotic thrombocytopenic purpura.

Bone marrow examination

This may be performed by aspiration or trephine biopsy (Fig. 2.18). During bone marrow aspiration a needle is inserted into the marrow and a liquid sample of marrow is sucked into a syringe. This is then spread on a slide for microscopy and stained by the usual Romanowsky technique. A great deal of morphological information can be obtained by examining aspirate slides. The detail of the developing cells can be examined (e.g. normoblastic or megaloblastic), the proportion of the different cell lines assessed (myeloid : erythroid ratio) and the presence of cells foreign to the marrow (e.g. secondary carcinoma) observed. The cellularity of the marrow can also be viewed provided fragments are obtained. An iron stain is performed routinely so that the amount of iron in reticuloendothelial stores (macrophages) and as fine granules ('siderotic' granules) in the developing erythroblasts can be assessed.

An aspirate sample may also be used for a number of other specialized investigations (Table 2.6).

A trephine biopsy provides a solid core of bone including marrow and is examined as a histological specimen after fixation in formalin, decalcification and sectioning. It is less valuable than aspiration when individual cell detail is to be examined but provides a panoramic view of the marrow from which overall marrow architecture, cellularity and presence of fibrosis or abnormal infiltrates can be reliably determined.

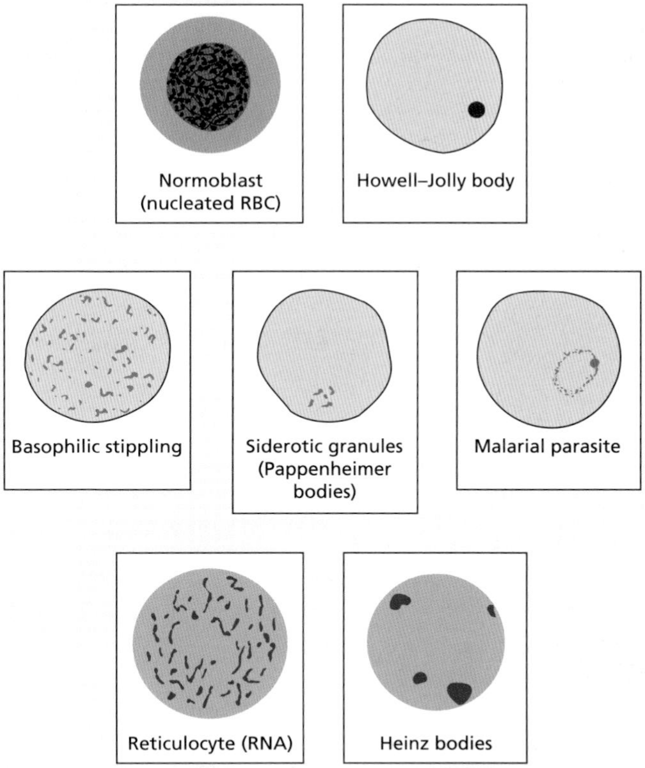

Fig. 2.17 Red blood cell (RBC) inclusions which may be seen in the peripheral blood film in various conditions. The reticulocyte RNA and Heinz bodies are only demonstrated by supravital staining (e.g. with new methylene blue). Heinz bodies are oxidized denatured haemoglobin. Siderotic granules (Pappenheimer bodies) contain iron. They are purple on conventional staining but blue with Perls' stain. The Howell–Jolly body is a DNA remnant. Basophilic stippling is denatured RNA.

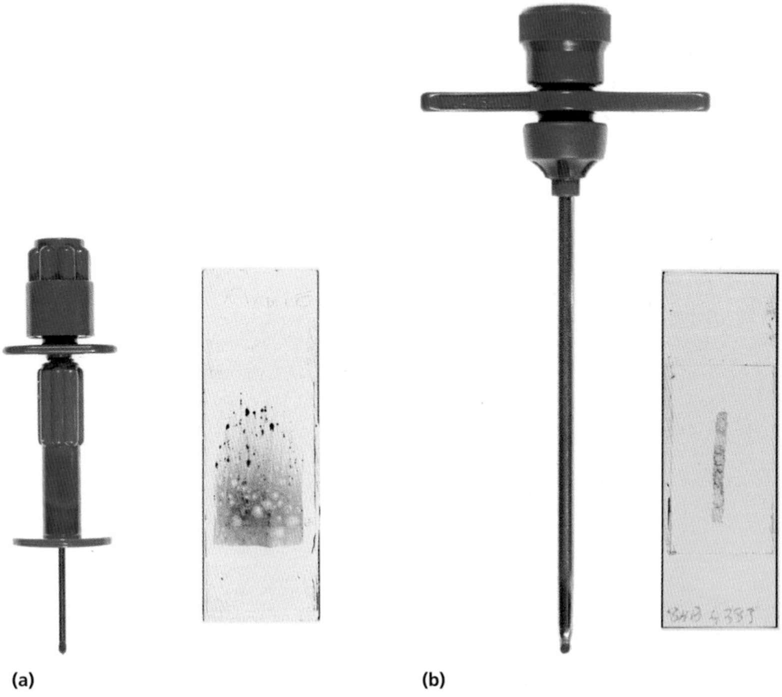

Fig. 2.18 **(a)** The bone marrow aspiration needle and a smear made from a bone marrow aspirate. **(b)** The bone marrow trephine (biopsy) needle and normal trephine section.

Table 2.6 Comparison of bone marrow aspiration and trephine biopsy.

	Aspiration	Trephine
Site	Posterior iliac crest or sternum (tibia in infants)	Posterior iliac crest
Stains	Romanowsky; Perls' reaction (for iron)	Haematoxylin and eosin; reticulin (silver stain)
Result available	1–2 h	1–7 days (according to decalcification method)
Main indications	Investigation of anaemia, pancytopenia, suspected leukaemia or myeloma, neutropenia, thrombocytopenia, etc.	Indications for additional trephine: suspicion of polycythaemia vera, myelofibrosis and other myeloproliferative disorders, aplastic anaemia, malignant lymphoma, secondary carcinoma, cases of splenomegaly or pyrexia of undetermined cause. Any case where aspiration gives a 'dry' tap
Special tests	Cytogenetics, microbiological culture, biochemical analysis, immunological and cytochemical markers, DNA or RNA analysis for gene abnormalities, progenitor cell culture	Immunological staining

Ineffective erythropoiesis

Erythropoiesis is not entirely efficient because approximately 10–15% of developing erythroblasts die within the marrow without producing mature cells. This is termed ineffective erythropoiesis and it is substantially increased in a number of chronic anaemias. The serum unconjugated bilirubin (derived from breaking down haemoglobin) and lactate dehydrogenase (LDH, derived from breaking down cells) are usually raised when ineffective erythropoiesis is marked. The reticulocyte count is low in relation to the degree of anaemia and to the proportion of erythroblasts in the marrow.

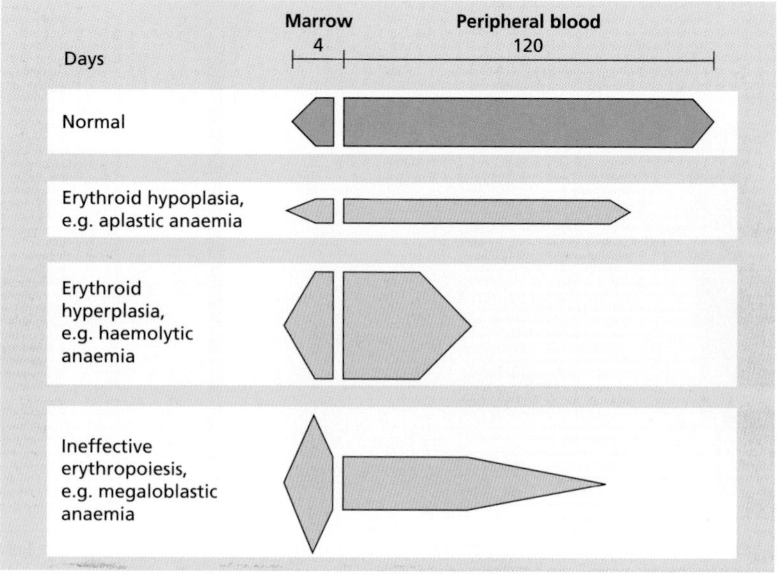

Fig. 2.19 The relative proportions of marrow erythroblastic activity, circulating red cell mass and red cell lifespan in normal subjects and in three types of anaemia.

Assessment of erythropoiesis

Total erythropoiesis and the amount of erythropoiesis that is effective in producing circulating red cells can be assessed by examining the bone marrow, haemoglobin level and reticulocyte count.

Total erythropoiesis is assessed from the marrow cellularity and the myeloid : erythroid ratio (i.e. the proportion of granulocyte precursors to red cell precursors in the bone marrow, normally 2.5 : 1 to 12 : 1). This ratio falls and may be reversed when total erythropoiesis is selectively increased.

Effective erythropoiesis is assessed by the reticulocyte count. This is raised in proportion to the degree of anaemia when erythropoiesis is effective, but is low when there is ineffective erythropoiesis or an abnormality preventing normal marrow response (Table 2.5).

Red cell lifespan

This used to be measured by ^{51}Cr-labelled red cell survival. A sample of the subject's blood was incubated with ^{51}Cr which binds firmly to haemoglobin and the labelled cells reinjected into the circulation. The disappearance of ^{51}Cr from the blood was measured sequentially over the next 3 weeks. The sites of red cell destruction were determined by surface counting over the spleen, liver and heart (as an index of blood activity). This test has now fallen out of routine use: Figure 2.19 shows typical changes in marrow erythropoiesis, circulating red cell mass and red cell life span in some of the different types of anaemia.

Bibliography

Bennett C.L., Luminari S., Nissenson A.R. *et al.* (2004) Pure red-cell aplasia and epoetin therapy. *N Engl J Med* **351**,1403–8.

Cantor A.B. and Orkin S.H. (2002) Transcriptional regulation of erythropoiesis: an affair involving multiple partners. *Oncogene* **21**,3368–76.

Eschbach J.W. (2005) Iron requirements in erythropoietin therapy. *Best Pract Res Clin Haematol* **18**,347–61.

Samol J. and Littlewood T.J. (2003) The efficacy of rHuEPO in cancer-related anaemia. *Br J Haematol* **121**,3–11.

CHAPTER 3

3 Hypochromic anaemias and iron overload

Iron deficiency is the most common cause of anaemia in every country of the world. It is the most important cause of a microcytic hypochromic anaemia, in which the two red cell indices MCV (mean corpuscular volume) and MCH (mean corpuscular haemoglobin) are reduced and the blood film shows small (microcytic) and pale (hypochromic) red cells. This appearance is caused by a defect in haemoglobin synthesis (Fig. 3.1). The major differential diagnosis in microcytic hypochromic anaemia is thalassaemia which is considered in Chapter 6 and anaemia of chronic disease which is dealt with in this chapter.

Nutritional and metabolic aspects of iron

Iron is one of the most common elements in the Earth's crust, yet iron deficiency is the most common cause of anaemia, affecting about 500 million people worldwide. This is because the body has a limited ability to absorb iron and excess loss of iron as a result of haemorrhage is frequent.

Body iron distribution and transport

The transport and storage of iron is largely mediated by three proteins: transferrin, the transferrin receptor 1 (TfR1) and ferritin.

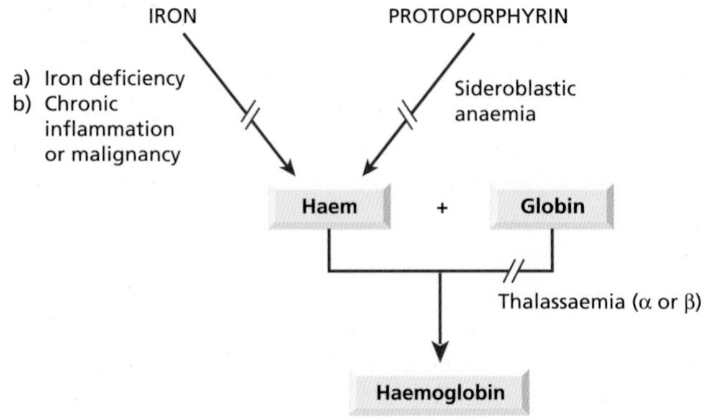

Fig. 3.1 The causes of a hypochromic, microcytic anaemia. These include lack of iron (iron deficiency) or of iron release from macrophages to serum (anaemia of chronic inflammation or malignancy), failure of protoporphyrin synthesis (sideroblastic anaemia) or of globin synthesis (α- or β-thalassaemia). Lead also inhibits haem and globin synthesis.

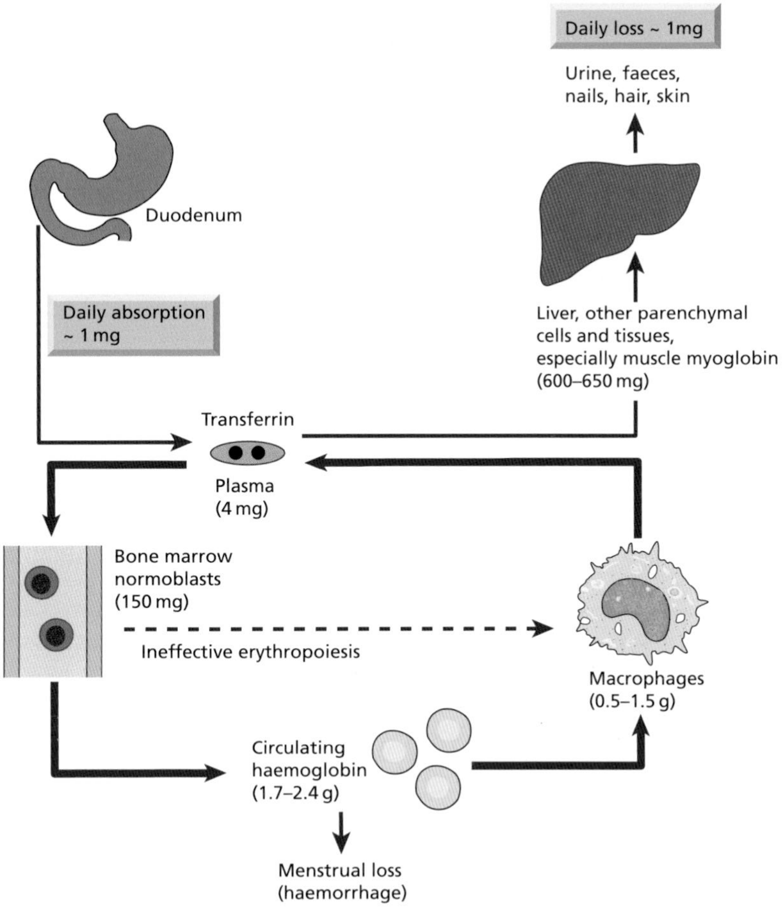

Fig. 3.2 Daily iron cycle. Most of the iron in the body is contained in circulating haemoglobin (Table 3.1) and is reutilized for haemoglobin synthesis after the red cells die. Iron is transferred from macrophages to plasma transferrin and so to bone marrow erythroblasts. Iron absorption is normally just sufficient to make up for iron loss. The dashed line indicates ineffective erythropoiesis.

Transferrin can contain up to two atoms of iron. It delivers iron to tissues that have transferrin receptors, especially erythroblasts in the bone marrow which incorporate the iron into haemoglobin (Fig. 3.2). The transferrin is then reutilized. At the end of their life, red cells are broken down in the macrophages of the reticuloendothelial system (RES) and the iron is released from haemoglobin, enters the plasma and provides most of the iron on transferrin. Only a small proportion of plasma transferrin iron comes from dietary iron, absorbed through the duodenum and jejunum.

Some iron is stored in the macrophages as ferritin and haemosiderin, the amount varying widely according to overall body iron status. Ferritin is a water-soluble protein–iron complex of molecular weight 465 000. It is made up of an outer protein shell, apoferritin, consisting of 22 subunits and an iron–phosphate–hydroxide core. It contains up to 20% of its weight as iron and is not visible by light microscopy. Each molecule of apoferritin may bind up to 4000–5000 atoms of iron.

Haemosiderin is an insoluble protein–iron complex of varying composition containing approximately 37% iron by weight. It is derived from partial lysosomal digestion of aggregates of ferritin molecules and is visible in macrophages and other cells by light microscopy after staining by Perls' (Prussian blue) reaction. Iron in ferritin and haemosiderin is in the ferric form. It is mobilized after reduction to the ferrous form, vitamin C being involved. A copper-containing enzyme, caeruloplasmin, catalyses oxidation of the iron to the ferric form for binding to plasma transferrin.

Iron is also present in muscle as myoglobin and in most cells of the body in iron-containing enzymes (e.g. cytochromes, succinic dehydrogenase, catalase) (Table 3.1). This tissue iron is less likely to

Table 3.1 The distribution of body iron.

Amount of iron in average adult	Male (g)	Female (g)	Percentage of total
Haemoglobin	2.4	1.7	65
Ferritin and haemosiderin	1.0 (0.3–1.5)	0.3 (0–1.0)	30
Myoglobin	0.15	0.12	3.5
Haem enzymes (e.g. cytochromes, catalase, peroxidases, flavoproteins)	0.02	0.015	0.5
Transferrin-bound iron	0.004	0.003	0.1

become depleted than haemosiderin, ferritin and haemoglobin in states of iron deficiency, but some reduction of haem-containing enzymes may occur.

Regulation of ferritin and transferrin receptor 1 synthesis

The levels of ferritin and TfR1 are linked to iron status so that iron overload causes a rise in tissue ferritin and a fall in TfR1, whereas in iron deficiency ferritin is low and TfR1 increased. This linkage arises through the binding of an iron regulatory protein (IRP) to iron response elements (IREs) on the ferritin and TfR1 mRNA molecules. Iron deficiency increases the ability of IRP to bind to the IREs whereas iron overload reduces the binding. The site of IRP binding to IREs, whether upstream (5′) or downstream (3′) from the coding gene, determines whether the amount of mRNA and so protein produced is increased or decreased (Fig. 3.3). Upstream binding reduces translation whereas downstream binding stabilizes the mRNA, increasing protein translation.

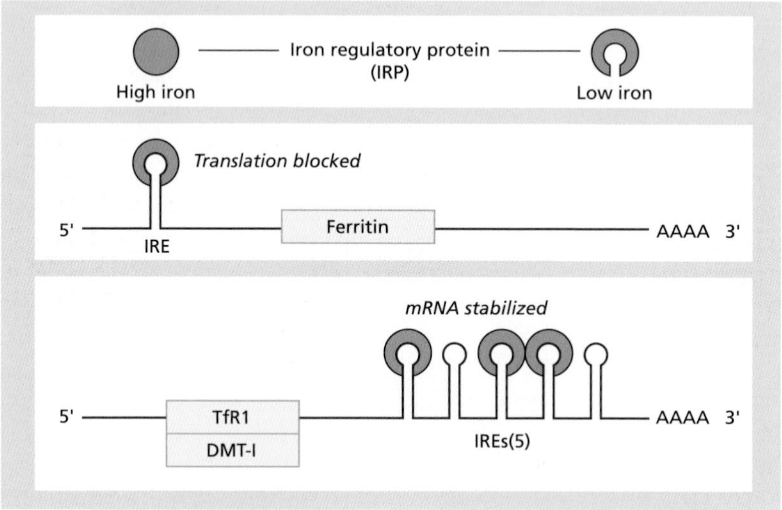

Fig. 3.3 Regulation of transferrin receptor 1 (TfR1), DMT-1 (divalent metal transporter) and ferritin expression by iron regulatory protein (IRP) sensing of intracellular iron levels. IRPs (●) are able to bind to stem-loop structures called iron response elements (IREs) in transferrin receptor or ferritin mRNAs. IRP binding to the IRE within the 3′ untranslated region of TfR or DMT-1 mRNA leads to stabilization of the mRNA and increased protein synthesis whereas IRP binding to the IRE within the 5′ untranslated region of ferritin mRNA reduces translation. IRPs can exist in two states: at times of high iron levels the IRP binds iron and exhibits a reduced affinity for the IREs whereas when iron levels are low the binding of IRPs to IREs is increased. In this way synthesis of TfR, DMT-1 and ferritin is coordinated to physiological requirements.

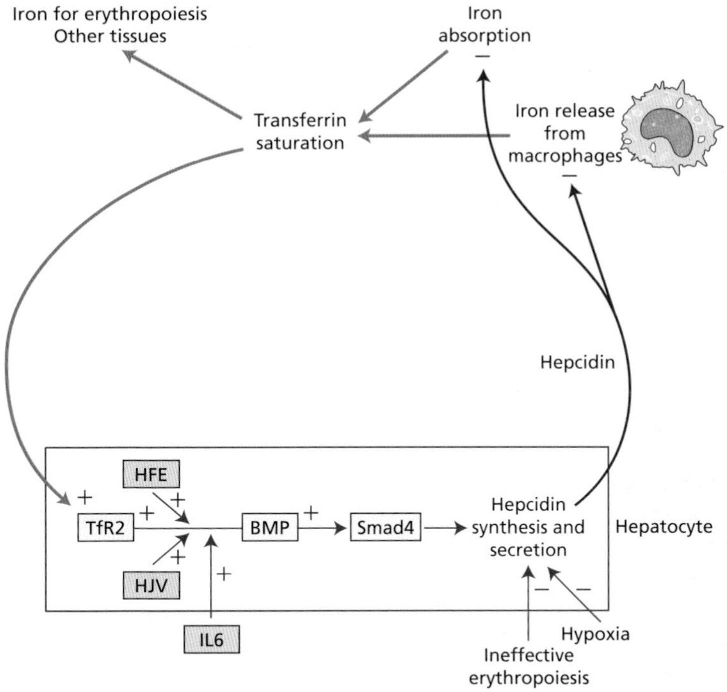

Fig. 3.4 The role of hepcidin in the regulation of iron-absorption and iron-release from macrophages. BMP, bone morphogenetic protein; HJV, hemojuvelin; Smad4, transcription factor Smad4 which stimulates hepcidin synthesis; TfR2, transferrin receptor 2.

When plasma iron is raised and transferrin is saturated the amount of iron transferred to parenchymal cells (e.g. those of the liver, endocrine organs, pancreas and heart) is increased and this is the basis of the pathological changes associated with iron loading conditions.

Hepcidin

Hepcidin is a 25-amino acid polypeptide produced by liver cells. It is both an acute phase protein and the major hormonal regulator of iron homeostasis (Fig. 3.4). It inhibits iron release from macrophages, intestinal epithelial cells and from placental syncytiotrophoblasts by its interaction with the transmembrane iron exporter ferroportin, accelerating degradation of ferroportin mRNA. Increased production of hepcidin is induced by inflammation via interleukin 6 (IL-6). Hepcidin synthesis and secretion are controlled by three proteins: HFE, hemojuvelin and transferrin receptor 2. Decreased production of hepcidin occurs in response to iron deficiency, hypoxia and ineffective erythropoiesis.

Transferrin receptor 2

This senses the degree of saturation of transferrin and is a key regulator of hepcidin synthesis (Fig. 3.4). High saturation levels of transferrin stimulate hepcidin synthesis by this pathway whereas low saturation levels as in iron deficiency reduce hepcidin synthesis. HFE and hemojuvelin are also involved in hepcidin synthesis. Transferrin receptor 2 is restricted to erythroid, duodenal crypt and liver cells.

Dietary iron

Iron is present in food as ferric hydroxides, ferric–protein and haem–protein complexes. Both the iron content and the proportion of iron absorbed differ from food to food; in general, meat—in particular liver—is a better source than vegetables, eggs or dairy foods. The average Western diet contains 10–15 mg iron daily from which only 5–10% is normally absorbed. The proportion can be increased to 20–30% in iron deficiency or pregnancy (Table 3.2)

Table 3.2 Iron absorption.

Factors favouring absorption	Factors reducing absorption
Haem iron	Inorganic iron
Ferrous form (Fe^{2+})	Ferric form (Fe^{3+})
Acids (HCl, vitamin C)	Alkalis—antacids, pancreatic secretions
Solubilizing agents (e.g. sugars, amino acids)	Precipitating agents—phytates, phosphates
Iron deficiency	Iron excess
Ineffective erythropoiesis	Decreased erythropoiesis
Pregnancy	Infection
Hereditary haemochromatosis	Tea
Increased expression of DMT-1 and ferroportin in duodenal enterocytes	Decreased expression of DMT-1 and ferroportin in duodenal enterocytes
	Increased hepcidin

but even in these situations most dietary iron remains unabsorbed.

Iron absorption

Organic dietary iron is partly absorbed as haem and partly broken down in the gut to inorganic iron. Absorption occurs through the duodenum. Haem is absorbed through a specific receptor, HCP-1, exposed on the apical membrane of the duodenal enterocyte. Haem is then digested to release iron. Inorganic iron absorption is favoured by factors such as acid and reducing agents that keep iron in the gut lumen in the Fe^{2+} rather than the Fe^{3+} state (Table 3.2). The protein DMT-1 (divalent metal transporter) is involved in transfer of iron from the lumen of the gut across the enterocyte microvilli (Fig. 3.5). Ferroportin at the basolateral surface controls exit of iron from the cell into portal plasma. The amount of iron absorbed is partly regulated

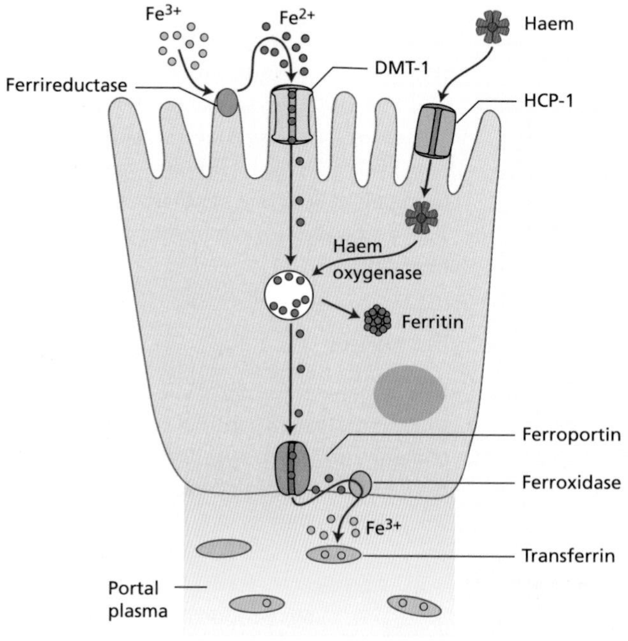

Fig. 3.5 The regulation of iron-absorption. Dietary ferric (Fe^{3+}) iron is reduced to Fe^{2+} and its entry to the enterocyte is through the divalent cation binder DMT-1. Its export into portal plasma is controlled by ferroportin. It is oxidized before binding to transferrin in plasma. Haem is absorbed after binding to its receptor protein HCP-1.

Table 3.3 Estimated daily iron requirements. Units are mg/day.

	Urine, sweat, faeces	Menses	Pregnancy	Growth	Total
Adult male	0.5–1				0.5–1
Postmenopausal female	0.5–1				0.5–1
Menstruating female*	0.5–1	0.5–1			1–2
Pregnant female*	0.5–1		1–2		1.5–3
Children (average)	0.5			0.6	1.1
Female (age 12–15)*	0.5–1	0.5–1		0.6	1.6–2.6

* These groups are more likely to develop iron deficiency.

according to the body's needs by changing the levels of DMT-1 according to the iron status of the duodenal villous crypt enterocyte. In iron deficiency less iron is delivered to the crypt cell from transferrin which is largely unsaturated with iron. The consequent iron deficiency in the crypt cell results in increased expresssion of DMT-1. This occurs by the same mechanism (IRP/IRE binding) by which transferrin receptor is increased in iron deficiency (Fig. 3.3). The increased expression of DMT-1 results, when the enterocyte reaches the apical absorptive surface of the duodenal villous 24–48 h later, in increased transfer of iron from the gut lumen into the enterocyte. Hepcidin is also a major regulator by affecting ferroportin concentration. Low hepcidin levels in iron deficiency increase ferroportin levels and allow more iron to enter portal plasma. Thus, less iron is lost when the enterocyte is shed into the gut lumen from the apex of the villous.

Ferrireductase present at the apical surface converts iron from the Fe^{3+} to Fe^{2+} state and another enzyme, hephaestin (which contains copper), converts Fe^{2+} to Fe^{3+} at the basal surface prior to binding to transferrin.

Iron requirements

The amount of iron required each day to compensate for losses from the body and for growth varies with age and sex; it is highest in pregnancy, adolescent and menstruating females (Table 3.3). Therefore these groups are particularly likely to develop iron deficiency if there is additional iron loss or prolonged reduced intake.

Iron deficiency

Clinical features

When iron deficiency is developing the reticuloendothelial stores (haemosiderin and ferritin) become completely depleted before anaemia occurs (Fig. 3.6).

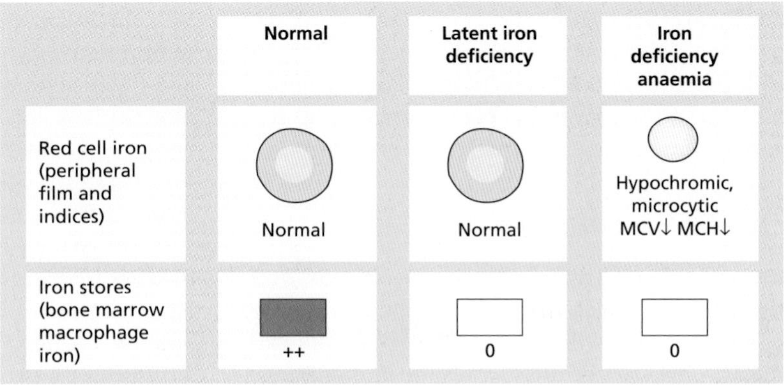

Fig. 3.6 The development of iron deficiency anaemia. Reticuloendothelial (macrophage) stores are lost completely before anaemia develops. MCH, mean corpuscular haemoglobin; MCV, mean corpuscular volume.

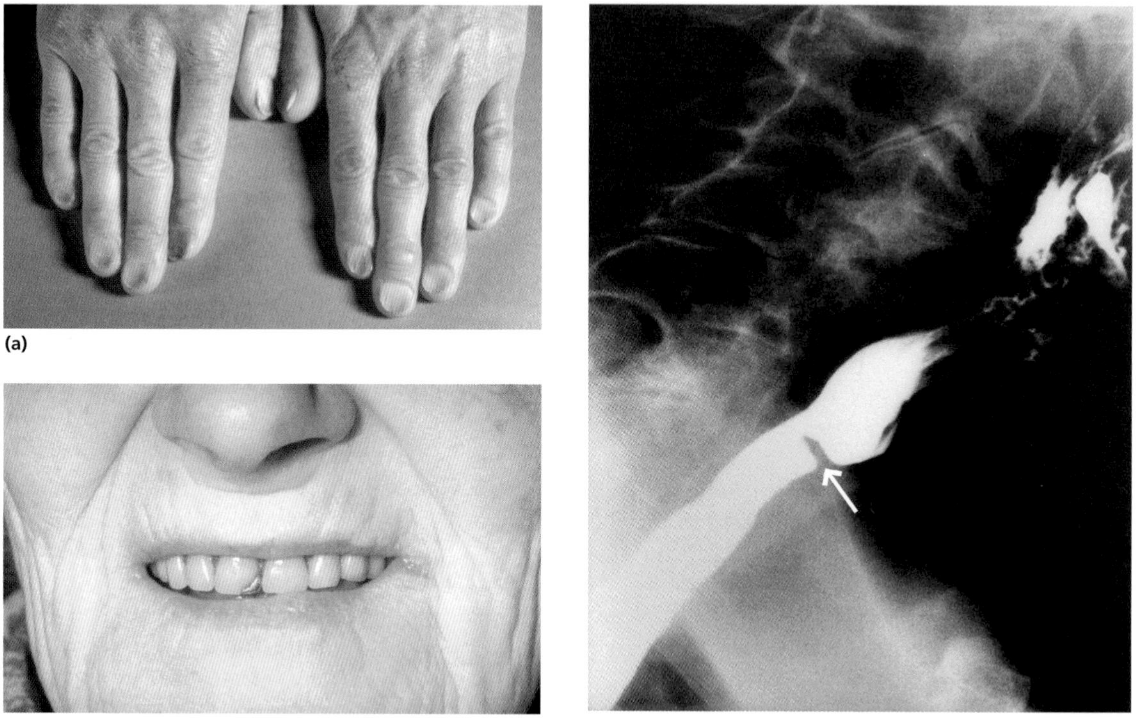

(a) (b) (c)

Fig. 3.7 Iron deficiency anaemia. **(a)** Koilonychia: typical 'spoon' nails. **(b)** Angular cheilosis: fissuring and ulceration of the corner of the mouth. **(c)** Paterson–Kelly (Plummer–Vinson) syndrome: barium swallow X-ray showing a filling defect (arrow) caused by a postcricoid web.

As the condition develops the patient may develop the general symptoms and signs of anaemia (p. 21) and also show a painless glossitis, angular stomatitis, brittle, ridged or spoon nails (koilonychia), dysphagia as a result of pharyngeal webs (Paterson–Kelly or Plummer–Vinson syndrome) (Fig. 3.7) and unusual dietary cravings (pica). The cause of the epithelial cell changes is not clear but may be related to reduction of iron in iron-containing enzymes. In children, iron deficiency is particularly significant as it can cause irritability, poor cognitive function and a decline in psychomotor development.

Causes of iron deficiency

Chronic blood loss, especially uterine or from the gastrointestinal tract, is the dominant cause (Table 3.4). In contrast, in developed countries dietary deficiency is rarely a cause on its own. Half a litre of whole blood contains approximately 250 mg of iron and, despite the increased absorption of food iron at an early stage of iron deficiency, negative iron balance is usual in chronic blood loss.

Increased demands during infancy, adolescence, pregnancy, lactation and in menstruating women account for the high risk of anaemia in these particular clinical groups. Newborn infants have a store of iron derived from delayed clamping of the cord and the breakdown of excess red cells. From 3 to 6 months there is a tendency for negative iron balance because of growth. From 6 months supplemented formula milk and mixed feeding, particularly with iron-fortified foods, prevents iron deficiency.

In pregnancy increased iron is needed for an increased maternal red cell mass of approximately 35%, transfer of 300 mg of iron to the fetus and because of blood loss at delivery. Although iron absorption is also increased, iron therapy is often

Table 3.4 Causes of iron deficiency.

Chronic blood loss
Uterine
Gastrointestinal, e.g. peptic ulcer, oesophageal varices, aspirin (or other non-steroidal anti-inflammatory drugs) ingestion, partial gastrectomy, carcinoma of the stomach, caecum, colon or rectum, hookworm, angiodysplasia, colitis, piles, diverticulosis
Rarely, haematuria, haemoglobinuria, pulmonary haemosiderosis, self-inflicted blood loss
Increased demands (see also Table 3.3)
Prematurity
Growth
Pregnancy
Erythropoietin therapy
Malabsorption
Gluten-induced enteropathy, gastrectomy
Poor diet
A contributory factor in many developing countries but rarely the sole cause except in infants and children

needed if the haemoglobin (Hb) falls below 10 g/dL or the mean cell volume (MCV) is below 82 fL in the third trimester.

Menorrhagia (a loss of 80 mL or more of blood at each cycle) is difficult to assess clinically, although the loss of clots, the use of large numbers of pads or tampons or prolonged periods all suggest excessive loss.

It has been estimated to take 8 years for a normal adult male to develop iron deficiency anaemia solely as a result of a poor diet or malabsorption resulting in no iron intake at all. In clinical practice inadequate intake or malabsorption are only rarely the sole cause of iron deficiency anaemia although in developing countries iron deficiency may occur as a result of a life-long poor diet, consisting mainly of cereals and vegetables. Gluten-induced enteropathy, partial or total gastrectomy and atrophic gastritis (often autoimmune and with *Helicobacter pylori* infection) may, however, predispose to iron deficiency.

Laboratory findings

These are summarized and contrasted with those in other hypochromic anaemias in Table 3.7.

Red cell indices and blood film

Even before anaemia occurs, the red cell indices fall and they fall progressively as the anaemia becomes more severe. The blood film shows hypochromic microcytic cells with occasional target cells and pencil-shaped poikilocytes (Fig. 3.8). The reticulocyte count is low in relation to the degree of anaemia. When iron deficiency is associated with severe folate or vitamin B_{12} deficiency a 'dimorphic' film

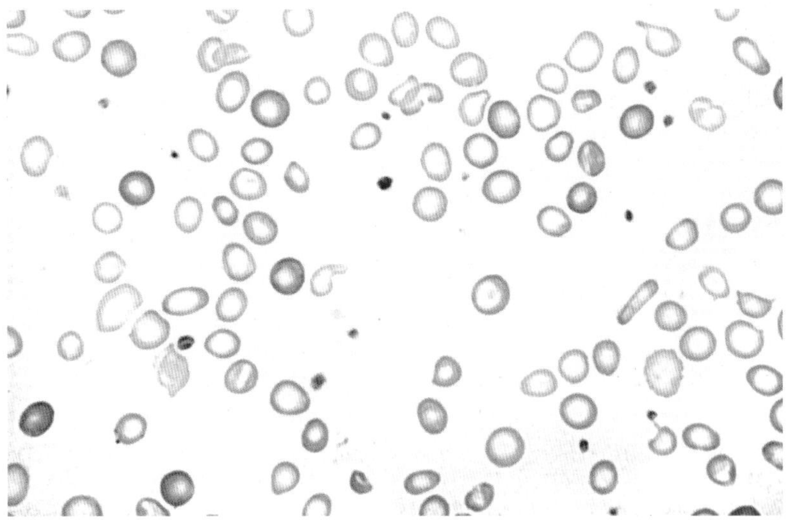

Fig. 3.8 The peripheral blood film in severe iron deficiency anaemia. The cells are microcytic and hypochromic with occasional target cells.

occurs with a dual population of red cells of which one is macrocytic and the other microcytic and hypochromic; the indices may be normal. A dimorphic blood film is also seen in patients with iron deficiency anaemia who have received recent iron therapy and produced a population of new haemoglobinized normal-sized red cells (Fig. 3.9) and when the patient has been transfused. The platelet count is often moderately raised in iron deficiency, particularly when haemorrhage is continuing.

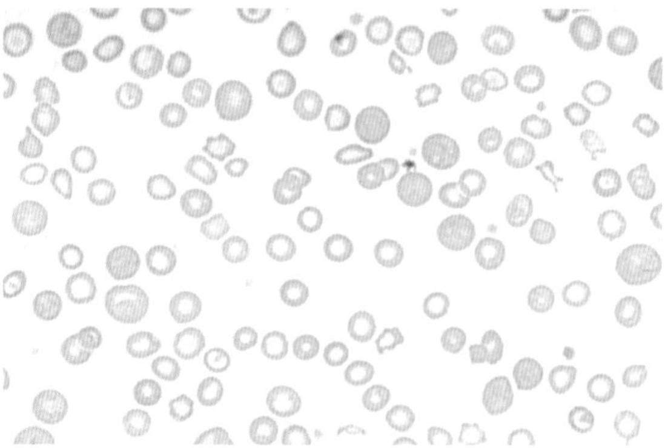

Fig. 3.9 Dimorphic blood film in iron deficiency anaemia responding to iron therapy. Two populations of red cells are present: one microcytic and hypochromic, the other normocytic and well haemoglobinized.

Bone marrow iron

Bone marrow examination is not essential to assess iron stores except in complicated cases. In iron deficiency anaemia there is a complete absence of iron from stores (macrophages) and from developing erythroblasts (Fig. 3.10). The erythroblasts are small and have a ragged cytoplasm.

Serum iron and total iron-binding capacity

The serum iron falls and total iron-binding capacity (TIBC) rises so that the TIBC is less than 10% saturated (Fig. 3.11). This contrasts both with the anaemia of chronic disorders (see below) when the serum iron and the TIBC are both reduced and with other hypochromic anaemias where the serum iron is normal or even raised.

Serum transferrin receptor

Transferrin receptor is shed from cells into plasma.

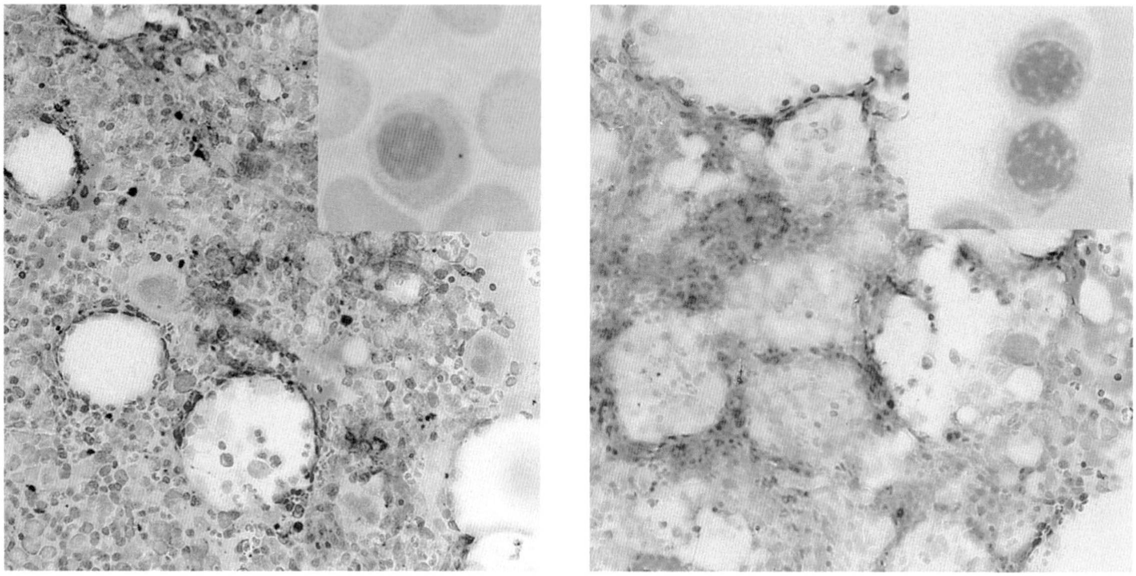

(a) (b)

Fig. 3.10 Bone marrow iron assessed by Perls' stain. **(a)** Normal iron stores indicated by blue staining in the macrophages. Inset: normal siderotic granule in erythroblast. **(b)** Absence of blue staining (absence of haemosiderin) in iron deficiency. Inset: absence of siderotic granules in erythroblasts.

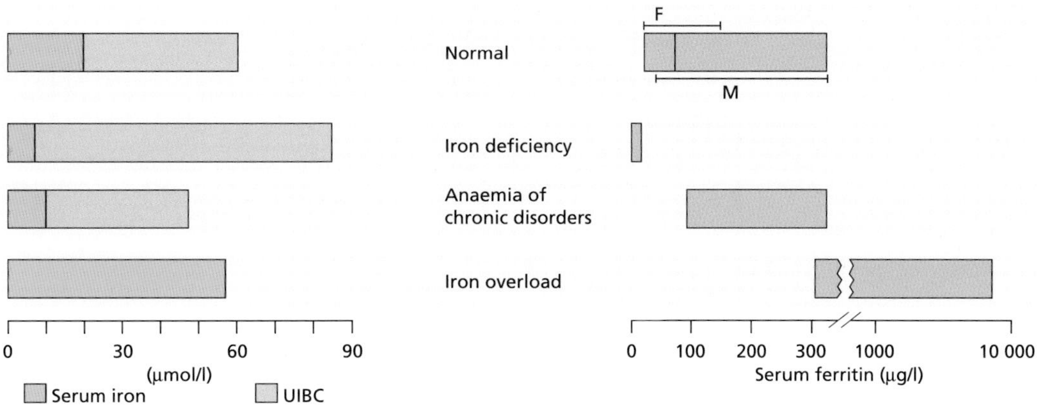

Fig. 3.11 The serum iron, unsaturated serum iron-binding capacity (UIBC) and serum ferritin in normal subjects and in those with iron deficiency, anaemia of chronic disorders and iron overload. The total iron-binding capacity (TIBC) is made up of the serum iron and the UIBC. In some laboratories, the transferrin content of serum is measured directly by immunodiffusion, rather than by its ability to bind iron, and is expressed in g/L. Normal serum contains 2–4 g/L transferrin (1 g/L transferrin = 20 μmol/L binding capacity). Normal ranges for serum iron are 10–30 μmol/L; for TIBC, 40–75 μmol/L; for serum ferritin, male, 40–340 μg/L; female, 14–150 μg/L.

The level of serum transferrin receptor (sTfR) is increased in iron deficiency anaemia but not in the anaemia of chronic disease or thalassaemia trait. The level is also raised if the overall level of erythropoiesis is increased.

Serum ferritin

A small fraction of body ferritin circulates in the serum, the concentration being related to tissue, particularly reticuloendothelial, iron stores. The normal range in men is higher than in women (Fig. 3.11). In iron deficiency anaemia the serum ferritin is very low while a raised serum ferritin indicates iron overload or excess release of ferritin from damaged tissues or an acute phase response (e.g. in inflammation). The serum ferritin is normal or raised in the anaemia of chronic disorders.

Investigation of the cause of iron deficiency

(Table 3.4)

In premenopausal women, menorrhagia and/or repeated pregnancies are the usual causes of the deficiency. If these are not present other causes must be sought. In some patients with menorrhagia a clotting or platelet abnormality (e.g. von Willebrand disease) is present. In men and post-menopausal women, gastrointestinal blood loss is the main cause of iron deficiency and the exact site is sought from the clinical history, physical and rectal examination, by occult blood tests, and by appropriate use of upper and lower gastrointestinal endoscopy and/or radiology (e.g. computed tomography (CT) of the pneumocolon) or virtual colonscopy using the 3D colon system (Figs 3.12 and 3.13). In difficult cases a camera in a capsule can be swallowed which relays pictures of the gastrointestinal tract electronically. Tests for endomysial and transglutaminase antibodies and duodenal biopsy to look for gluten-induced enteropathy can be valuable. Hookworm ova are sought in stools of subjects from areas where this infestation occurs. Rarely, a coeliac axis angiogram is needed to demonstrate angiodysplasia.

If gastrointestinal blood loss is excluded, loss of iron in the urine as haematuria or haemosiderinuria (resulting from chronic intravascular haemolysis) is considered. A normal chest X-ray excludes the rare condition of pulmonary haemosiderosis. Rarely, patients bleed themselves producing iron deficiency.

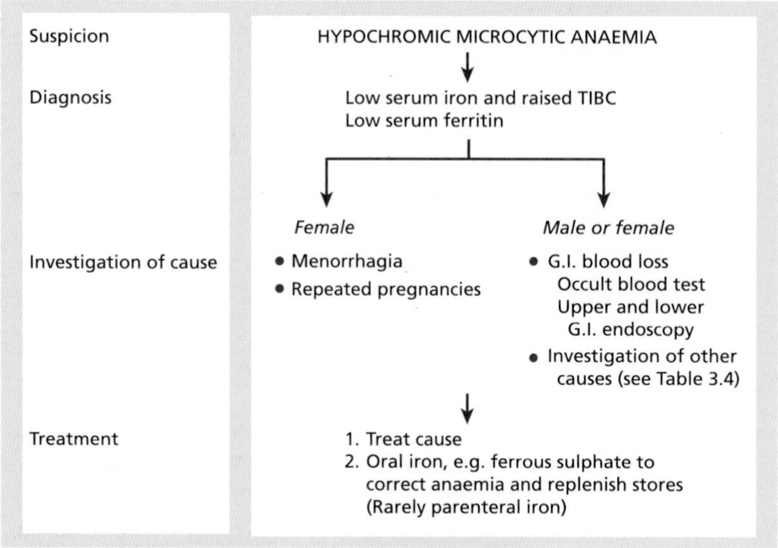

Fig. 3.12 Investigation and management of iron deficiency anaemia. GI, gastrointestinal; TIBC, total iron-binding capacity.

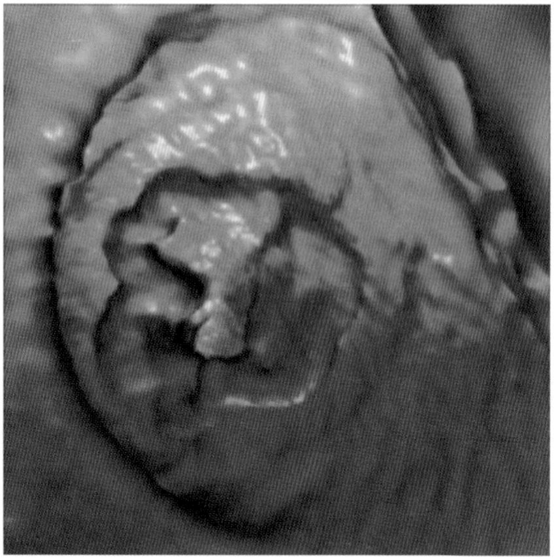

Fig. 3.13 Virtual colonoscopy to show carcinoma of colon causing colonic obstruction and iron deficiency.

Treatment

The underlying cause is treated as far as possible. In addition, iron is given to correct the anaemia and replenish iron stores.

Oral iron

The best preparation is ferrous sulphate which is cheap, contains 67 mg of iron in each 200 mg tablet and is best given on an empty stomach in doses spaced by at least 6 h. If side-effects occur (e.g. nausea, abdominal pain, constipation or diarrhoea), these can be reduced by giving iron with food or by using a preparation of lower iron content (e.g. ferrous gluconate which contains less iron (37 mg) per 300 mg tablet). An elixir is available for children. Slow-release preparations should not be used.

Oral iron therapy should be given for long enough both to correct the anaemia and to replenish body iron stores, which usually means for at least 6 months. The haemoglobin should rise at the rate of approximately 2 g/dL every 3 weeks. Failure of response to oral iron has several possible causes (Table 3.5) which should all be considered before parenteral iron is used.

Iron fortification of the duct in infants in Africa reduces the incidence of anaemia but increases suceptibility to malaria.

Parenteral iron

Ferric hydroxide-sucrose (Venofer®) is the safest form. It is administered by slow intravenous injection or infusion, usually 200 mg iron in each infusion. Iron dextran (CosmoFer®) can be given as slow injection or infusion either in small single doses or as a total dose infusion given in one day. Iron sorbitol (Jectofer®) is given by deep intramuscular injection but not intravenously. There may be hypersensitivity or anaphylactoid reactions so

Table 3.5 Failure of response to oral iron.

Continuing haemorrhage
Failure to take tablets
Wrong diagnosis—especially thalassaemia trait, sideroblastic anaemia
Mixed deficiency—associated folate or vitamin B_{12} deficiency
Another cause for anaemia (e.g. malignancy, inflammation)
Malabsorption—coeliac disease, atrophic gastritis
Use of slow-release preparation

Table 3.6 Causes of the anaemia of chronic disorders.

Chronic inflammatory diseases
Infections (e.g. pulmonary abscess, tuberculosis, osteomyelitis, pneumonia, bacterial endocarditis)
Non-infectious (e.g. rheumatoid arthritis, systemic lupus erythematosus and other connective tissue diseases, sarcoidosis, Crohn's disease)
Malignant diseases
Carcinoma, lymphoma, sarcoma

parenteral iron is only given when there are high iron requirements as in gastrointestinal bleeding, severe menorrhagia, chronic haemodialysis, with erythropoietin therapy, and when oral iron is ineffective (e.g. iron malabsorption resulting from gluten-induced enteropathy or atrophic gastritis) or impractical (e.g. active Crohn's disease). The haematological response to parenteral iron is no faster than to adequate dosage of oral iron but the stores are replenished faster.

Anaemia of chronic disorders

One of the most common anaemias occurs in patients with a variety of chronic inflammatory and malignant diseases (Table 3.6). The characteristic features are:

1 Normochromic, normocytic or mildly hypochromic (MCV rarely <75 fL) indices and red cell morphology.

2 Mild and non-progressive anaemia (haemoglobin rarely <9.0 g/dL)—the severity being related to the severity of the disease.

3 Both the serum iron and TIBC are reduced; sTfR levels are normal.

4 The serum ferritin is normal or raised.

5 Bone marrow storage (reticuloendothelial) iron is normal but erythroblast iron is reduced (Table 3.7).

Table 3.7 Laboratory diagnosis of a hypochromic anaemia.

	Iron deficiency	Chronic inflammation or malignancy	Thalassaemia trait (α or β)	Sideroblastic anaemia
MCV MCH	Reduced in relation to severity of anaemia	Normal or mild reduction	Reduced; very low for degree of anaemia	Usually low in congenital type but MCV often raised in acquired type
Serum iron	Reduced	Reduced	Normal	Raised
TIBC	Raised	Reduced	Normal	Normal
Serum transferrin receptor	Raised	Normal/low	Variable	Normal
Serum ferritin	Reduced	Normal or raised	Normal	Raised
Bone marrow iron stores	Absent	Present	Present	Present
Erythroblast iron	Absent	Absent	Present	Ring forms
Haemoglobin electrophoresis	Normal	Normal	Hb A_2 raised in β form	Normal

MCH, mean corpuscular haemoglobin; MCV, mean corpuscular volume; TIBC, total iron-binding capacity.

The pathogenesis of this anaemia appears to be related to decreased release of iron from macrophages to plasma, reduced red cell lifespan and an inadequate erythropoietin response to anaemia caused by the effects of cytokines such as IL-1 and tumour necrosis factor (TNF) on erythropoiesis.

Hepcidin, released by the liver in response to inflammation, inhibits macrophage release of iron as well as iron absorption. The anaemia is corrected by successful treatment of the underlying disease and does not respond to iron therapy. Recombinant erythropoietin improves the anaemia in some cases. In many conditions this anaemia is complicated by anaemia resulting from other causes (e.g. iron, vitamin B_{12} or folate deficiency, renal failure, bone marrow failure, hypersplenism, endocrine abnormality, leucoerythroblastic anaemia) and these are discussed in Chapter 26.

Sideroblastic anaemia

This is a refractory anaemia with hypochromic cells in the peripheral blood and increased marrow iron; it is defined by the presence of many pathological ring sideroblasts in the bone marrow (Fig. 3.14). These are abnormal erythroblasts containing numerous iron granules arranged in a ring or collar around the nucleus instead of the few randomly distributed iron granules seen when normal erythroblasts are stained for iron. Sideroblastic anaemia is diagnosed when 15% or more of marrow erythroblasts are ring sideroblasts but they can be found at lower numbers in a variety of haematological conditions.

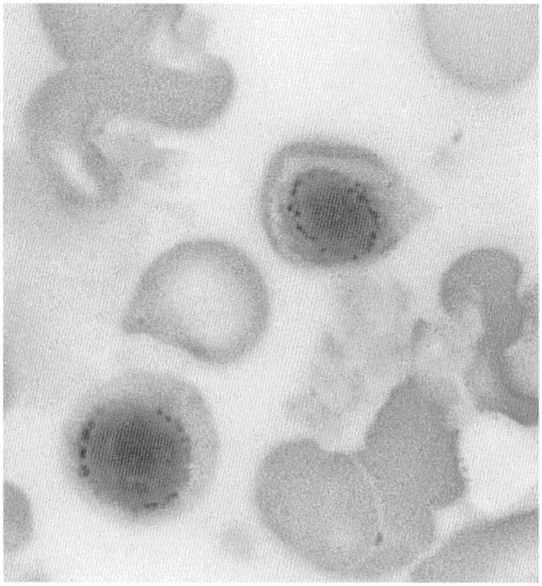

Fig. 3.14 Ring sideroblasts with a perinuclear ring of iron granules in sideroblastic anaemia.

Table 3.8 Classification of sideroblastic anaemia.

Hereditary

Usually occurs in males, transmitted by females; also occurs rarely in females (see text)

Acquired

Primary

Myelodysplasia (refractory anaemia with ring sideroblasts) (p. 185)

Secondary

Ring sideroblast formation may also occur in the bone marrow in:

Other malignant diseases of the marrow (e.g. other types of myelodysplasia, myelofibrosis, myeloid leukaemia, myeloma)

Drugs, e.g. antituberculous (isoniazid, cycloserine), alcohol, lead

Other benign conditions (e.g. haemolytic anaemia, megaloblastic anaemia, malabsorption, rheumatoid arthritis)

Sideroblastic anaemia is classified into different types (Table 3.8) and the common link is a defect in haem synthesis. In the hereditary forms the anaemia is usually characterized by a markedly hypochromic and microcytic blood picture. The most common mutations are in the δ-aminolaevulinic acid synthase (ALA-S) gene which is on the X chromosome. Pyridoxal-6-phosphate is a coenzyme for ALA-S. Other rare types include mitochondrial defects, thiamine-responsive and other autosomal defects. The much more common primary acquired form is one subtype of myelodysplasia. It is also termed 'refractory anaemia with ring sideroblasts'. This condition is discussed together with the other types of myelodysplasia in Chapter 14.

In some patients, particularly with the hereditary type, there is a response to pyridoxine therapy. Folate deficiency may occur and folic acid therapy may also be tried. Other treatments that have been tried in myelodysplasia (e.g. erythropoietin) may be tried in the primary acquired form (Chapter 14). In many severe cases, however, repeated blood transfusions are the only method of maintaining a satisfactory haemoglobin concentration and transfusional iron overload becomes a major problem.

Lead poisoning

Lead inhibits both haem and globin synthesis at a number of points. In addition it interferes with the breakdown of RNA by inhibiting the enzyme pyrimidine 5′ nucleotidase, causing accumulation of denatured RNA in red cells, the RNA giving an appearance called basophilic stippling on the ordinary (Romanowsky) stain (see Fig. 2.17). The anaemia may be hypochromic or predominantly haemolytic, and the bone marrow may show ring sideroblasts. Free erythrocyte protoporphyrin is raised.

Differential diagnosis of hypochromic anaemia

Table 3.7 lists the laboratory investigations that may be necessary. The clinical history is particularly important as the source of the haemorrhage leading to iron deficiency or the presence of a chronic disease may be revealed. The country of origin and the family history may suggest a possible diagnosis of thalassaemia or other haemoglobinopathy. Physical examination may also be helpful in determining a site of haemorrhage, features of a chronic inflammatory or malignant disease, koilonychia or, in some haemoglobinopathies, an enlarged spleen or bony deformities.

In thalassaemia trait the red cells tend to be small, often with an MCV of 70 fL or less, even when anaemia is mild or absent; the red cell count is usually over 5.5×10^{12}/L. Conversely, in iron deficiency anaemia the indices fall progressively with the degree of anaemia and when anaemia is mild the indices are often only just reduced below normal (e.g. MCV 75–80 fL). In the anaemia of chronic disorders the indices are also not markedly low, an MCV in the range 75–82 fL being usual.

It is usual to perform a serum iron and TIBC measurement, or alternatively serum ferritin estimation, to confirm a diagnosis of iron deficiency. sTfR assay is also useful in distinguishing iron deficiency anaemia from anaemia of chronic disease but not widely available. Haemoglobin electrophoresis with an estimation of Hb A_2 and Hb F is carried out in all patients suspected of thalassaemia or other haemoglobinopathy because of the family history, country of origin, red cell indices and blood film. Iron deficiency or the anaemia of chronic disorders may also occur in these subjects. β-Thalassaemia trait is characterized by a raised Hb A_2 above 3.5%, but in α-thalassaemia trait there is no abnormality on simple haemoglobin studies so the diagnosis is usually made by exclusion of all other causes of hypochromic red cells and by the presence of a red cell count $>5.5 \times 10^{12}$/L. DNA studies can be used to confirm the diagnosis. In some α-thalassaemia patients, however, occasional red cells show deposits of Hb H (β_4) in reticulocyte preparations (Chapter 6).

Bone marrow examination is essential if a diagnosis of sideroblastic anaemia is suspected but is not usually needed in diagnosis of the other hypochromic anaemias.

Iron overload

There is no physiological mechanism for eliminating excess iron from the body and so iron absorption is normally carefully regulated to avoid accumulation. Iron overload can occur in disorders associated with excessive absorption or chronic blood transfusion. Excessive iron deposition in tissues can cause serious damage to organs, particularly the heart, liver and endocrine organs. The causes of iron overload are listed in Tables 3.9 and 3.10. Transfusional iron overload and iron chelation therapy are discussed in Chapter 6.

Hereditary (genetic, primary) haemochromatosis

This is a group of diseases in which there is excessive absorption of iron from the gastrointestinal tract leading to iron overload of the parenchymal cells of the liver (Fig. 3.15), of the endocrine organs and, in severe cases, of the heart.

The most common gene involved is *HFE* and most patients are homozygous for a missense mutation (845 G to A) which leads to insertion of a tyrosine residue rather than cysteine in the mature

Table 3.9 The causes of iron overload.

Increased iron absorption	Hereditary (primary) haemochromatosis Ineffective erythropoiesis, e.g. thalassaemia intermedia, sideroblastic anaemia Chronic liver disease
Increased iron intake	African siderosis (dietary and genetic)
Repeated red cell transfusions	Transfusion siderosis

Table 3.10 Genetic causes of haemochromatosis, iron overload and hyperferritinaemia.

Type	Inheritance	Clinical condition	Defect in
I	AR	Classical hereditary haemochromatosis	HFE
II	AR	Juvenile haemochromatosis	Hemojuvelin Hepcidin
III	AR	Hereditary haemochromatosis	Transferrin receptor 2
IV	AD	Marked increase in RE iron, less hepatic iron	Ferroportin 1
V	AD	Hereditary hyperferritinaemia—cataract syndrome (no iron deposition)	Low molecular weight ferritin

AD, autosomal dominant; AR, autosomal recessive; RE, reticuloendothelial.

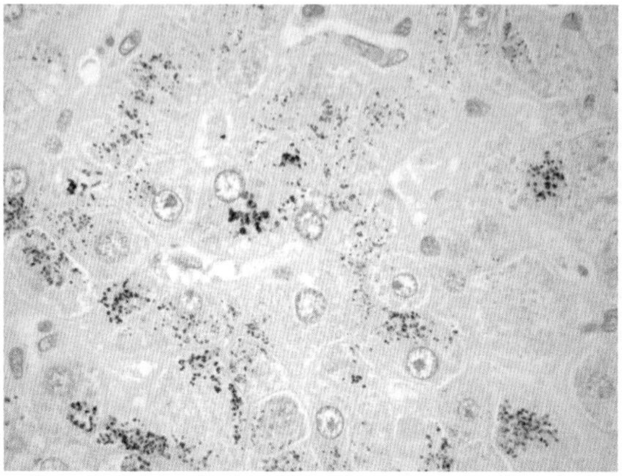

Fig. 3.15 Liver biopsy. Iron loading of hepatic parenchymal cells (Perls' stain). (Courtesy of Professor A.P. Dhillon)

protein (C282Y). This allele has a prevalence of approximately 1 in 300 within the white North European population. The *HFE* gene is situated close to the major histocompatibility complex (MHC) locus on chromosome 6. The abnormal allele is associated with HLA-A3 and -B8. Only a small proportion of those homozygous for the mutation present with clinical features of the disease. A second mutation resulting in a histidine to aspartic acid substitution H63D is found with the C282Y mutation in approximately 5% of patients but homozygotes for the H63D mutation do not have the disease.

Serum hepcidin levels are low in patients with mutated *HFE* implying *HFE* is involved in hepcidin synthesis or secretion (Fig. 3.4). Low serum hepcidin levels lead to high levels of ferroportin on the basolateral surface of the duodenal enterocyte and so increased iron absorption. Low levels of hepcidin also lead by the same mechanism to increased release of iron from macrophages.

The consequent iron overload damages parenchymal cells and patients present usually in adult life with hepatic disease, endocrine disturbances such as diabetes mellitus or impotence, melanin skin pigmentation and arthropathy (resulting from pyrophosphate deposition). In some severe cases there is cardiac failure or arrhythmia (Chapter 6). Diagnosis is suspected by increased serum iron, increased serum transferrin saturation and ferritin. It is confirmed by testing for the *HFE* mutation. Liver biopsy may quantify the degree of iron overload and assess liver damage. Magnetic resonance imaging (MRI) can also be used to measure liver and cardiac iron. Treatment is with regular venesection, initially at 1–2 week intervals, each unit of blood lost removing 200–250 mg iron. It is monitored by serum iron, TIBC, serum ferritin and by tests of organ function.

Rarer forms of genetic haemochromatosis are caused by mutations in the genes for hemojuvelin, transferrin receptor 2 and hepcidin (Table 3.10). All three are associated with low levels of hepcidin in serum. They often present as severe iron overload with cardiomyopathy in children, adolescents or young adults. On the other hand, ferroportin mutations cause reticuloendothelial but not parenchymal cell iron overload. Mutations of the ferritin light chain gene cause a raised monoclonal serum ferritin with cataracts resulting from ferritin deposition in the eye but no tissue iron overload.

Bibliography

Adams P.C., Reboussin D.M., Barton J.C. *et al.* (2005) Hemachromatosis and iron-overload screening in a racially diverse population. *N Engl J Med* **352**,1769–78.

Andrews N.C. (2005) Understanding heme transport. *N Engl J Med* **353**,2508–9.

Bomford A. (2002) Genetics of haemochromatosis. *Lancet* **360**,1673–4.

Camaschella C. (2005) Understanding iron homeostasis through genetic analysis of hemochromatosis and related disorders. *Blood* **106**,3710–7.

De Domenico I., Ward D.M., Musci G. and Kaplan J. (2006) Iron overload due to mutations in ferroportin. *Haematologica* **91**,92–5.

Fleming R.E. and Bacon B.R. (2005) Orchestration of iron homeostasis. *N Engl J Med* **352**,1741–4.

Ganz T. (2005) Hepcidin: a regulator of intestinal iron absorption and iron recycling by macrophages. *Clin Haematol* **18**,171–82.

Hentze M.W., Muckenthaler M.U., Andrews N.C. (2004) Balancing acts: molecular control of mammalian iron metabolism. *Cell* **117**,285–97.

Hershko C. (ed.) (2005) Iron diseases. *Best Pract Res Clin Haematol* **18**,157–380.

Hershko C., Hoffbrand A.V., Keret D. *et al.* (2005) Role of autoimmune gastritis, *Helicobacter pylori* and celiac disease in refractory or unexplained iron deficiency anemia. *Haematologica* **90**,585–95.

Lee P.L., Beutler E., Rao S.V. *et al.* (2004) Genetic abnormalities and juvenile hemochromatosis: mutations of the *HJV* gene encoding hemojuvelin. *Blood* **103**,4669–71.

Nemeth E. and Ganz T. (2006) Hepcidin and iron-loading anemias. *Haematologica* **91**, 727–32.

Nemeth E., Rivera S., Gabayan V. *et al.* (2004) IL-6 mediates hypoferremia of inflammation by inducing the synthesis of the iron regulatory hormone hepcidin. *J Clin Invest* **113**,1271–6.

Papanikolaou G., Tzilianos M., Christakis J.I. *et al.* (2005) Hepcidin in iron overload disorders. *Blood* **105**,4103–5.

Pietrangelo A. (2004) Hereditary hemochromatosis: a new look at an old disease. *N Engl J Med* **350**,2383–97.

Shayeghi M., Latunde-Dada G.O., Oakhill J.S. *et al.* (2005) Identification of an intestinal heme transporter. *Cell* **122**,789–801.

Wang R.H., Li C., Xu X. *et al.* (2005) A role of SMAD4 in iron metabolism through the positive regulation of hepcidin expression. *Cell Metab* **2**,399–409.

Weiss G. and Goodnough L. (2005) Anemia of chronic disorders. *N Engl J Med* **352**,1011–22.

CHAPTER 4

4 Megaloblastic anaemias and other macrocytic anaemias

Introduction to macrocytic anaemia

In macrocytic anaemia the red cells are abnormally large (mean corpuscular volume, MCV >95 fL). There are several causes (see Table 2.4) but they can be broadly subdivided into megaloblastic and non-megaloblastic, based on the appearance of developing erythroblasts in the bone marrow.

Megaloblastic anaemias

This is a group of anaemias in which the erythroblasts in the bone marrow show a characteristic abnormality—maturation of the nucleus being delayed relative to that of the cytoplasm. The underlying defect accounting for the asynchronous maturation of the nucleus is defective DNA synthesis and in clinical practice this is usually caused by deficiency of vitamin B_{12} or folate. Less commonly, abnormalities of metabolism of these vitamins or other lesions in DNA synthesis may cause an identical haematological appearance (Table 4.1). Dietary and metabolic aspects of the two vitamins are reviewed before considering the anaemia.

Table 4.1 Causes of megaloblastic anaemia.

Vitamin B_{12} deficiency
Folate deficiency
Abnormalities of vitamin B_{12} or folate metabolism
(e.g. transcobalamin deficiency, nitrous oxide, antifolate drugs)
Other defects of DNA synthesis
congenital enzyme deficiencies (e.g. orotic aciduria)
acquired enzyme deficiencies (e.g. alcohol, therapy with hydroxyurea, cytosine arabinoside)

Vitamin B_{12} (B_{12}, cobalamin)

This vitamin is synthesized in nature by micro-organisms; animals acquire it by eating other animal foods, by internal production from intestinal bacteria (not in humans) or by eating bacterially contaminated foods. The vitamin consists of a small group of compounds, the cobalamins, which have the same basic structure, with a cobalt atom at the centre of a corrin ring which is attached to a nucleotide portion (Fig. 4.1). The vitamin is found in foods of animal origin such as liver, meat, fish and dairy produce but does not occur in fruit, cereals or vegetables. Table 4.2 compares nutritional aspects of B_{12} and folate.

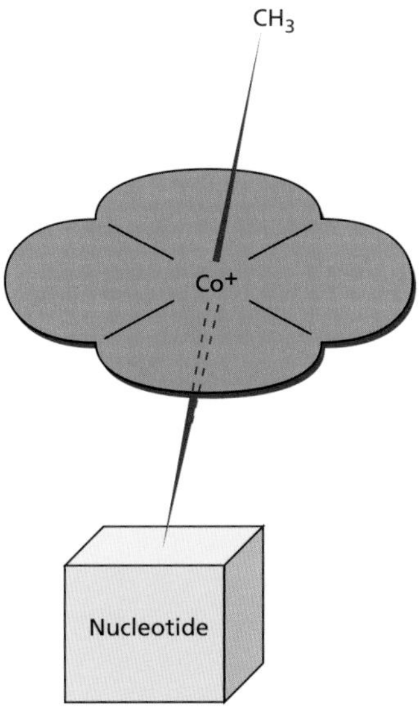

Fig. 4.1 The structure of methylcobalamin (methyl B_{12}), the main form of vitamin B_{12} in human plasma. Other forms include deoxyadenosylcobalamin (ado B_{12}), the main form in human tissues; hydroxocobalamin (hydroxo B_{12}), the main form in treatment; and cyanocobalamin (cyano B_{12}), the radioactively labelled (^{57}Co or ^{58}Co) form used to study vitamin B_{12} absorption or metabolism.

Absorption

A normal diet contains a large excess of B_{12} compared with daily needs (Table 4.2). B_{12} is combined with the glycoprotein intrinsic factor (IF) (molecular weight, MW 45 000) which is synthesized by the gastric parietal cells. The IF–B_{12} complex can then bind to a specific surface receptor for IF, cubilin, which then binds to a second protein, amnionless which directs endocytosis of the cubilin IF–B_{12} complex in the distal ileum where B_{12} is absorbed and IF destroyed (Fig. 4.2).

Transport: the transcobalamins

Vitamin B_{12} is absorbed into portal blood where it becomes attached to the plasma-binding protein transcobalamin (TC, previously called transcobalamin II) which delivers B_{12} to bone marrow and other tissues. Although TC is the essential plasma protein for transferring B_{12} into the cells of the body, the amount of B_{12} on TC is normally very low (<50 ng/L). TC deficiency causes megaloblastic anaemia because of failure of B_{12} to enter marrow (and other cells) from plasma but the serum B_{12} level

Table 4.2 Vitamin B_{12} and folate: nutritional aspects.

	Vitamin B_{12}	Folate
Normal daily dietary intake	7–30 μg	200–250 μg
Main foods	Animal produce only	Most, especially liver, greens and yeast
Cooking	Little effect	Easily destroyed
Minimal adult daily requirement	1–2 μg	100–150 μg
Body stores	2–3 mg (sufficient for 2–4 years)	10–12 mg (sufficient for 4 months)
Absorption		
Site	Ileum	Duodenum and jejunum
Mechanism	Intrinsic factor	Conversion to methyltetrahydrofolate
Limit	2–3 μg/day	50–80% of dietary content
Enterohepatic circulation	5–10 μg/day	90 μg/day
Transport in plasma	Most bound to haptocorrin; TC essential for cell uptake	Weakly bound to albumin
Major intracellular physiological forms	Methyl- and deoxyadenosylcobalamin	Reduced polyglutamate derivatives
Usual therapeutic form	Hydroxocobalamin	Folic (pteroylglutamic) acid

TC, transcobalamin.

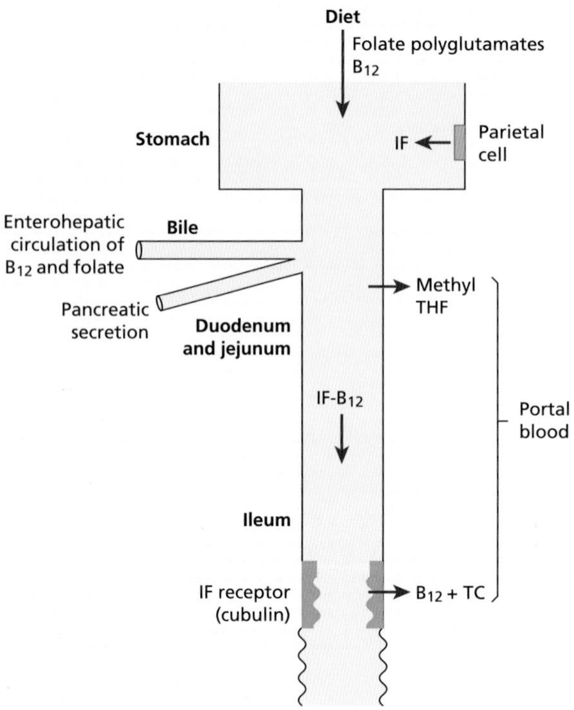

Fig. 4.2 The absorption of dietary vitamin B_{12} after combination with intrinsic factor (IF), through the ileum. Folate absorption occurs through the duodenum and jejunum after conversion of all dietary forms to methyltetrahydrofolate (methyl THF). TC, transcobalamin.

in TC deficiency is normal. This is because most B_{12} in plasma is bound to another transport protein, haptocorrin (previously called transcobalamin I). This is a glycoprotein largely synthesized by granulocytes and macrophages. In myeloproliferative diseases where granulocyte production is greatly increased, the haptocorrin and B_{12} levels in serum both rise considerably. B_{12} bound to haptocorrin does not transfer to marrow; it appears to be functionally 'dead'. Closely related glycoproteins to plasma haptocorrin are present in gastric juice, milk and other body fluids.

Biochemical function

Vitamin B_{12} is a coenzyme for two biochemical reactions in the body: first, as methyl B_{12} it is a cofactor for methionine synthase, the enzyme responsible for methylation of homocysteine to methionine using methyl tetrahydrofolate (methyl THF) as methyl donor (Fig. 4.3a); and, secondly, as deoxyadenosyl B_{12} (ado B_{12}) it assists in conversion of methylmalonyl coenzyme A (CoA) to succinyl CoA (Fig. 4.3b). Assay of homocysteine and methylmalonic acid in plasma may be used as tests for B_{12} deficiency (p. 52).

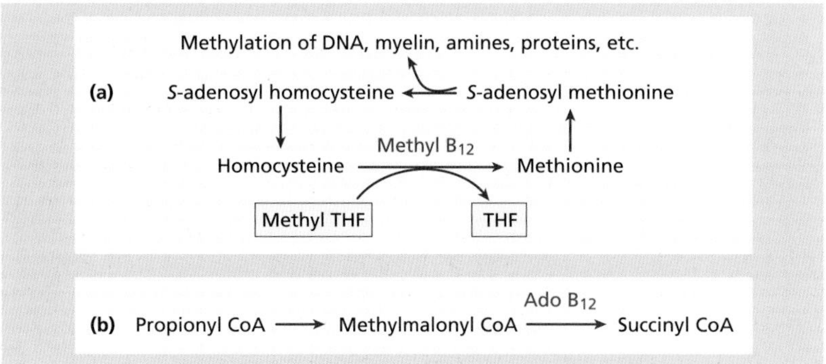

Fig. 4.3 The biochemical reactions of vitamin B_{12} in humans. Ado B_{12}, deoxyadenosylcobalamin; CoA, coenzyme A; THF, tetrahydrofolate.

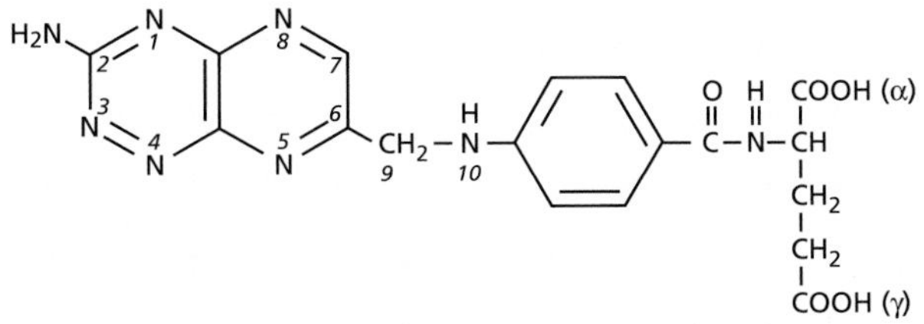

Fig. 4.4 The structure of folic (pteroylglutamic) acid. Dietary folates may contain: (a) additional hydrogen atoms at positions 7 and 8 (dihydrofolate) or 5, 6, 7 and 8 (tetrahydrofolate); (b) a formyl group at N_5 or N_{10}, a methyl group at N_5 or other 1-carbon groups; and (c) additional glutamate moiety attached to the γ-carboxyl group of the glutamate moiety.

Folate

Folic (pteroylglutamic) acid is the parent compound of a large group of compounds, the folates, that are derived from it (Fig. 4.4). Humans are unable to synthesize the folate structure and thus require preformed folate as a vitamin.

Absorption, transport and function

Dietary folates are converted to methyl THF (which, like folic acid, contains only one glutamate moiety) during absorption through the upper small intestine. Once inside the cell they are converted to folate polyglutamates (Fig. 4.5). Folate binding proteins are present on cell surfaces including the enterocyte and facilitate entry of reduced folates into cells. There is no specific plasma protein that enhances cellular folate uptake.

Folates are needed in a variety of biochemical reactions in the body involving single carbon unit transfer, in amino acid interconversions (e.g. homocysteine conversion to methionine) (Fig. 4.5) and serine to glycine or in synthesis of purine precursors of DNA.

Biochemical basis for megaloblastic anaemia (Fig. 4.5)

DNA is formed by polymerization of the four deoxyribonucleoside triphosphates. Folate deficiency is thought to cause megaloblastic anaemia by inhibiting thymidylate synthesis, a rate-limiting step in DNA synthesis in which thymidine monophosphate (dTMP) is synthesized, as this reaction needs 5,10-methylene THF polyglutamate as coenzyme.

All body cells, including those of the bone marrow, receive folate from plasma as methyl

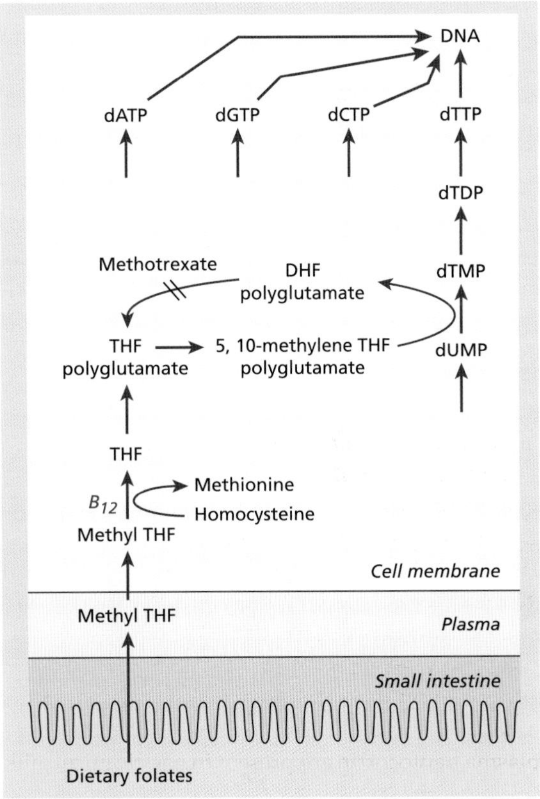

Fig. 4.5 The biochemical basis of megaloblastic anaemia caused by vitamin B_{12} or folate deficiency. Folate is required in one of its coenzyme forms, 5,10-methylene tetrahydrofolate (THF) polyglutamate, in the synthesis of thymidine monophosphate from its precursor deoxyuridine monophosphate. Vitamin B_{12} is needed to convert methyl THF, which enters the cells from plasma, to THF, from which polyglutamate forms of folate are synthesized. Dietary folates are all converted to methyl THF (a monoglutamate) by the small intestine. A, adenine; C, cytosine; d, deoxyribose; DHF, dihydrofolate; DP, diphosphate; G, guanine; MP, monophosphate; T, thymine; TP, triphosphate; U, uracil.

THF. B_{12} is needed in the conversion of this methyl THF to THF, a reaction in which homocysteine is methylated to methionine. THF (but not methyl THF) is a substrate for folate polyglutamate synthesis inside cells. The folate polyglutamates act as intracellular folate coenzymes, including 5,10-methylene THF polyglutamate, the coenzyme form of folate involved in the thymidylate synthetase reaction (Fig. 4.5). Lack of B_{12} prevents the demethylation of methyl THF, thus depriving cells of THF and so of folate polyglutamate coenzymes.

Other congenital or acquired causes of megaloblastic anaemia (e.g. antimetabolite drug therapy) inhibit purine or pyrimidine synthesis at one or other step. The result is a reduced supply of one or other of the four precursors needed for DNA synthesis.

Folate reduction

During thymidylate synthesis, the folate polyglutamate coenzyme becomes oxidized from the THF state to dihydrofolate (DHF) (Fig. 4.5). Regeneration of active THF requires the enzyme DHF reductase. Inhibitors of this enzyme (e.g. methotrexate) therefore inhibit all folate coenzyme reactions, and so DNA synthesis (Fig. 4.5). Methotrexate is a useful drug, mainly in the treatment of malignant or inflammatory disease (e.g. of the skin) with excessive cell turnover. The weaker antagonist, pyrimethamine, is used primarily against malaria. Trimethoprim, active against bacterial DHF reductase but only very weakly against the human enzyme, is used alone or in combination with a sulphonamide, as co-trimoxazole. Toxicity caused by methotrexate or pyrimethamine is reversed by giving the reduced folate, folinic acid (5-formyl THF).

Vitamin B_{12} deficiency

In Western countries, severe deficiency is usually caused by (Addisonian) pernicious anaemia (Table 4.3). Less commonly, it may be caused by veganism in which the diet lacks B_{12} (usually in Hindu Indians), gastrectomy or small intestinal lesions. There is no syndrome of B_{12} deficiency as a result of increased utilization or loss of the vitamin. The deficiency takes at least 2 years to develop (i.e. the time needed for body stores to deplete at the rate of 1–2 μg/day) when there is severe malabsorption of B_{12} from the diet. Nitrous oxide, however, may rapidly inactivate body B_{12} (p. 56).

Table 4.3 Causes of severe vitamin B_{12} deficiency.

Nutritional
Especially vegans
Malabsorption
Gastric causes
Pernicious anaemia
Congenital lack or abnormality of intrinsic factor
Total or partial gastrectomy
Intestinal causes
Intestinal stagnant loop syndrome—jejunal diverticulosis, blind-loop, stricture, etc.
Chronic tropical sprue
Ileal resection and Crohn's disease
Congenital selective malabsorption with proteinuria (autosomal recessive megaloblastic anaemia)
Fish tapeworm

Causes of mild vitamin B_{12} deficiency; other causes of malabsorption of vitamin B_{12} (e.g. malabsorption, atrophic gastritis, severe pancreatitis, gluten-induced enteropathy, HIV infection or therapy with metformin) do not usually lead to food vitamin B_{12} deficiency sufficient to cause anaemia or neuropathy.

Pernicious anaemia

This is caused by autoimmune attack on the gastric mucosa leading to atrophy of the stomach. The wall of the stomach becomes thin, with a plasma cell and lymphoid infiltrate of the lamina propria. Intestinal metaplasia may occur. There is achlorhydria and secretion of IF is absent or almost absent. Serum gastrin levels are raised. *Helicobater pylori* infection may initiate an autoimmune gastritis which presents in younger subjects as iron deficiency and in the elderly as pernicious anaemia.

More females than males are affected (1.6 : 1), with a peak occurrence at 60 years, and there may be associated autoimmune disease including the autoimmune polyendocrine syndrome (Table 4.4). The disease is found in all races but is most common in northern Europeans and tends to occur in families. There is also an increased incidence of carcinoma of the stomach (approximately 2–3% of all cases of pernicious anaemia).

Table 4.4 Pernicious anaemia: associations.

Female	Vitiligo
Blue eyes	Myxoedema
Early greying	Hashimoto's disease
Northern European	Thyrotoxicosis
Familial	Addison's disease
Blood group A	Hypoparathyroidism
	Hypogammaglobulinaemia
	Carcinoma of the stomach

Antibodies

Ninety per cent of patients show parietal cell antibody in the serum directed against gastric H^+/K^+-ATPase, and 50% type I or blocking antibody to IF which inhibits IF binding to B_{12}. Thirty-five per cent show a second (type II or precipitating) antibody to IF which inhibits its ileal binding site. IF antibodies are virtually specific for pernicious anaemia but occur in the serum of only half of patients, whereas the more common parietal cell antibody is less specific and occurs quite commonly in older subjects (e.g. 16% of normal women over 60 years).

Other causes of vitamin B_{12} deficiency

Congenital lack or abnormality of IF usually presents at approximately 2 years of age when stores of B_{12} that were derived from the mother *in utero* have been used up. There is also a form of autoimmune pernicious anaemia that presents in childhood. Specific malabsorption of B_{12} is brought about by genetic mutation of the IF–B_{12} receptor, cubilin or of amnionless which is involved in processing the IF–B_{12} complex. It usually presents in infancy or childhood and is associated with proteinuria in 90% of cases.

Lesser degrees of B_{12} deficiency occur resulting from inadequate intake of B_{12}, malabsorption of food B_{12}, atrophic gastritis (possibly triggered by *Helicobacter pylori*) without IF antibodies and other conditions listed in Table 4.3. Serum homocysteine and methylmalonic acid levels may be mildly raised and serum B_{12} levels subnormal but megaloblastic anaemia or neuropathy rarely occur.

Table 4.5 Causes of folate deficiency.

Nutritional
Especially old age, institutions, poverty, famine, special diets, goat's milk anaemia, etc.

Malabsorption
Tropical sprue, gluten-induced enteropathy (adult or child). Possible contributory factor to folate deficiency in some patients with partial gastrectomy, extensive jejunal resection or Crohn's disease

Excess utilization
Physiological
Pregnancy and lactation, prematurity

Pathological
Haematological diseases: haemolytic anaemias, myelofibrosis
Malignant disease: carcinoma, lymphoma, myeloma
Inflammatory diseases: Crohn's disease, tuberculosis, rheumatoid arthritis, psoriasis, exfoliative dermatitis, malaria

Excess urinary folate loss
Active liver disease, congestive heart failure

Drugs
Anticonvulsants, sulfasalazine

Mixed
Liver disease, alcoholism, intensive care

Folate deficiency

This is most often a result of a poor dietary intake of folate alone or in combination with a condition of increased folate utilization or malabsorption (Table 4.5). Excess cell turnover of any sort, including pregnancy, is the main cause of an increased need for folate, because the folate molecule becomes degraded when DNA synthesis is increased. The mechanism by which anticonvulsants and barbiturates cause the deficiency is still controversial. Alcohol, sulfasalazine and other drugs may have multiple effects on folate metabolism.

Clinical features of megaloblastic anaemia

The onset is usually insidious with gradually progressive symptoms and signs of anaemia (Chapter 2).

The patient may be mildly jaundiced (lemon yellow tint) (Fig. 4.6) because of the excess breakdown of haemoglobin resulting from increased ineffective erythropoiesis in the bone marrow. Glossitis (a beefy-red sore tongue) (Fig. 4.7), angular stomatitis (Fig. 4.8) and mild symptoms of malabsorption with loss of weight may be present because of the epithelial abnormality. Purpura as a result of thrombocytopenia and widespread melanin pigmentation (the cause of which is unclear) are less frequent presenting features (Table 4.6). Many asymptomatic patients are diagnosed when a blood count that has been performed for another reason reveals macrocytosis.

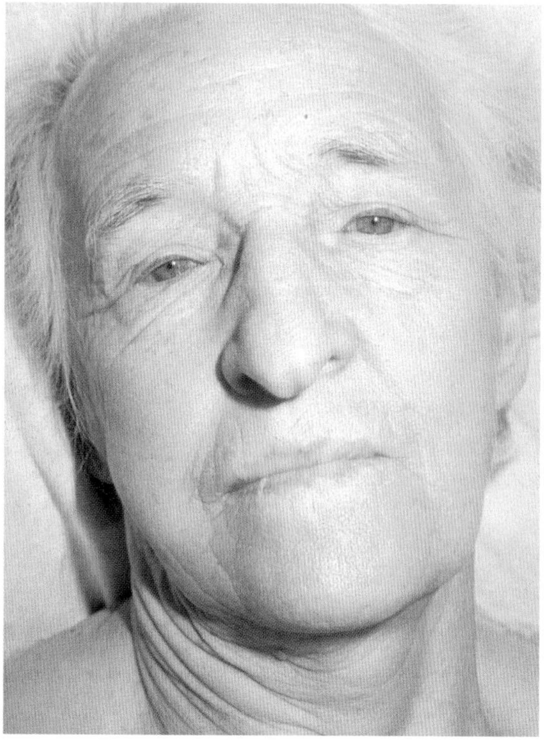

Fig. 4.6 Megaloblastic anaemia: pallor and mild icterus in a patient with a haemoglobin count of 7.0 g/dL and a mean corpuscular volume of 132 fL.

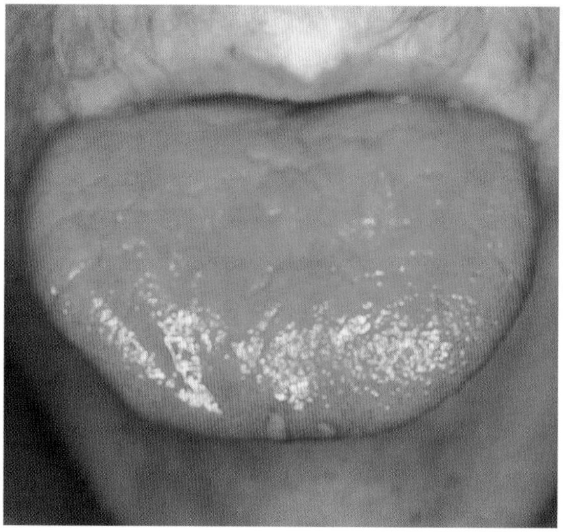

Fig. 4.7 Megaloblastic anaemia: glossitis—the tongue is beefy-red and painful.

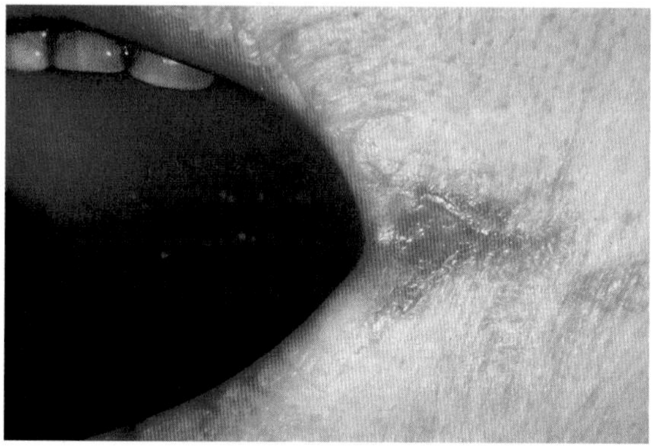

Fig. 4.8 Megaloblastic anaemia: angular cheilosis (stomatitis).

Table 4.6 Effects of vitamin B_{12} or folate deficiency.

Megaloblastic anaemia
Macrocytosis of epithelial cell surfaces
Neuropathy (for vitamin B_{12} only)
Sterility
Rarely, reversible melanin skin pigmentation
Decreased osteoblast activity
Neural tube defects in the fetus are related to folate or B_{12} deficiency
Cardiovascular disease (see text and Chapter 25)

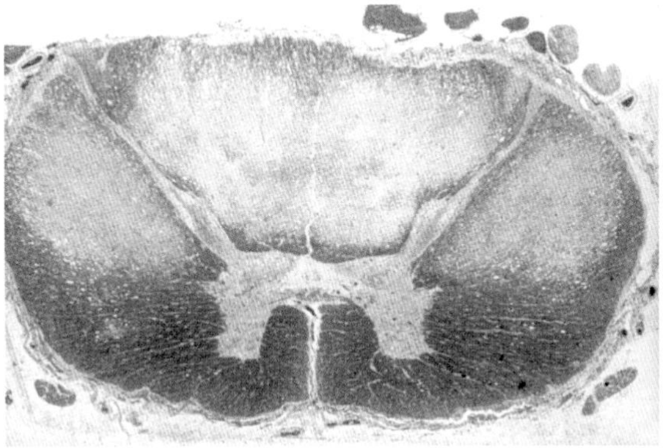

Fig. 4.9 Cross-section of the spinal cord in a patient who died with subacute combined degeneration of the cord (Weigert–Pal stain). There is demyelination of the dorsal and dorsolateral columns.

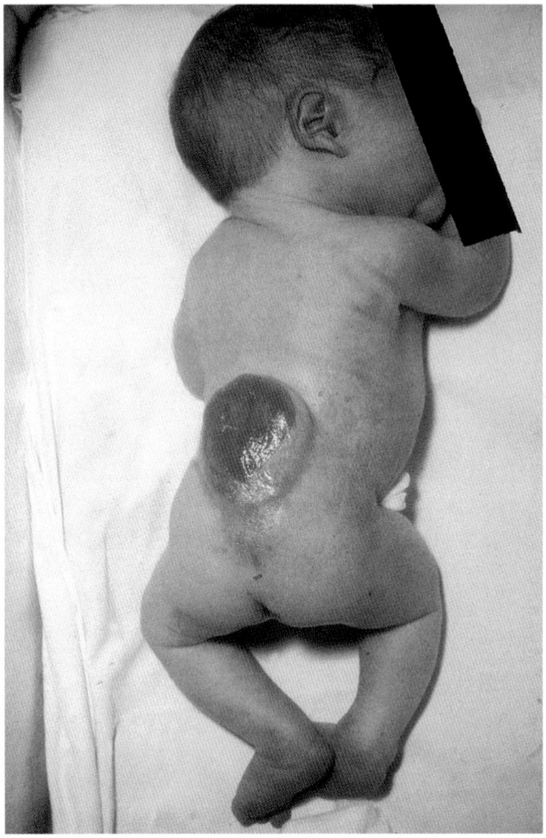

Fig. 4.10 A baby with neural tube defect (spina bifida). (Courtesy of Professor C.J. Schorah)

Vitamin B_{12} neuropathy (subacute combined degeneration of the cord)

Severe B_{12} deficiency can cause a progressive neuropathy affecting the peripheral sensory nerves and posterior and lateral columns (Fig. 4.9). The neuropathy is symmetrical and affects the lower limbs more than the upper limbs. The patient notices tingling in the feet, difficulty in walking and may fall over in the dark. Rarely, optic atrophy or severe psychiatric symptoms are present. Anaemia may be severe, mild or even absent, but the blood film and bone marrow appearances are always abnormal. The cause of the neuropathy is likely to be related to the accumulation of *S*-adenosyl homocysteine and reduced levels of *S*-adenosyl methionine in nervous tissue resulting in defective methylation of myelin and other substrates. The evidence that folate deficiency in the adult can cause a neuropathy is conflicting although there are some data suggesting it causes psychiatric changes.

Neural tube defect

Folate or B_{12} deficiency in the mother predisposes to neural tube defect (NTD) (anencephaly, spina bifida or encephalocoele) in the fetus (Fig. 4.10). The lower the maternal serum or red cell folate or serum B_{12} levels (even when these are in the normal range), the higher the incidence of NTDs. Moreover, supplementation of the diet with folic acid at the time of conception and in early pregnancy reduces the incidence of NTD by 75%. The exact mechanism is uncertain but is thought to be related to build-up of homocysteine and *S*-adenosyl homocysteine in the fetus which may impair methylation of various proteins and lipids. A common polymorphism in the enzyme 5,10-methylene tetrahydrofolate reductase (5,10-MTHFR) (677C $\rightarrow$ T) (p. 308) results in higher serum homocysteine and lower serum and red cell folate levels compared with controls. The incidence of the mutation is higher in the parents and fetus with NTD than in controls. Other studies suggest that an autoantibody against folate cell membrane receptors may occur more frequently than in controls in the sera of women who have a baby with NTD.

Other tissue abnormalities

Sterility is frequent in either sex with severe B_{12} or folate deficiency. Macrocytosis, excess apoptosis and other morphological abnormalities of cervical, buccal, bladder and other epithelia occur. Widespread reversible melanin pigmentation may also occur. B_{12} deficiency is associated with reduced osteoblastic activity. The associations of folate deficiency with cardiovascular and malignant diseases are discussed on page 56.

Laboratory findings

The anaemia is macrocytic (MCV >95 fL and often as high as 120–140 fL in severe cases) and the macrocytes are typically oval in shape (Fig. 4.11). The reticulocyte count is low and the total white cell and platelet counts may be moderately reduced, especially in severely anaemic patients. A proportion of the neutrophils show hypersegmented nuclei (with six or more lobes). The bone marrow is usually hypercellular and the erythroblasts are large and show failure of nuclear maturation maintaining an open, fine, lacy primitive chromatin pattern but normal haemoglobinization (Fig. 4.12). Giant and abnormally shaped metamyelocytes are characteristic.

The serum unconjugated bilirubin and lactate dehydrogenase (LDH) are raised as a result of marrow cell breakdown.

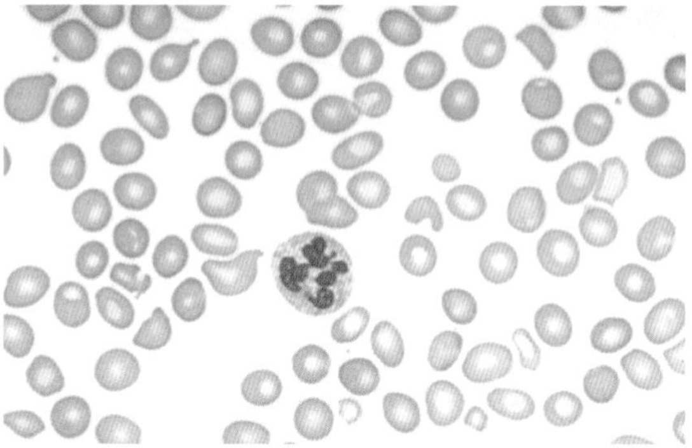

Fig. 4.11 Megaloblastic anaemia: peripheral blood film showing oval macrocytes.

Diagnosis of vitamin B_{12} or folate deficiency

It is usual to assay serum B_{12}, and serum and red cell folate (Table 4.7). The serum B_{12} is low in megaloblastic anaemia or neuropathy caused by B_{12} deficiency. The serum and red cell folate are both low in megaloblastic anaemia caused by folate deficiency. In B_{12} deficiency, the serum folate tends to rise but the red cell folate falls. In the absence of B_{12} deficiency, however, the red cell folate is a more accurate guide than the serum folate of tissue folate status. Measurement of serum methylmalonic acid is a test for B_{12} deficiency and of homocysteine for folate or B_{12} deficiency. These are not specific and it is difficult to establish normal levels in different age groups. These tests are not widely available.

Tests for cause of vitamin B_{12} or folate deficiency

For B_{12} deficiency, absorption tests (Table 4.8) using an oral dose of radioactive cobalt (^{57}Co)-labelled cyanocobalamin are valuable in distinguishing malabsorption from an inadequate diet. When the test is repeated with an active IF preparation, gastric lesions

Table 4.7 Laboratory tests for vitamin B_{12} and folate deficiency.

Test	Normal values*		Result in: Vitamin B_{12} deficiency	Result in: Folate deficiency
Serum vitamin B_{12}	160–925 ng/L	120–680 pmol/L	Low	Normal or borderline
Serum folate	3.0–15.0 μg/L	4–30 nmol/L	Normal or raised	Low
Red cell folate	160–640 μg/L	360–1460 nmol/L	Normal or low	Low

* Normal values differ slightly with different commercial kits.

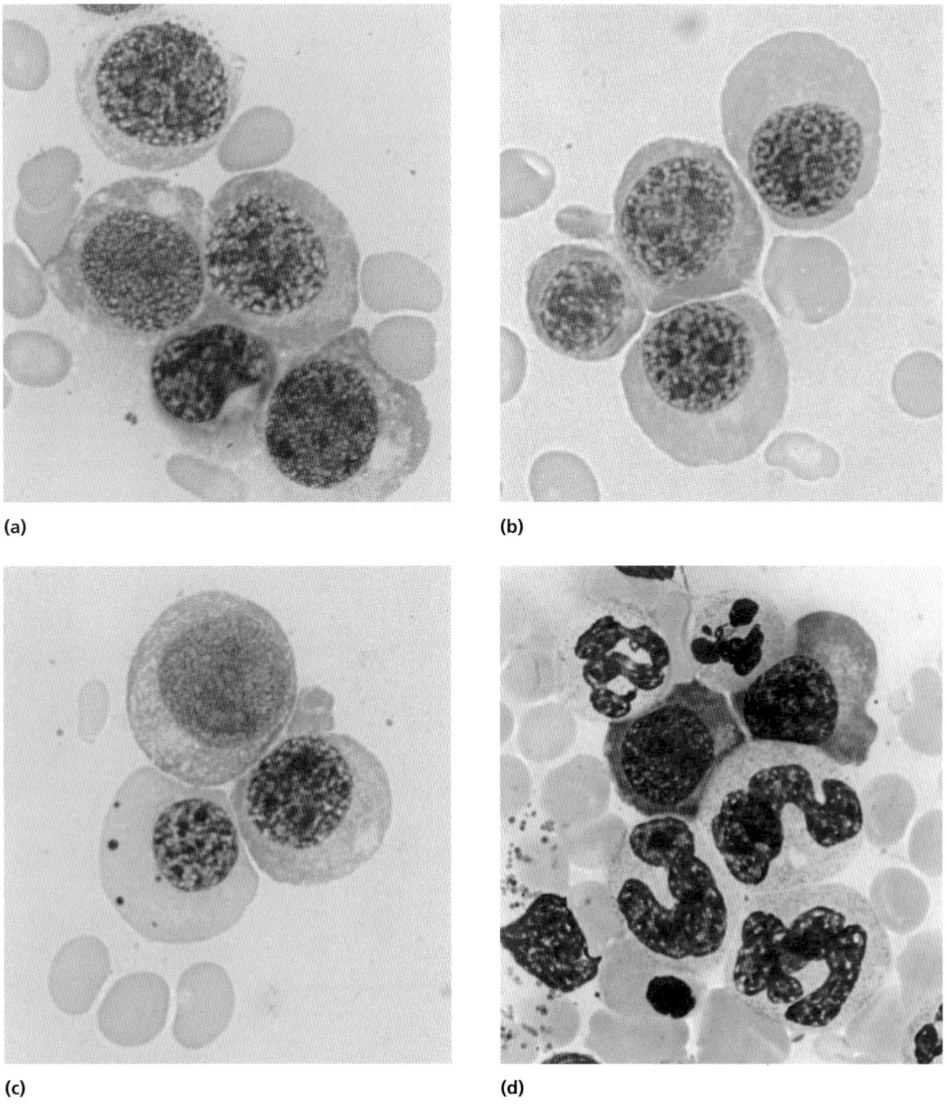

Fig. 4.12 Megaloblastic changes in the bone marrow in a patient with severe megaloblastic anaemia. **(a–c)** Erythroblasts showing fine, open stippled (primitive) appearance of the nuclear chromatin even in late cells (pale cytoplasm with some haemoglobin formation). **(d)** Abnormal giant metamyelocytes and band forms.

such as those associated with pernicious anaemia can be distinguished from intestinal lesions (Table 4.9). Absorption is most frequently measured indirectly by the urinary excretion (Schilling) technique in which absorbed radiolabelled B_{12} is 'flushed' into a 24-h urine sample by a large (1 mg) dose of non-radioactive B_{12} given simultaneously with the labelled oral dose. Problems with using human IF, non-virally inactivated and availability of radioactive B_{12} have led to less frequent use of the test.

Other useful tests are listed in Table 4.8. These are mainly concerned with assessing gastric function and testing for antibodies to gastric antigens. In all cases of pernicious anaemia endoscopy studies should be performed to confirm the presence of gastric atrophy and exclude carcinoma of the stomach.

Table 4.8 Tests for cause of vitamin B_{12} or folate deficiency.

Vitamin B_{12}	Folate
Diet history	Diet history
B_{12} absorption ± IF	Tests for intestinal malabsorption
IF, parietal cell antibodies	Anti-transglutaminase and endomysial antibodies
Endoscopy or barium meal and follow through	Duodenal biopsy
	Underlying disease

IF, intrinsic factor.

Table 4.9 Results of absorption tests of radioactive vitamin B_{12}.

	Dose of labelled B_{12} given alone	Dose of labelled B_{12} given with IF
Vegan	Normal	Normal
Pernicious anaemia or gastrectomy	Low	Normal
Ileal lesion	Low	Low
Intestinal blind-loop syndrome	Low*	Low*

IF, intrinsic factor.
* Corrected by antibiotic therapy.

For folate deficiency, the dietary history is most important, although it is difficult to estimate folate intake accurately. Unsuspected gluten-induced enteropathy or other underlying conditions should also be considered (Table 4.5).

Treatment

Most cases only need therapy with the appropriate vitamin (Table 4.10). If large doses of folic acid (e.g. 5 mg/day) are given in B_{12} deficiency they cause a haematological response but may aggravate the neuropathy. They should therefore not be given alone unless B_{12} deficiency has been excluded. In severely anaemic patients who need treatment urgently it may be safer to initiate treatment with both vitamins after blood has been taken for B_{12} and folate examinations and a bone marrow test has

Table 4.10 Treatment of megaloblastic anaemia.

	Vitamin B_{12} deficiency	Folate deficiency
Compound	Hydroxocobalamin	Folic acid
Route	Intramuscular*	Oral
Dose	1000 μg	5 mg
Initial dose	6 × 1000 μg over 2–3 weeks	Daily for 4 months
Maintenance	1000 μg every 3 months	Depends on underlying disease; life-long therapy may be needed in chronic inherited haemolytic anaemias, myelofibrosis, renal dialysis
Prophylactic	Total gastrectomy Ileal resection	Pregnancy, severe haemolytic anaemias, dialysis, prematurity

* Some authors have recommended daily oral or sublingual therapy of vitamin B_{12} deficiency.

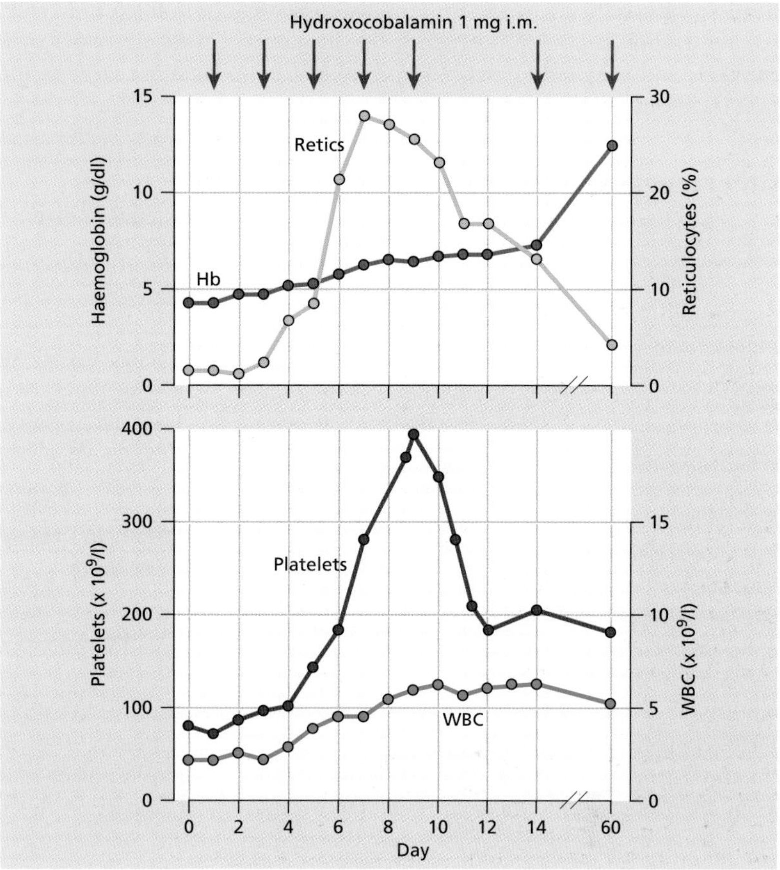

Fig. 4.13 Typical haematological response to vitamin B_{12} (hydroxocobalamin) therapy in pernicious anaemia. Hb, haemoglobin; Retics, reticulocytes; WBC, white blood cells.

been performed. In the elderly, the presence of heart failure should be corrected with diuretics and oral potassium supplements given for 10 days (because hypokalaemia has been found to occur during the response in some cases). Blood transfusion should be avoided if possible as it may cause circulatory overload.

Response to therapy

The patient feels better after 24–48 h of correct vitamin therapy with increased appetite and well-being. The haemoglobin should rise by 2–3 g/dL each fortnight. The white cell and platelet counts become normal in 7–10 days (Fig. 4.13) and the marrow is normoblastic in about 48 h, although giant metamyelocytes persist for up to 12 days.

The peripheral neuropathy may partly improve but spinal cord damage is irreversible. The shorter the history of neurological symptoms, the greater the chance of recovery.

Prophylactic therapy

Vitamin B_{12} is given to patients who have total gastrectomy or ileal resection. Folic acid is given in pregnancy at a recommended dosage of 400 μg/day and all women of child-bearing age are recommended to have an intake of at least 400 μg/day (by increased intake of folate-rich or folate-supplemented foods or as folic acid) to prevent a first occurrence of an NTD in the fetus. Folic acid is also given to patients undergoing chronic dialysis and with severe haemolytic anaemias and chronic myelofibrosis, and to premature babies. Food fortification with folic acid (e.g. in flour) is currently recommended in the UK to reduce the incidence of NTDs and is already practised in over 40 countries including North America.

Other megaloblastic anaemias

See Table 4.1.

Abnormalities of vitamin B_{12} or folate metabolism

These include congenital deficiencies of enzymes concerned in B_{12} or folate metabolism or of the serum transport protein for B_{12}, TC. Nitrous oxide (N_2O) anaesthesia causes rapid inactivation of body B_{12} by oxidizing the reduced cobalt atom of methyl B_{12}. Megaloblastic marrow changes occur with several days of N_2O administration and can cause pancytopenia. Chronic exposure (as in dentists and anaesthetists) has been associated with neurological damage resembling B_{12} deficiency neuropathy. Antifolate drugs, particularly those which inhibit DHF reductase (e.g. methotrexate and pyrimethamine) may also cause megaloblastic change. Trimethoprim, which inhibits bacterial DHF reductase, has only a slight action against the human enzyme and causes megaloblastic change only in patients already B_{12} or folate deficient.

Systemic diseases associated with folate or vitamin B_{12} deficiency

Cardiovascular diseases

Raised serum homocysteine levels are associated with an increased incidence of myocardial infarct, peripheral and cerebral vascular disease and venous thrombosis (Chapter 25). Raised serum homocysteine levels are associated with low serum and red cell folate and low serum B_{12} or vitamin B_6 levels. In addition, homocysteine levels tend to be higher in men than in premenopausal women, in old age, in heavy smokers and those with excess alcohol consumption, with impaired renal function and with some drugs. Although folate deficiency (and in some studies, the presence of the polymorphism in the 5,10-MTHFR gene) has been associated with an increased incidence of cardiovascular disease, recent large randomised studies have not shown a reduction in the rate of myocardial infarction or stroke by the use of prophylactic folic acid.

Malignant diseases

Various associations have been found between folate status or polymorphisms in folate metabolizing enzymes and malignant diseases such as colon or breast cancer and acute lymphoblastic leukaemia in childhood. In most but not all, reduced folate status has been associated with an increased risk of malignancy.

Defects of DNA synthesis not related to vitamin B_{12} or folate

Congenital deficiency of one or other enzyme concerned in purine or pyrimidine synthesis can cause megaloblastic anaemia identical in appearance to that caused by a deficiency of B_{12} or folate. The best known is orotic aciduria. Therapy with drugs that inhibit purine or pyrimidine synthesis (such as hydroxyurea, cytosine arabinoside, 6-mercaptopurine and zidovudine (AZT)) and some forms of acute myeloid leukaemia or myelodysplasia also cause megaloblastic anaemia.

Other macrocytic anaemias

There are many non-megaloblastic causes of macrocytic anaemia (Table 4.11). The exact mechanisms creating large red cells in each of these conditions is not clear although increased lipid deposition on the red cell membrane or alterations of erythroblast maturation time in the marrow may be im-plicated. Alcohol is the most frequent cause of a raised MCV in the absence of anaemia. Reticulocytes are bigger than mature red cells and so haemolytic anaemia is an important cause of macrocytic anaemia. The other underlying conditions listed in Table 4.11 are usually easily diagnosed provided that they are considered and the appropriate investigations to exclude B_{12} or folate deficiency are carried out.

Table 4.11 Causes of macrocytosis other than megaloblastic anaemia.

Alcohol
Liver disease
Myxoedema
Myelodysplastic syndromes
Cytotoxic drugs
Aplastic anaemia
Pregnancy
Smoking
Reticulocytosis
Myeloma and paraproteinaemia
Neonatal

Differential diagnosis of macrocytic anaemias

The clinical history and physical examination may suggest B_{12} or folate deficiency as the cause. Diet, drugs, alcohol intake, family history, history suggestive of malabsorption, presence of autoimmune diseases or other associations with pernicious anaemia (Table 4.4), previous gastrointestinal disease or operations are all important. The presence of jaundice, glossitis or a neuropathy are also valuable indications of megaloblastic anaemia.

The laboratory features of particular importance are the shape of macrocytes (oval in megaloblastic anaemia), the presence of hypersegmented neutrophils and of leucopenia and thrombocytopenia in megaloblastic anaemia and the bone marrow appearance. Assay of B_{12} and folate is straightforward. Exclusion of alcoholism (particularly if the patient is not anaemic), liver and thyroid function tests, and bone marrow examination for myelodysplasia, aplasia or myeloma are important in the investigation of macrocytosis not caused by B_{12} or folate deficiency.

Bibliography

Chan J.C.W., Liu H.S.Y., Kho B.C.S. *et al.* (2006) Pernicious anemia in Chinese: A study of 181 patients in a Hong Kong hospital. *Medicine* **85**,129–38.

Clarke R., Grimley Evans J., Schneede J. *et al.* (2004) Vitamin B_{12} and folate deficiency in later life. *Age Ageing* **33**,34–41.

Czeizel A.E., Dobo M. and Vargha P. (2004) Hungarian cohort controlled trial of periconceptional multivitamin supplementation shows a reduction in certain congenital abnormalities. *Birth Defects Research* **70**,853–61.

Eicholzer M., Tonz O. and Zimmerman R. (2006) Folic acid: a public health challenge. *Lancet* **367**,1352–61.

Fyfe J.C., Madsen M., Hojrup P. *et al.* (2004) The functional cobalamin (vitamin B_{12})-intrinsic factor receptor is a novel complex of cubilin and amnionless. *Blood* **103**,1573–9.

He Q., Masden M., Kilkenney A. *et al.* (2005) Amnionless function is required for cubilin brush-border expression and intrinsic factor-cobalamin (vitamin B_{12}) absorption *in vivo*. *Blood* **106**,1447–53.

Hershko C., Ronson A, Souroujon M. *et al.* (2006) Variable hematologic presentation of autoimmune gastritis: age-related progression from iron deficiency to cobalamin depletion. *Blood* **107**,1673–9.

The Hope Investigators (2006) Homocysteine lowering with folic acid and B vitamins in vascular disease. *N Engl J Med* **354**,1567–77.

Hvas A.-M., Buhl T., Laursen N.B. *et al.* (2006) The effect of recombinant human intrinsic factor on the uptake of vitamin B_{12} in patients with evident vitamin B_{12} deficency. *Haematologica* **91**,805–8.

Marks P.W. and Zukerberg L.R. (2004) Case records of Massachusetts General Hospital. Weekly clinicopathological exercises. Case 30-2004. A 37-year-old woman with paresthesiae of the arms and legs. *N Engl J Med* **351**,1333–41.

Rothenberg S.P., da Costa M.P., Sequeira J.M. *et al.* (2004) Autoantibodies against folate receptors in women with a pregnancy complicated by a neural-tube defect. *N Engl J Med* **350**,134–42.

Solomon L.R. (2005) Cobalamin-responsive disorders in the ambulatory care setting: unreliability of cobalamin, methylmalonic acid, and homocysteine testing. *Blood* **105**,978–85.

Whitehead V.M. (2006) Acquired and inherited disorders of cobalamin and folate in children. *Br J Haematol* **134**,125–36.

Wickramasinghe S.N. (ed.) (1995) Megaloblastic anaemia. *Clin Haematol* **8**,441–703.

CHAPTER 5

5 Haemolytic anaemias

Normal red cell destruction

Red cell destruction usually occurs after a mean lifespan of 120 days when the cells are removed extravascularly by the macrophages of the reticuloendothelial (RE) system, especially in the marrow but also in the liver and spleen. As the cells have no nucleus, red cell metabolism gradually deteriorates as enzymes are degraded and not replaced and the cells become non-viable. The breakdown of haem from red cells liberates iron for recirculation via plasma transferrin to marrow erythroblasts, and protoporphyrin which is broken down to bilirubin. Bilirubin circulates to the liver where it is conjugated to glucuronides which are excreted into the gut via bile and converted to stercobilinogen and stercobilin (excreted in faeces) (Fig. 5.1). Stercobilinogen and stercobilin are partly reabsorbed and excreted in urine as urobilinogen and urobilin. Globin chains are broken down to amino acids which are reutilized for general protein synthesis in the body. Haptoglobins are proteins present in normal plasma capable of binding haemoglobin. The haemoglobin–haptoglobin complex is removed from plasma by the RE system. Intravascular haemolysis (breakdown of red cells within blood vessels) plays little or no part in normal red cell destruction.

Introduction to haemolytic anaemias

Haemolytic anaemias are defined as those anaemias that result from an increase in the rate of red cell destruction. Because of erythropoietic hyperplasia and anatomical extension of bone marrow, red cell destruction may be increased several-fold before the patient becomes anaemic—compensated haemolytic disease. The normal adult marrow, after full expansion, is able to produce red cells at 6–8 times the normal rate provided this is 'effective'. It leads to a marked reticulocytosis, particularly in the more anaemic cases. Therefore, haemolytic anaemia may not be seen until the red cell lifespan is less than 30 days.

Classification

Table 5.1 is a simplified classification of the haemolytic anaemias. Hereditary haemolytic anaemias are the result of 'intrinsic' red cell defects whereas acquired haemolytic anaemias are usually the result of an 'extracorpuscular' or 'environmental' change. Paroxysmal nocturnal haemoglobinuria (PNH) is the exception because although it is an acquired disorder the PNH red cells have an intrinsic defect.

Clinical features

The patient may show pallor of the mucous membranes, mild fluctuating jaundice and splenomegaly. There is no bilirubin in urine but this may turn dark on standing because of excess urobilinogen. Pigment (bilirubin) gallstones may complicate

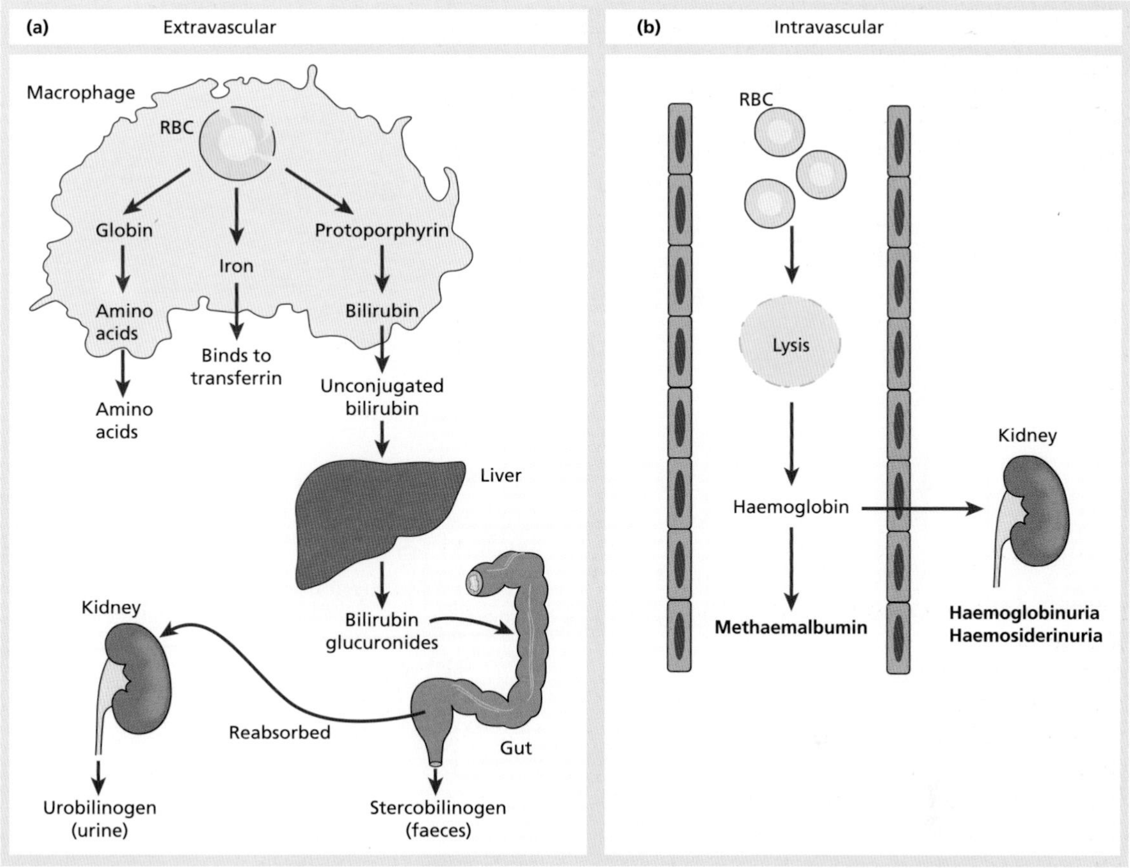

Fig. 5.1 **(a)** Normal red blood cell (RBC) breakdown. This takes place extravascularly in the macrophages of the reticuloendothelial system. **(b)** Intravascular haemolysis occurs in some pathological disorders.

the condition (Fig. 5.2) and some patients (particularly with sickle cell disease) develop ulcers around the ankle. Aplastic crises may occur, usually precipitated by infection with parvovirus which 'switches off' erythropoiesis, and are characterized by a sudden increase in anaemia and drop in reticulocyte count (see Fig. 20.4).

Rarely, folate deficiency may cause an aplastic crisis in which the bone marrow is megaloblastic.

Laboratory findings

The laboratory findings are conveniently divided into three groups.

1 Features of increased red cell breakdown:
(a) serum bilirubin raised, unconjugated and bound to albumin;
(b) urine urinobilinogen increased;
(c) faecal stercobilinogen increased;
(d) serum haptoglobins absent because the haptoglobins become saturated with haemoglobin and the complex is removed by RE cells.

2 Features of increased red cell production:
(a) reticulocytosis;
(b) bone marrow erythroid hyperplasia; the normal marrow myeloid : erythoid ratio of 2 : 1 to 12 : 1 is reduced to 1 : 1 or reversed.

3 Damaged red cells:
(a) morphology (e.g. microspherocytes, elliptocytes, fragments);
(b) osmotic fragility, autohaemolysis, etc.;
(c) red cell survival shortened; this was shown by ^{51}Cr labelling with study of the sites of destruction. This test is now not widely available.

Table 5.1 Classification of haemolytic anaemias.

Hereditary	Acquired
Membrane Hereditary spherocytosis, hereditary elliptocytosis **Metabolism** G6PD deficiency, pyruvate kinase deficiency **Haemoglobin** Genetic abnormalities (Hb S, Hb C, unstable); see Chapter 6	**Immune** *Autoimmune* Warm antibody type (see Table 5.5) Cold antibody type *Alloimmune* Haemolytic transfusion reactions Haemolytic disease of the newborn Allografts, especially marrow transplantation *Drug associated* **Red cell fragmentation syndromes** See Table 5.6 **March haemoglobinuria** **Infections** Malaria, clostridia **Chemical and physical agents** Especially drugs, industrial/domestic substances, burns **Secondary** Liver and renal disease **Paroxysmal nocturnal haemoglobinuria**

G6PD, glucose-6-phosphate dehydrogenase; Hb, haemoglobin.

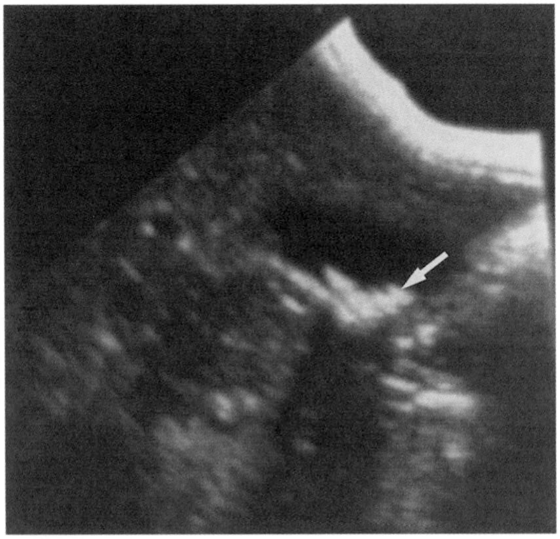

Fig. 5.2 Ultrasound of pigment gallstones (arrowed) in a 16-year-old male patient with hereditary spherocytosis. (Courtesy of L. Berger)

Intravascular and extravascular haemolysis

There are two main mechanisms whereby red cells are destroyed in haemolytic anaemia. There may be excessive removal of red cells by cells of the RE system (extravascular haemolysis) or they may be broken down directly in the circulation in a process known as intravascular haemolysis (Fig. 5.1; Table 5.2). Whichever mechanism dominates will depend on the pathology involved. In intravascular haemolysis, free haemoglobin is released which rapidly saturates plasma haptoglobins and the excess free haemoglobin is filtered by the glomerulus. If the rate of haemolysis saturates the renal tubular reabsorptive capacity, free haemoglobin enters urine (Fig. 5.3) and, as iron is released, the renal tubules become loaded with haemosiderin. Methaemalbumin and haemopexin are also formed from the process of intravascular haemolysis.

Table 5.2 Causes of intravascular haemolysis.

Mismatched blood transfusion (usually ABO)
G6PD deficiency with oxidant stress
Red cell fragmentation syndromes
Some autoimmune haemolytic anaemias
Some drug- and infection-induced haemolytic anaemias
Paroxysmal nocturnal haemoglobinuria
March haemoglobinuria
Unstable haemoglobin

G6PD, glucose-6-phosphate dehydrogenase

The main laboratory features of intravascular haemolysis are as follows.

1 Haemoglobinaemia and haemoglobinuria.

2 Haemosiderinuria (iron storage protein in the spun deposit of urine).

3 Methaemalbuminaemia (detected spectrophotometrically by Schumm's test).

Hereditary haemolytic anaemias

Membrane defects

Hereditary spherocytosis

Hereditary spherocytosis (HS) is the most common hereditary haemolytic anaemia in northern Europeans.

Pathogenesis

HS is usually caused by defects in the proteins involved in the vertical interactions between the membrane skeleton and the lipid bilayer of the red cell (Table 5.3; see Fig. 2.12). The loss of membrane may be caused by the release of parts of the lipid

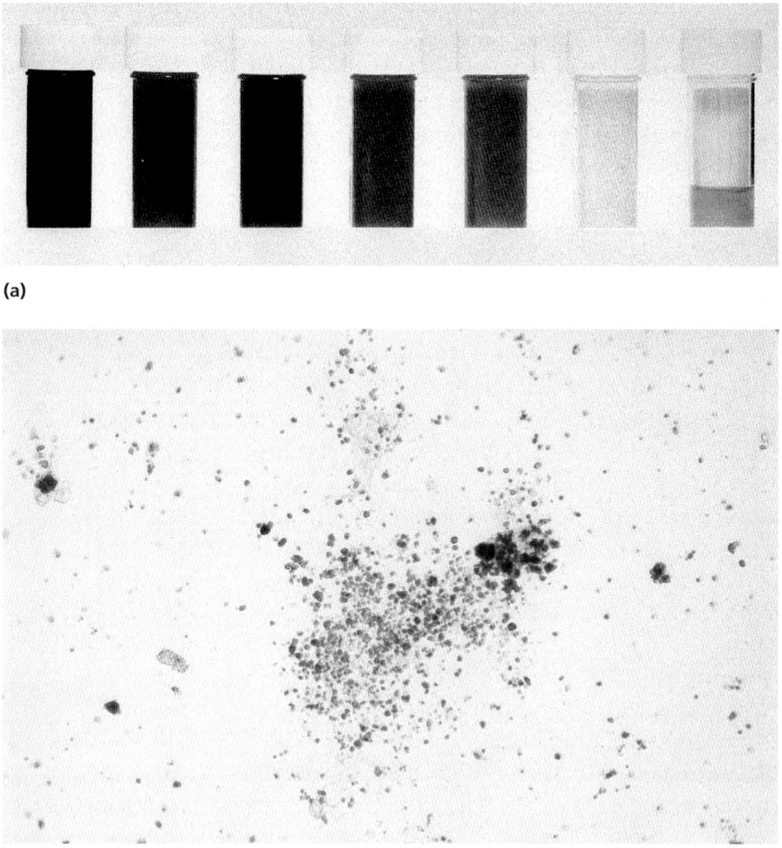

(a)

(b)

Fig. 5.3 **(a)** Progressive urine samples in an acute episode of intravascular haemolysis showing haemoglobinuria of decreasing severity. **(b)** Prussian blue-positive deposits of haemosiderin in a urine spun deposit (Perls' stain).

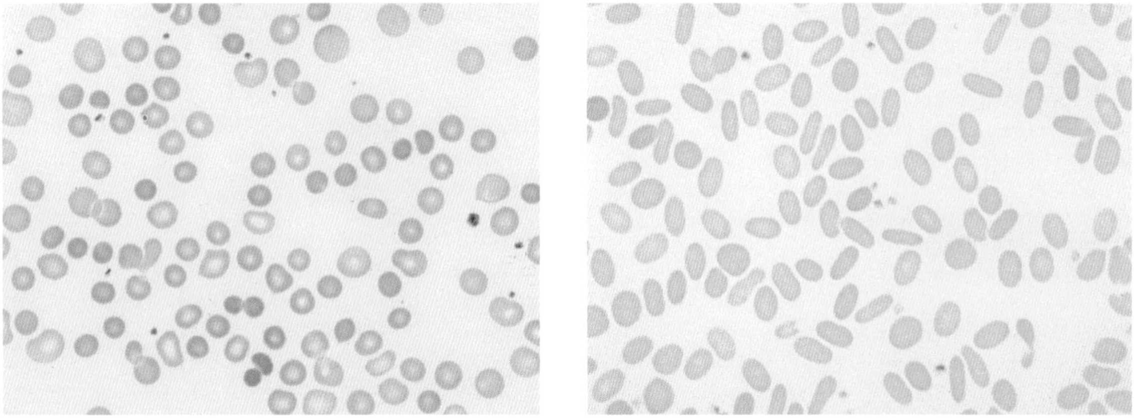

(a) (b)

Fig. 5.4 **(a)** Blood film in hereditary spherocytosis. The spherocytes are deeply staining and of small diameter. Larger polychromatic cells are reticulocytes (confirmed by supravital staining). **(b)** Blood film in hereditary elliptocytosis.

bilayer that are not supported by the skeleton. The marrow produces red cells of normal biconcave shape but these lose membrane and become increasingly spherical (loss of surface area relative to volume) as they circulate through the spleen and the rest of the RE system. Ultimately, the spherocytes are unable to pass through the splenic microcirculation where they die prematurely.

Clinical features

The inheritance is autosomal dominant with variable expression; rarely it may be autosomal recessive. The anaemia can present at any age from infancy to old age. Jaundice is typically fluctuating and is particularly marked if the haemolytic anaemia is associated with Gilbert's disease (a defect of hepatic conjugation of bilirubin); splenomegaly occurs in most patients. Pigment gallstones are frequent (Fig. 5.2); aplastic crises, usually precipitated by parvovirus infection, may cause a sudden increase in severity of anaemia (see Fig. 20.4).

Haematological findings

Anaemia is usual but not invariable; its severity tends to be similar in members of the same family. Reticulocytes are usually 5–20%. The blood film shows microspherocytes (Fig. 5.4a) which are densely staining with smaller diameters than normal red cells.

Investigation and treatment

The classic finding is that the osmotic fragility is increased (Fig. 5.5). The abnormality may require 24-h incubation at 37°C to become obvious. Autohaemolysis is increased and corrected by glucose. The cells are incubated with their own plasma for 48 h with or without glucose. The direct antiglobulin (Coombs') test is normal, excluding an autoimmune cause of spherocytosis and haemolysis.

The principal form of treatment is splenectomy

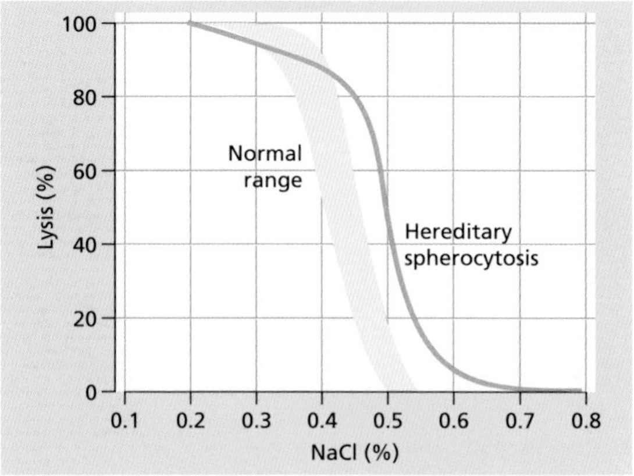

Fig. 5.5 The osmotic fragility in hereditary spherocytosis. The curve is shifted to the right of the normal range (in yellow), but a tail of more resistant cells (reticulocytes) is also present.

although this should not be performed unless clinically indicated because of anaemia or gallstones because of the risk of post-splenectomy sepsis, particularly in early childhood (p. 127). Splenectomy should always produce a rise in the haemoglobin level to normal, even though microspherocytes formed in the rest of the RE system will remain. Folic acid is given in severe cases to prevent folate deficiency.

Hereditary elliptocytosis

This has similar clinical and laboratory features to HS except for the appearance of the blood film (Fig. 5.4b), but it is usually a clinically milder disorder. It is usually discovered by chance on a blood film and there may be no evidence of haemolysis. Occasional patients require splenectomy. The basic defect is a failure of spectrin heterodimers to self-associate into heterotetramers. A number of genetic mutations affecting horizontal interactions have been detected (Table 5.3). Patients with homozygous or doubly heterozygous elliptocytosis present with a severe haemolytic anaemia with microspherocytes, poikilocytes and splenomegaly (hereditary pyropoikilocytosis).

South-East Asian ovalocytosis

This is common in Melanesia, Malaysia, Indonesia and the Philippines and is caused by a nine amino acid deletion at the junction of the cytoplasmic and transmembrane domains of the band 3 protein. The cells are rigid and resist invasion by malarial parasites. Most cases are not anaemic and are asymptomatic.

Table 5.3 Molecular basis of hereditary spherocytosis and elliptocytosis.

Hereditary spherocytosis
Ankyrin deficiency or abnormalities
Spectrin deficiency or abnormalities
Band 3 abnormalities
Pallidin (protein 4.2) abnormalities
Hereditary elliptocytosis
α- or β-spectrin mutants leading to defective spectrin dimer formation
α- or β-spectrin mutants leading to defective spectrin–ankyrin associations
Protein 4.1 deficiency or abnormality
South-East Asian ovalocytosis band 3 deletion

Defective red cell metabolism

Glucose-6-phosphate dehydrogenase deficiency

Glucose-6-phosphate dehydrogenase (G6PD) functions to reduce nicotinamide adenine dinucleotide phosphate (NADP) while oxidizing glucose-6-phosphate. It is the only source of NADP in red cells and as NADP is needed for the production of reduced glutathione a deficiency renders the red cell susceptible to oxidant stress (Fig. 5.6).

Epidemiology

There is a wide variety of normal genetic variants of the enzyme G6PD, the most common being type B (Western) and type A in Africans. In addition, more than 400 variants caused by point mutations or deletions of the enzyme G6PD have been characterized

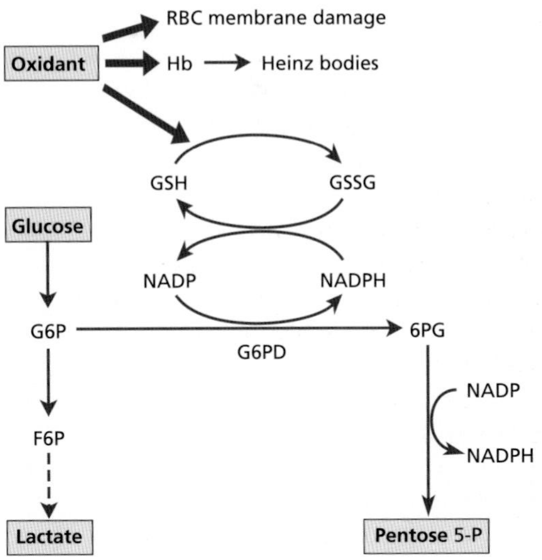

Fig. 5.6 Haemoglobin and red blood cell (RBC) membranes are usually protected from oxidant stress by reduced glutathione (GSH). In G6PD deficiency, NADPH and GSH synthesis is impaired. F6P, fructose-6-phosphate; G6P, glucose-6-phosphate; G6PD, glucose-6-phosphate dehydrogenase; GSSG, glutathione (oxidized form); NADP, NADPH, nicotinamide adenine dinucleotide phosphate.

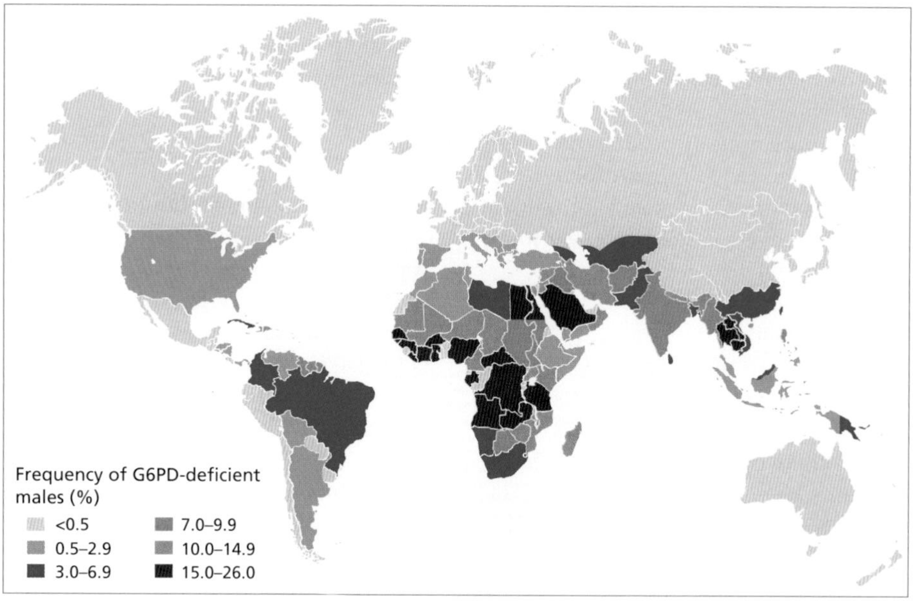

Fig. 5.7 Global distribution of *G6PD* gene variants causing G6PD deficiency. Shaded areas indicate the prevalence of G6PD deficiency. (From Luzzatto & Notaro 2001, *Science* **293**: 442, with permission)

which show less activity than normal and worldwide over 400 million people are G6PD deficient in enzyme activity (Fig. 5.7).

The inheritance is sex-linked, affecting males, and carried by females who show approximately half the normal red cell G6PD values. The female heterozygotes have an advantage of resistance to *Falciparum* malaria. The main races affected are in West Africa, the Mediterranean, the Middle East and South-East Asia. The degree of deficiency varies, often being mild (10–15% of normal activity) in black Africans, more severe in Orientals and most severe in Mediterraneans. Severe deficiency occurs occasionally in white people.

Clinical features

G6PD deficiency is usually asymptomatic. Although G6PD is present in all cells, the main syndromes that occur are as follows. (i) Acute haemolytic anaemia in response to oxidant stress, e.g. drugs, fava beans or infections (Table 5.4). The acute haemolytic anaemia is caused by rapidly developing intravascular haemolysis with haemoglobinuria (Fig. 5.3a). The anaemia may be self-limiting as new young red

Table 5.4 Agents that may cause haemolytic anaemia in glucose-6-phosphate dehydrogenase (G6PD) deficiency.

Infections and other acute illnesses (e.g. diabetic ketoacidosis)

Drugs

Antimalarials (e.g. primaquine, pamaquine, chloroquine, Fansidar, Maloprim)
Sulphonamides and sulphones (e.g. co-trimoxazole, sulfanilamide, dapsone, Salazopyrin)
Other antibacterial agents (e.g. nitrofurans, chloramphenicol)
Analgesics (e.g. aspirin), moderate doses are safe
Antihelminths (e.g. β-naphthol, stibophen)
Miscellaneous (e.g. vitamin K analogues, naphthalene (mothballs), probenecid)
Fava beans (possibly other vegetables)

NB. Many common drugs have been reported to precipitate haemolysis in G6PD deficiency in some patients (e.g. aspirin, quinine and penicillin) but not at conventional dosage.

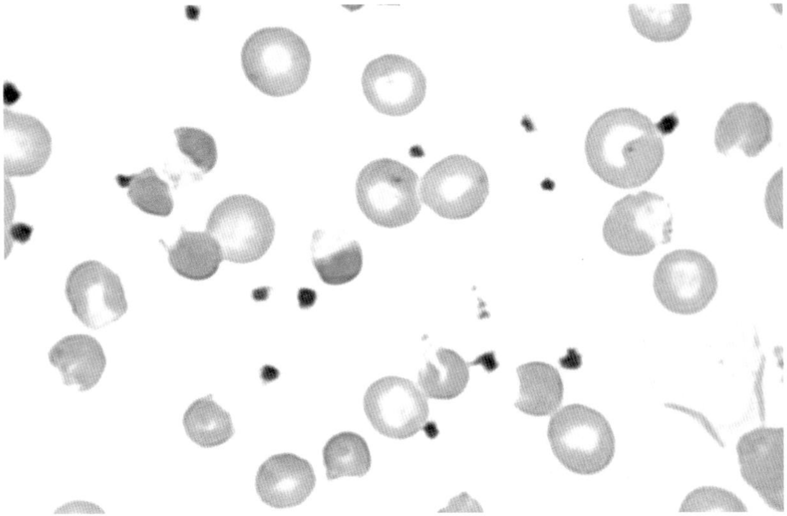

Fig. 5.8 Blood film in G6PD deficiency with acute haemolysis after an oxidant stress. Some of the cells show loss of cytoplasm with separation of remaining haemoglobin from the cell membrane ('blister' cells). There are also numerous contracted and deeply staining cells. Supravital staining (as for reticulocytes) showed the presence of Heinz bodies (see Fig. 2.17).

cells are made with near normal enzyme levels. (ii) Neonatal jaundice. (iii) Rarely, a congenital non-spherocytic haemolytic anaemia. These may result from different types of enzyme deficiency.

Diagnosis

Between crises the blood count is normal. The enzyme deficiency is detected by one of a number of screening tests or by direct enzyme assay on red cells. During a crisis the blood film may show contracted and fragmented cells, 'bite' cells and 'blister' cells (Fig. 5.8) which have had Heinz bodies removed by the spleen. Heinz bodies (oxidized, denatured haemoglobin) may be seen in the reticulocyte preparation, particularly if the spleen is absent. There are also features of intravascular haemolysis. Because of the higher enzyme level in young red cells, red cell enzyme assay may give a 'false' normal level in the phase of acute haemolysis with a reticulocyte response. Subsequent assay after the acute phase reveals the low G6PD level when the red cell population is of normal age distribution.

Treatment

The offending drug is stopped, any underlying infection is treated, a high urine output is maintained and blood transfusion undertaken where necessary for severe anaemia. G6PD-deficient babies are prone to neonatal jaundice and in severe cases phototherapy and exchange transfusion may be needed. The jaundice is usually not caused by excess haemolysis but by deficiency of G6PD affecting neonatal liver function.

Glutathione deficiency and other syndromes

Other defects in the pentose phosphate pathway leading to similar syndromes to G6PD deficiency have been described—particularly glutathione deficiency.

Glycolytic (Embden–Meyerhof) pathway defects

These are all uncommon and lead to a congenital non-spherocytic haemolytic anaemia. In some there are defects of other systems (e.g. a myopathy). The most frequently encountered is pyruvate kinase (PK) deficiency.

Pyruvate kinase deficiency

This is inherited as an autosomal recessive, the affected patients being homozygous or doubly heterozygous. Over 100 different mutations have been described. The red cells become rigid as a result of reduced adenosine triphosphate (ATP) formation. The severity of the anaemia varies widely (haemoglobin 4–10 g/dL) and causes relatively mild symptoms because of a shift to the right in the oxygen (O_2) dissociation curve caused by a rise in intracellular 2,3-diphosphoglycerate (2,3-DPG). Clinically, jaundice is usual and gallstones frequent. Frontal bossing may be present. The blood

Table 5.5 Immune haemolytic anaemias: classification.

Warm type	Cold type
Autoimmune	
Idiopathic	*Idiopathic*
Secondary	*Secondary*
SLE, other 'autoimmune' diseases	Infections—*Mycoplasma* pneumonia, infectious mononucleosis
CLL, lymphomas	Lymphoma
Drugs (e.g. methyldopa)	Paroxysmal cold haemoglobinuria (rare, sometimes associated with infections, e.g. syphilis)
Alloimmune	
Induced by red cell antigens	
Haemolytic transfusion reactions	
Haemolytic disease of the newborn post stem cell grafts	
Drug induced	
Drug–red cell membrane complex	
Immune complex	

CLL, chronic lymphocytic leukaemia; SLE, systemic lupus erythematosus.

film shows poikilocytosis and distorted 'prickle' cells, particularly post-splenectomy. Laboratory tests show that autohaemolysis is increased but, in contrast to HS, it is not corrected by glucose; direct enzyme assay is needed to make the diagnosis. Splenectomy may alleviate the anaemia but does not cure it and is indicated in those patients who need frequent transfusions.

Hereditary disorders of haemoglobin synthesis

Several of these cause clinical haemolysis. They are discussed in Chapter 6.

Acquired haemolytic anaemias

Immune haemolytic anaemias

Autoimmune haemolytic anaemias

Autoimmune haemolytic anaemias (AIHAs) are caused by antibody production by the body against its own red cells. They are characterized by a positive direct antiglobulin test (DAT) also known as the Coombs' test (see Fig. 27.5) and divided into 'warm' and 'cold' types (Table 5.5) according to whether the antibody reacts more strongly with red cells at 37°C or 4°C.

Warm autoimmune haemolytic anaemias

The red cells are coated with immunoglobulin (Ig), usually immunoglobulin G (IgG) alone or with complement, and are therefore taken up by RE macrophages which have receptors for the Ig Fc fragment. Part of the coated membrane is lost so the cell becomes progressively more spherical to maintain the same volume and is ultimately prematurely destroyed, predominantly in the spleen. When the cells are coated with IgG and complement (C3d, the degraded fragment of C3) or complement alone, red cell destruction occurs more generally in the RE system.

Clinical features

The disease may occur at any age, in either sex, and presents as a haemolytic anaemia of varying severity. The spleen is often enlarged. The disease tends to remit and relapse. It may occur alone or in association with other diseases, or arise in some patients as a result of methyldopa therapy (Table 5.5). When associated with idiopathic thrombocytopenic purpura (ITP), which is a similar condition affecting platelets (p. 281), it is known as Evans' syndrome. When secondary to systemic lupus erythematosus the cells typically are coated with immunoglobulin and complement.

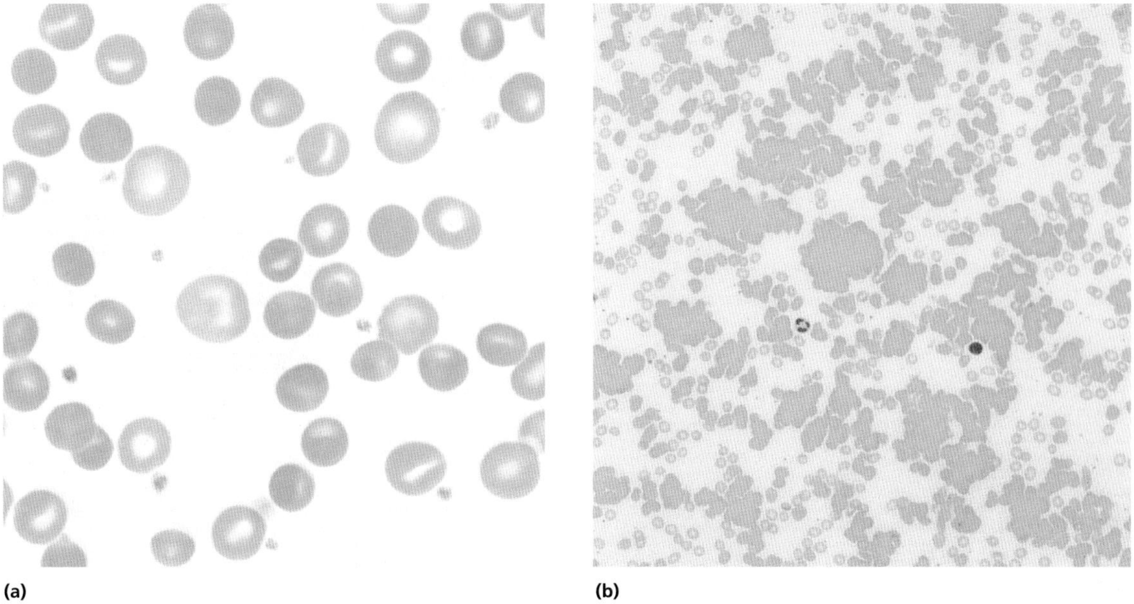

Fig. 5.9 **(a)** Blood film in warm autoimmune haemolytic anaemia. Numerous microspherocytes are present and larger polychromatic cells (reticulocytes). **(b)** Blood film in cold autoimmune haemolytic anaemia. Marked red cell agglutination is present in films made at room temperature. The background is caused by the raised plasma protein concentration.

Laboratory findings

The haematological and biochemical findings are typical of an extravascular haemolytic anaemia with spherocytosis prominent in the peripheral blood (Fig. 5.9a). The DAT is positive as a result of IgG, IgG and complement or IgA on the cells and, in some cases, the autoantibody shows specificity within the rhesus system. The antibodies both on the cell surface and free in serum are best detected at 37°C.

Treatment

1 Remove the underlying cause (e.g. methyldopa).

2 Corticosteroids. Prednisolone is the usual first-line treatment; 60 mg/day is a typical starting dose in adults and should then be tapered down. Those with predominantly IgG on red cells do best whereas those with complement often respond poorly, both to corticosteroids and splenectomy.

3 Splenectomy may be of value in those who fail to respond well or fail to maintain a satisfactory haemoglobin level on an acceptably small steroid dosage.

4 Immunosuppression may be tried after other measures have failed. Azathioprine, cyclophosphamide, chlorambucil, ciclosporin and mycophenolate mofetil have been tried.

5 Monoclonal antibodies. Anti-CD20 (rituximab) has produced prolonged remissions in a proportion of cases and anti-CD52 (Campath-1H) has been tried successfully in a few cases.

6 Folic acid is given to severe cases.

7 Blood transfusion may be needed if anaemia is severe and causing symptoms. The blood should be the least incompatible and if the specificity of the autoantibody is known, donor blood is chosen that lacks the relevant antigen(s). The patients also readily make alloantibodies against donor red cells.

8 High-dose immunoglobulin has been used but with less success than in ITP (p. 283).

Cold autoimmune haemolytic anaemias

In these syndromes the autoantibody, whether monoclonal (as in the idiopathic cold haemagglutinin syndrome or associated with lymphoproliferative disorders) or polyclonal (as following infection, e.g. infectious mononucleosis or *Mycoplasma* pneumonia) attaches to red cells mainly in the peripheral circulation where the blood temperature is cooled

(Table 5.5). The antibody is usually IgM and binds to red cells best at 4°C. IgM antibodies are highly efficient at fixing complement and both intravascular and extravascular haemolysis can occur. Complement alone is usually detected on the red cells, the antibody having eluted off the cells in warmer parts of the circulation. Interestingly, in nearly all these cold AIHA syndrome the antibody is directed against the 'I' antigen on the red cell surface. In infectious mononucleosis it is anti-i.

Clinical features

The patient may have a chronic haemolytic anaemia aggravated by the cold and often associated with intravascular haemolysis. Mild jaundice and splenomegaly may be present. The patient may develop acrocyanosis (purplish skin discoloration) at the tip of the nose, ears, fingers and toes caused by the agglutination of red cells in small vessels.

Laboratory findings are similar to those of warm AIHA except that spherocytosis is less marked, red cells agglutinate in the cold (Fig. 5.9b) and the DAT reveals complement (C3d) only on the red cell surface.

Treatment consists of keeping the patient warm and treating the underlying cause, if present. Alkylating agents such as chlorambucil may be helpful in the chronic varieties. Both anti-CD20 (rituximab) and anti-CD52 (Campath-1H) have been used. Rituximab is particularly effective when there is an associated B-lymphoproliferative disease. Splenectomy does not usually help unless massive splenomegaly is present, and steroids are not helpful. Underlying lymphoma should be excluded in 'idiopathic' cases.

Paroxysmal cold haemoglobinuria is a rare syndrome of acute intravascular haemolysis after exposure to the cold. It is caused by the Donath–Landsteiner antibody, an IgG antibody with specificity for the P blood group antigens, which binds to red cells in the cold but causes lysis with complement in warm conditions. Viral infections and syphilis are predisposing causes and the condition is usually self-limiting.

Alloimmune haemolytic anaemias

In these anaemias, antibody produced by one individual reacts with red cells of another. Two important situations are transfusion of ABO-incompatible blood and rhesus disease of the newborn which are considered in Chapters 27 and 28. The increased use of allogeneic transplantation for renal, hepatic, cardiac and bone marrow diseases has led to the recognition of alloimmune haemolytic anaemia resulting from the production of red cell antibodies in the recipient by donor lymphocytes transferred in the allograft.

Drug-induced immune haemolytic anaemias

Drugs may cause immune haemolytic anaemias via three mechanisms (Fig. 5.10):

1 Antibody directed against a drug–red cell membrane complex (e.g. penicillin, ampicillin);

2 Deposition of complement via a drug–protein (antigen)–antibody complex onto the red cell surface (e.g. quinidine, rifampicin); or

3 A true autoimmune haemolytic anaemia in which the role of the drug is unclear (e.g. methyldopa).

In each case, the haemolytic anaemia gradually disappears when the drug is discontinued but with methyldopa the autoantibody may persist for several months. The penicillin-induced immune haemolytic anaemias only occur with massive doses of the antibiotic.

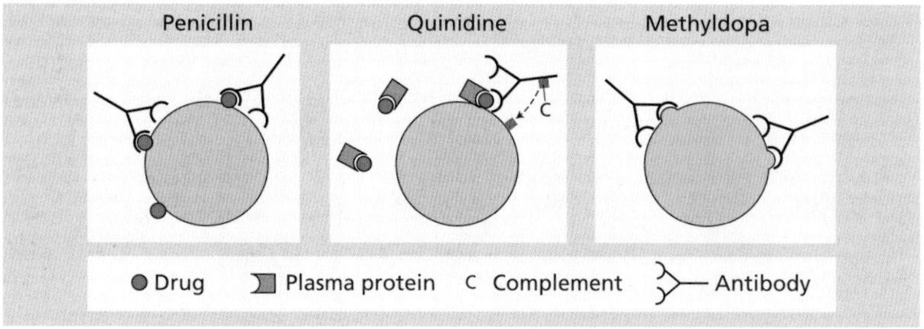

Fig. 5.10 Three different mechanisms of drug-induced immune haemolytic anaemia. In each case the coated (opsonized) cells are destroyed in the reticuloendothelial system.

Red cell fragmentation syndromes

These arise through physical damage to red cells either on abnormal surfaces (e.g. artificial heart valves or arterial grafts), arteriovenous malformations or as a microangiopathic haemolytic anaemia. This is caused by red cells passing through abnormal small vessels. The latter may be caused by deposition of fibrin strands often associated with disseminated intravascular coagulation (DIC) or platelet adherence as in thrombotic thrombocytopenic purpura (TTP) (p. 284) or vasculitis (e.g. polyarteritis nodosa; Table 5.6). The peripheral blood contains many deeply staining red cell fragments (Fig. 5.11). Clotting abnormalities typical of DIC (p. 298) with a low platelet count are also present when DIC underlies the haemolysis. TTP is discussed in detail on page 284.

Table 5.6 Red cell fragmentation syndromes.

Cardiac haemolysis	Prosthetic heart valves
	Patches, grafts
	Perivalvular leaks
Arteriovenous malformations	
Microangiopathic	TTP-HUS
	Disseminated intravascular coagulation
	Malignant disease
	Vasculitis (e.g. polyarteritis nodosa)
	Malignant hypertension
	Pre-eclampsia/HELLP
	Renal vascular disorders/HELLP syndrome
	Ciclosporin
	Homograft rejection

HELLP, haemolysis with elevated liver function tests and low platelets; HUS, haemolytic uraemic syndrome; TTP, thrombotic thrombocytopenic purpura.

March haemoglobinuria

This is caused by damage to red cells between the small bones of the feet, usually during prolonged marching or running. The blood film does not show fragments.

Infections

Infections can cause haemolysis in a variety of ways. They may precipitate an acute haemolytic crisis in G6PD deficiency or cause microangiopathic haemolytic anaemia (e.g. with meningococcal or pneumococcal septicaemia). Malaria causes haemolysis by extravascular destruction of parasitized red cells as well as by direct intravascular lysis. Blackwater fever is an acute intravascular haemolysis accompanied by acute renal failure caused by *Falciparum* malaria. *Clostridium perfringens* septicaemia

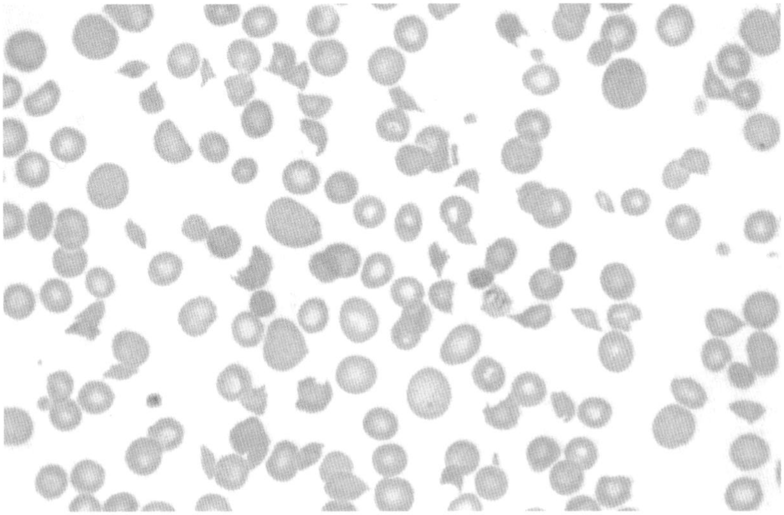

Fig. 5.11 Blood film in microangiopathic haemolytic anaemia (in this patient Gram-negative septicaemia). Numerous contracted and deeply staining cells and cell fragments are present.

can cause intravascular haemolysis with marked microspherocytosis.

Chemical and physical agents

Certain drugs (e.g. dapsone and Salazopyrin) in high doses cause oxidative intravascular haemolysis with Heinz body formation in normal subjects. In Wilson's disease an acute haemolytic anaemia can occur as a result of high levels of copper in the blood. Chemical poisoning (e.g. with lead, chlorate or arsine) can cause severe haemolysis. Severe burns damage red cells causing acanthocytosis or spherocytosis.

Secondary haemolytic anaemias

In many systemic disorders red cell survival is shortened. This may contribute to anaemia (Chapter 26).

Paroxysmal nocturnal haemoglobinuria

PNH is a rare, acquired, clonal disorder of marrow stem cells in which there is deficient synthesis of the glycosylphosphatidylinositol (GPI) anchor, a structure that attaches several surface proteins to the cell membrane. It results from mutations in the X chromosome gene coding for phosphatidylinositol glycan protein A (PIG-A) which is essential for the formation of the GPI anchor. The net result is that GPI-linked proteins (such as CD55 and CD59) are absent from the cell surface of all the cells derived from the abnormal stem cell (Fig. 5.12). The lack of surface molecules decay-activating factor (DAF, CD55) and membrane inhibitor of reactive lysis (MIRL, CD59) render red cells sensitive to lysis by complement and the result is chronic intravascular haemolysis. Haemosiderinuria is a constant feature and can give rise to iron deficiency which may exacerbate the anaemia. CD55 and CD59 are also present on white cells and platelets. The other main clinical problem seen in PNH is thrombosis and patients may develop recurrent thromboses of large veins including portal and hepatic veins, as well as intermittent abdominal pain brought about by thrombosis of mesenteric veins.

PNH is almost invariably associated with some form of bone marrow hypoplasia, often frank aplastic anaemia. It appears that the PNH clone may expand as a result of a selective pressure, possibly immunologically mediated, against cells that have normal GPI-linked membrane proteins.

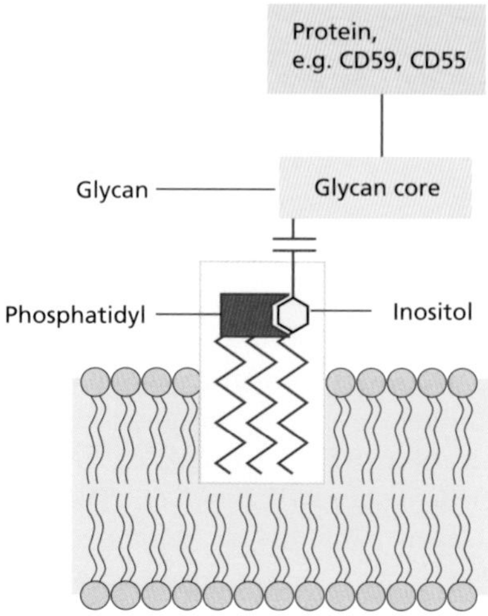

Fig. 5.12 Schematic representation of the phosphatidylinositol glycan which anchors many different proteins to the cell membrane, e.g. CD59 (MIRL, membrane inhibitor of reactive lysis).

PNH may be diagnosed by flow cytometry which shows loss of expression of the GPI-linked proteins, CD55 (DAF) and CD59 (MIRL). This has replaced the demonstration of red cell lysis in serum at low pH—the Ham's test.

Eculizumab, a humanized antibody against complement C5, inhibits the activation of terminal components of complement, reduces haemolysis and reduces transfusion requirements. Iron therapy is used for iron deficiency and long-term anticoagulation with warfarin may be needed. Immunosuppression can be useful and allogeneic stem cell transplantation is a definitive treatment. The disease occasionally remits but the median survival is approximately 10 years.

Bibliography

Beutler E. (1996) Glucose-6-phosphate-dehydrogenase: population genetics and clinical manifestations. *Blood Rev* **10**,45–52.

Bolton-Maggs P.H.B. (2000) The diagnosis and management of hereditary spherocytosis. *Clin Haematol* **13**,327–42.

Dacie J.V. (1988, 1999) *The Haemolytic Anaemias*. Vol. 2, *The Hereditary Haemolytic Anaemias*; Vol. 3, *The Haemolylic Anaemias of Immune Origin*; Vol. 4, *Secondary and Symptomatic Haemolytic Anaemias*; Vol. 5, *Drug and Chemical-induced Haemolytic Anaemias; PNH; Haemolytic Disease of the Newborn*, 3rd edn. Churchill Livingstone, Edinburgh.

Delaunay J. (2003) Red cell membrane and erythropoiesis genetic defects. *Hematol J* **4**,225–32.

Ekvall H. (2003) Malaria and anemia. *Curr Opin Hematol* **10**,108–14.

Gertz M.A. (2006) Cold agglutinin disease. *Haematologica* **91**,439–45.

Hillmen P., Hall C., Marsh J.C. *et al.* (2004) Effect of eculizumab on hemolysis and transfusion requirements in patients with paroxysmal nocturnal hemoglobinuria. *N Engl J Med* **350**,552–9.

Luzzatto L. and Notaro R. (2001) Malaria: protecting against bad air. *Science* **293**,442–3.

Parker C., Omine M., Richards S. *et al.* (2005) Diagnosis and management of paroxysmal nocturnal hemoglobinuria. *Blood* **106**,3699–709.

Rees D.C., Duley J.A., Marinaki A.M. (2003) Pyrimidine 5′ nucleotidase deficiency. *Br J Haematol* **120**,375–83.

Zanella A. (ed.) (2000) Inherited disorders of red cell metabolism. *Clin Haematol* **13**,1–150.

Zanella A., Fermo E., Bianchi P., Valentini G. (2005) Red cell pyruvate kinase deficiency: molecular and clinical aspects. *Br J Haematol* **130**,11–25.

CHAPTER 6

6 Genetic disorders of haemoglobin

This chapter deals with inherited diseases caused by reduced or abnormal synthesis of globin. Mutations in the globin genes are the most prevalent monogenic disorders worldwide and affect approximately 7% of the world's population. The synthesis of normal haemoglobin in the fetus and adult is described first.

Haemoglobin synthesis

Normal adult blood contains three types of haemoglobin (see Table 2.2). The major component is haemoglobin A with the molecular structure $\alpha_2\beta_2$. The minor haemoglobins contain γ (fetal Hb or Hb F) or δ (Hb A_2) globin chains instead of β chains. In the embryo and fetus, Gower 1, Portland, Gower 2 and fetal Hb dominate at different stages (Fig. 6.1). The genes for the globin chains occur in two clusters: ε, γ, δ and β on chromosome 11 and ζ and α on chromosome 16. Two types of γ chain occur, G_γ and A_γ, which differ by a glycine or alanine amino acid at position 136 in the polypeptide chain. The α-chain gene is duplicated and both α genes (α_1 and α_2) on each chromosome are active (Fig. 6.1).

Molecular aspects

All the globin genes have three exons (coding regions) and two introns (non-coding regions whose DNA is not represented in the finished protein). The initial RNA is transcribed from both introns and exons, and from this transcript the RNA derived from introns is removed by a process known as splicing (Fig. 6.2). The introns always begin with a G-T dinucleotide and end with an A-G dinucleotide. The splicing machinery recognizes these sequences as well as neighbouring conserved sequences. The RNA in the nucleus is also 'capped' by addition of a structure at the 5′ end which contains a seven methyl-guanosine group. The cap structure may be important for attachment of the mRNA to ribosomes. The newly formed mRNA is also polyadenylated at the 3′ end (Fig. 6.2). This stabilizes it. Thalassaemia may arise from mutations or deletions of any of these sequences.

A number of other conserved sequences are important in globin synthesis and mutations at these sites may also give rise to thalassaemia. These sequences influence gene transcription, ensure its fidelity, specify sites for the initiation and termination of translation, and ensure the stability of newly synthesized mRNA. Promoters are found 5′ of the gene, either close to the initiation site or more distally. They are the sites where RNA polymerases bind and catalyse gene transcription (see Fig. 1.9). Enhancers occur either 5′ or 3′ to the gene (Fig. 6.2). Enhancers are important in the tissue-specific regulation of globin gene expression and in regulation of the synthesis of the various globin chains during fetal and postnatal life. The locus control region (LCR) is a genetic regulatory element, situated a long way upstream of the β-globin cluster,

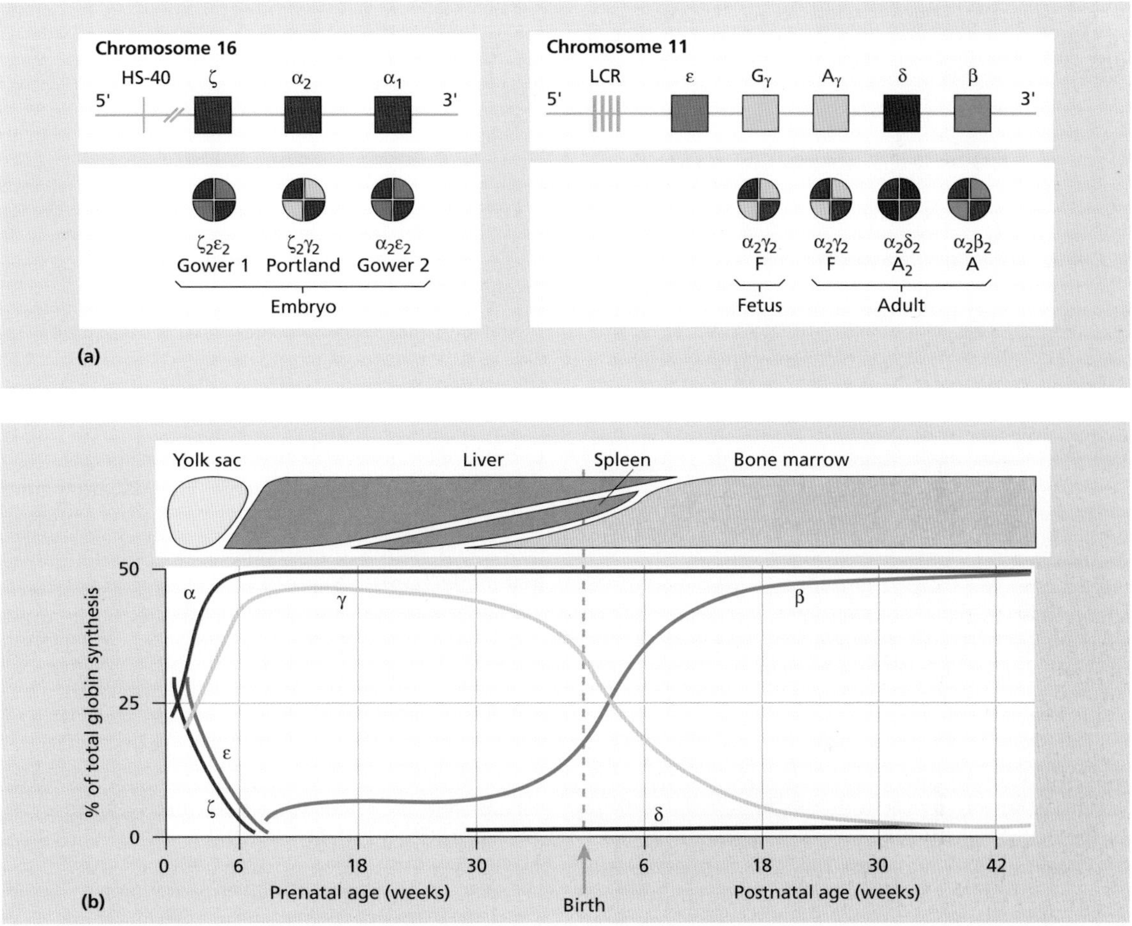

Fig. 6.1 **(a)** The globin gene clusters on chromosomes 16 and 11. In embryonic, fetal and adult life different genes are activated or suppressed. The different globin chains are synthesized independently and then combine with each other to produce the different haemoglobins. The γ gene may have two sequences, which code for either a glutamic acid or alanine residue at position 136 (G_γ or A_γ, respectively). LCR, locus control region, HS-40, see text below. **(b)** Synthesis of individual globin chains in prenatal and postnatal life.

that controls the genetic activity of each domain, probably by physically interacting with the promoter region and opening up the chromatin to allow transcription factors to bind. The α-globin gene cluster also contains an LCR-like region termed HS40. GATA-1, FoG and NF-E2 transcription factors, expressed mainly in erythroid precursors, are important in determining the expression of globin genes in erythroid cells.

Globin mRNA enters the cytoplasm and attaches to ribosomes (translation) where the synthesis of globin chains takes place. This occurs by attachment of transfer RNAs, each with its individual amino acid, by codon–anticodon base pairing to an appropriate position on the mRNA template.

Switch from fetal to adult haemoglobin

The globin genes are arranged on chromosomes 11 and 16 in the order in which they are expressed (Fig. 6.1). Certain embryonic haemoglobins are usually only expressed in yolk sac erythroblasts. The β-globin gene is expressed at a low level in early fetal life, but the main switch to adult haemoglobin

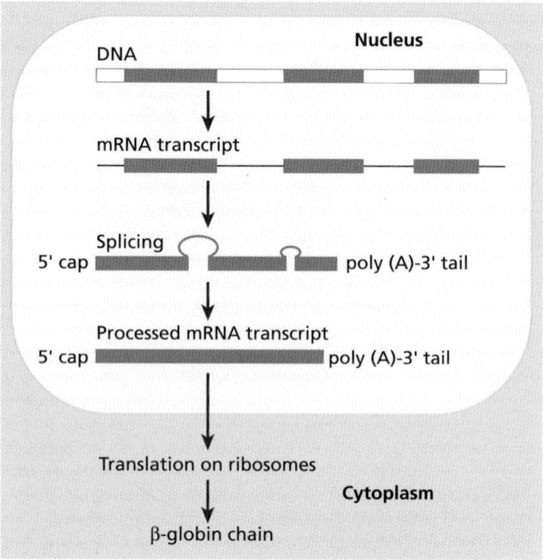

Fig. 6.2 The expression of a human globin gene from transcription, excision of introns, splicing of exons and translation to ribosomes. The primary transcript is 'capped' at the 5′ end and a poly A tail is then added.

occurs 3–6 months after birth when synthesis of the γ chain is largely replaced by the β chain. How this switch comes about is largely unknown. However, it is clear that the methylation state of the gene (expressed genes tend to be hypomethylated, non-expressed hypermethylated), the state of the chromosome packaging and various enhancer sequences all play a part in determining whether a particular gene will be transcribed.

Haemoglobin abnormalities

These result from the following:

1 Synthesis of an abnormal haemoglobin.

2 Reduced rate of synthesis of normal α- or β-globin chains (the α- and β-thalassaemias).

Table 6.1 shows some of the first group of syndromes that arise from synthesis of an α or β chain with an amino acid substitution. In many cases, however, the abnormality is completely silent. The clinically most important abnormality is sickle cell anaemia. Haemoglobin (Hb) C, D and E are also common and, like Hb S, are substitutions in the β chain. Unstable haemoglobins are rare and cause a

Table 6.1 The clinical syndromes produced by haemoglobin abnormalities.

Syndrome	Abnormality
Haemolysis	Crystalline haemoglobins (Hb S, C, D, E, etc.)
	Unstable haemoglobin
Thalassaemia	α or β resulting from reduced globin chain synthesis
Familial polycythaemia	Altered oxygen affinity
Methaemoglobinaemia	Failure of reduction (Hb Ms)

chronic haemolytic anaemia of varying severity with intravascular haemolysis (see Table 5.2). Abnormal haemoglobins may also cause (familial) polycythaemia (Chapter 19) or congenital methaemoglobinaemia (Chapter 2).

The genetic defects of haemoglobin are the most common genetic disorders worldwide. They occur in tropical and subtropical areas (Fig. 6.3) and most appear to have been selected because the carrier state affords some protection against malaria. β-Thalassaemia is more common in the Mediterranean region while α-thalassaemia is more common in the Far East.

Thalassaemias

These are a heterogeneous group of genetic disorders that result from a reduced rate of synthesis of α or β chains.

α-Thalassaemia syndromes

These are usually caused by gene deletions and are listed in Table 6.2. As there are normally four copies of the α-globin gene, the clinical severity can be classified according to the number of genes that are missing or inactive. Loss of all four genes completely suppresses α-chain synthesis (Fig. 6.4) and because the α chain is essential in fetal as well as in adult haemoglobin this is incompatible with life and leads to death *in utero* (hydrops fetalis; Fig. 6.5). Three α gene deletions leads to a moderately severe (haemoglobin 7–11 g/dL) microcytic, hypochromic anaemia (Fig. 6.6) with splenomegaly. This is

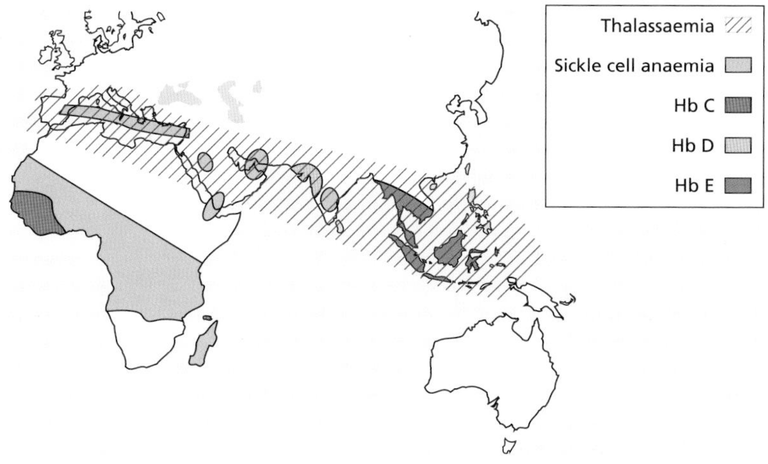

Fig. 6.3 The geographical distribution of the thalassaemias and the more common, inherited, structural haemoglobin abnormalities.

Table 6.2 Classification of thalassaemia.

Clinical

Hydrops fetalis
Four gene deletion α-thalassaemia

Thalassaemia major
Transfusion dependent, homozygous β^0-thalassaemia or other combinations of β-thalassaemia trait

Thalassaemia intermedia
See Table 6.5

Thalassaemia minor
β^0-Thalassaemia trait

β^+-Thalassaemia trait
Hereditary persistence of fetal haemoglobin
δβ-Thalassaemia trait

α^0-Thalassaemia trait
α^+-Thalassaemia trait

Genetic

Type	Haplotype	Heterozygous thalassaemia trait (minor)*	Homozygous
α-Thalassaemias†			
α^0	– –/	MCV, MCH low	Hydrops fetalis
α^+	–α/	MCV, MCH minimally reduced	As heterozygous α^0-thalassaemia
β-Thalassaemias			
β^0		MCV, MCH low (Hb A_2 >3.5%)	Thalassaemia major (Hb F 98%, Hb A_2 2%)
β^+		MCV, MCH low (Hb A_2 >3.5%)	Thalassaemia major or intermedia (Hb F 70–80%, Hb A 10–20%, Hb A_2 variable)
δβ-Thalassaemia and hereditary persistence of fetal haemoglobin		MCV, MCH low (Hb F 5–20%, Hb A_2 normal)	Thalassaemia intermedia (Hb F 100%)
Hb Lepore		MCV, MCH low (Hb A 80–90%, Hb Lepore 10%, Hb A_2 reduced)	Thalassaemia major or intermedia (Hb F 80%, Hb Lepore 10–20%, Hb A, Hb A_2 absent)

MCH, mean corpuscular haemoglobin; MCV, mean corpuscular volume.
* Occasionally heterozygous β-thalassaemia is dominant (associated with the clinical picture of thalassaemia intermedia). There are several explanations.
† Compound heterozygote $\alpha^0\alpha^+$ (– –/–α) is haemoglobin H disease.

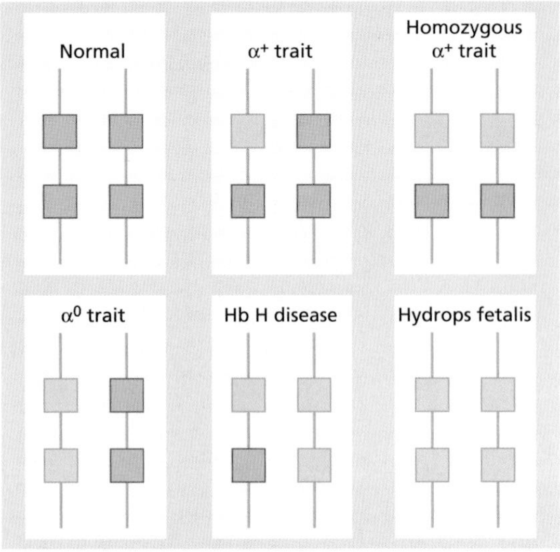

Fig. 6.4 The genetics of α-thalassaemia. Each α gene may be deleted or (less frequently) dysfunctional. The orange boxes represent normal genes, and the blue boxes represent gene deletions or dysfunctional genes.

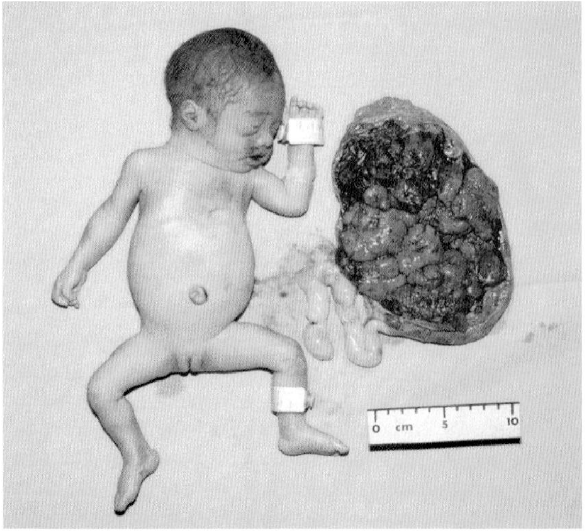

Fig. 6.5 α-Thalassaemia: hydrops fetalis, the result of deletion of all four α-globin genes (homozygous α^0-thalassaemia). The main haemoglobin present is Hb Barts (γ_4). The condition is incompatible with life beyond the fetal stage. (Courtesy of Professor D. Todd)

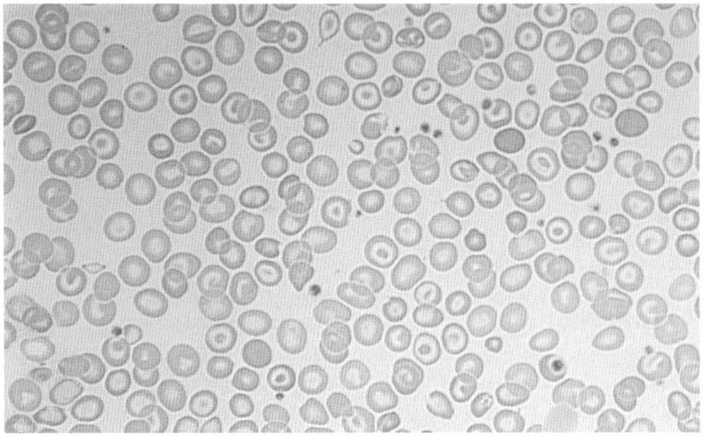

(a)

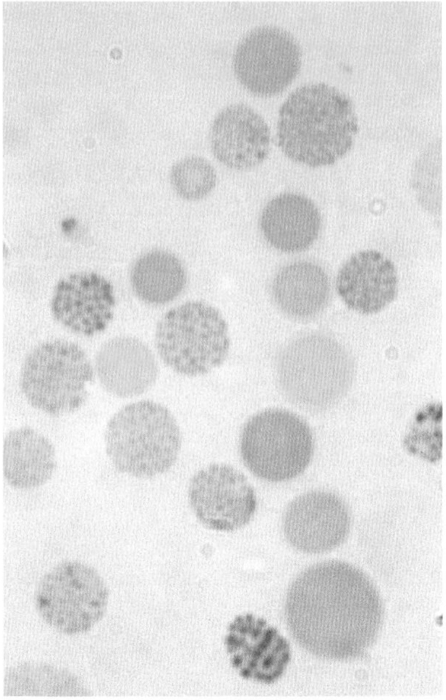

(b)

Fig. 6.6 **(a)** α-Thalassaemia: haemoglobin H disease (three α-globin gene deletion). The blood film shows marked hypochromic, microcytic cells with target cells and poikilocytosis. **(b)** α-Thalassaemia: haemoglobin H disease. Supravital staining with brilliant cresyl blue reveals multiple fine, deeply stained deposits ('golf ball' cells) caused by precipitation of aggregates of β-globin chains. Hb H can also be detected as a fast-moving band on haemoglobin electrophoresis (see Fig. 6.14).

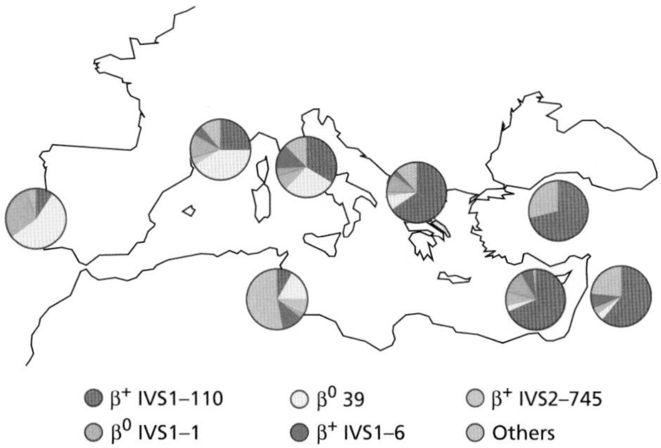

Fig. 6.7 Distribution of different mutations of β-thalassaemia major in the Mediterranean area. IVSI, IVS2 intervening sequences; 1, 6, 39, 110, 745 are mutations of corresponding codons. (Courtesy of Professor A. Cao)

known as Hb H disease because haemoglobin H (β_4) can be detected in red cells of these patients by electrophoresis or in reticulocyte preparations (Fig. 6.6). In fetal life, Hb Barts (γ_4) occurs.

The α-thalassaemia traits are caused by loss of one or two genes and are usually not associated with anaemia, although the mean corpuscular volume (MCV) and mean corpuscular haemoglobin (MCH) are low and the red cell count is over 5.5×10^{12}/L. Haemoglobin electrophoresis is normal and α/β-chain synthesis studies or DNA analyses are needed to be certain of the diagnosis. The normal α/β-synthesis ratio is 1 : 1 and this is reduced in the α-thalassaemias and raised in β-thalassaemias. Uncommon non-deletional forms of α-thalassaemia are caused by point mutations producing dysfunction of the genes or rarely by mutations affecting termination of translation which give rise to an elongated but unstable chain (e.g. Hb Constant Spring). Two rare forms of α-thalassaemia are associated with mental retardation. They are caused by mutation in a gene on chromosome 16 (ATR-16) or on chromosome X (ATR-X) which control the transcription of the α globin and other genes.

β-Thalassaemia syndromes

β-Thalassaemia major

This condition occurs on average in one in four offspring if both parents are carriers of the β-thalassaemia trait. Either no β chain (β^0) or small amounts (β^+) are synthesized. Excess α chains precipitate in erythroblasts and in mature red cells causing the severe ineffective erythropoiesis and haemolysis that are typical of this disease. The greater the α-chain excess, the more severe the anaemia. Production of γ chains helps to 'mop up' excess α chains and to ameliorate the condition. Over 200 different genetic defects have now been detected (Figs 6.7 and 6.8).

Unlike α-thalassaemia, the majority of genetic lesions are point mutations rather than gene deletions. These mutations may be within the gene complex itself or in promoter or enhancer regions. Certain mutations are particularly frequent in some communities (Fig. 6.7) and this may simplify antenatal diagnosis aimed at detecting the mutations in fetal DNA. Thalassaemia major is often a result of inheritance of two different mutations, each affecting β-globin synthesis (compound heterozygotes). In some cases, deletion of the β gene, δ and β genes or even δ, β and γ genes occurs. In others, unequal crossing-over has produced δβ fusion genes (so called Lepore syndrome named after the first family in which this was diagnosed) (p. 84).

Clinical features

1 Severe anaemia becomes apparent at 3–6 months after birth when the switch from γ- to β-chain production should take place.

2 Enlargement of the liver and spleen occurs as a result of excessive red cell destruction, extramedullary haemopoiesis and later because of iron overload. The large spleen increases blood requirements by

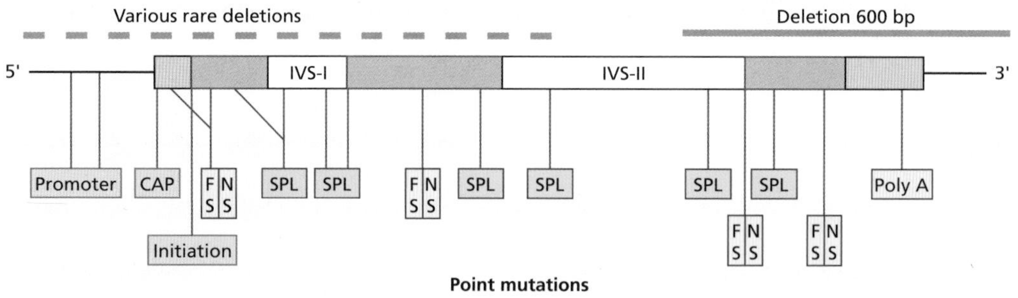

Fig. 6.8 Examples of mutations that produce β-thalassaemia. These include single base changes, small deletions and insertions of one or two bases affecting introns, exons or the flanking regions of the β-globin gene. FS, 'frameshifts': deletion of nucleotide(s) that places the reading frame out of phase downstream of the lesion; NS, 'non-sense': premature chain termination as a result of a new translational stop codon (e.g. UAA); SPL, 'splicing': inactivation of splicing or new splice sites generated (aberrant splicing) in exons or introns; promoter, CAP, initiation: reduction of transcription or translation as a result of lesion in promoter, CAP or initiation regions; Poly A, mutations on the poly A addition signal resulting in failure of poly A addition and an unstable mRNA.

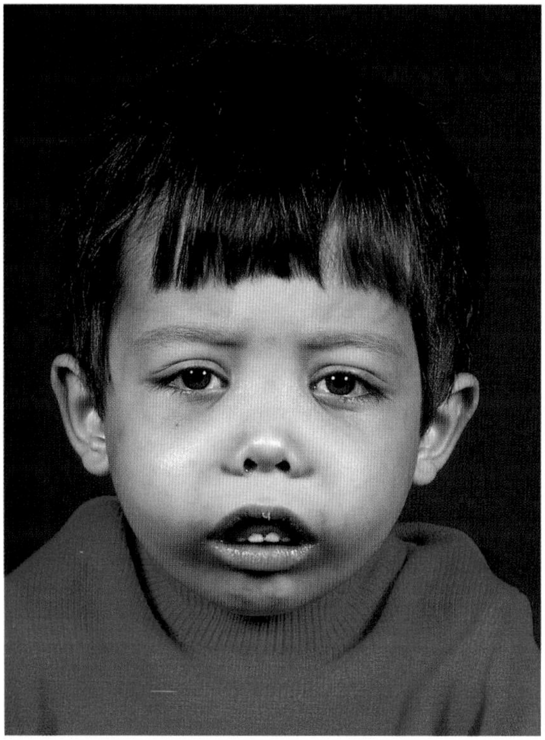

Fig. 6.9 The facial appearance of a child with β-thalassaemia major. The skull is bossed with prominent frontal and parietal bones; the maxilla is enlarged.

increasing red cell destruction and pooling, and by causing expansion of the plasma volume.

3 Expansion of bones caused by intense marrow hyperplasia leads to a thalassaemic facies (Fig. 6.9) and to thinning of the cortex of many bones with a tendency to fractures and bossing of the skull with a 'hair-on-end' appearance on X-ray (Fig. 6.10).

4 The patient can be sustained by blood transfusions but iron overload caused by repeated transfusions is inevitable unless chelation therapy is given (Table 6.3). Each 500 mL of transfused blood contains approximately 250 mg iron. To make matters worse, iron absorption from food is *increased* in β-thalassaemia, probably secondary

Table 6.3 Causes of refractory anaemia that may lead to transfusional iron overload.

Congenital	Acquired
β-Thalassaemia major	Myelodysplasia
β-Thalassaemia/Hb E disease	Red cell aplasia
Sickle cell anaemia (some cases)	Aplastic anaemia
Red cell aplasia (Diamond–Blackfan)	Myelofibrosis
Sideroblastic anaemia	
Dyserythropoietic anaemia	

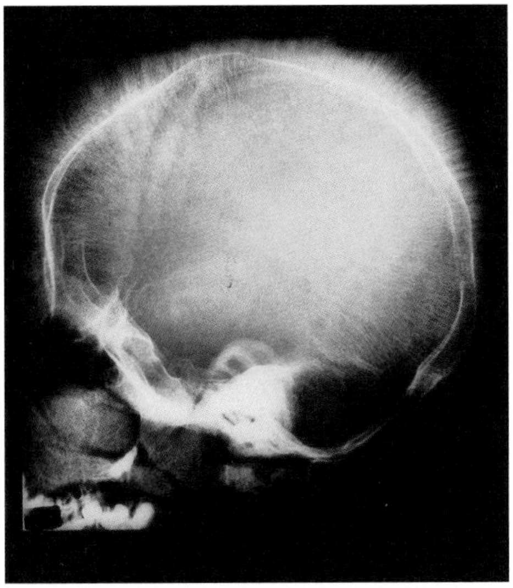

Fig. 6.10 The skull X-ray in β-thalassaemia major. There is a 'hair-on-end' appearance as a result of expansion of the bone marrow into cortical bone.

to ineffective erythropoiesis and inappropriately low serum hepcidin levels. Iron damages the liver (Fig. 6.11) and the endocrine organs with failure of growth, delayed or absent puberty, diabetes mellitus, hypothyroidism and hypoparathyroidism.

Skin pigmentation as a result of excess melanin and haemosiderin gives a slately grey appearance at an early stage of iron overload.

Most importantly, iron damages the heart. In the absence of intensive iron chelation, death occurs in the second or third decade, usually from congestive heart failure or cardiac arrhythmias. T_2* magnetic resonance imaging (MRI) is a valuable measure of cardiac (or liver) iron (Fig. 6.12). It can detect increased cardiac iron before sensitive tests detect impaired cardiac function. Serum ferritin and liver iron show poor correlation with cardiac iron estimated by T_2* MRI (Fig. 6.12).

5 Infections can occur for a variety of reasons. In infancy, without adequate transfusion, the anaemic

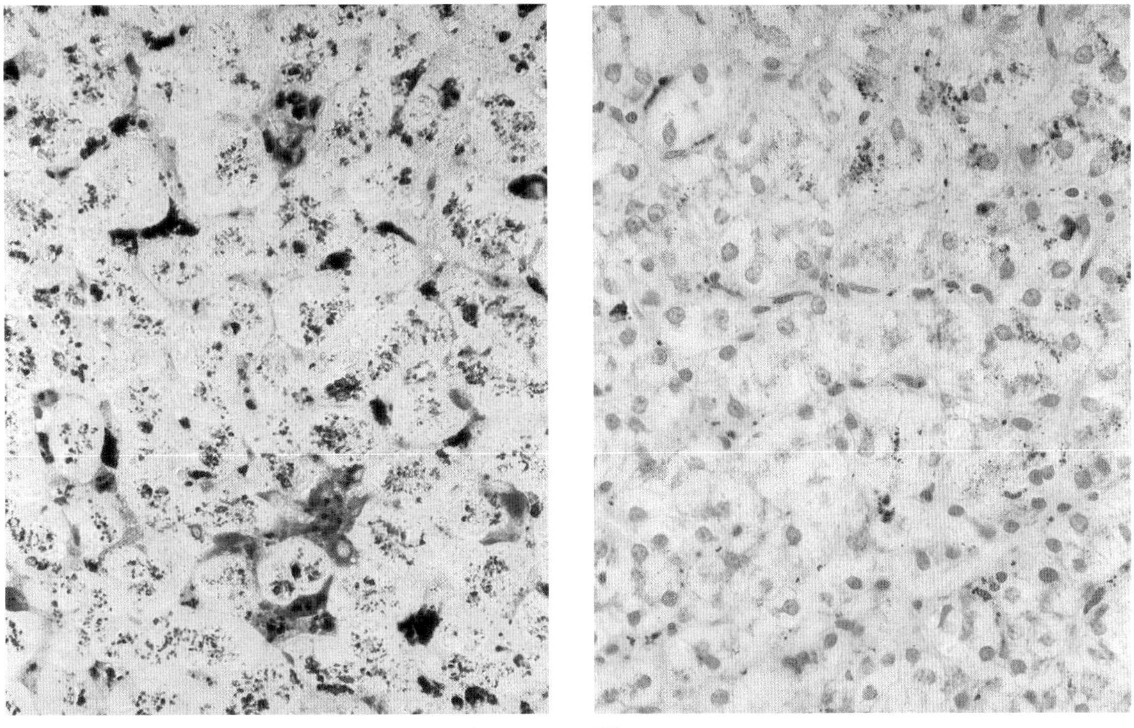

(a) (b)

Fig. 6.11 β-Thalassaemia major: needle biopsy of liver. **(a)** Grade IV siderosis with iron deposition in the hepatic parenchymal cells, bile duct epithelium, macrophages and fibroblasts (Perls' stain). **(b)** Reduction of iron excess in liver after intensive chelation therapy.

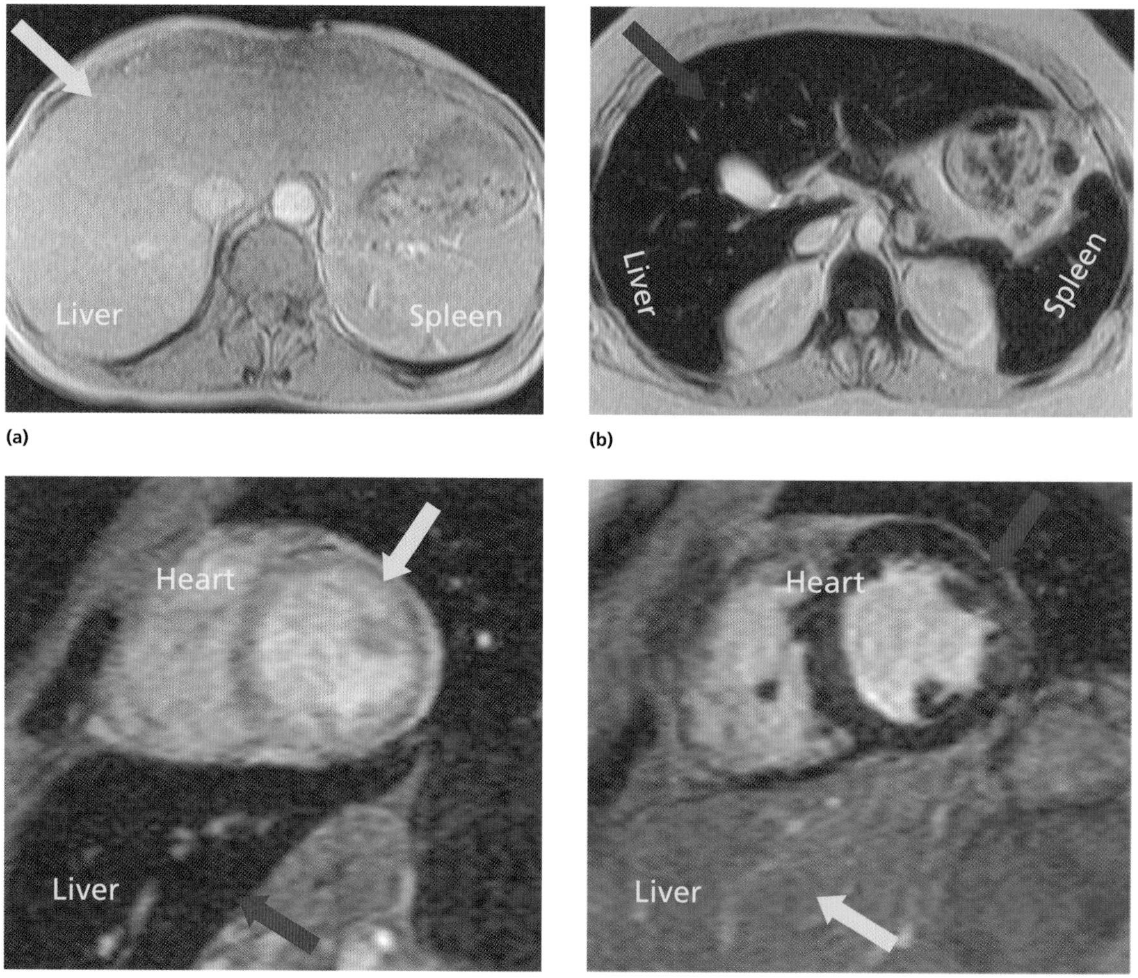

(a) (b) (c) (d)

Fig. 6.12 T_2* magnetic resonance images (MRIs) showing tissue appearance in iron overload **(a)** normal volunteer, **(b)** severe iron overload. Green arrow, normal appearance; red arrow, iron overload. Lack of correlation: liver and cardiac iron in two cases of thalassaemia major **(c)** and **(d)**.

child is prone to bacterial infections. Pneumococcal, *Haemophilus* and meningococcal infections are likely if splenectomy has been carried out and prophylactic penicillin is not taken. *Yersinia enterocolitica* occurs, particularly in iron-loaded patients being treated with deferoxamine; it may cause severe gastroenteritis. Transfusion of viruses by blood transfusion may occur. Liver disease in thalassaemia is most frequently a result of hepatitis C but hepatitis B is also common where the virus is endemic. Human immunodeficiency virus (HIV) has been transmitted to some patients by blood transfusion.

6 Osteoporosis may occur in well-transfused patients. It is more common in diabetic patients with endocrine abnormalities and with marrow expansion resulting from ineffective erythopoiesis.

Laboratory diagnosis

1 There is a severe hypochromic, microcytic anaemia, raised reticulocyte percentage with normoblasts, target cells and basophilic stippling in the blood film (Fig. 6.13).

2 Haemoglobin electrophoresis reveals absence or almost complete absence of Hb A, with almost all the circulating haemoglobin being Hb F. The Hb A_2 percentage is normal, low or slightly raised

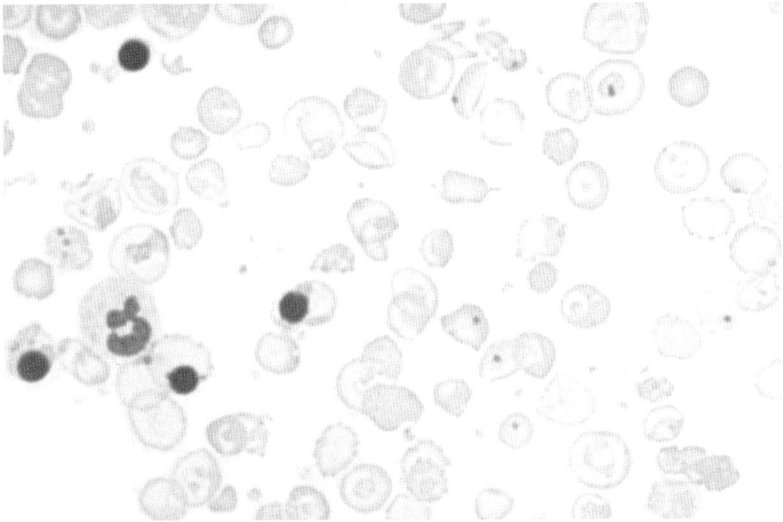

Fig. 6.13 Blood film in β-thalassaemia major post-splenectomy. There are hypochromic cells, target cells and many nucleated red cells (normoblasts). Howell–Jolly bodies are seen in same red cells.

(Fig. 6.14a). High performance liquid chromatography is now usually used as first-line method to diagnose haemoglobin disorders (Fig. 16.14b). α/β-Globin chain synthesis studies on reticulocytes show an increased α : β ratio with reduced or absent β-chain synthesis. DNA analysis is used to identify the defect on each allele.

Assessment of iron status

The tests that can be performed to assess iron overload are listed in Table 6.4. Tests may also be carried out to determine the degree of organ damage caused by iron. The serum ferritin is the most widely used test. It is usual in thalassaemia major to attempt to keep the level between 1000 and 1500 μg/L, when

Table 6.4 Assessment of iron overload.

Assessment of iron stores	
Serum ferritin	
Serum iron and percentage saturation of transferrin (iron-binding capacity)	
Serum non-transferrin bound iron	
Bone marrow biopsy (Perls' stain) for reticuloendothelial stores	
DNA test for mutation resulting in Cys282Tyr in the *HFE* gene	
Liver biopsy (parenchymal and reticuloendothelial stores)	
Liver CT scan or MRI	
Cardiac MRI (T_2* technique)	
Deferoxamine or deferiprone iron excretion test (chelatable iron)	
Repeated phlebotomy until iron deficiency occurs	
Assessment of tissue damage caused by iron overload	
Cardiac	Clinical; chest X-ray; ECG; 24-h monitor; echocardiography; radionuclide (MUGA) scan to check left ventricular ejection fraction at rest and with stress
Liver	Liver function tests; liver biopsy; CT scan or MRI
Endocrine	Clinical examination (growth and sexual development); glucose tolerance test; pituitary gonadotrophin release tests; thyroid, parathyroid, gonadal, adrenal function, growth hormone assays; radiology for bone age; isotopic bone density study

CT, computed tomography; ECG, electrocardiography; MRI, magnetic resonance imaging; MUGA, multiple gated acquisition.

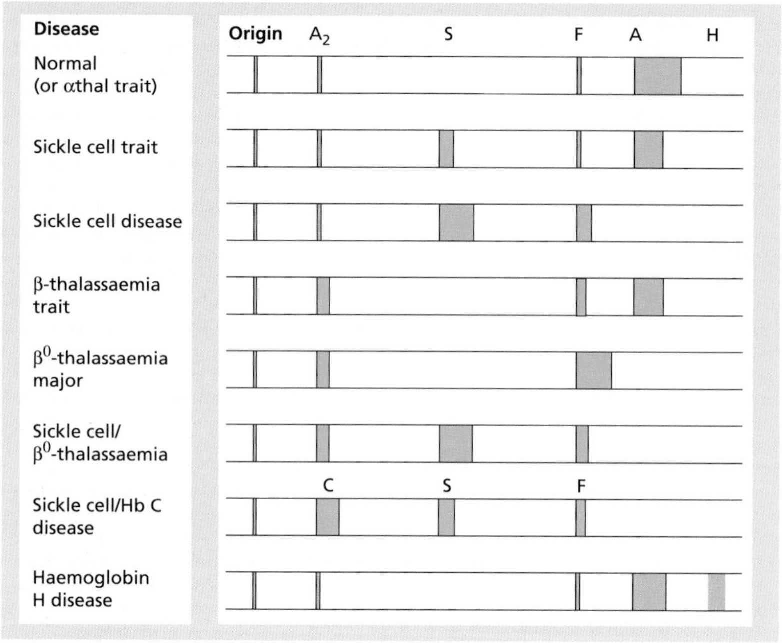

(a)

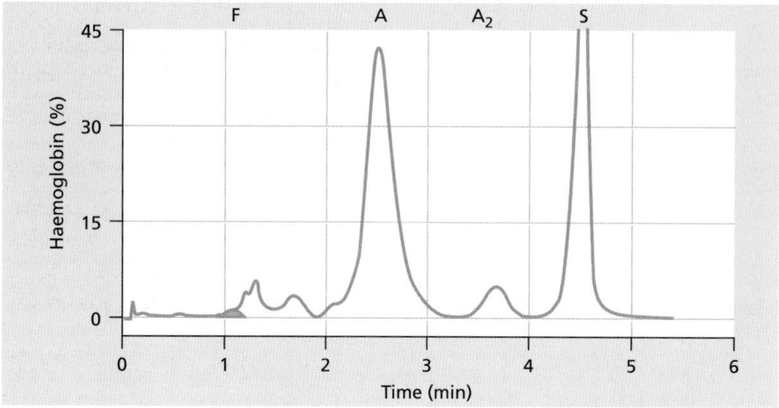

(b)

Fig. 6.14 **(a)** Haemoglobin electrophoretic patterns in normal adult human blood and in subjects with sickle cell (Hb S) trait or disease, β-thalassaemia trait, β-thalassaemia major, Hb S/β-thalassaemia or Hb S/Hb C disease and Hb H disease. **(b)** High performance liquid chromatography. The different haemoglobins elute at different times from the column and their concentrations are read automatically. In this example, the patient is a carrier of sickle cell disease.

the body iron stores are approximately 5–10 times normal. However, the serum ferritin correlates poorly with cardiac iron and is raised in relation to iron status in viral hepatitis and other inflammatory disorders and should therefore be interpreted in conjunction with other tests such as T_2* MRI assessment of cardiac iron, liver biopsy iron (Fig. 6.11) and urine excretion of iron in response to deferoxamine or deferiprone. The function of the heart, liver and endocrine organs are also needed to determine the efficacy of chelation therapy (Table 6.4).

Treatment

1 Regular blood transfusions are needed to maintain the haemoglobin over 10 g/dL at all times. This usually requires 2–3 units every 4–6 weeks. Fresh blood, filtered to remove white cells, gives the best red cell survival with the fewest reactions. The patients should be genotyped at the start of the transfusion programme in case red cell antibodies against transfused red cells develop.

2 Regular folic acid (e.g. 5 mg/day) is given if the diet is poor.

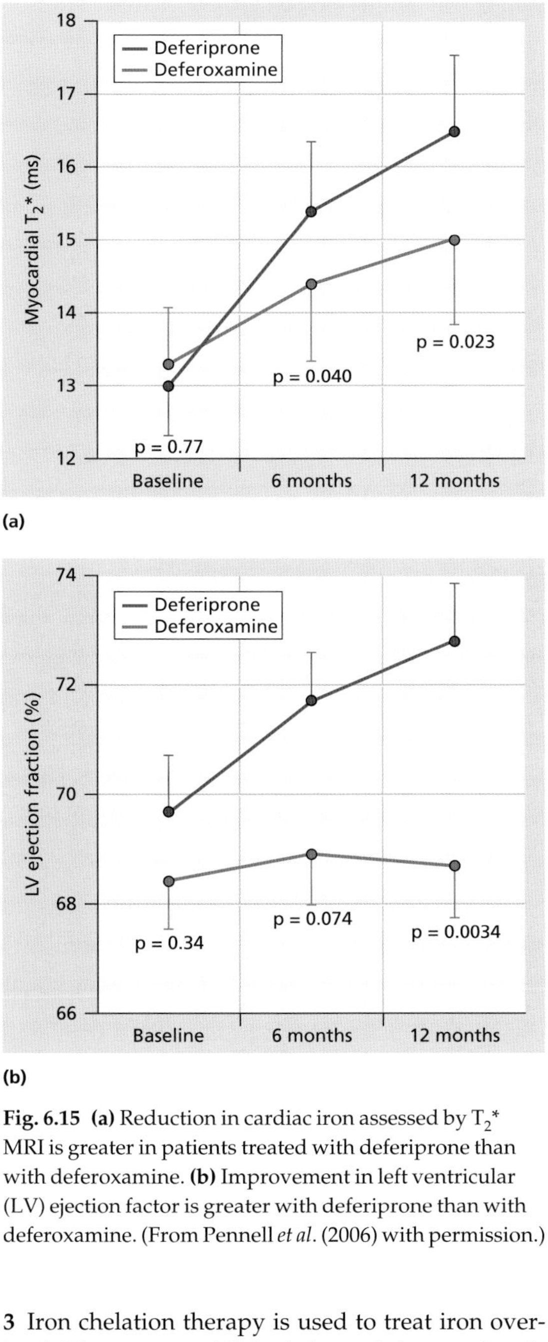

Fig. 6.15 (a) Reduction in cardiac iron assessed by T_2* MRI is greater in patients treated with deferiprone than with deferoxamine. **(b)** Improvement in left ventricular (LV) ejection factor is greater with deferiprone than with deferoxamine. (From Pennell *et al.* (2006) with permission.)

3 Iron chelation therapy is used to treat iron overload. The most established drug, deferoxamine, is inactive orally. It may be given by a separate infusion bag 1–2 g with each unit of blood transfused and by subcutaneous infusion 40 mg/kg over 8–12 h, 5–7 days weekly. It is commenced in infants after 10–15 units of blood have been transfused. Iron chelated by deferoxamine is mainly excreted in the urine but up to one-third is also excreted in the stools. If patients comply with this intensive iron chelation regime, life expectancy for patients with thalassaemia major and other chronic refractory anaemias receiving regular blood transfusion (Table 6.3) improves considerably. In some cases, intensive continuous chelation therapy with intravenous deferoxamine can reverse heart damage caused by iron overload. However, lack of compliance is frequent and the drug is costly. In addition, deferoxamine may have side-effects, especially in children with relatively low serum ferritin levels. These include high tone deafness, retinal damage, bone abnormalities and growth retardation. Patients should have auditory and fundoscopic examinations at regular intervals.

Deferiprone is an orally active iron chelator which causes predominantly urine iron excretion. It is usually given in three doses daily. It may be used alone or in combination with deferoxamine. The drugs have an additive effect on iron excretion. Deferiprone is more effective than deferoxamine at removing cardiac iron (Fig. 6.15a). Compliance is also better. Side-effects include an arthropathy, agranulocytosis (in about 1%), neutropenia, gastrointestinal disturbance and zinc deficiency.

Deferasirox (ICL670, Exjade) is the newest oral chelator. It is given once daily and causes faecal iron excretion only. Skin rashes and transient changes in liver enzymes have been reported. The ease of administration and its lack of major side-effects are likely to result in its widespread use.

4 Vitamin C, 200 mg/day, increases excretion of iron produced by deferoxamine.

5 Splenectomy may be needed to reduce blood requirements. This should be delayed until the patient is over 6 years old because of the high risk of dangerous infections post-splenectomy. The vaccinations and antibiotics to be given are described in Chapter 9.

6 Endocrine therapy is given either as replacement because of end-organ failure or to stimulate the pituitary if puberty is delayed. Diabetics will require insulin therapy. Patients with osteoporosis may need additional therapy with increased calcium and vitamin D in their diet, together with a bisphosphonate and appropriate endocrine therapy.

7 Immunization against hepatitis B should be carried out in all non-immune patients. Treatment for transfusion-transmitted hepatitis C with α-interferon and ribavirin is needed if viral genomes are detected in plasma.
8 Allogeneic bone marrow transplantation offers the prospect of permanent cure. The success rate (long-term thalassaemia major-free survival) is over 80% in well-chelated younger patients without liver fibrosis or hepatomegaly. A human leucocyte antigen (HLA) matching sibling (or rarely other family member or matching unrelated donor) acts as donor. Failure is mainly a result of recurrence of thalassaemia, death (e.g. from infection) or severe chronic graft-versus-host disease.

β-Thalassaemia trait (minor)

This is a common, usually symptomless, abnormality characterized like α-thalassaemia trait by a hypochromic, microcytic blood picture (MCV and MCH very low) but high red cell count ($>5.5 \times 10^{12}/L$) and mild anaemia (haemoglobin 10–12 g/dL). It is usually more severe than α trait. A raised Hb A_2 (>3.5%) confirms the diagnosis. One of the most important indications for making the diagnosis is that it allows the possibility of prenatal counselling to patients with a partner who also has a significant haemoglobin disorder. If both carry β-thalassaemia trait there is a 25% risk of a thalassaemia major child.

Thalassaemia intermedia

Cases of thalassaemia of moderate severity (haemoglobin 7.0–10.0 g/dL) who do not need regular transfusions are called thalassaemia intermedia (Table 6.5). This is a *clinical* syndrome which may be caused by a variety of genetic defects: homozygous β-thalassaemia with production of more Hb F than usual or with mild defects in β-chain synthesis, by β-thalassaemia trait alone of unusual severity ('dominant' β-thalassaemia) or β-thalassaemia trait in association with mild globin abnormalities such as Hb Lepore. The coexistence of α-thalassaemia trait improves the haemoglobin level in homozygous β-thalassaemia by reducing the degree of chain imbalance and thus of α-chain precipitation and ineffective erythropoiesis. Conversely, patients with β-thalassaemia trait who also have excess (five or six) α genes tend to be more anaemic than usual. The patient with thalassaemia intermedia may show bone deformity, enlarged liver and spleen, extramedullary erythropoiesis (Fig. 6.16) and features of iron overload caused by increased iron absorption. Hb H disease (three-gene deletion α-thalassaemia) is a type of thalassaemia intermedia without iron overload or extramedullary haemopoiesis.

Table 6.5 Thalassaemia intermedia.

Homozygous β-thalassaemia
Homozygous mild β^+-thalassaemia
Coinheritance of α-thalassaemia
Enhanced ability to make fetal haemoglobin (γ-chain production)
Heterozygous β-thalassaemia
Coinheritance of additional α-globin genes (ααα/αα or ααα/ααα)
Dominant β-thalassaemia trait
δβ-Thalassaemia and hereditary persistence of fetal haemoglobin
Homozygous δβ-thalassaemia
Heterozygous δβ-thalassaemia/β-thalassaemia
Homozygous Hb Lepore (some cases)
Haemoglobin H disease

δβ-Thalassaemia

This involves failure of production of both β and δ chains. Fetal haemoglobin production is increased to 5–20% in the heterozygous state which resembles thalassaemia minor haematologically. In the homozygous state only Hb F is present and haematologically the picture is of thalassaemia intermedia.

Haemoglobin Lepore

This is an abnormal haemoglobin caused by unequal crossing-over of the β and δ genes to produce a polypeptide chain consisting of the δ chain at its amino end and β chain at its carboxyl end. The δβ-fusion chain is synthesized inefficiently and normal δ- and β-chain production is abolished. The homozygotes show thalassaemia intermedia and the heterozygotes thalassaemia trait.

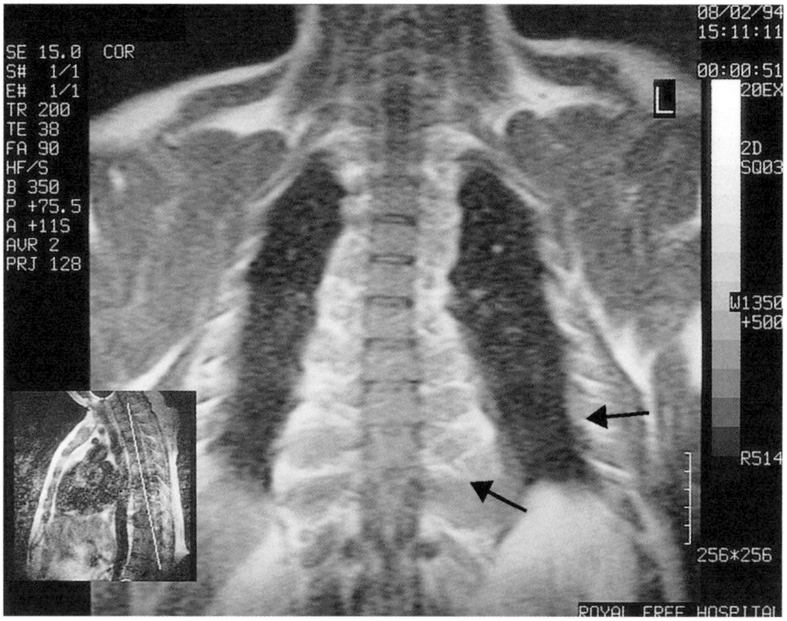

Fig. 6.16 β-Thalassaemia intermedia: MRI scan showing masses of extramedullary haemopoietic tissue arising from the ribs and in the paravertebral region without encroachment of the spinal cord.

Hereditary persistence of fetal haemoglobin

These are a heterogeneous group of genetic conditions caused by deletions or cross-overs affecting the production of β and γ chains or, in non-deletion forms, by point mutations upstream from the γ-globin genes.

Association of β-thalassaemia trait with other genetic disorders of haemoglobin

The combination of β-thalassaemia trait with Hb E trait usually causes a transfusion-dependent thalassaemia major syndrome, but some cases are intermediate. β-Thalassaemia trait with Hb S trait produces the clinical picture of sickle cell anaemia rather than of thalassaemia (p. 90). β-Thalassaemia trait with Hb D trait causes a hypochromic, microcytic anaemia of varying severity.

Sickle cell anaemia

Sickle cell disease is a group of haemoglobin disorders in which the sickle β-globin gene is inherited. Homozygous sickle cell anaemia (Hb SS) is the most common while the doubly heterozygote conditions of Hb SC and Hb Sβthal also cause sickling disease. Hb S (Hb $\alpha_2\beta_2^S$) is insoluble and forms crystals when exposed to low oxygen tension. Deoxygenated sickle haemoglobin polymerizes into long fibres, each consisting of seven intertwined double strands with cross-linking. The red cells sickle and may block different areas of the microcirculation or large vessels causing infarcts of various organs. The sickle β-globin abnormality is caused by substitution of valine for glutamic acid in position 6 in the β chain (Fig. 6.17). It is very widespread and is found in up to one in four West Africans, maintained at this level because of the protection against malaria that is afforded by the carrier state.

Normal β- chain	Amino acid	pro	glu	glu
	Base composition	CCT	GAG	GAG
Sickle β- chain	Base composition	CCT	GTG	GAG
	Amino acid	pro	val	glu

Fig. 6.17 Molecular pathology of sickle cell anaemia. There is a single base change in the DNA coding for the amino acid in the sixth position in the β-globin chain (adenine is replaced by thymine). This leads to an amino acid change from glutamic acid to valine. A, adenine; C, cytosine; G, guanine; glu, glutamic acid; pro, proline; T, thymine; val, valine.

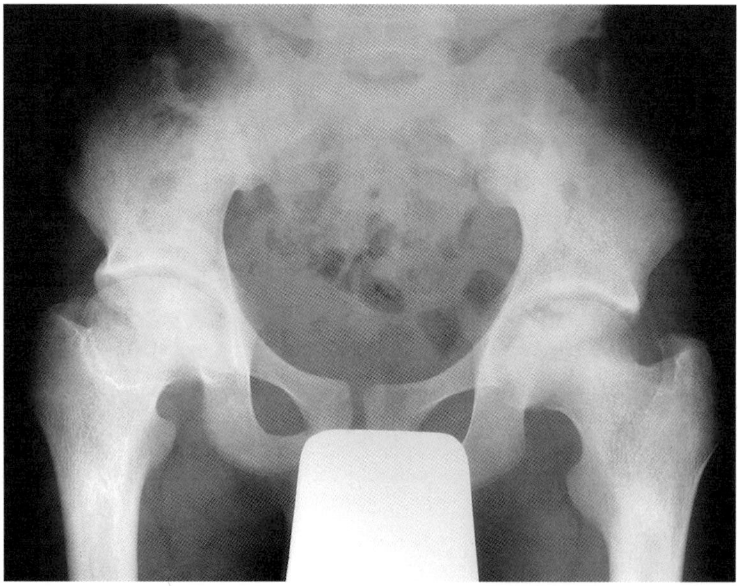

(a)

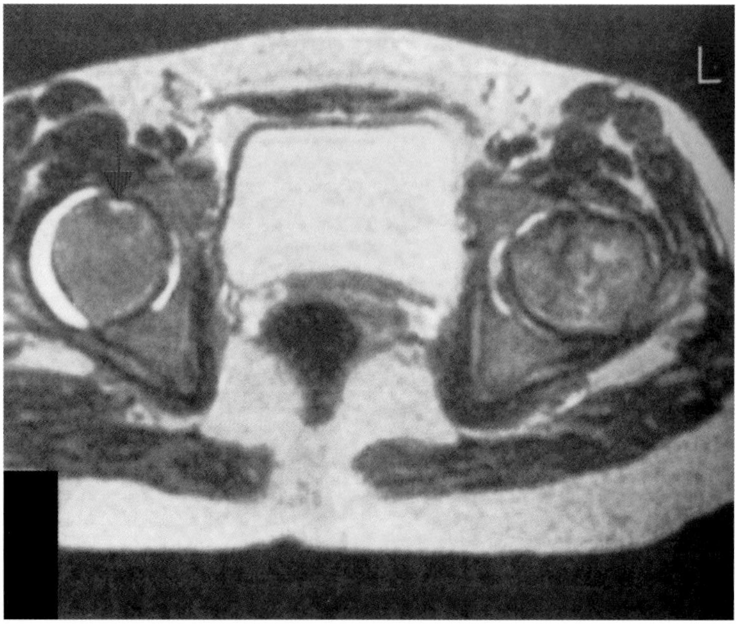

(b)

Fig. 6.18 Sickle cell anaemia. **(a)** Radiograph of the pelvis of a young man of West Indian origin which shows avascular necrosis with flattening of the femoral heads, more marked on the right, coarsening of the bone architecture and cystic areas in the right femoral neck caused by previous infarcts. **(b)** MRI scan of the hips of a 17-year-old female, showing a small area of high signal in the anterior portion of the right hip (arrowed) with a low intensity rim. This is typical of early avascular necrosis. The irregular outline and signal in the left hip results from more advanced avascular necrosis. Joint fluid is shown as a high signal (white rim) surrounding the femoral head. (Courtesy of Dr L. Berger)

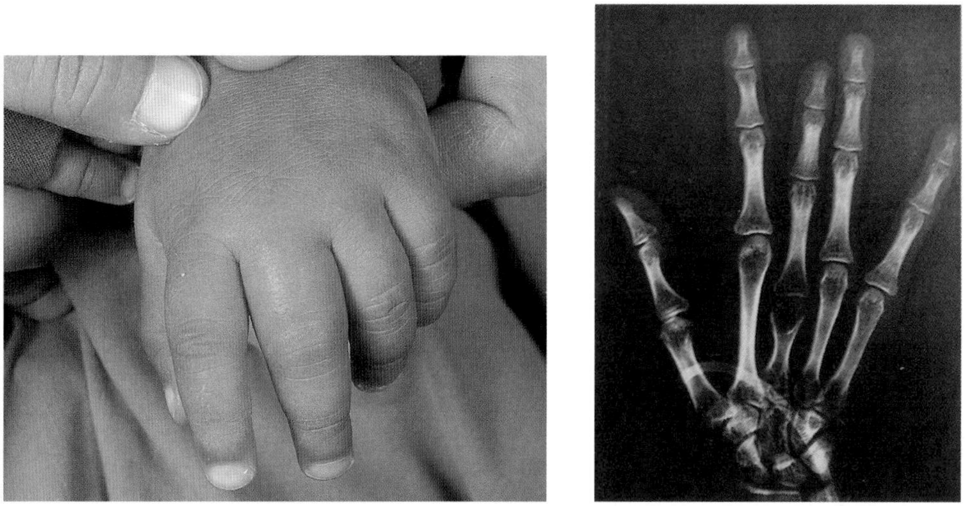

(a) (b)

Fig. 6.19 Sickle cell anaemia: **(a)** painful swollen fingers (dactylitis) in a child and **(b)** the hand of an 18-year-old Nigerian boy with the 'hand–foot' syndrome. There is marked shortening of the right middle finger because of dactylitis in childhood affecting the growth of the epiphysis.

Homozygous disease

Clinical features

Clinical features are of a severe haemolytic anaemia punctuated by crises. The symptoms of anaemia are often mild in relation to the severity of the anaemia because Hb S gives up oxygen (O_2) to tissues relatively easily compared with Hb A, its O_2 dissociation curve being shifted to the right (see Fig. 2.9). The clinical expression of Hb SS is very variable, some patients having an almost normal life, free of crises but others develop severe crises even as infants and may die in early childhood or as young adults. Crises may be vaso-occlusive, visceral, aplastic or haemolytic.

Painful vaso-occlusive crises

These are the most frequent and are precipitated by such factors as infection, acidosis, dehydration or deoxygenation (e.g. altitude, operations, obstetric delivery, stasis of the circulation, exposure to cold, violent exercise). Infarcts can occur in a variety of organs including the bones (hips, shoulders and vertebrae are commonly affected) (Fig. 6.18), the lungs and the spleen. The most serious vaso-occlusive crisis is of the brain (a stroke occurs in 7% of all patients) or spinal cord. Transcranial Doppler ultrasonography detects abnormal blood flow indicative of arterial stenosis. This predicts for strokes in children. This can be largely prevented by regular blood transfusions in these cases. The 'hand–foot' syndrome (painful dactylitis caused by infarcts of the small bones) is frequently the first presentation of the disease and may lead to digits of varying lengths (Fig. 6.19).

Visceral sequestration crises

These are caused by sickling within organs and pooling of blood, often with a severe exacerbation of anaemia. The acute sickle chest syndrome is a feared complication and the most common cause of death after puberty. It presents with dyspnoea, falling arterial Po_2, chest pain and pulmonary infiltrates on chest X-ray. Treatment is with analgesia, oxygen, exchange transfusion and ventilatory support if necessary. Hepatic and girdle sequestration crises and splenic sequestration may lead to severe illness requiring exchange transfusions. Splenic sequestration is typically seen in infants and presents with an enlarging spleen, falling haemoglobin and abdominal pain. Treatment is with transfusion and patients must be monitored at regular intervals as progression may be rapid. Attacks tend to be recurrent and splenectomy is often needed.

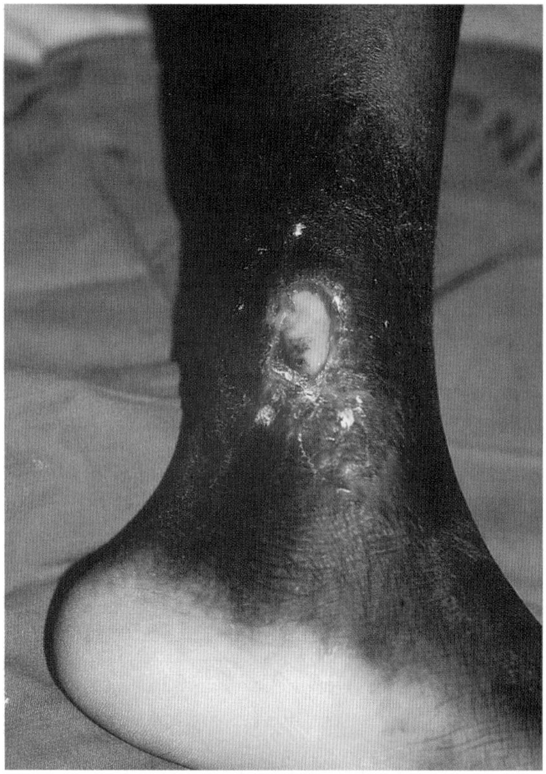

Fig. 6.20 Sickle cell anaemia: medial aspect of the ankle of a 15-year-old Nigerian boy showing necrosis and ulceration.

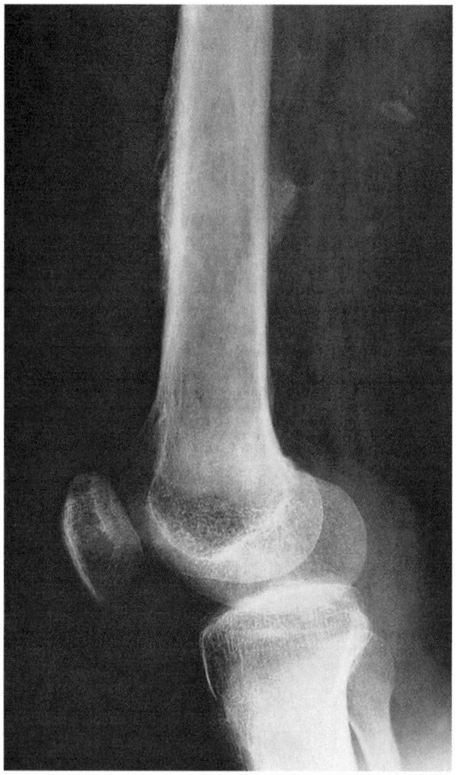

Fig. 6.21 *Salmonella* osteomyelitis: lateral radiograph of the lower femur and knee. The periosteum is irregularly raised in the lower third of the femur.

Aplastic crises

These occur as a result of infection with parvovirus or from folate deficiency and are characterized by a sudden fall in haemoglobin, usually requiring transfusion. They are characterized by a fall in reticulocytes as well as haemoglobin (see Fig. 20.4).

Haemolytic crises

These are characterized by an increased rate of haemolysis with a fall in haemoglobin but rise in reticulocytes and usually accompany a painful crisis.

Other clinical features

Ulcers of the lower legs are common, as a result of vascular stasis and local ischaemia (Fig. 6.20). The spleen is enlarged in infancy and early childhood but later is often reduced in size as a result of infarcts (autosplenectomy). Pulmonary hypertension detected by Doppler echocardiography and an increased tricuspid regurgitant velocity are common and increases the risk of death. A proliferative retinopathy and priapism are other clinical complications. Chronic damage to the liver may occur through microinfarcts. Pigment (bilirubin) gallstones are frequent. The kidneys are vulnerable to infarctions of the medulla with papillary necrosis. Failure to concentrate urine aggravates the tendency to dehydration and crisis, and nocturnal enuresis is common. Osteomyelitis may also occur, usually from *Salmonella* spp. (Fig. 6.21).

Laboratory findings

1 The haemoglobin is usually 6–9 g/dL—low in comparison to symptoms of anaemia.

2 Sickle cells and target cells occur in the blood (Fig. 6.22). Features of splenic atrophy (e.g. Howell–Jolly bodies) may also be present.

3 Screening tests for sickling are positive when the

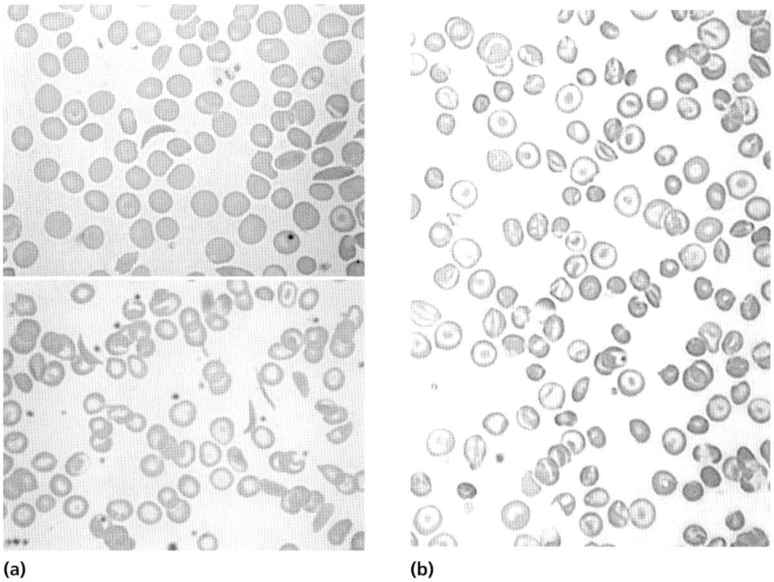

Fig. 6.22 **(a)** Sickle cell anaemia: peripheral blood film showing deeply staining sickle cells, target cells and polychromasia. **(b)** Homozygous Hb C disease: peripheral blood film showing many target cells, deeply staining rhomboidal and spherocytic cells.

blood is deoxygenated (e.g. with dithionate and Na_2HPO_4).

4 Haemoglobin electrophoresis (Fig. 6.14): in Hb SS, no Hb A is detected. The amount of Hb F is variable and is usually 5–15%, larger amounts are normally associated with a milder disorder.

Treatment

1 Prophylactic—avoid those factors known to precipitate crises, especially dehydration, anoxia, infections, stasis of the circulation and cooling of the skin surface.

2 Folic acid (e.g. 5 mg once weekly).

3 Good general nutrition and hygiene.

4 Pneumococcal, *Haemophilus* and meningococcal vaccination and regular oral penicillin are effective at reducing the infection rate with these organisms and should be strongly encouraged. Oral penicillin should start at diagnosis and continue at least until puberty. Hepatitis B vaccination is also given as transfusions may be needed.

5 Crises—treat by rest, warmth, rehydration by oral fluids and/or intravenous normal saline (3 L in 24 h) and antibiotics if infection is present. Analgesia at the appropriate level should be given. Suitable drugs are paracetamol, a non-steroidal anti-inflammatory agent and opiates (e.g. continuous subcutaneous diamorphine). Blood transfusion is given only if there is very severe anaemia with symptoms. Exchange transfusion may be needed particularly if there is neurological damage, a visceral sequestration crisis or repeated painful crises. This is aimed at achieving an Hb S percentage of less than 30 in severe cases and after a stroke is continued for at least 2 years.

6 Particular care is needed in pregnancy and anaesthesia. There is debate as to whether or not patients need transfusions with normal blood to reduce Hb S levels during pregnancy or before delivery or for minor operations. Careful anaesthetic and recovery techniques must be used to avoid hypoxaemia or acidosis. Routine transfusions throughout pregnancy are given to those with a poor obstetric history or a history of frequent crises.

7 Transfusions—these are also sometimes given repeatedly as prophylaxis to patients having frequent crises or who have had major organ damage (e.g. of the brain) or show abnormal transcranial Doppler studies. The aim is to suppress Hb S production over a period of several months or even years. Iron overload, which may need iron chelation therapy, and alloimmunization against donated blood are common problems.

8 Hydroxyurea (15.0–20.0 mg/kg) can increase Hb F levels and has been shown to improve the clinical course of children or adults who are having three or more painful crises each year. It should not be used during pregnancy.

9 Stem cell transplantation can cure the disease and many patients have now been successfully treated. The mortality rate is less than 10%. Transplantation is only indicated in the severest of cases whose quality of life or life expectancy are substantially impaired.

10 Research into other drugs (e.g. butyrates) to enhance Hb F synthesis or to increase the solubility of Hb S is taking place. 'Gene therapy' is a distant prospect not yet available (Chapter 21).

Sickle cell trait

This is a benign condition with no anaemia and normal appearance of red cells on a blood film. Haematuria is the most common symptom and is thought to be caused by minor infarcts of the renal papillae. Hb S varies from 25 to 45% of the total haemoglobin (Fig. 6.14a). Care must be taken with anaesthesia, pregnancy and at high altitudes.

Combination of haemoglobin S with other genetic defects of haemoglobin

The most common of these are Hb S/β-thalassaemia, and sickle cell/C disease. In Hb S/β-thalassaemia, the MCV and MCH are lower than in homozygous Hb SS. The clinical picture is of sickle cell anaemia; splenomegaly is usual. Patients with Hb SC disease have a particular tendency to thrombosis and pulmonary embolism, especially in pregnancy. In general, when compared with Hb SS disease, they have a higher incidence of retinal abnormalities, milder anaemia, splenomegaly and generally a longer life expectancy. Diagnosis is made by haemoglobin electrophoresis, particularly with family studies.

Haemoglobin C disease

This genetic defect of haemoglobin is frequent in West Africa and is caused by substitution of lysine for glutamic acid in the β-globin chain at the same point as the substitution in Hb S. Hb C tends to form rhomboidal crystals and in the homozygous state there is a mild haemolytic anaemia with marked target cell formation, cells with rhomboidal shape and microspherocytes (Fig. 6.22b). The spleen is enlarged. The carriers show a few target cells only.

Haemoglobin D disease

This is a group of variants all with the same electrophoretic mobility. Heterozygotes show no haematological abnormality while homozygotes have a mild haemolytic anaemia.

Haemoglobin E disease

This is the most common haemoglobin variant in South-East Asia. In the homozygous state, there is a mild microcytic, hypochromic anaemia. Haemoglobin E/β^0-thalassaemia, however, resembles homozygous β^0-thalassaemia both clinically and haematologically.

Prenatal diagnosis of genetic haemoglobin disorders

It is important to give genetic counselling to couples at risk of having a child with a major haemoglobin defect. If a pregnant woman is found to have a haemoglobin abnormality, her partner should be

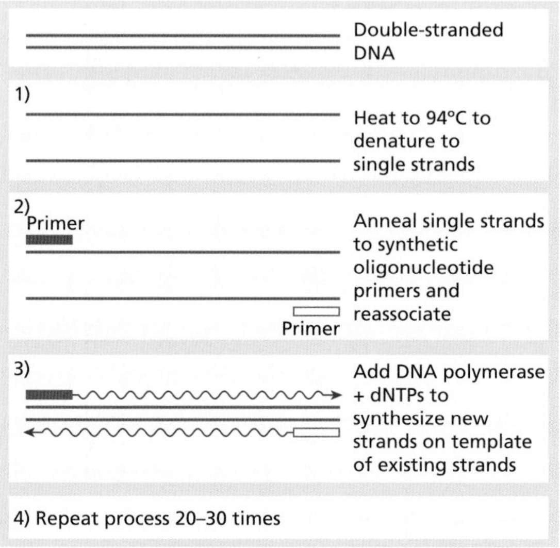

Fig. 6.23 Polymerase chain reaction. The primers hybridize to DNA on either side of the piece of DNA to be analysed. Repeated cycles of denaturation, association with the primers, incubation with a DNA polymerase and deoxyribonucleotides (dNTPs) results in amplification of the DNA over a million times within a few hours.

tested to determine whether he also carries a defect. When both partners show an abnormality and there is a risk of a serious defect in the offspring, particularly β-thalassaemia major, it is important to offer antenatal diagnosis. Several techniques are available, the choice depending on the stage of pregnancy and the potential nature of the defect.

DNA diagnosis

The majority of samples are obtained by chorionic villus biopsy although amniotic fluid cells are sometimes used. Techniques to sample maternal blood for fetal cells or fetal DNA are being developed. The DNA is then analysed using one of the following methods.

Polymerase chain reaction (PCR) is the most commonly used technique (Fig. 6.23) and may be performed by using primer pairs that only amplify individual alleles ('allele-specific priming') (Fig. 6.24) or by using consensus primers that amplify all the alleles followed by restriction digestion to detect a particular allele. This is best illustrated by Hb S in which the enzyme DdeI detects the A-T change (Fig. 6.25).

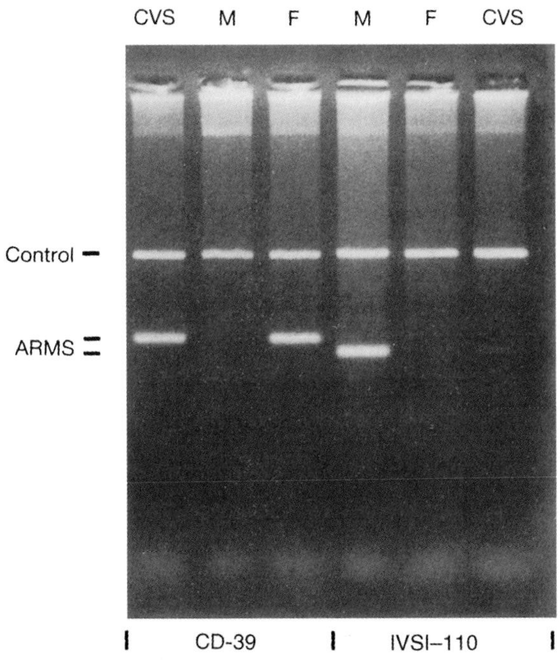

Fig. 6.24 The rapid prenatal diagnosis of β-thalassaemia by amplification refractory mutation system (ARMS). The father has the common Mediterranean codon 39 (CD39) mutation, the mother the IVS1–110 G → A mutation. The fetus is heterozygous for the CD39 mutation. CVS, fetal DNA from chorionic villus sampling; F, father; M, mother. (Courtesy of Dr J. Old and Professor D.J. Weatherall)

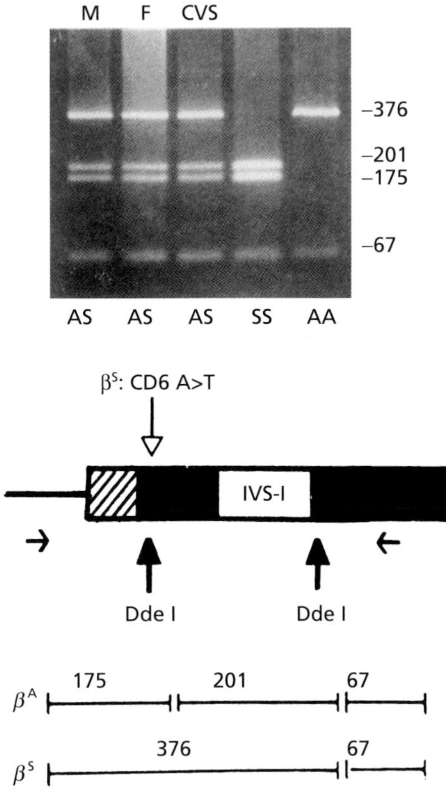

Fig. 6.25 Sickle cell anaemia: antenatal diagnosis by DdeI-PCR analysis. The DNA is amplified by two primers that span the sickle cell gene mutation site and produces a product of 473 base pairs (bp) in size. The product is digested with the restriction enzyme DdeI and the resulting fragments analysed by agarose gel electrophoresis. The replacement of an adenine base in the normal β-globin gene by thymine results in Hb S and removes a normal restriction site for DdeI, producing a larger 376 bp fragment than the normal 175 and 201 bp fragments in the digested amplified product. In this case, the CVS DNA shows both the normal fragments and the larger sickle cell product and so is AS. The gel shows DNA from the mother (M), father (F), fetal DNA from a chorionic villus sample (CVS), a normal DNA control (AA) and a homozygous sickle cell DNA control (SS). (Courtesy of Dr. J. Old)

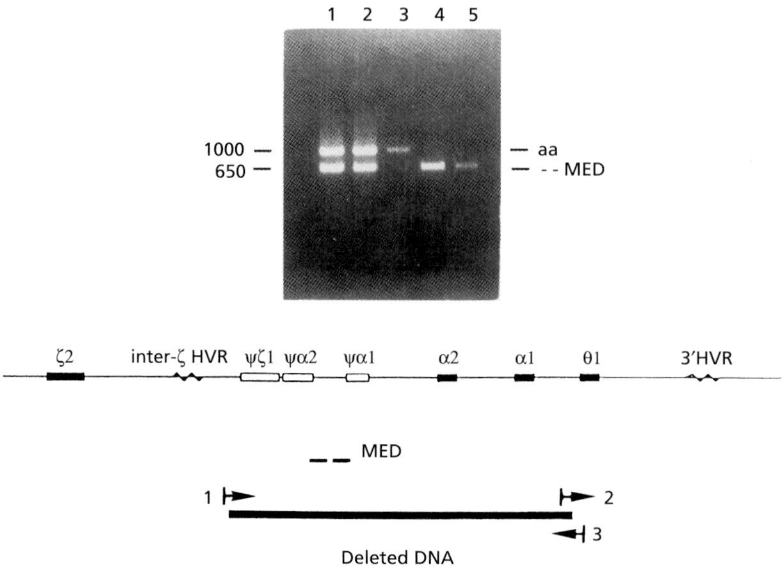

Fig. 6.26 α^0-Thalassaemia: antenatal diagnosis by gap-PCR analysis. The common α^0-thalassaemia deletion mutations are diagnosed using primers which bind to flanking sequences on either side of the deletion breakpoint. For the $-^{MED}$ deletion, the primer pair (1 & 2) produce an amplified product of 650 base pairs (bp) in size. The primers are too far apart to amplify the normal DNA sequence, so a third primer (3) is included that is complementary to the deleted sequence near one of the breakpoints. This produces a normal fragment of 1000 bp. The gel electrophoresis photograph shows the mother's DNA (lane 1, heterozygous), father's DNA (lane 2, heterozygous), CVS DNA (lane 3, normal) and two homozygous control DNAs (lanes 4 & 5). (Courtesy of Dr. J. Old)

Gap-PCR analysis is useful for detecting gene deletions in α-thalassaemia (Fig. 6.26), for δβ-thalassaemia, and Hb Lepore. Small deletions and point mutations are diagnosed by cycle-sequencing of PCR product using fluorescent labels and analysis of the fragments on a capillary-based automatic sequencer. This approach is useful for rare and unknown mutations, for confirming prenatal diagnosis of β-thalassaemia and sickle cell disorders by other PCR methods, and for the rare non-deletion α^+-thalassaemia mutations that result in severe Hb H hydrops fetalis syndrome.

Pre-implantation genetic diagnosis which avoids the need for pregnancy termination involves performing conventional *in vitro* fertilization, followed by removing one or two cells from the blastomeres on day 3. PCR is used to detect thalassaemia mutations so that unaffected blastomeres can be selected for implantation. HLA typing can also be used to select an HLA matching blastomere matching a previous thalassaemia major child. Ethical considerations are important in deciding to use these applications.

Fetal blood sampling

Fetal blood sampling may be performed in mid-second trimester and allows DNA study and protein synthesis studies.

Bibliography

Adams R.J., Brambilla D., Optimizing Primary Stroke Prevention in Sickle Cell Anemia (STOP 2) Trial Investigators (2005) Discontinuing prophylactic transfusions used to prevent stroke in sickle cell disease. *N Engl J Med* **353**,2769–78.

Ahmed S., Saleem M., Modell B., Petrou M. (2002) Screening extended families for genetic hemoglobin disorders in Pakistan. *N Engl J Med* **347**,1162–8.

Anderson L.J., Holden S., Davis B. *et al.* (2001) Cardiovascular T2-star (T2*) magnetic resonance for the early diagnosis of myocardial iron overload. *Eur Heart J* **22**,2171–9.

Bain B.J. (2005) *Haemoglobinopathy Diagnosis*, 2nd edn. Blackwell Publishing, Oxford.

Borgna-Pignatti C., Cappellini M.D., De Stefano P. *et al.* (2006) Cardiac morbidity and mortality in deferoxaine- or deferiprone-treated patients with thalassemia major. *Blood* **107**,3733–7.

Borgna-Pignatti C., Rugolotto S., De Stefano P. *et al.* (2004) Survival and complications in patients with thalassemia major treated with transfusion and deferoxamine. *Haematologica* **89**,1187–93.

Gladwin M.T., Sachdev V., Jison M.L. *et al.* (2004) Pulmonary hypertension as a risk factor for death in patients with sickle cell disease. *N Engl J Med* **350**,886–95.

Hankins J.S., Ware R.E., Rogers Z.R. *et al.* (2005) Long-term hydroxyurea therapy for infants with sickle cell anemia: the HUSOFT extension study. *Blood* **106**,2269–75.

Hoffbrand A.V. (2005) Deferiprone therapy for transfusional iron overload. *Best Pract Res Clin Haematol* **18**,299–317.

Kattamis A., Papassotiriai I., Palaiologu D. *et al.* (2006) The effects of erythropoiedic activity and iron burden on hepcidin expression in patients with thalassemia major. *Haematologica* **91**,809–12.

Origa R., Bina P., Agus A. *et al.* (2005) Combined therapy with deferiprone and desferrioxamine in thalassemia major. *Haematologica* **90**,1309–14.

Papanikolaou G., Tzilianos M., Christakis J.I. *et al.* (2005) Hepcidin in iron overload disorders. *Blood* **105**,4103–5.

Pennell D.J., Berdoukas V., Karagiorga M. *et al.* (2006) Randomized controlled trial of deferiprone or deferoxamine in β-thalassemia major patients with asymptomatic myocardial siderosis. *Blood* **107**,3738–44.

Rund D. and Rachmilewitz E. (2005) Beta-thalassemia. *N Engl J Med* **353**,1135–46.

Steinberg M.H., Barton F., Castro O. *et al.* (2003) Effect of hydroxyurea on mortality and morbidity in adult sickle cell anemia: risks and benefits up to 9 years of treatment. *JAMA* **289**,1645–51. Erratum in *JAMA* **290**,756.

Thein S.L. (2004) Genetic insights into the clinical diversity of beta thalassaemia. *Br J Haematol* **124**,264–74.

Weatherall D.J. and Clegg J.B. (2001) *The Thalassaemia Syndromes*, 4th edn. Blackwell Science, Oxford.

CHAPTER 7

7 The white cells 1: granulocytes, monocytes and their benign disorders

The white blood cells (leucocytes) may be divided into two broad groups: the phagocytes and the immunocytes. Granulocytes, which include three types of cell—neutrophils (polymorphs), eosinophils and basophils—together with monocytes comprise the phagocytes. Their normal development and function, and benign disorders of white blood cells, are dealt with in this chapter. Only mature phagocytic cells and lymphocytes are found in normal peripheral blood (Table 7.1; Fig. 7.1). The lymphocytes, their precursor cells and plasma cells, which make up the immunocyte population, are considered in Chapter 8.

The function of phagocytes and immunocytes in protecting the body against infection is closely connected with two soluble protein systems of the body: immunoglobulins and complement. These proteins, which may also be involved in blood cell destruction in a number of diseases, are discussed together with the lymphocytes in Chapter 8.

Granulocytes

Neutrophil (polymorph)

This cell has a characteristic dense nucleus consisting of between two and five lobes, and a pale

Table 7.1 White cells: normal blood counts.

Adults	Blood count	Children	Blood count
Total leucocytes	$4.00–11.0 \times 10^9/L$*	*Total leucocytes*	
Neutrophils	$2.5–7.5 \times 10^9/L$*	Neonates	$10.0–25.0 \times 10^9/L$
Eosinophils	$0.04–0.4 \times 10^9/L$	1 year	$6.0–18.0 \times 10^9/L$
Monocytes	$0.2–0.8 \times 10^9/L$	4–7 years	$6.0–15.0 \times 10^9/L$
Basophils	$0.01–0.1 \times 10^9/L$	8–12 years	$4.5–13.5 \times 10^9/L$
Lymphocytes	$1.5–3.5 \times 10^9/L$		

* Normal black and Middle Eastern subjects may have lower counts. In normal pregnancy the upper limits are: total leucocytes $14.5 \times 10^9/L$, neutrophils $11 \times 10^9/L$.

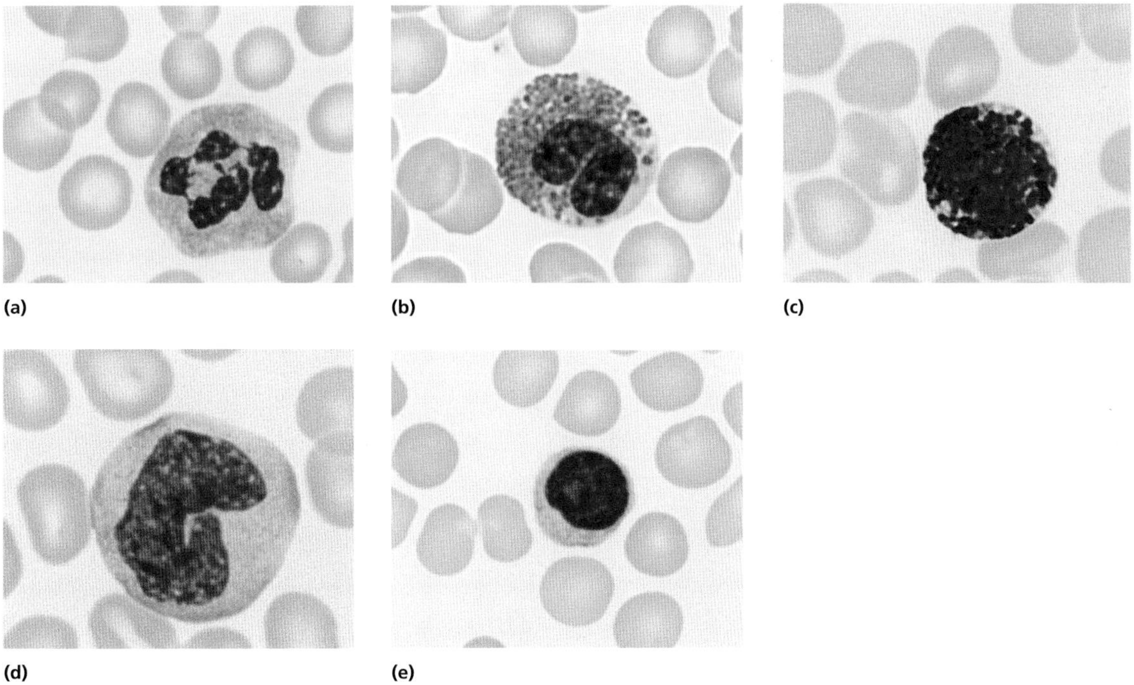

Fig. 7.1 White blood cells (leucocytes): **(a)** neutrophil (polymorph); **(b)** eosinophil; **(c)** basophil; **(d)** monocyte; **(e)** lymphocyte.

cytoplasm with an irregular outline containing many fine pink–blue (azurophilic) or grey–blue granules (Fig. 7.1a). The granules are divided into primary, which appear at the promyelocyte stage, and secondary (specific) which appear at the myelocyte stage and predominate in the mature neutrophil. Both types of granule are lysosomal in origin: the primary contains myeloperoxidase, acid phosphatase and other acid hydrolases; the secondary contains collagenase, lactoferrin and lysozyme (see Fig. 7.7). The lifespan of neutrophils in the blood is only 6–10 h.

Neutrophil precursors

These do not normally appear in normal peripheral blood but are present in the marrow (Fig. 7.2). The earliest recognizable precursor is the myeloblast, a cell of variable size which has a large nucleus with fine chromatin and usually two to five nucleoli. The cytoplasm is basophilic and no cytoplasmic granules are present. The normal bone marrow contains up to 4% of myeloblasts. Myeloblasts give rise by cell division to promyelocytes which are slightly larger cells and have developed primary granules in the cytoplasm. These cells then produce myelocytes which have specific or secondary granules. The nuclear chromatin is now more condensed and nucleoli are not visible. Separate myelocytes of the neutrophil, eosinophil and basophil series can be indentified. The myelocytes give rise by cell division to metamyelocytes, non-dividing cells, which have an indented or horseshoe-shaped nucleus and a cytoplasm filled with primary and secondary granules. Neutrophil forms between the metamyelocyte and fully mature neutrophil are termed 'band', 'stab' or 'juvenile'. These cells may occur in normal peripheral blood. They do not contain the clear, fine filamentous distinction between nuclear lobes that is seen in mature neutrophils.

Monocytes

These are usually larger than other peripheral blood leucocytes and possess a large central oval or indented nucleus with clumped chromatin (Fig. 7.1d). The

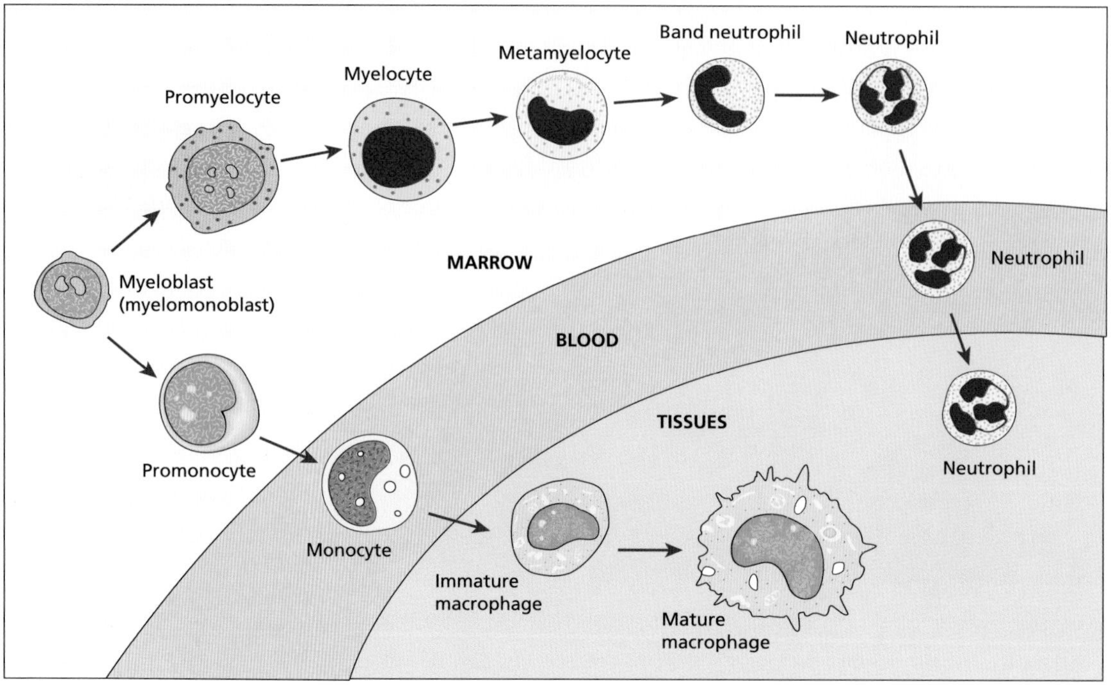

Fig. 7.2 The formation of the neutrophil and monocyte phagocytes. Eosinophils and basophils are also formed in the marrow in a process similar to that for neutrophils.

abundant cytoplasm stains blue and contains many fine vacuoles, giving a ground-glass appearance. Cytoplasmic granules are also often present. The monocyte precursors in the marrow (monoblasts and promonocytes) are difficult to distinguish from myeloblasts and monocytes.

Eosinophils

These cells are similar to neutrophils, except that the cytoplasmic granules are coarser and more deeply red staining and there are rarely more than three nuclear lobes (Fig. 7.1b). Eosinophil myelocytes can be recognized but earlier stages are indistinguishable from neutrophil precursors. The blood transit time for eosinophils is longer than for neutrophils. They enter inflammatory exudates and have a special role in allergic responses, defence against parasites and removal of fibrin formed during inflammation.

Basophils

These are only occasionally seen in normal peripheral blood. They have many dark cytoplasmic granules which overlie the nucleus and contain heparin and histamine (Fig. 7.1c). In the tissues they become mast cells. They have immunoglobulin E (IgE) attachment sites and their degranulation is associated with histamine release.

Granulopoiesis

The blood granulocytes and monocytes are formed in the bone marrow from a common precursor cell (see Fig. 1.2). In the granulopoietic series progenitor cells, myeloblasts, promyelocytes and myelocytes form a proliferative or mitotic pool of cells while the metamyelocytes, band and segmented granulocytes make up a post-mitotic maturation compartment (Fig. 7.3). Large numbers of band and segmented neutrophils are held in the marrow as a 'reserve pool' or storage compartment. The bone marrow normally contains more myeloid cells than erythroid cells in the ratio of 2 : 1 to 12 : 1, the largest proportion being neutrophils and metamyelocytes. In the stable or normal state, the bone marrow

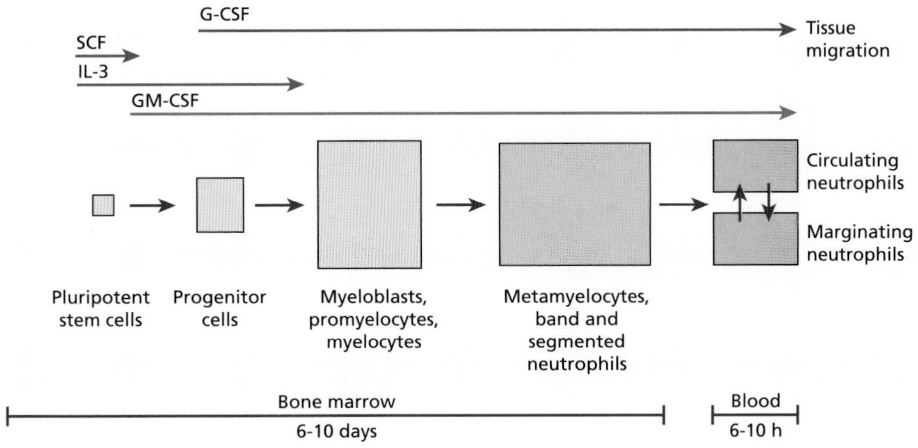

Fig. 7.3 Neutrophil kinetics. CSF, colony-stimulating factor; G, granulocyte; IL, interleukin; M, monocyte; SCF, stem cell factor.

storage compartment contains 10–15 times the number of granulocytes found in the peripheral blood. Following their release from the bone marrow, granulocytes spend only 6–10 h in the circulation before moving into the tissues where they perform their phagocytic function. In the bloodstream there are two pools usually of about equal size: the circulating pool (included in the blood count) and the marginating pool (not included in the blood count). It has been estimated that they spend on average 4–5 days in the tissues before they are destroyed during defensive action or as the result of senescence.

Control of granulopoiesis: myeloid growth factors

The granulocyte series arises from bone marrow progenitor cells which are increasingly specialized. Many growth factors are involved in this maturation process including interleukin-1 (IL-1), IL-3, IL-5 (for eosinophils), IL-6, IL-11, granulocyte–macrophage colony-stimulating factor (GM-CSF), granulocyte CSF (G-CSF) and monocyte CSF (M-CSF) (see Fig. 1.7). The growth factors stimulate proliferation and differentiation and also affect the function of the mature cells on which they act (e.g. phagocytosis, superoxide generation and cytotoxicity in the case of neutrophils; phagocytosis, cytotoxicity and production of other cytokines by monocytes).

Increased granulocyte and monocyte production in response to an infection is induced by increased production of growth factors from stromal cells and T lymphocytes, stimulated by endotoxin, IL-1 or tumour necrosis factor (TNF) (Fig. 7.4).

Clinical applications of myeloid growth factors

Clinical administration of G-CSF intravenously or subcutaneously has been found to produce a rise in neutrophils whereas administration of GM-CSF increases neutrophils, eosinophils and monocytes. G-CSF has become widely used in clinical practice and some of the indications are as follows. Short-acting G-CSF is given daily. There is also a longer acting pegolated (PEG) G-CSF which can be given once weekly.

Post-chemotherapy, radiotherapy or bone marrow transplantation In these situations, G-CSF accelerates haemopoietic recovery and shortens the period of neutropenia (Fig. 7.5). This may translate into a reduction of length of time in hospital, antibiotic usage and frequency of infection but periods of extreme neutropenia after intensive chemotherapy cannot be prevented.

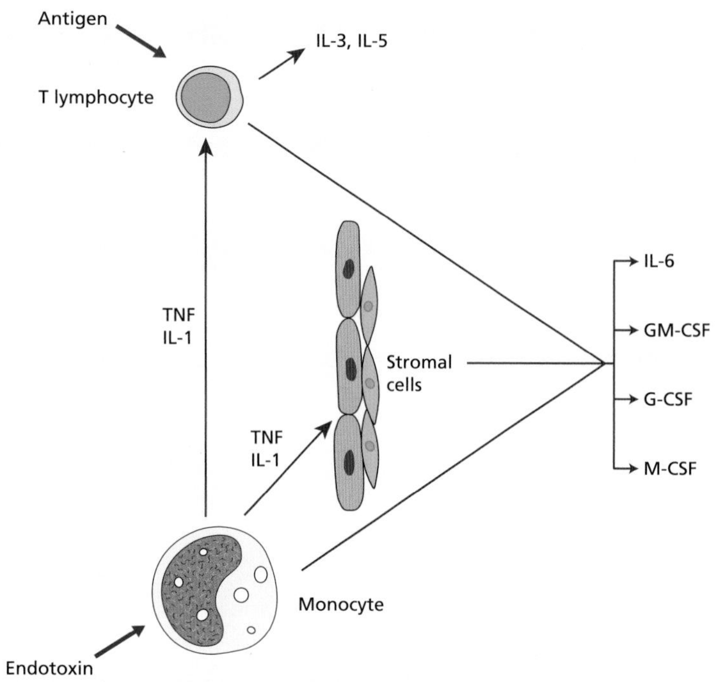

Fig. 7.4 Regulation of haemopoiesis; pathways of stimulation of leucopoiesis by endotoxin, for example from infection. It is likely that endothelial and fibroblast cells release basal quantities of granulocyte–macrophage colony-stimulating factor (GM-CSF) and granulocyte colony-stimulating factor (G-CSF) in the normal resting state and that this is enhanced substantially by the monokine's tumour necrosis factor (TNF) and interleukin-1 (IL-1).

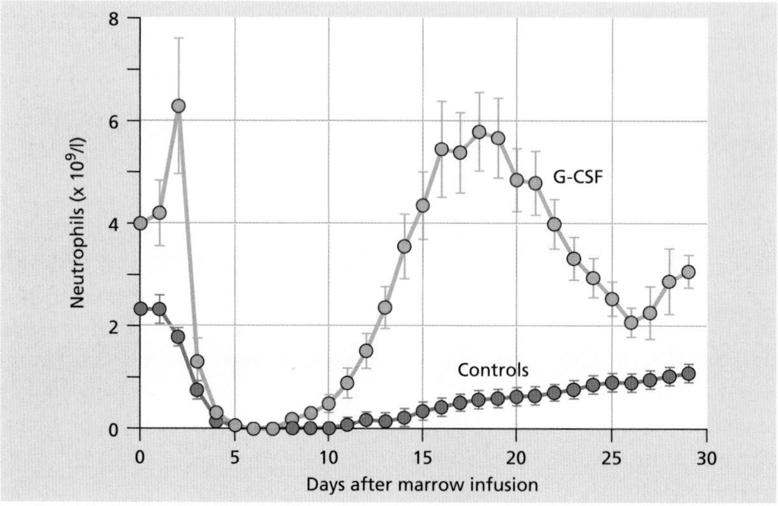

Fig. 7.5 Typical effect of granulocyte colony-stimulating factor (G-CSF) on recovery of neutrophils following autologous bone marrow transplantation.

Acute myeloid leukaemia G-CSF may be used after induction and consolidation chemotherapy to reduce hospital stay and antibiotic usage. In some protocols it is given with initial induction chemotherapy to mobilize blast cells into cell cycle, enhancing their sensitivity to chemotherapy.

Acute lymphoblastic leukaemia G-CSF is indicated to reduce the severity of neutropenia after intensive phases of therapy.

Myelodysplasia G-CSF has been given alone or in conjunction with erythropoietin in an attempt to improve bone marrow function without accelerating leukaemic transformation. It is also used after intensive chemotherapy.

Severe neutropenia Both congenital and acquired neutropenia, including cyclical and drug-induced neutropenia, have been found to respond well to G-CSF.

Severe infection G-CSF has been used as an adjuvant to antimicrobial therapy.

Peripheral blood stem cell transplants G-CSF is used to increase the number of circulating multipotent progenitors, improving the harvest of sufficient peripheral blood stem cells for transplantation. It is also used to accelerate reconstitution after allogeneic or autologous transplantation.

Lymphomas G-CSF is given to reduce infection, delay in giving chemotherapy and hospitalization after chemotherapy. A single injection of pegolated G-CSF immediately after chemotherapy is often used.

Monocytes

Monocytes spend only a short time in the marrow and, after circulating for 20–40 h, leave the blood to enter the tissues where they mature and carry out their principal functions. Their extravascular lifespan after their transformation to macrophages may be as long as several months or even years. They may assume specific functions in different tissues (e.g. skin, gut, liver) (Fig. 7.6). One particularly important lineage is that of dendritic cells which are involved in antigen presentation to T cells (Chapter 8). GM-CSF and M-CSF are involved in their production and activation.

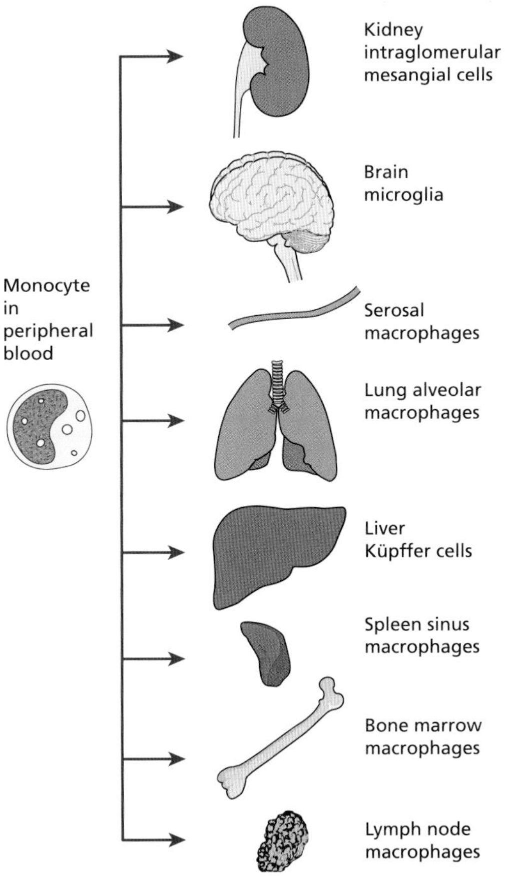

Fig. 7.6 Reticuloendothelial system: distribution of macrophages.

Disorders of neutrophil and monocyte function

The normal function of neutrophils and monocytes may be divided into three phases.

Chemotaxis (cell mobilization and migration) The phagocyte is attracted to bacteria or the site of inflammation by chemotactic substances released from damaged tissues or by complement components and also by the interaction of leucocyte adhesion molecules with ligands on the damaged tissues. The leucocyte adhesion molecules also mediate recruitment, migration and interaction with other immune cells. They are also variously expressed on endothelial cells and platelets (Chapter 1).

Phagocytosis The foreign material (e.g. bacteria, fungi) or dead or damaged cells of the host are phagocytosed (Fig. 7.7). Recognition of a foreign particle is aided by opsonization with immunoglobulin or complement because both neutrophils and monocytes have Fc and C3b receptors. Opsonization of normal body cells (e.g. red cells or platelets) also makes them liable to destruction

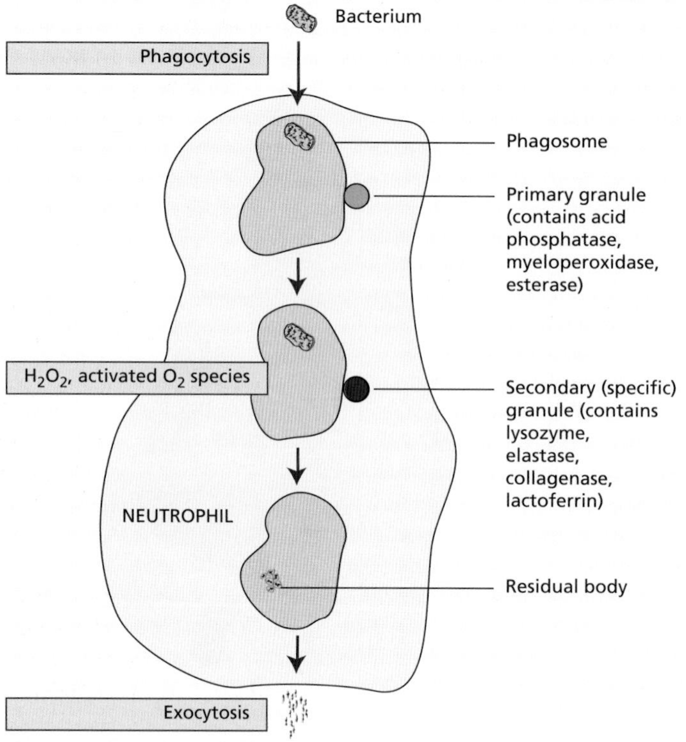

Fig. 7.7 Phagocytosis and bacterial destruction. On entering the neutrophil, the bacterium is surrounded by an invaginated surface membrane and fuses with a primary lysosome to form a phagosome. Enzymes from the lysosome attack the bacterium. Secondary granules also fuse with the phagosomes, and new enzymes from these granules including lactoferrin attack the organism. Various types of activated oxygen, generated by glucose metabolism, also help to kill bacteria. Undigested residual bacterial products are excreted by exocytosis.

by macrophages of the reticuloendothelial system, as in autoimmune haemolysis, idiopathic (autoimmune) thrombocytopenic purpura or many of the drug-induced cytopenias.

Macrophages have a central role in antigen presentation: processing and presenting foreign antigens on human leucocyte antigen (HLA) molecules to the immune system. They also secrete a large number of growth factors and chemokines which regulate inflammation and immune responses.

Chemokines are chemotactic cytokines of which there are two main classes: CXC (α) chemokines, small (8–10 000 MW) pro-inflammatory cytokines which mainly act on neutrophils, and CC (β) chemokines such as macrophage inflammatory protein-1α (MIP-1α) and RANTES which act on monocytes, basophils, eosinophils and natural killer (NK) cells. Chemokines may be produced constitutively and control lymphocyte traffic under physiological conditions; inflammatory chemokines are induced or up-regulated by inflammatory stimuli. They bind to and activate cells via chemokine receptors and play an important part in recruiting appropriate cells to the sites of inflammation. Chemokine receptors have been identified as co-receptors for human immunodeficiency virus (HIV) entry into cells.

Killing and digestion This occurs by oxygen-dependent and oxygen-independent pathways. In the oxygen-dependent reactions, superoxide (O_2^-), hydrogen peroxide (H_2O_2) and other activated oxygen (O_2) species, are generated from O_2 and reduced nicotinamide adenine dinucleotide phosphate (NADPH). In neutrophils, H_2O_2 reacts with myeloperoxidase and intracellular halide to kill bacteria; activated oxygen may also be involved. The non-oxidative microbicidal mechanisms involve microbicidal proteins. These may act alone (e.g. cathepsin G) or in conjunction with H_2O_2 (e.g. lysozyme, elastase). They may also act with a fall in pH within phagocytic vacuoles into which lysosomal enzymes are released. An additional factor, lactoferrin—an iron-binding protein present in neutrophil granules—is bacteriostatic by depriving bacteria of iron and generating free radicals (Fig. 7.7). Finally, nitric oxide (NO) generated through NO synthase from L-arginine is another mechanism by which phagocytes kill microbes.

Defects of phagocytic cell function

Chemotaxis These defects occur in rare congenital abnormalities (e.g. 'lazy leucocyte' syndrome) and in more common acquired abnormalities either of the environment (e.g. corticosteroid therapy) or of the leucocytes themselves (e.g. in acute or chronic myeloid leukaemia, myelodysplasia and the myeloproliferative syndromes).

Phagocytosis These defects usually arise because of a lack of opsonization which may be caused by congenital or acquired causes of hypogammaglobulinaemia or lack of complement components.

Killing This abnormality is clearly illustrated by the rare X-linked or autosomal recessive chronic granulomatous disease that results from abnormal leucocyte oxidative metabolism. There is an abnormality affecting different elements of the respiratory burst oxidase or its activating mechanism. The patients have recurring infections, usually bacterial but sometimes fungal, which present in infancy or early childhood in most cases.

Other rare congenital abnormalities may also result in defects of bacterial killing (e.g. myeloperoxidase deficiency and the Chédiak–Higashi syndrome; see below). Acute or chronic myeloid leukaemia and myelodysplastic syndromes may also be associated with defective killing of ingested microorganisms.

Benign disorders

A number of the hereditary conditions may give rise to changes in granulocyte morphology.

Pelger–Huët anomaly In this uncommon condition bilobed neutrophils are found in the peripheral blood. Occasional unsegmented neutrophils are also seen. Inheritance is autosomal dominant.

May–Hegglin anomaly In this rare condition the neutrophils contain basophilic inclusions of RNA (resembling Döhle bodies) in the cytoplasm. There is an associated mild thrombocytopenia with giant platelets. Inheritance is autosomal dominant.

Other rare disorders In contrast to these two relatively benign anomalies, other rare congenital leucocyte disorders may be associated with severe disease. The Chédiak–Higashi syndrome is inherited in an autosomal recessive manner, and there are giant granules in the neutrophils, eosinophils, monocytes and lymphocytes accompanied by neutropenia, thrombocytopenia and marked hepatosplenomegaly. Abnormal leucocyte granulation or vacuolation is also seen in patients with rare mucopolysaccharide disorders (e.g. Hurler's syndrome).

Common morphological abnormalities Figure 7.8 shows some of the more common abnormalities of neutrophil morphology that can be seen in peripheral blood. Hypersegmented forms occur in megaloblastic anaemia, Döhle bodies and toxic changes in infection. The 'drumstick' appears on the nucleus of a proportion of the neutrophils in normal females and is caused by the presence of two X chromosomes. Pelger cells are seen in the benign congenital abnormality but also in patients with acute myeloid leukaemia or myelodysplasia.

Causes of leucocytosis and monocytosis

Neutrophil leucocytosis

An increase in circulating neutrophils to levels greater than 7.5×10^9/L is one of the most frequently observed blood count changes. The causes of neutrophil leucocytosis are given in Table 7.2. Neutrophil leucocytosis is sometimes accompanied by fever as a result of the release of leucocyte pyrogens. Other characteristic features of reactive neutrophilia may include: (a) a 'shift to the left' in the peripheral blood differential white cell count (i.e. an increase in the number of band forms) and the occasional presence of more primitive cells such as metamyelocytes and myelocytes; (b) the presence of cytoplasmic toxic granulation

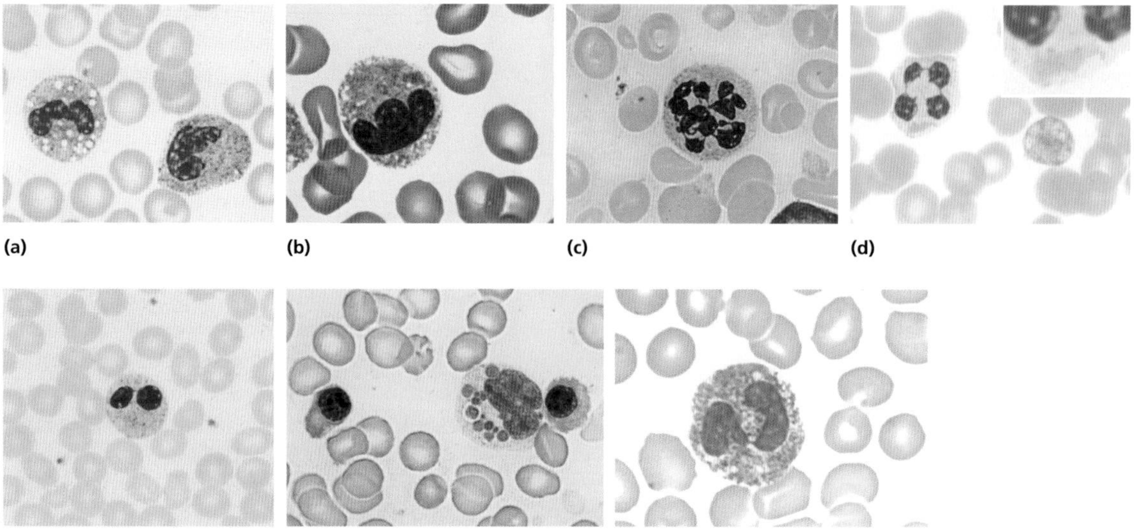

(a) (b) (c) (d) (e) (f) (g)

Fig. 7.8 Abnormal white blood cells. **(a)** Neutrophil leucocytosis: toxic changes shown by the presence of red–purple granules in the band form neutrophils. **(b)** Neutrophil leucocytosis: a Döhle body can be seen in the cytoplasm of the neutrophil. **(c)** Megaloblastic anaemia: hypersegmented oversized neutrophil in peripheral blood. **(d)** May–Hegglin anomaly: the neutrophils contain basophilic inclusions 2–5 μm in diameter; there is an associated mild thrombocytopenia with giant platelets. **(e)** Pelger–Huët anomaly: coarse clumping of the chromatin in *pince nez* configuration. **(f)** Chédiak–Higashi syndrome: bizarre giant granules in the cytoplasm of a monocyte. **(g)** Alder's anomaly: coarse violet granules in the cytoplasm of a neutrophil.

Table 7.2 Causes of neutrophil leucocytosis.

Bacterial infections (especially pyogenic bacterial, localized or generalized)
Inflammation and tissue necrosis (e.g. myositis, vasculitis, cardiac infarct, trauma)
Metabolic disorders (e.g. uraemia, eclampsia, acidosis, gout)
Neoplasms of all types (e.g. carcinoma, lymphoma, melanoma)
Acute haemorrhage or haemolysis
Drugs (e.g. corticosteroid therapy (inhibits margination): lithium, tetracycline)
Chronic myeloid leukaemia, myeloproliferative disease, polycythaemia vera, myelofibrosis, essential thrombocythaemia
Treatment with myeloid growth factors (e.g. G-CSF, GM-CSF)
Rare inherited disorders
Asplenia

G- and GM-CSF, granulocyte and granulocyte–macrophage colony-stimulating factor.

and Döhle bodies (Fig. 7.8a,b); and (c) an elevated neutrophil alkaline phosphatase (NAP) score. For this the strength of the staining of each of 100 neutrophils is scored between 0 and 4. The maximum score is therefore 400; a normal score is between 20 and 100.

The leukaemoid reaction

The leukaemoid reaction is a reactive and excessive leucocytosis usually characterized by the presence of immature cells (e.g. myeloblasts, promyelocytes and myelocytes) in the peripheral blood. Occasionally,

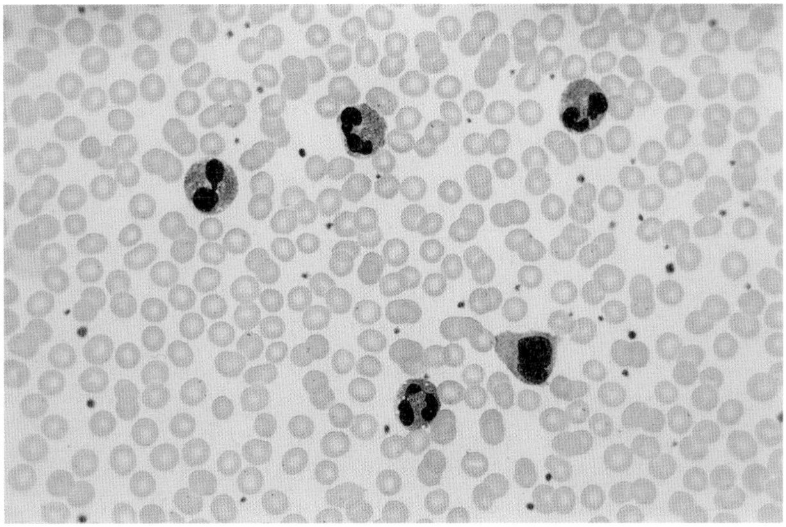

Fig. 7.9 Eosinophilia.

Table 7.3 Causes of eosinophilia.

Allergic diseases, especially hypersensitivity of the atopic type (e.g. bronchial asthma, hay fever, urticaria and food sensitivity)
Parasitic diseases (e.g. amoebiasis, hookworm, ascariasis, tapeworm infestation, filariasis, schistosomiasis and trichinosis)
Recovery from acute infection
Certain skin diseases (e.g. psoriasis, pemphigus and dermatitis herpetiformis, urticaria and angioedema, atopic dermatitis)
Drug sensitivity
Polyarteritis nodosa, vasculitis, serum sickness
Graft-versus-host disease
Hodgkin's disease and some other tumours, especially clonal T-cell disorders
Metastatic malignancy with tumour necrosis
Hypereosinophilic syndrome
Chronic eosinophilic leukaemia
Myeloproliferative including systemic mastocytosis
Treatment with GM-CSF
Pulmonary syndromes
Eosinophilic pneumonia, transient pulmonary infiltrates (Loeffler's syndrome), allergic granulomatosis (Churg–Strauss syndrome), tropical pulmonary eosinophilia

GM-CSF, granulocyte–macrophage colony-stimulating factor.

lymphocytic reactions occur. Associated disorders include severe or chronic infections, severe haemolysis or metastatic cancer. Leukaemoid reactions are often particularly marked in children. Granulocyte changes such as toxic granulation and Döhle bodies and a high NAP score help to differentiate the leukaemoid reaction from chronic myeloid leukaemia (in which the NAP score is low).

Eosinophilic leucocytosis (eosinophilia)

The causes of an increase in blood eosinophils (Fig. 7.9) above 0.4×10^9/L are listed in Table 7.3. Sometimes no underlying cause is found and if the eosinophil count is elevated ($>1.5 \times 10^9$/L) for over 6 months and associated with tissue damage then the hypereosinophilic syndrome is diagnosed. The

Table 7.4 Causes of monocytosis.

Chronic bacterial infections: tuberculosis, brucellosis, bacterial endocarditis, typhoid
Connective tissue diseases—SLE, temporal arteritis, rheumatoid arthritis
Protozoan infections
Chronic neutropenia
Hodgkin's disease, AML, and other malignancies
Myelodysplasia (especially chronic myelomonocytic leukaemia)
Treatment with GM-CSF or M-CSF

AML, acute myeloblastic leukemia; GM- and M-CSF, granulocyte–macrophage and macrophage colony-stimulating factor; SLE, systemic lupus erythematosus.

heart valves, skin and lungs may be affected and treatment is usually with steroids or cytotoxic drugs. In 25% of cases a clonal T-cell population is present. In other cases of chronic eosinophilia, a clonal cytogenetic abnormality is present in the bone marrow and the term chronic eosinophilic leukaemia is used. In 50% of cases there is a novel fusion gene on chromosome 4q caused by deletion of part of the long arm causing joining of the fragments of FIPILI and PDGFRA. This creates an active tyrosine kinase and the condition responds to imatinib (p. 181).

Basophil leucocytosis (basophilia)

An increase in blood basophils above 0.1×10^9/L is uncommon. The usual cause is a myeloproliferative disorder such as chronic myeloid leukaemia or polycythaemia vera. Reactive basophil increases are sometimes seen in myxoedema, during smallpox or chickenpox infection and in ulcerative colitis.

Monocytosis

A rise in blood monocyte count above 0.8×10^9/L is infrequent. The conditions listed in Table 7.4 may be responsible.

Neutropenia

The lower limit of the normal neutrophil count is 2.5×10^9/L except in black people and in the Middle East where 1.5×10^9/L is normal. When the absolute neutrophil level falls below 0.5×10^9/L the patient is likely to have recurrent infections and when the count falls to less than 0.2×10^9/L the risks are very serious, particularly if there is also a functional defect. Neutropenia may be selective or part of a general pancytopenia (Table 7.5).

Table 7.5 Causes of neutropenia.

Selective neutropenia
Congenital
Kostmann's syndrome
Acquired
Drug-induced
Anti-inflammatory drugs (phenylbutazone)
Antibacterial drugs (chloramphenicol, co-trimoxazole, sulfasalazine, imipenem)
Anticonvulsants (phenytoin, carbamazepine)
Antithyroids (carbimazole)
Hypoglycaemics (tolbutamide)
Phenothiazines (chlorpromazine, thioridazine)
Psychotropics and antidepressants (clozapine, mianserin, imipramine)
Miscellaneous (gold, penicillamine, mepacrine, frusemide, deferiprone)
Benign (racial or familial)
Cyclical
Immune
Autoimmune
Systemic lupus erythematosus
Felty's syndrome
Hypersensitivity and anaphylaxis
Large granular lymphocytic leukaemia (p. 195)
Infections
Viral (e.g. hepatitis, influenza, HIV)
Fulminant bacterial infection (e.g. typhoid, miliary tuberculosis)
Part of general pancytopenia (see Table 20.1)
Bone marrow failure
Splenomegaly

HIV, human immunodeficiency virus.

Congenital neutropenia

Kostmann's syndrome is an autosomal recessive disease presenting in the first year of life with life-threatening infections. Most cases are caused by mutations of the gene coding for neutrophil elastase. G-CSF produces a clinical response although marrow fibrosis and acute myeloid leukaemia may supervene.

Drug-induced neutropenia

A large number of drugs have been implicated (Table 7.5) and may induce neutropenia either by direct toxicity or immune-mediated damage.

Cyclical neutropenia

This is a rare syndrome with 3–4-week periodicity. Severe but temporary neutropenia occurs. Monocytes tend to rise as the neutrophils fall. Mutation of the gene for neutrophil elastase underlies some cases.

Autoimmune neutropenia

In some cases of chronic neutropenia an autoimmune mechanism can be demonstrated. The antibody may be directed against one of the neutrophil-specific antigens (e.g. NA, NB).

Idiopathic benign neutropenia

An increase in the marginating fraction of blood neutrophils and a corresponding reduction in the circulating fraction is one cause of benign neutropenia. Many normal Africans and other races, especially in the Middle East, have a low peripheral blood neutrophil count without excess margination. These subjects have no increased susceptibility to infection and the bone marrow appears normal although there is diminished neutrophil production.

Finally, the term chronic idiopathic neutropenia is used for unexplained acquired neutropenia (neutrophil count below normal for the ethnic group), without phasic variations or underlying disease. It is more common in females and thought to be brought about by immune cells causing inhibition of myelopoiesis in the bone marrow.

Clinical features

Severe neutropenia is particularly associated with infections of the mouth and throat. Painful and often intractable ulceration may occur at these sites (Fig. 7.10), on the skin or at the anus. Septicaemia rapidly supervenes. Organisms carried as commensals by normal individuals, such as *Staphylococcus epidermidis* or Gram-negative organisms in the bowel, may become pathogens. Other features of infections associated with severe neutropenia are described on p. 149.

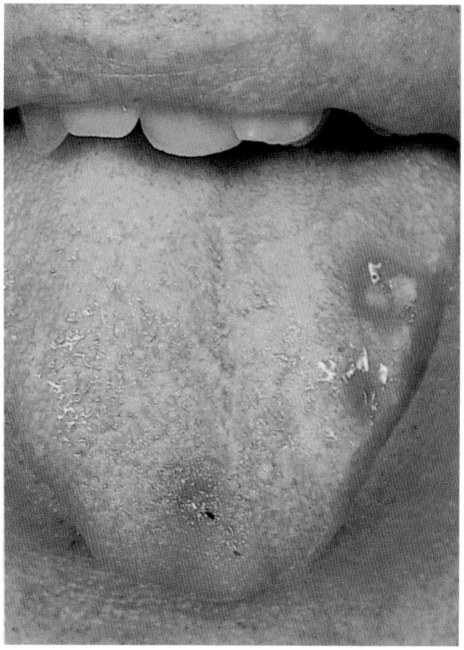

Fig. 7.10 Ulceration of the tongue in severe neutropenia.

Diagnosis

Bone marrow examination is useful in determining the level of damage in granulopoiesis (i.e. whether there is reduction in early precursors or whether there is reduction only of circulating and marrow neutrophils with late precursors remaining in the marrow). Marrow aspiration and trephine biopsy may also provide evidence of leukaemia, myelodysplasia or other infiltration.

Management

The treatment of patients with acute severe neutropenia is described on p. 150. In many patients with drug-induced neutropenia spontaneous recovery occurs within 1–2 weeks after stopping the drug. Patients with chronic neutropenia have recurrent infections which are mainly bacterial in origin although fungal and viral infections (especially herpes) also occur. Early recognition and vigorous treatment with antibiotics, antifungal or antiviral agents, as appropriate, is essential. Prophylactic antibacterial agents (e.g. oral co-trimoxazole or ciprofloxacin and colistin) and antifungal agents (e.g. oral amphotericin and fluconazole or itraconazole) may be of value in reducing the incidence and severity of infections caused by severe neutropenia. The haemopoietic growth factor G-CSF may be used to stimulate neutrophil production and is effective in a variety of benign chronic neutropenic states. Corticosteroid therapy or splenectomy has been associated with good results in some patients with autoimmune neutropenia. Rituximab (anti-CD20) may also be effective. Conversely, corticosteroids impair neutrophil function and should not be used indiscriminately in patients with neutropenia.

Histiocytic disorders

A classification of the histiocytic disorders is given in Table 7.6.

Dendritic cells

These are specialized antigen-presenting cells found mainly in the skin, lymph nodes, spleen and thymus. They comprise myeloid- and monocyte-derived cells including Langerhans' cells and a lymphocyte-derived subset. Their primary role is in antigen presentation to T and B lymphocytes (p. 115).

Table 7.6 Classification of histiocytic disorders.

Dendritic cell-related
Langerhans' cell histiocytosis
Solitary dendritic cell histiocytoma
Macrophage-related
Haemophagocytic lymphohistiocytosis
primary (familial)
secondary—infection, drug, tumour
Sinus histiocytosis with massive lymphadenopathy
Malignancies
AML FAB type M4 and M5 (p. 158)
Chronic myelomonocytic leukaemia (p. 186)
Dendritic and macrophage-related sarcomas (localized or disseminated)

AML, acute myeloid leukaemia;
FAB, French–American–British.

Langerhans' cell histiocytes

Langerhans' cell histiocytosis (LCH) includes diseases previously called histiocytosis X, Letterer–Siwe disease, Hand–Schüller–Christian disease and eosinophilic granuloma. The disease may be single organ or multisystem. There is a clonal proliferation of CD1a-positive cells. The multisystem disease affects children in the first 3 years of life with hepatosplenomegaly, lymphadenopathy and eczematous skin symptoms. Localized lesions may occur especially in the skull, ribs and long bones, the posterior pituitary causing diabetes insipidus, the central nervous system, gastrointestinal tract and lungs. The lesions include Langerhans' cells (characterized by the presence of tennis racquet-shaped Birbeck granules in electron-microscopy sections), eosinophils, lymphocytes, neutrophils and macrophages.

Haemophagocytic lymphohistiocytosis (haemophagocytic syndrome)

This is a rare, recessively inherited or more frequently acquired disease, usually precipitated by a viral (especially Epstein–Barr or herpes viruses), bacterial or fungal infection or occuring in association with tumours. Often the patient is immunocompromised. Patients present with fever and pancytopenia, often with splenomegaly and liver dysfunction. There are increased numbers of histiocytes in the bone marrow which ingest red cells, white cells and platelets (Fig. 7.11). Clinical features are fever, pancytopenia and multiorgan dysfunction often with lymphadenopathy, hepatic and splenic enlargement, coagulopathy and CNS signs. Treatment is of the underlying infection, if known, with support care. T-cell activation is implicated in the aetiology. Chemotherapy with etoposide, corticosteroids, ciclosporin or Rituximab (anti-CD20) may be tried. The condition is often fatal.

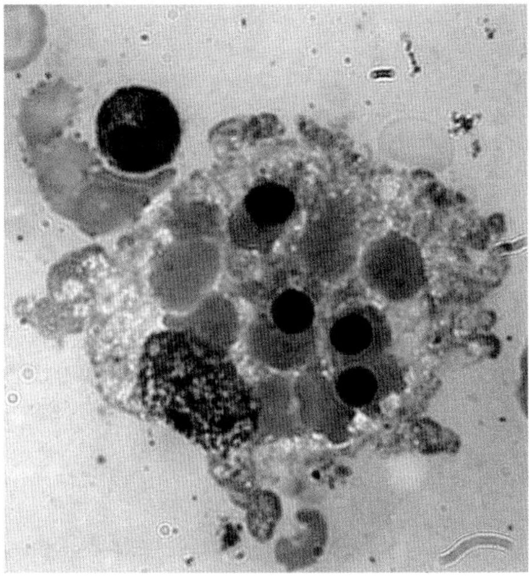

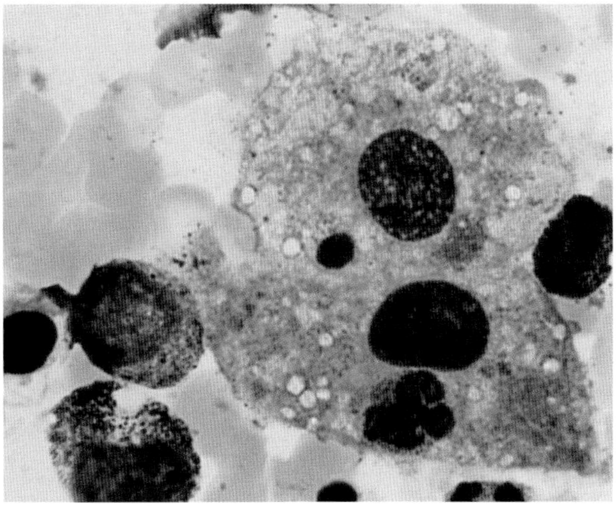

Fig. 7.11 Haemophagocytic lymphohistiocytosis: bone marrow aspirates showing histiocytes that have ingested red cells, erythroblasts and neutrophils.

Sinus histiocytosis with massive lymphadenopathy

This is also known as the Rosai–Dorfman syndrome. There is painless, chronic cervical lymphadenopathy. There may be fever and weight loss. The histology is typical and the condition subsides over months or years.

Bibliography

Brito-Babapulle F. (2003) The eosinophilias, including the idiopathic hypereosinophilic syndrome. *Br J Haematol* **121**,203–23.

Charo I.F. and Ransohoff R.M. (2006) The many roles of chemokines and chemokine receptors in inflammation. *N Engl J Med* **354**,610–21.

Dale D.C. (ed.) (2002) Severe chronic neutropenia. *Semin Hematol* **39**,73–141.

Duffield J.S. (2003) The inflammatory macrophage: a story of Jekyll and Hyde. *Clin Sci (Lond)* **104**,27–38.

Kyono W. and Coates T.D. (2002) A practical approach to neutrophil disorders. *Pediatr Clin North Am* **49**,929–71.

Lakshman R. and Finn A. (2001) Neutrophil disorders and their management. *J Clin Pathol* **54**,7–19.

Ozer H., Armitage J.O., Bennett C.L. *et al.* (2000) 2000 update of recommendations for the use of hematopoietic colony-stimulating factors: evidence-based, clinical practice guidelines. American Society of Clinical Oncology Growth Factors Expert Panel. *J Clin Oncol* **18**,3558–85.

Stock W. and Hoffman R. (2000) White blood cells 1: non-malignant disorders. *Lancet* **355**,1351–7.

Tefferi A. (ed.) (2005) Eosinophilic and mast cell disorders. *Acta Haematol* **114**,52–60.

Tefferi A., Patnaik M.M. and Pardanani A. (2006) Eosinophilia: secondary, clonal and idiopathic. *Br J Haematol* **133**,468–92.

Zeidler C. and Welte K. (2002) Kostmann syndrome and severe congenital neutropenia. *Semin Hematol* **39**,82–8.

CHAPTER 8

8 The white cells 2: lymphocytes and their benign disorders

Lymphocytes are the immunologically competent cells that assist the phagocytes in defence of the body against infection and other foreign invasion (Fig. 8.1). Two unique features characteristic of the immune system are the ability to generate ***antigenic specificity*** and the phenomenon of ***immunological memory***. A complete description of the functions of lymphocytes is beyond the scope of this book, but information essential to an understanding of the diseases of the lymphoid system, and of the role of lymphocytes in haematological diseases, is included here.

Lymphocytes

In postnatal life, the bone marrow and thymus are the ***primary lymphoid organs*** in which lymphocytes develop (Fig. 8.2). The ***secondary lymphoid organs*** in which specific immune responses are generated are the lymph nodes, spleen and lymphoid tissues of the alimentary and respiratory tracts.

B and T lymphocytes

The immune response depends upon two types of lymphocytes, B and T cells (Table 8.1), which derive from the haemopoietic stem cell. B cells mature in the bone marrow and circulate in the peripheral blood until they undergo recognition of antigen. The B-cell receptor is membrane-bound immunoglobulin and after activation this is secreted as free soluble immunoglobulin. At this point they mature into memory B cells or plasma cells. The latter home to the bone marrow and have a characteristic morphology with an eccentric round nucleus with a 'clock-face' chromatin pattern and strongly basophilic cytoplasm (Fig. 8.1d).

T cells develop from cells that have migrated to the thymus where they differentiate into mature T cells during passage from the cortex to the medulla. During this process, self-reactive T cells are deleted (negative selection) whereas T cells with some specificity for host human leucocyte antigen (HLA) molecules are selected (positive selection). The mature helper cells express CD4 and cytotoxic cells express CD8 (Table 8.1). The cells also express one of two T-cell antigen receptor heterodimers, $\alpha\beta$ (>90%) or $\gamma\delta$ (<10%), and recognize antigen only when it is presented at a cell surface (see below).

Natural killer cells

Natural killer (NK) cells are cytotoxic $CD8^+$ cells that lack the T-cell receptor (TCR). They are large cells with cytoplasmic granules and typically express surface molecules CD16 (Fc receptor), CD56 and CD57. NK cells are designed to kill target cells that have a low level of expression of HLA class I

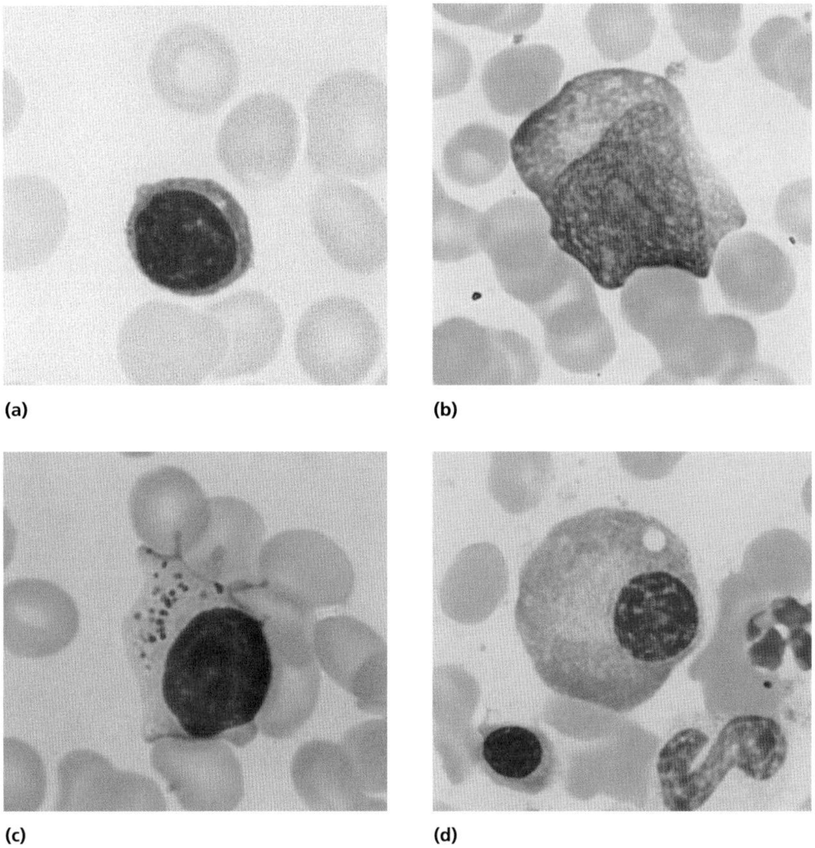

Fig. 8.1 Lymphocytes:
(a) small lymphocyte;
(b) activated lymphocyte;
(c) large granular lymphocyte;
(d) plasma cell.

molecules such as may occur during viral infection or on a malignant cell. NK cells do this by displaying a number of receptors for HLA molecules on their surface. When HLA is expressed on the target cell these deliver an inhibitory signal into the NK cell. When HLA molecules are absent on the target cell this inhibitory signal is lost and the NK cell can then kill its target. In addition, NK cells display antibody-dependent cell-mediated cytotoxicity (ADCC). In this, antibody binds to antigen on the surface of the target cell and then NK cells bind to the Fc portion of the bound antibody and kill the target cell.

Lymphocyte circulation

Lymphocytes in the peripheral blood migrate through ***post-capillary venules*** into the substance of the lymph nodes or into the spleen or bone marrow. T cells home to the perifollicular zones of the cortical areas of lymph nodes (paracortical areas) (Fig. 8.2) and to the periarteriolar sheaths surrounding the central arterioles of the spleen. B cells selectively accumulate in follicles of the lymph nodes and spleen. Lymphocytes return to the peripheral blood via the efferent lymphatic stream and the thoracic duct. CD4 helper cells predominate in normal peripheral blood and germinal centres, but in the marrow and gut the major T-cell subpopulation is CD8 positive.

Immunoglobulins

These are a group of proteins produced by plasma cells and B lymphocytes that bind to antigen. They are divided into five subclasses or ***isotypes***: immunoglobulin G (IgG), IgA, IgM, IgD and IgE. IgG, the most common, contributes approximately 80% of normal serum immunoglobulin and is further

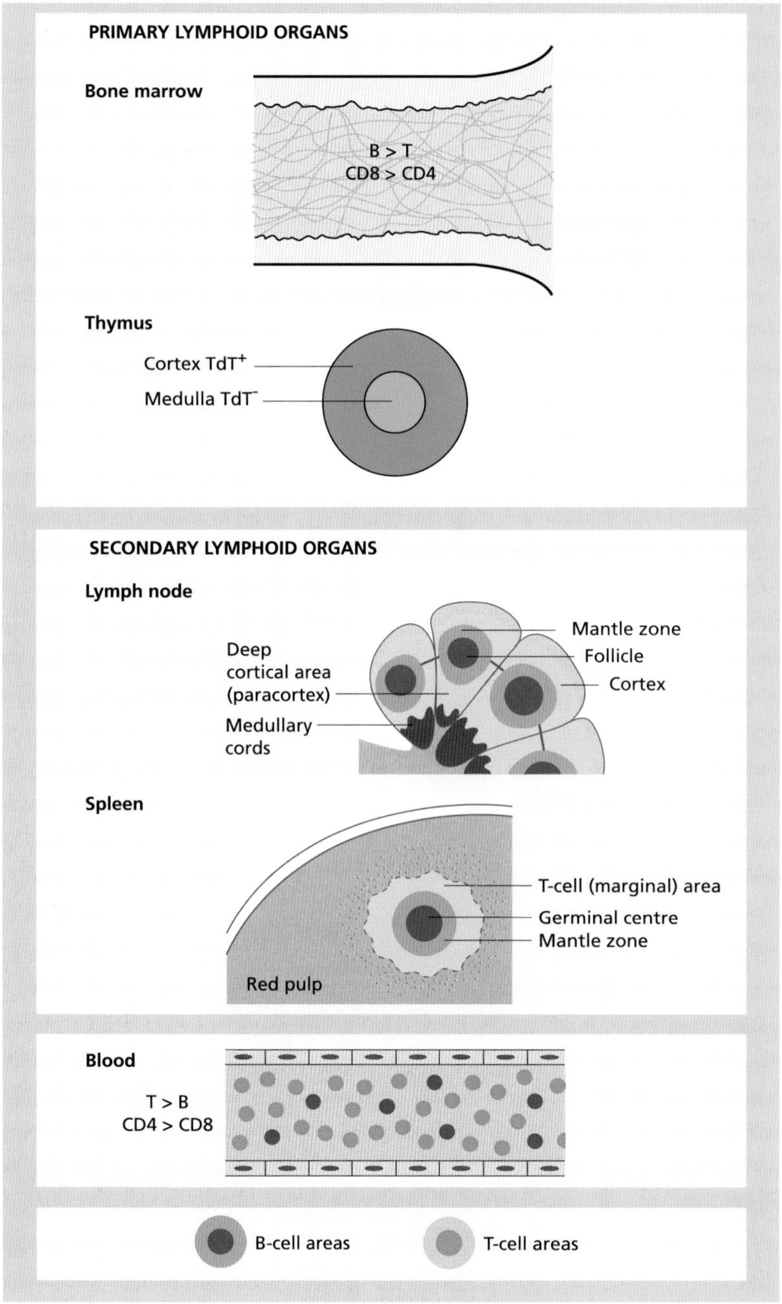

Fig. 8.2 Primary and secondary lymphoid organs and blood.

subdivided into four ***subclasses***: IgG_1, IgG_2, IgG_3 and IgG_4. IgA is subdivided into two types. IgM is usually produced first in response to antigen, IgG subsequently and for a more prolonged period. The same cell can switch from IgM to IgG, or to IgA or IgE synthesis. IgA is the main immunoglobulin in secretions, particularly of the gastrointestinal tract. IgD and IgE (involved in delayed hypersensitivity reactions) are minor fractions. Some important biochemical and biological properties of the three

Table 8.1 Functional aspects of T and B cells.

	T cells	B cells
Origin	Thymus	Bone marrow
Tissue distribution	Parafollicular areas of cortex in nodes, peri-arteriolar in spleen	Germinal centres of lymph nodes, spleen, gut, respiratory tract; also subcapsular and medullary cords of lymph nodes
Blood	80% of lymphocytes; CD4 > CD8	20% of lymphocytes
Membrane receptors	TCR for antigen	BCR (= immunoglobulin) for antigen
Function	$CD8^+$: CMI against intracellular organisms $CD4^+$: T-cell help for antibody production and generation of CMI	Humoral immunity by generation of antibodies
Characteristic surface markers	CD1 CD2 CD3 CD4 or 8 CD5 CD6 CD7 MHC class I MHC class II when activated	CD19 CD20 CD22 CD9 (pre B cells) CD10 (precursor B cells) CD79 MHC class I and II
Genes rearranged	TCR α, β, γ, δ	IgH, Igκ, Igλ

BCR, B-cell receptor; C, complement; CMI, cell-mediated immunity; IFN, interferon; Ig, immunoglobulin; MHC, major histocompatibility complex; TCR, T-cell receptor; TNF, tumour necrosis factor.

Table 8.2 Some properties of the three main classes of immunoglobulin (Ig).

	IgG	IgA	IgM
Molecular weight	140 000	140 000	900 000
Sedimentation constant	7S	7S	19S
Normal serum level (g/L)	6.0–16.0	1.5–4.5	0.5–1.5
Present in	Serum and extracellular fluid	Serum and other body fluids (e.g. of bronchi and gut)	Serum only
Complement fixation	Usual	Yes (alternative pathway)	Usual and very efficient
Placental transfer	Yes	No	No
Heavy chain	(γ_{1-4})	α (α_1 or α_2)	μ

main immunoglobulin subclasses are summarized in Table 8.2.

The immunoglobulins are all made up of the same basic structure (Fig. 8.3) consisting of two heavy chains which are called gamma (γ) in IgG, alpha (α) in IgA, mu (μ) in IgM, delta (δ) in IgD and epsilon (ε) in IgE, and two light chains—kappa (κ) or lambda (λ)—which are common to all five immunoglobulins. The heavy and light chains each have highly variable regions which give the immunoglobulin specificity, and constant regions in which there is virtual complete correspondence in amino acid sequence in all antibodies of a given isotype (e.g. IgA, IgG) or isotype subclass (e.g. IgG_1, IgG_2). IgG antibody can be broken into a constant Fc fragment and two highly variable Fab fragments. IgM molecules are much larger because they consist of five subunits.

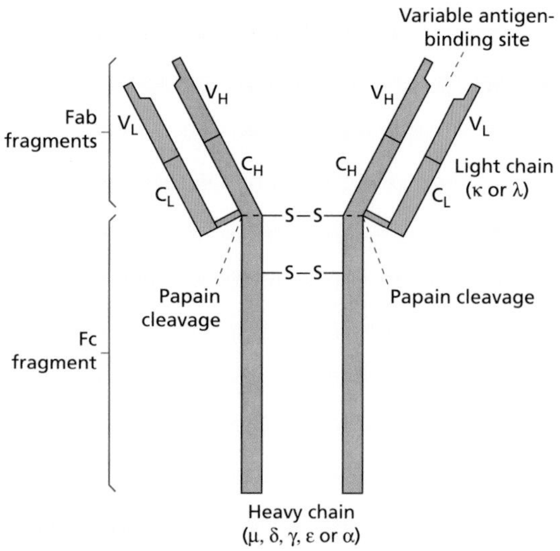

Fig. 8.3 Basic structure of an immunoglobulin molecule. Each molecule is made up of two light (κ or λ) (blue areas) and two heavy (purple) chains, and each chain is made up of variable (V) and constant (C) portions, the V portions including the antigen-binding site. The heavy chain (μ, δ, γ, ε or α) varies according to the immunoglobulin class. IgA molecules form dimers, while IgM forms a ring of five molecules. Papain cleaves the molecules into an Fc fragment and two Fab fragments.

The main role of immunoglobulins is defence of the body against foreign organisms. However, they also have a vital role in the pathogenesis of a number of haematological disorders. Secretion of a specific immunoglobulin from a monoclonal population of lymphocytes or plasma cells causes ***paraproteinaemia*** (p. 216). Bence-Jones protein found in the urine in some cases of myeloma consists of a monoclonal secretion of light chains or light-chain fragments (either κ or λ). Immunoglobulins may bind to blood cells in a variety of immune disorders and cause their agglutination (e.g. in cold agglutinin disease; p. 67) or destruction following direct complement lysis or after elimination by the reticuloendothelial system.

Antigen–receptor gene arrangements

Immunoglobulin gene rearrangements

The immunoglobulin heavy-chain and κ and λ light-chain genes occur on chromosomes 14, 2 and 22, respectively. In the germline state, the heavy-chain gene consists of separate segments for variable (V), diversity (D), joining (J) and constant (C) regions. Each of the V, D and J regions contain a number (*n*) of different ***gene segments*** (Fig. 8.4). In cells not committed to immunoglobulin synthesis these gene segments remain in their separate germline state. During early differentiation of B cells there is rearrangement of heavy-chain genes so that one of the V heavy-chain segments combines with one of the D segments, which has itself already combined with one of the J segments. Thus, they form a transcriptionally active gene for the heavy chain. The protein coding segments of the C region mRNA

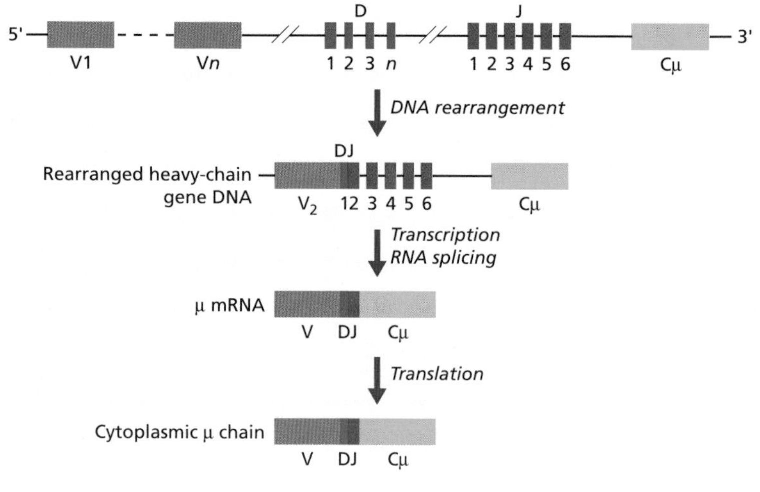

Fig. 8.4 Rearrangement of a heavy-chain immunoglobulin gene. One of the V segments is brought into contact with a D, a J and a C (in this case Cμ) segment, forming an active transcriptional gene from which the corresponding mRNA is produced. The DJ rearrangement precedes VDJ joining. The class of immunoglobin depends on which of the nine constant regions (1μ, 1δ, 4γ, 2α, 1ε) is used.

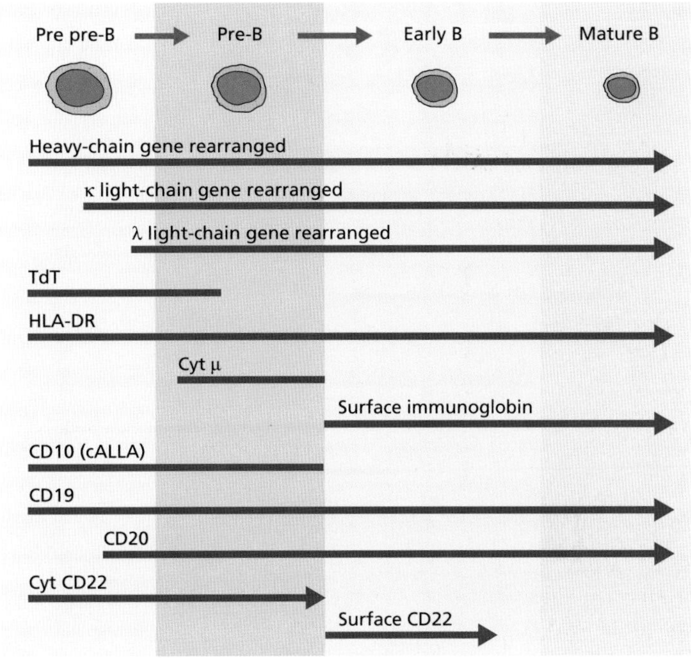

Fig. 8.5 The sequence of immunoglobulin gene rearrangement, antigen and immunoglobulin expression during early B-cell development. Intracytoplasmic CD22 is a feature of very early B cells. HLA, human leucocyte antigen; TdT, terminal deoxynucleotidyl transferase.

are joined to the V region after splicing out intervening RNA. The class of immunoglobulin that is secreted depends on which of the nine (4γ, 2α, 1μ, 1δ and 1ε) constant regions is used. Diversity is introduced by the variability of which V segment joins with which D and with which J segment. In the arbitrary example shown in Fig. 8.4, V_2 joins with D_1 and J_2. Additional diversity is generated by the enzyme terminal deoxynucleotidyl transferase (TdT), which inserts a variable number of new bases into the DNA of the D region at the time of gene rearrangement.

Similar rearrangements occur during generation of the light-chain gene (Fig. 8.5). Enzymes called ***recombinases*** are needed both in B and T cells to join up the adjacent pieces of DNA after excision of intervening sequences. These recognize certain heptamer- and nonamer-conserved sequences flanking the various gene segments. Mistakes in recombinase activity play an important part in the chromosome translocations of B- or T-cell malignancy.

T-cell receptor gene rearrangements

The vast majority of T cells contain a TCR composed of a heterodimer of α and β chain. In a minority of T cells, the TCR is composed of γ and δ chains. The α, β, γ and δ genes of the TCRs each include V, D, J and C regions. During T-cell ontogeny, rearrangements of these gene segments occur in a similar fashion to those for immunoglobulin genes, thus creating T cells expressing a wide variety (10^8 or more) of TCR structures (Fig. 8.6). TdT is involved in creating additional diversity and the same recombinase enzymes used in B cells are involved in joining up TCR gene segments.

Complement

This consists of a series of plasma proteins constituting an ***amplification enzyme system*** which is capable of lysis of bacteria (or of blood cells) or can 'opsonize' (coat) bacteria or cells so that they are phagocytosed. The complement sequence consists of nine major components—C1, C2, etc.—which are activated in turn (denoted thus C1—) and form a cascade, resembling the coagulation sequence (Fig. 8.7). The most abundant and pivotal protein is C3, which is present in plasma at a level of approximately 1.2 g/L. The early (opsonizing) stages leading to coating of the cells with C3b can occur by two different pathways:

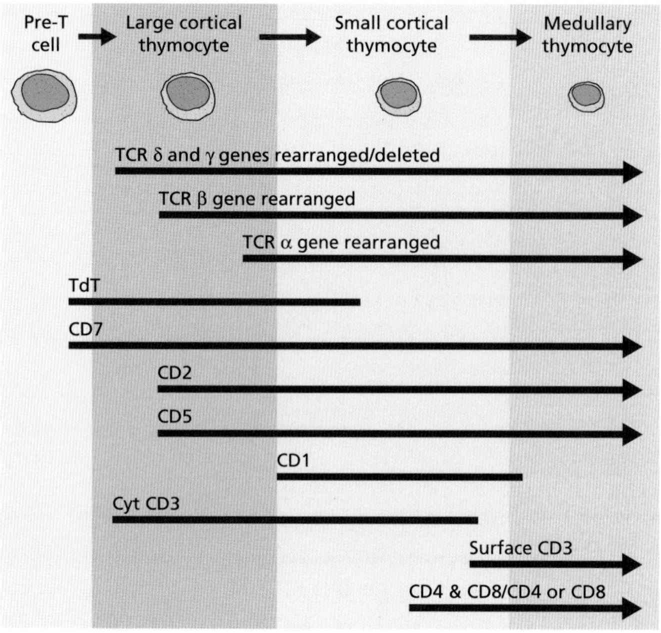

Fig. 8.6 The sequence of events during early T-cell development. The earliest events appear to be the expression of surface CD7, intranuclear terminal deoxynucleotidyl transferase (TdT) and intracytoplasmic CD3 followed by T-cell receptor (TCR) gene rearrangement. Early medullary thymocytes may express both CD4 and CD8, but they then lose one or other of these structures.

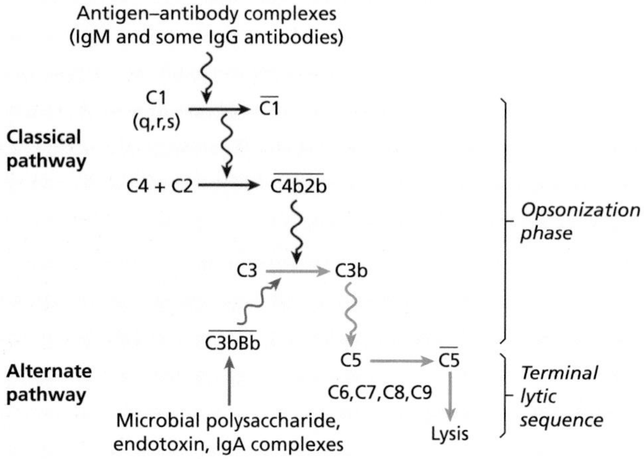

Fig. 8.7 The complement (C) sequence. The activated factors are denoted by a bar over the number. Both pathways generate a C3 convertase. In the classic pathway, the convertase is the major (b) component of C4 and C2 ($\overline{\text{C4b2b}}$). In the alternate pathway, it is the combination of C3b and the major fragment (b) of factor B ($\overline{\text{C3bBb}}$).

1 The ***classical pathway*** usually activated by IgG or IgM coating of cells; or
2 The ***alternate pathway***, which is more rapid and activated by IgA, endotoxin (from Gram-negative bacteria) and other factors (Fig. 8.7).

Macrophages and neutrophils have C3b receptors and they phagocytose C3b-coated cells. C3b is degraded to C3d detected in the direct antiglobulin (Coombs') test using an anticomplement agent (p. 343). If the complement sequence goes to completion there is generation of an active phospholipase that punches holes in the cell membrane (e.g. of the red cell or bacterium), causing direct lysis. The complement pathway also generates the biologically active fragments C3a and C5a which act directly on phagocytes to stimulate the respiratory burst (p. 100). Both may trigger anaphylaxis by release of mediators from tissue mast cells and basophils which causes vasodilatation and increased permeability.

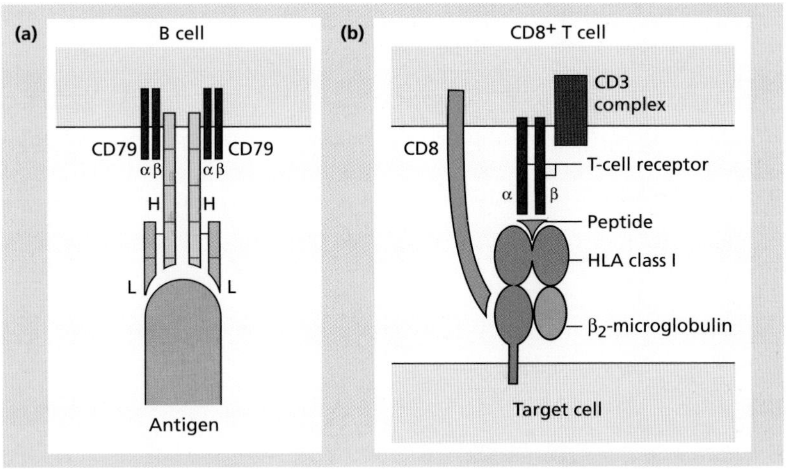

Fig. 8.8 Antigen receptors on lymphocytes and their interaction with antigen. **(a)** The B-cell antigen receptor is membrane-bound immunoglobulin. Two heavy chains (H) are covalently bonded to two light chains (L). This antigen-binding unit is associated with the CD79 heterodimer which acts as a signal transduction unit. **(b)** The T-cell receptor consists of a number of components that together constitute the CD3 complex. Two antigen-binding chains (α, β) are associated with several proteins (γ, δ, ε, ζ) that mediate signal transduction. Antigen is recognized in the form of short peptides held on the surface of HLA molecules. $CD8^+$ T cells interact with peptide on a class I HLA molecule and the CD8 heterodimer interacts with the α_3 domain of the class I protein.

The immune response

One of the most striking features of the immune system is its capacity to produce a highly *specific* response. For both T and B cells this specificity is achieved by the presence of a particular receptor on the lymphocyte surface (Fig. 8.8). Naïve (or virgin) B and T lymphocytes which leave the bone marrow and thymus are resting cells that are not in cell division. They recirculate in the lymphatic system. Specialized macrophages called dendritic cells (DCs; p. 99) process antigens before presenting them to B and T lymphocytes—they are therefore known as ***antigen-presenting cells*** (APCs). The immune system contains many different lymphocytes. Each of these lymphocytes has a receptor that shows differences in structure from that of any other lymphocyte, and consequently will bind to only a restricted number of antigens. T and B cells undergo clonal expansion if they meet an APC that is presenting an antigen that can trigger their antigen receptor molecules. At this stage, lymphocytes may develop into effector cells (such as plasma cells or cytotoxic T cells) or memory cells.

DC precursors constitutively migrate at low levels from blood into tissues but their rate of migration is increased at the site of inflammation. Immature DCs are efficient at macropinocytosis which allows them to capture antigens from the environment. DCs can be matured by a variety of stimuli such as inflammatory cytokines—tumour necrosis factor-α (TNF-α) and interleukin-1 (IL-1)—and viral and bacterial products such as lipopolysaccharide (LPS) or double-stranded (ds) RNA. Mature DCs express high levels of co-stimulatory molecules and can efficiently present antigen to naïve antigen-specific T cells.

T cells are unable to bind antigen free in solution and require it to be presented on APCs in the form of peptides held on the surface of HLA molecules (Fig. 8.8b). T cells therefore recognize not only the antigen, but also 'self' HLA molecules and are known as ***HLA-restricted***. The CD4 molecule on helper cells recognizes class II (HLA-DP, -DQ and -DR) molecules, whereas the CD8 molecule recognizes class I (HLA-A, -B and -C) molecules (Fig. 21.5). The antigen recognition site of the TCR is joined to several other subunits in the CD3 complex which together mediate signal transduction. During these structural interactions the cells release cytokines such as IL-1, -2, -4 and -10 which act to modify expansion of activated cells. Depending on their cytokine production, $CD4^+$ T cells can be broadly subdivided into T helper type 1 (Th1) and Th2 cells. Th1 cells produce mainly IL-2, TNF-β and γ-interferon (IFN-γ), and are important in boosting cell-mediated immunity (and granuloma formation), whereas Th2 cells produce IL-4 and IL-10 and are mainly responsible for providing help for antibody production. An imbalance in the ratio of these two subsets may be partly responsible for some forms of immunodeficiency.

Antigen-specific immune responses are generated in ***secondary lymphoid organs*** and commence when antigen is carried into a lymph node (Fig. 8.9)

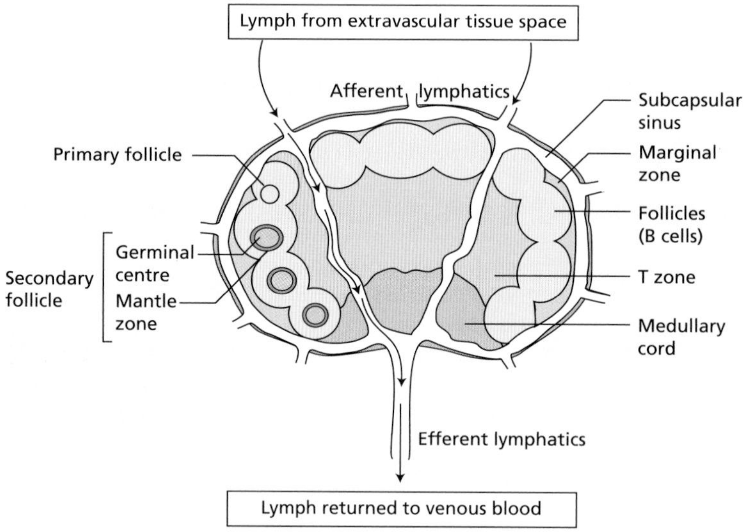

(a)

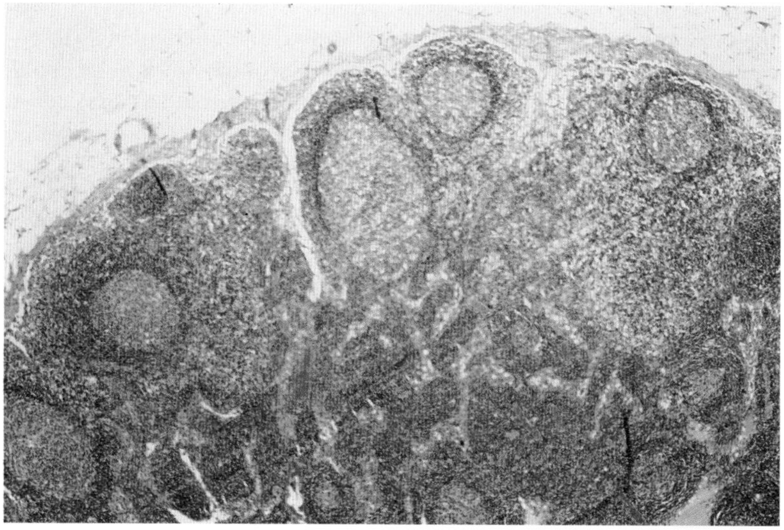

(b)

Fig. 8.9 **(a)** Structure of a lymph node. **(b)** Lymph node showing germinal follicles surrounded by a darker mantle zone rim and lighter, more diffuse marginal and T-zone areas.

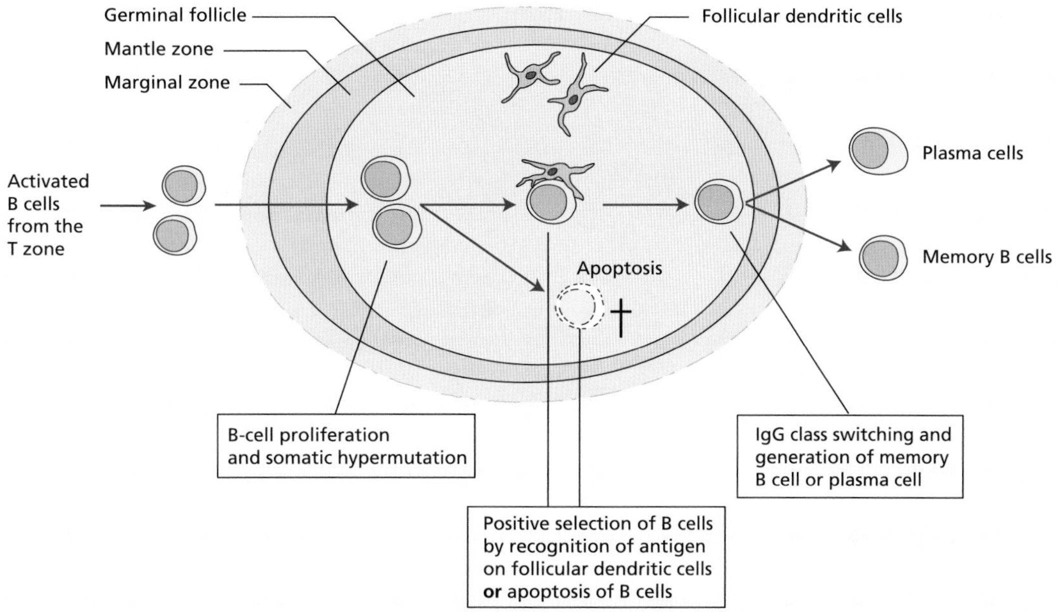

Fig. 8.10 Generation of a germinal centre. B cells activated by antigen migrate from the T zone to the follicle where they undergo massive proliferation. Cells enter the dark zone as centroblasts and accumulate mutations in their immunoglobulin V genes. Cells then pass back into the light zone (Fig. 8.8a) as centrocytes. Only those cells that can interact with antigen on follicular dendritic cells and receive signals from antigen-specific T cells (Fig. 8.8) are selected and migrate out as plasma cells and memory cells. Cells not selected die by apoptosis.

on dendritic cells. B cells recognize antigen through their surface immunoglobulin and although most antibody responses require help from antigen-specific T cells, some antigens such as polysaccharides can lead to T-cell independent antibody production. T cells are screened for recognition of antigen and if a T cell makes an interaction it migrates into the follicle. In the follicle, germinal centres arise as a result of continuing response to antigenic stimulation (Fig. 8.10). These consist of follicular dendritic cells (FDCs), which are loaded with antigen, B cells and activated T cells which have migrated up from the T zone. Proliferating B cells move to the dark zone of the germinal centre as ***centroblasts*** where they undergo somatic mutation of their immunoglobulin variable-region genes. Their progeny are known as ***centrocytes*** and these must be selected by antigen on FDCs otherwise they will undergo apoptosis. If selected they become memory B cells or plasma cells (Fig. 8.10). Plasma cells migrate to the bone marrow and produce high affinity antibody. Although they contain intracellular immunoglobulin they do not express surface immunoglobulin.

Lymphocytosis

Lymphocytosis often occurs in infants and young children in response to infections that produce a neutrophil reaction in adults. Conditions particularly associated with lymphocytosis are listed in Table 8.3.

Glandular fever is a general term for a disease characterized by fever, sore throat, lymphadenopathy and atypical lymphocytes in the blood. It may be caused by primary infection with Epstein–Barr virus (EBV), cytomegalovirus, human immunodeficiency virus (HIV) or toxoplasma. EBV infection, otherwise known as infectious mononucleosis, is the most common cause.

Table 8.3 Causes of lymphocytosis.

Infections
acute: infectious mononucleosis, rubella, pertussis, mumps, acute infectious lymphocytosis, infectious hepatitis, cytomegalovirus, HIV, herpes simplex or zoster
chronic: tuberculosis, toxoplasmosis, brucellosis, syphilis
Chronic lymphoid leukaemias (Chapter 15)
Acute lymphoblastic leukaemia
Non-Hodgkin's lymphoma (some)
Thyrotoxicosis

HIV, human immunodeficiency virus.

Infectious mononucleosis

This is caused by primary infection with EBV and occurs only in a minority of infected individuals—in most cases infection is subclinical. The disease is characterized by a lymphocytosis caused by clonal expansions of T cells reacting against B lymphocytes infected with EBV. The disease is associated with a high titre of heterophile ('reacting with cells of another species') antibody which reacts with sheep, horse or ox red cells.

Clinical features

The majority of patients are between the ages of 15 and 40 years. A prodromal period of a few days occurs with lethargy, malaise, headaches, stiff neck and a dry cough. In established disease the following features may be found.

1 Bilateral cervical lymphadenopathy is present in 75% of cases. Symmetrical generalized lymphadenopathy occurs in 50% of cases. The nodes are discrete and may be tender.

2 Over half of patients have a sore throat with inflamed oral and pharyngeal surfaces. Follicular tonsillitis is frequently seen.

3 Fever may be mild or severe.

4 A morbilliform rash, severe headache and eye signs (e.g. photophobia, conjunctivitis and periorbital oedema) are not uncommon. The rash may follow therapy with amoxicillin or ampicillin.

5 Palpable splenomegaly occurs in over half of patients and hepatomegaly in approximately 15%. Approximately 5% of patients are jaundiced.

6 Peripheral neuropathy, severe anaemia (caused by autoimmune haemolysis) or purpura (caused by thrombocytopenia) are less frequent complications.

Diagnosis

Pleomorphic atypical lymphocytosis A moderate rise in white cell count (e.g. $10–20 \times 10^9/L$) with an absolute lymphocytosis is usual, and some patients have even higher counts. Large numbers of atypical lymphocytes are seen in the peripheral blood film (Fig. 8.11). These T cells are variable in appearance but most have nuclear and cytoplasmic features similar to those seen during reactive lymphocyte transformation. The greatest number of atypical lymphocytes are usually found between the seventh and 10th day of the illness.

Heterophile antibodies Heterophile antibodies against sheep red cells may be found in the serum at high titres. These form the basis of the Paul–Bunnell test—the antibodies are not absorbed by guinea-pig kidney cells but are absorbed by ox red cells (Fig. 8.12). Modern slide screening tests, such as the ***monospot test***, substitute formalinized horse red cells for the sheep cells used in the Paul–Bunnell test. Highest titres occur during the second and third week and the antibody persists in most patients for 6 weeks.

EBV antibody If viral diagnostic facilities are available, a rise in the titre of antibody against the EBV capsid antigen may be demonstrated during the first 2–3 weeks. Specific antibody to the EBV nuclear antigen develops later and persists for life.

Haematological abnormalities other than the atypical lymphocytosis are frequent. Occasional patients develop an autoimmune haemolytic anaemia. The IgM autoantibody is typically of the 'cold' type and usually shows 'i' blood group specificity. Thrombocytopenia is frequent and an autoimmune thrombocytopenic purpura occurs in a smaller number of patients.

Differential diagnosis

The differential diagnosis of infectious mononucleosis includes cytomegalovirus, HIV or toxoplasmosis infection; acute leukaemia; influenza; rubella; bacterial tonsillitis; and infectious hepatitis.

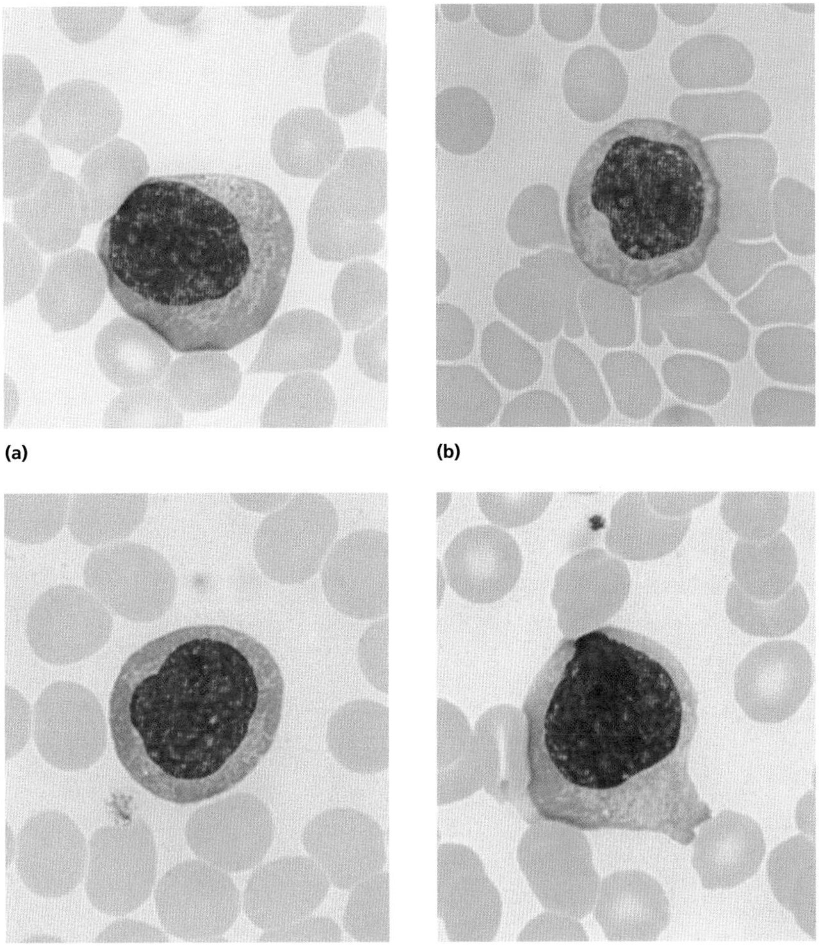

(a) (b) (c) (d)

Fig. 8.11 Infectious mononucleosis: representative 'reactive' T lymphocytes in the peripheral blood film of a 21-year-old man (see also Fig. 8.1b).

Treatment

In the great majority of patients only symptomatic treatment is required. Corticosteroids are sometimes given to those with severe systemic symptoms. Patients characteristically develop an erythematous rash if given ampicillin therapy. Most patients recover fully 4–6 weeks after initial symptoms. However, convalescence may be slow and associated with severe malaise and lethargy.

Lymphopenia

Lymphopenia may occur in severe bone marrow failure, with corticosteroid and other immunosuppressive therapy, in Hodgkin's disease and with widespread irradiation. It also occurs in a variety of immunodeficiency syndromes, the most important of which is HIV infection (p. 328).

Immunodeficiency

A large number of inherited or acquired deficits in any of the components of the immune system can cause an impaired immune response with increased susceptibility to infection (Table 8.4). A primary lack of T cells (as in AIDS) leads not only to bacterial infections, but also to viral, protozoal, fungal and mycobacterial infections. In some cases, however, lack of specific subsets of T cells which control B-cell maturation may lead to a secondary lack of B-cell

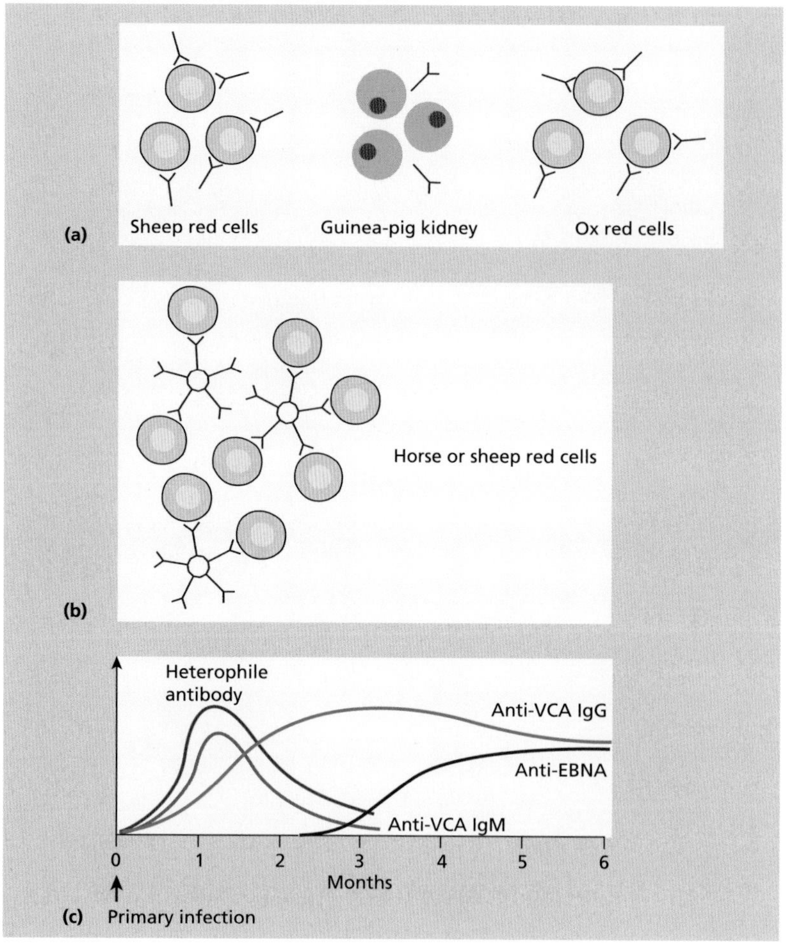

Fig. 8.12 Serological diagnosis of acute Epstein–Barr virus (EBV) infection. **(a)** IgM heterophile antibodies (shown here as antibody monomers for ease of illustration) against sheep red cells are used in the Paul–Bunnell test. These are not absorbed out by guinea-pig kidney but do react with ox red cells. A positive Paul–Bunnell test should show a titre of sheep red cell agglutination that is at least fourfold lower after absorption with ox red cells but not greater than threefold lower after absorption with guinea-pig kidney. **(b)** The commonly used monospot test detects agglutination of sheep red cells or formalized horse red cells only. **(c)** After acute infection heterophile and EBV-specific IgM are present for approximately 3 months. IgG antibodies to viral capsid antigen (VCA) and EBV nuclear antigen (EBNA) remain elevated for years.

Table 8.4 Classification of immunodeficiencies.

Primary	
B cell (antibody deficiency)	X-linked agammaglobulinaemia, acquired common variable hypogammaglobulinaemia, selective IgA or IgG subclass deficiencies
T cell	Thymic aplasia (DiGeorge's syndrome), PNP deficiency
Mixed B and T cell	Severe combined immune deficiency (as a result of ADA deficiency or other causes); Bloom's syndrome; ataxia-telangiectasia; Wiskott–Aldrich syndrome
Secondary	
B cell (antibody deficiency)	Myeloma; nephrotic syndrome, protein-losing enteropathy
T cell	AIDS; Hodgkin's lymphoma, non-Hodgkin's lymphoma; drugs: steroids, ciclosporin, azathioprine, fludarabine, etc.
T and B cell	Chronic lymphocytic leukaemia, post-bone marrow transplantation and post-chemotherapy/radiotherapy

ADA, adenosine deaminase; AIDS, acquired immune deficiency syndrome; Ig, immunoglobulin; PNP, purine nucleoside phosphorylase.

function as in many cases of common variable immunodeficiency, which may develop in children or adults of either sex. In others, a primary defect of B cells or of APCs is present. X-linked agammaglobulinaemia is caused by a failure of B-cell development and pyogenic bacterial infections dominate the clinical course. Immunoglobulin replacement therapy can be given by monthly courses of intravenous immunoglobulin. Rare syndromes include aplasia of the thymus, severe combined (T and B) immunodeficiency as a result of adenosine deaminase deficiency and selective deficiencies of IgA or IgM. Acquired immune deficiency occurs after cytotoxic chemotherapy or radiotherapy and is particularly pronounced after stem cell transplantation where dysregulation of the immune system persists for 1 year or more and is responsible for a high incidence of serious viral infections (e.g. with cytomegalovirus or herpes zoster). Immunodeficiency is also frequently associated with tumours of the lymphoid system including chronic lymphocytic leukaemia and myeloma.

Differential diagnosis of lymphadenopathy

The principal causes of lymphadenopathy are listed in Fig. 8.13. The clinical history and examination give essential information. The age of the patient, length of history, associated symptoms of possible infectious or malignant disease, whether the nodes are painful or tender, consistency of the nodes and whether there is generalized or local lymphadenopathy are all important. The size of the liver and spleen are assessed. In the case of local node enlargement, inflammatory or malignant disease in the associated lymphatic drainage area are particularly considered.

Localized

Local infection
- pyogenic infection, e.g. pharyngitis, dental abscess, otitis media, actinomyces
- viral infection
- cat scratch fever
- lymphogranuloma venereum
- tuberculosis

Lymphoma
- Hodgkin's lymphoma
- non-Hodgkin's lymphoma

Carcinoma (secondary)

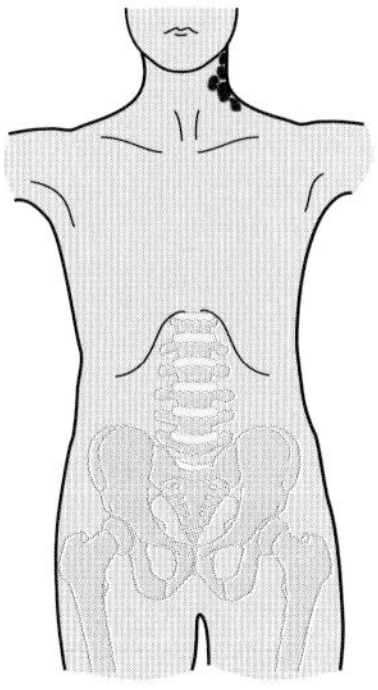

Generalized

Infection
- viral, e.g. infectious mononucleosis, measles, rubella, viral hepatitis, HIV
- bacterial, e.g. syphilis, brucellosis,tuberculosis, *Salmonella*, bacterial endocarditis
- fungal, e.g. histoplasmosis
- protozoal, e.g. toxoplasmosis

Non-infectious inflammatory diseases, e.g. sarcoidosis, rheumatoid arthritis, SLE, other connective tissue diseases, serum sickness

Malignant
- leukaemias, especially CLL, ALL
- lymphoma: non-Hodgkin's lymphoma, Hodgkin's lymphoma
- Waldenström's macroglobulinaemia
- rarely secondary carcinoma
- angioimmunoblastic lymphadenopathy

Miscellaneous
- sinus histocytosis with massive lymphadenopathy
- reaction to drugs and chemicals, e.g. hydantoins and related chemicals, beryllium
- hyperthyroidism

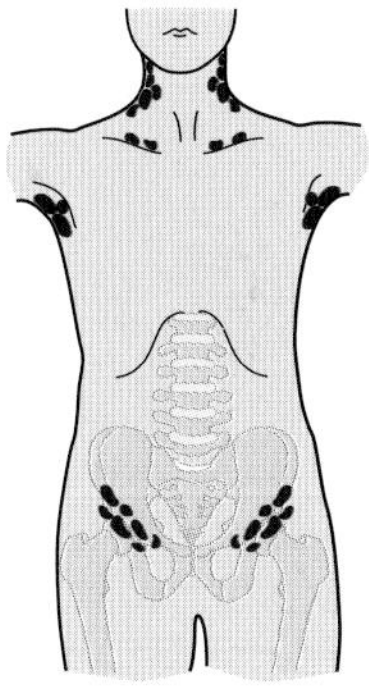

Fig. 8.13 Causes of lymphadenopathy. ALL, acute lymphoblastic leukaemia; CLL, chronic lymphocytic leukaemia; SLE, systemic lupus erythematosus. Malignancies are listed in red.

Further investigations will depend on the initial clinical diagnosis but it is usual to include a full blood count, blood film and erythrocyte sedimentation rate (ESR). Chest X-ray, monospot test, cytomegalovirus and *Toxoplasma* titres, and anti-HIV and Mantoux (Heaf) tests are frequently needed. In many cases, it will be essential to make a histological diagnosis by node biopsy but a fine needle aspirate may sometimes avoid the need for this. Computed tomography (CT) scanning is valuable in determining the presence and extent of deep node enlargement. Subsequent investigations will depend on the diagnosis made and the patient's particular features. In some cases of deep node enlargement, where enlarged superficial nodes are not available for biopsy, bone marrow, liver biopsies, CT or ultrasound guided trucut node biopsy may be needed in an attempt to reach a histological diagnosis and avoid the need for a diagnostic laparotomy.

Bibliography

Hsu K.C. and Dupont B. (2005) Natural killer cell receptors: regulating innate immune responses to hematologic malignancy. *Semin Hematol* **42**,91–103.

Janeway C.A., Travers P., Walport M., Shlomchik M.J. (eds) (2004) *Immunobiology*, 6th edn. Garland Science, New York and Oxford.

Krogsgaard M. and Davis M.M. (2005) How T cells 'see' antigen. *Nat Immunol* **3**,239–45.

Randolph G.J., Angeli V., Swartz M.A. (2005) Dendritic-cell trafficking to lymph nodes through lymphatic vessels. *Nat Rev Immunol* **8**,617–28.

Webster A.D.B. (2005) Immunodeficiency diseases. In: Hoffbrand A.V., Catovsky D., Tuddenham E.G.D. (eds) *Postgraduate Haematology*, 5th edn. Blackwell Publishing, Oxford: 370–9.

CHAPTER 9

9 The spleen

The spleen has an important and unique role in the function of the haemopoietic and immune systems. As well as being directly involved in many diseases of these systems, a number of important clinical features are associated with hypersplenic and hyposplenic states.

The anatomy and circulation of the spleen

The spleen lies under the left costal margin, has a normal weight of 150–250 g and a length of between 5 and 13 cm. It is normally not palpable but becomes palpable when the size is increased to over 14 cm.

Blood enters the spleen through the splenic artery which then divides into ***trabecular arteries*** which permeate the organ and give rise to ***central arterioles*** (Fig. 9.1). The majority of the arterioles end in ***cords*** which lack an endothelial lining and form an open blood system unique to the spleen with a loose reticular connective tissue network lined by fibroblasts and many macrophages. The blood re-enters the circulation by passing across the endothelium into venous ***sinuses.*** Blood then passes into the splenic vein and so back into the general circulation. The cords and sinuses form the ***red pulp*** which forms 75% of the spleen and has an essential role in monitoring the integrity of red blood cells (see below). A minority of the splenic vasculature is closed in which the arterial and venous systems are connected by a continuous endothelial layer.

The central arterioles are surrounded by a core of lymphatic tissue known as ***white pulp*** which has an organization similar to lymph nodes (Fig. 9.1). The ***periarteriolar lymphatic sheath*** (PALS) lies directly around the arteriole and is equivalent to the T zone of the lymph node (p. 116). B cell follicles are found adjacent to the PALS and these are surrounded by the ***marginal zone*** and ***perifollicular zone*** which are rich in macrophages and dendritic cells. Lymphocytes migrate into white pulp from the sinuses of the red pulp or from vessels that end directly in the marginal and perifollicular zones.

There are both rapid (1–2 min) and slow (30–60 min) blood circulations through the spleen. The slow circulation becomes increasingly important in splenomegaly.

The functions of the spleen

The spleen is the largest filter of the blood in the body and several of its functions are derived from this.

Control of red cell integrity

The spleen has an essential role in the 'quality control' of red cells. Excess DNA, nuclear remnants (Howell–Jolly bodies) and siderotic granules are

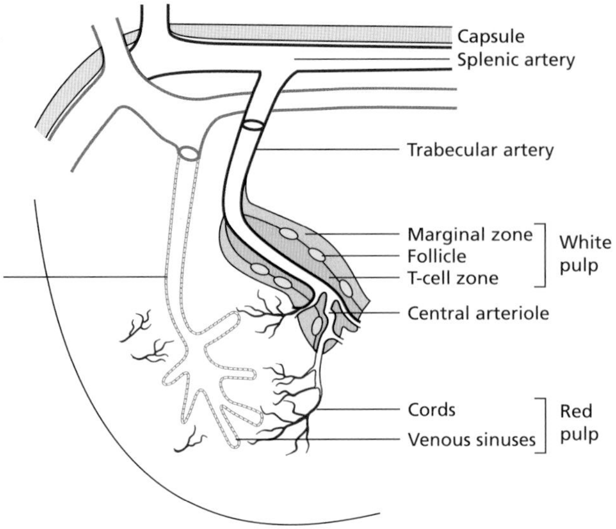

Fig. 9.1 Schematic representation of the blood circulation in the spleen. Most blood flows in an 'open' circulation through splenic cords and regains entry into the circulation through the venous sinuses.

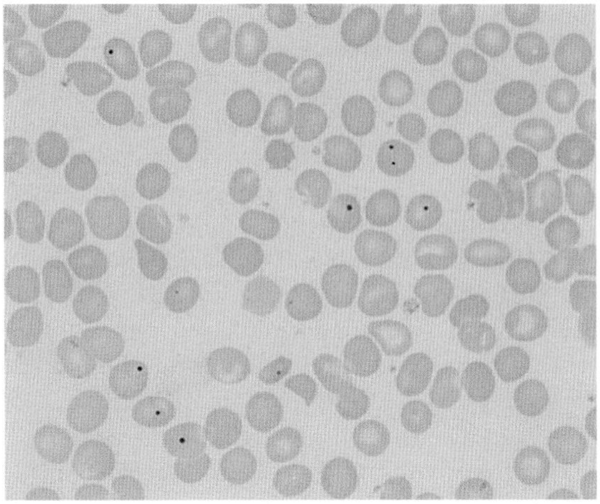

Fig. 9.2 Splenic atrophy: peripheral blood film showing Howell–Jolly bodies, Pappenheimer bodies (siderotic granules; see p. 25) and misshapen cells.

removed (Fig. 9.2). Aged or abnormal red cells are also removed from the circulation. In the relatively hypoxic environment of the red pulp, and because of plasma skimming in the cords, the membrane flexibility of aged and abnormal red cells is impaired and they are retained within the sinus where they are ingested by macrophages.

Immune function

The lymphoid tissue in the spleen is in a unique position to respond to antigens filtered from the blood and entering the white pulp. Macrophages and dendritic cells in the marginal zone initiate an immune response and then present antigen to B and T cells to start adaptive immune responses. This arrangement is highly efficient at initiating immune responses to encapsulated bacteria and explains the susceptibility of hyposplenic patients to these organisms.

Extramedullary haemopoiesis

The spleen, like the liver, undergoes a transient period of haemopoiesis at around 3–7 months of fetal life but is not a site of erythropoiesis in the adult. However, haemopoiesis may be re-established in both organs as ***extramedually haemopoiesis***, in disorders such as myelofibrosis or in chronic severe haemolytic and megaloblastic anaemias. Extramedullary haemopoiesis may result either from reactivation of dormant stem cells within the spleen or homing of stem cells from the bone marrow to the spleen.

Imaging the spleen

Ultrasound is the most frequently used technique to image the spleen (Fig. 9.3). This can also detect whether or not blood flow in the splenic, portal and hepatic veins is normal, as well as liver size and consistency. Computed tomography (CT) is preferable for detecting structural detail and any associated lymphadenopathy (e.g. for lymphoma staging). Magnetic resonance imaging (MRI) also gives improved fine detail structure. Positron emission tomography (PET) is used particularly for detecting residual disease after treatment of lymphoma.

Splenomegaly

Splenic size is increased in a wide range of conditions (Table 9.1). Splenomegaly is usually apparent under the left costal margin but massive splenomegaly may be felt in the right iliac fossa (see Fig. 19.4). The spleen moves with respiration and a medial splenic notch may be palpable in some cases. In developed countries the most common causes of splenomegaly are infectious mononucleosis, haematological malignancy and portal hypertension, whereas malaria and schistosomiasis are more prevalent on a global scale (Table 9.1). Chronic myeloid leukaemia, myelofibrosis, lymphoma, Gaucher's disease, malaria, leishmaniasis and schistosomiasis are potential causes of massive splenomegaly.

Tropical splenomegaly syndrome

A syndrome of massive splenomegaly of uncertain aetiology has been found frequently in many malarious zones of the tropics including Uganda, Nigeria, New Guinea and the Congo. Smaller numbers of patients with this disorder are seen in southern

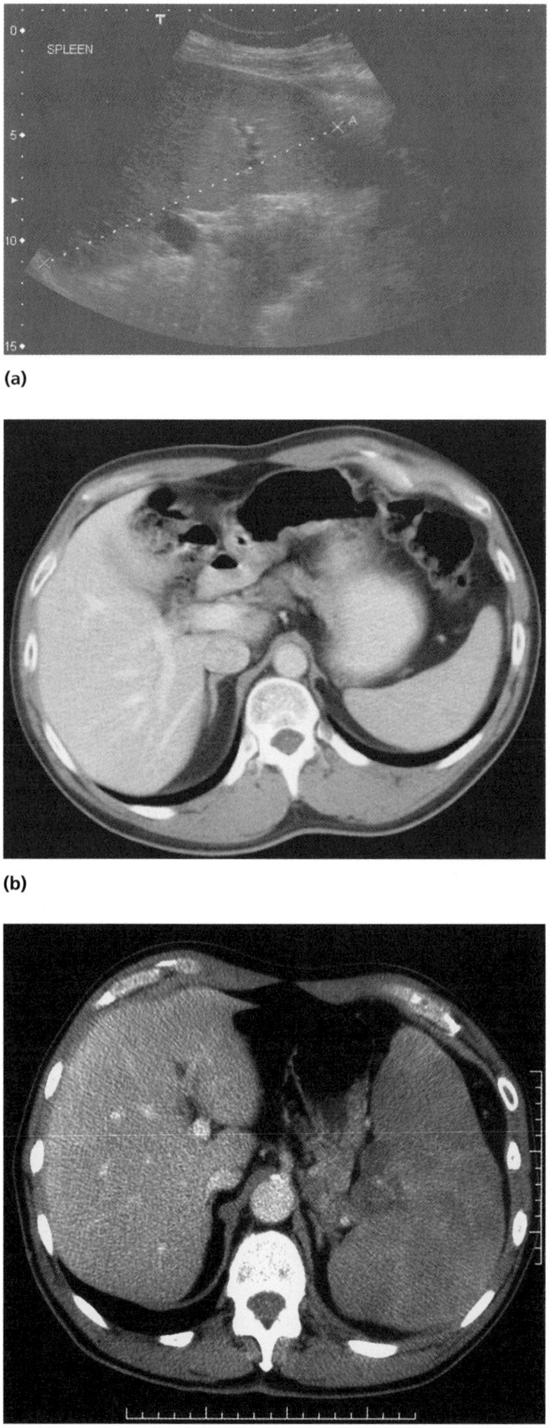

(a)

(b)

(c)

Fig. 9.3 Imaging the spleen. **(a)** Ultrasound of spleen showing splenomegaly (15.3 cm). **(b)** Normal spleen (10 cm) on computed tomography (CT) scan. **(c)** CT scan: The spleen is enlarged and shows multiple low density areas. A diagnosis of diffuse large cell B lymphoma was made histologically after splenectomy. (Figs (a) and (b) courtesy of Dr T. Ogunremi)

Table 9.1 Causes of splenomegaly.

Haematological
Chronic myeloid leukaemia*
Chronic lymphocytic leukaemia
Acute leukaemia
Malignant lymphoma*
Chronic myelofibrosis*
Polycythaemia vera
Hairy cell leukaemia
Thalassaemia major or intermedia*
Sickle cell anaemia (before splenic infarction)
Haemolytic anaemias
Megaloblastic anaemia
Portal hypertension
Cirrhosis
Hepatic, portal, splenic vein thrombosis
Storage diseases
Gaucher's disease*
Niemann–Pick disease
Histiocytosis X
Systemic diseases
Sarcoidosis
Amyloidosis
Collagen diseases—systemic lupus erythematosus, rheumatoid arthritis
Systemic mastocytosis
Infections
Acute: septicaemia, bacterial endocarditis, typhoid, infectious mononucleosis
Chronic: tuberculosis, brucellosis, syphilis, malaria, leishmaniasis,* schistosomiasis*
*Tropical**
Possibly caused by malaria

* Possible causes of massive (>20 cm) splenomegaly.

Arabia, the Sudan and Zambia. Previously, such terms as 'big spleen disease', 'cryptogenic splenomegaly' and 'African macroglobulinaemia' have been used to describe this syndrome.

While it seems probable that malaria is the fundamental cause of tropical splenomegaly syndrome, this disease is not the result of active malarial infection as parasitaemia is usually scanty and malarial pigment is not found in biopsy material from the liver and spleen. The available evidence suggests that an abnormal host response to the continual presence of malarial antigen results in a reactive and relatively benign lymphoproliferative disorder that predominantly affects the liver and spleen.

Splenomegaly is usually gross and the liver is also enlarged. Portal hypertension may be a feature. The anaemia is often severe and the lowest haemoglobin levels are found in subjects with the largest spleens. While leucopenia is usual, some patients develop a marked lymphocytosis. The moderate degree of thrombocytopenia present does not often cause spontaneous bleeding. Serum IgM levels are high and fluorescent techniques reveal high titres of malarial antibody.

Although splenectomy corrects the pancytopenia, there is an increased risk of fulminant malarial infection. Trials of antimalarial prophylaxis (e.g. proguanil and other antimalarial drugs) have proved successful in the management of many affected patients, supporting the view that a continuing presence of malarial antigen is needed for the perpetuation of the lymphoproliferation associated with this syndrome. Resistant cases have also been treated successfully with chemotherapy.

Hypersplenism

Normally, only approximately 5% (30–70 mL) of the total red cell mass is present in the spleen although up to half of the total marginating neutrophil pool and 30% of the platelet mass may be located there. As the spleen enlarges, the proportion of haemopoietic cells within the organ increases such that up to 40% of the red cell mass, and 90% of platelets (Fig. 23.9), may be pooled in an enlarged spleen. ***Hypersplenism*** is a clinical syndrome that can be seen in any form of splenomegaly. It is characterized by:

- Enlargement of the spleen;
- Reduction of at least one cell line in the blood in the presence of normal bone marrow function; and
- Evidence of increased release of premature cells, such as reticulocytes or immature platelets, from the bone marrow into the blood.

Splenectomy may be indicated if the hypersplenism is symptomatic. It is followed by a rapid improvement in the peripheral blood count.

Table 9.2 Causes of hyposplenism and blood film features.

Causes	Blood film features
Splenectomy Sickle cell disease Essential thrombocythaemia Adult gluten-induced enteropathy Dermatitis herpetiformis Rarely inflammatory bowel disease splenic arterial venous thrombosis	*Red cells* Target cells Acanthocytes Irregularly contracted or crenated cells Howell–Jolly bodies (DNA remnants) Siderotic (iron) granules (Pappenheimer bodies) *White cells* ± Mild lymphocytosis, monocytosis *Platelets* ± Thrombocytosis

Hyposplenism

Functional hyposplenism is revealed by the blood film findings of Howell–Jolly bodies or Pappenheimer bodies (siderotic granules on iron staining; Fig. 9.2). The most obvious cause is surgical removal of the spleen but hyposplenism can also occur in sickle cell anaemia, gluten-induced enteropathy, inflammatory bowel disease and splenic arterial thrombosis (Table 9.2).

Splenectomy

Surgical removal of the spleen may be indicated for treatment of haematological disorders as well as after splenic rupture or for splenic tumours or cysts (Table 9.3). Splenectomy is usually performed by open abdominal laparotomy but it is also possible to remove the spleen by laparoscopic surgery.

The platelet count can often rise dramatically in the early postoperative period, reaching levels of up to 1000×10^9/L and peaking at 1–2 weeks. Thrombotic complications are seen in some patients and prophylactic aspirin or heparin are often required during this period. Long-term alterations in the peripheral blood cell count may also be seen, including a persistent thrombocytosis, lymphocytosis or monocytosis.

Table 9.3 Indications for splenectomy.

Splenic rupture
Chronic immune thrombocytopenia
Haemolytic anaemia (some cases), e.g. hereditary spherocytosis, autoimmune haemolytic anaemia, thalassaemia major or intermedia
Chronic lymphocytic leukaemia and lymphomas
Myelofibrosis
Tropical splenomegaly

Prevention of infection in hyposplenic patients

Patients with hyposplenism are at lifelong increased risk of infection from a variety of organisms. This is seen particularly in children under the age of 5 years and those with sickle cell anaemia. The most characteristic susceptibility is to encapsulated bacteria such as *Streptococcus pneumoniae*, *Haemophilus influenzae* type B and *Neisseria meningitidis*. *Streptococcus pneumoniae* is a particular concern and can cause a rapid and fulminant disease. Malaria tends to be more severe in splenectomized individuals. Measures to reduce the risk of serious infection include the following:

1 The patient should be informed about the increased susceptibility to infection and advised to carry

Table 9.4 Recommendations for vaccination of patients with hyposplenism.

Vaccine	Time of vaccination	Revaccination schedule	Comments
1 Pneumoccal polyvalent vaccine	If possible, at least 2 weeks prior to splenectomy. Alternatively, 2 weeks post-splenectomy for all 3 vaccines	5 yearly	Assessment of antibody response may be useful
2 Haemophilus influenzae Type b conjugate		Not required	
3 Meningococcal C conjugate		Not required	Not required if previously vaccinated
4 Influenza	As soon as available for seasonal protection	Annual	Standard killed vaccine

a card about their condition. They should be counselled about the increased risk of infection on foreign travel, including that from malaria and tick bites.

2 Prophylactic oral phenoxymethylpenicillin is recommended for life. Erythromycin may be prescribed for patients allergic to penicillin. A supply of tablets may also be given to the patient to take in the event of onset of fever before medical care is available.

3 Vaccination against pneumococcus, haemophilus, meningococcus and influenza infection is recommended (Table 9.4). All types of vaccine, including live vaccines, can be given safely to hyposplenic individuals although the immune response to vaccination may be impaired.

Bibliography

Bowdler A.J. (ed.) (2002) *The Complete Spleen: Structure, Function and Clinical Disorders*, 2nd edn. Humana Press, Towota, NJ.

Davies J.M., Barnes R., Milligan D. *et al.* for the British Committee for Standards in Haematology. Working Party of the Haematology/Oncology Task Force. (2002) Update of guidelines for the prevention and treatment of infection in patients with an absent or dysfunctional spleen. *Clin Med* **2**,440–3.

Giebink G.S. (2001) The prevention of pneumococcal disease in children. *N Engl J Med* **345**,1177–83.

Mebius R.E. and Kraal G. (2005) Structure and function of the spleen. *Nat Rev Immunol* **5**,606–16.

Shadbolt C. and Peters A.M. (2003) The spleen. In: Peters A.M. (ed.) *Nuclear Medicine in Radiological Diagnosis*. Martin Dunitz, London.

CHAPTER 10

10 The aetiology and genetics of haematological malignancies

The haemopoietic malignancies are clonal diseases that derive from a single cell in the marrow or peripheral lymphoid tissue which has undergone a genetic alteration (Fig. 10.1). In this chapter we discuss the aetiology and genetic basis of haematological malignancy and subsequent chapters discuss the diagnosis and management of these conditions.

The aetiology of haemopoietic malignancy

Exactly how genetic mutations accumulate in haemopoietic malignancies is largely unknown. As in most diseases it is the combination of genetic background and environmental influence that determines the risk of developing a malignancy. However, in the majority of individual cases neither a genetic susceptibility nor an environmental agent is apparent.

Inherited factors

The incidence of leukaemia is greatly increased in some genetic diseases, particularly Down's syndrome (where acute leukaemia occurs with a 20–30-fold increased frequency), Bloom's syndrome, Fanconi's anaemia, ataxia telangiectasia, Klinefelter's syndrome and Wiskott–Aldrich syndrome. There is also a weak familial tendency in diseases such as acute myeloid leukaemia (AML), B-cell chronic lymphocytic leukaemia (CLL), Hodgkin's lymphoma and non-Hodgkin's lymphoma (NHL) although the genes predisposing to this risk are largely unknown.

Environmental influences

Chemicals

Chronic exposure to benzene may cause bone marrow hypoplasia, dysplasia and chromosome abnormalities and is an unusual cause of myelodysplasia or AML. Other industrial solvents and chemicals less commonly cause leukaemia.

Drugs

The alkylating agents (e.g. chlorambucil, mustine (chlormethine), melphalan, procarbazine and nitrosoureas—BCNU, CCNU) predispose to AML, especially if combined with radiotherapy or if used to treat patients with lymphocytic or plasmacytic disorders. Epipodophyllotoxins such as etoposide are powerful antileukaemic agents but their use is associated with a risk of the development of

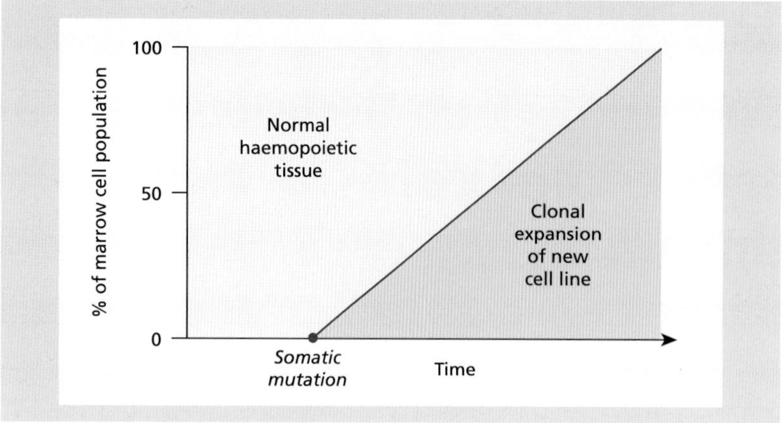

Fig. 10.1 Theoretical graph to show the replacement of normal bone marrow cells by a clonal population of malignant cells arising by successive mitotic divisions from a single cell with an acquired genetic alteration.

secondary leukaemias associated with balanced translocations including that of the *MLL* gene at 11q23.

Radiation

Radiation, especially to the marrow, is leukaemogenic. This is illustrated by an increased incidence of all types of leukaemia (except CLL) in survivors of the atom bomb explosions in Japan.

Infection

A proportion of cases of childhood acute lymphoblastic leukaemia (ALL) are initiated by genetic mutations that occur during development *in utero* (Fig. 10.2). Studies in identical twins have shown that both may be born with the same chromosomal abnormality (e.g. t(12; 21)). This has presumably arisen spontaneously in a progenitor cell that has

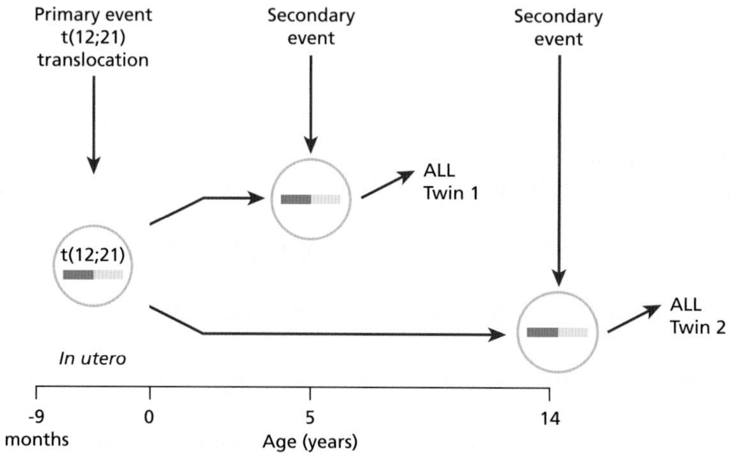

Fig. 10.2 Prenatal origin of acute lymphoblastic leukaemia (ALL) in a pair of identical twins. ALL was diagnosed in the first twin at age 5 years and in the second at age 14 years. Both tumours had an identical t(12; 21) translocation indicating probable origin of the leukaemic clone *in utero* and dissemination to both twins via a shared placental blood supply. Because of the prolonged latency of the ALL it is presumed that a secondary event is required to initiate the development of frank leukaemia. At the time of the diagnosis of ALL in twin 1 the t(12; 21) translocation could be detected in the bone marrow of twin 2. It is likely that such a 'fetal origin' of childhood ALL occurs in a significant number of sporadic ALL cases. (After J.L. Wiemels *et al*. 1999)

Table 10.1 Infections associated with haemopoietic malignancies.

Infection	Tumour
Virus	
HTLV-1	Adult T-cell leukaemia/lymphoma
Epstein–Barr virus	Burkitt's and Hodgkin's lymphomas; PTLD
HHV-8	Primary effusion lymphoma; multicentric Castleman's disease
HIV-1	High-grade B-cell lymphoma
Bacteria	
Helicobacter pylori	Gastric lymphoma (MALT)
Protozoa	
Malaria	Burkitt's lymphoma

HHV-8, human herpes virus 8; HIV, human immunodeficiency virus; HTLV-1, human T-lymphotropic virus type 1; MALT, mucosa-associated lymphoid tissue; PTLD, post-transplant lymphoproliferative disease.

passed from one twin to the other as a result of the shared placental circulation. Environmental exposure during pregnancy may be important for this first event. One twin may develop ALL early (e.g. at age 4) because of a second transforming event while the other remains well or develops ALL later. The *TEL-AML1* translocation is present in the blood of approximately 10% of newborn infants but only 1 in 100 of these go on to develop ALL at a later date. The mechanism of the 'second genetic hit' within the tumour cell is unclear but an abnormal response of the immune system to infection is suggested by epidemiological studies. Children with a high level of social activity, notably those attending early nursery daycare, have a reduced incidence of ALL, whereas those living in more isolated communities and who have a reduced exposure to common infections in the first years of life have a higher risk.

Viruses (Table 10.1)

Viral infection is associated with several types of haemopoietic malignancy. The retrovirus human T-lymphotropic virus type 1 (HTLV-1) is the cause of adult T-cell leukaemia/lymphoma (ATLL) (p. 214) although most people infected with this virus do not develop the tumour. Epstein–Barr virus (EBV) DNA is integrated into the genome of endemic (African) Burkitt's lymphoma cells but rarely in sporadic Burkitt's lymphoma cells. It is also the cause of post-transplant lymphoproliferative disease (PTLD) which develops during immunosuppressive therapy after solid organ transplantation, of many cases of lymphoma associated with HIV infection and is present in a proportion of patients with Hodgkin's disease. Human herpes virus 8 (HHV-8; Kaposi's sarcoma-associated virus (KSHV)) is associated with Kaposi's sarcoma and primary effusion lymphoma (PEL).

HIV infection is associated with an increased incidence of lymphomas at unusual sites such as the central nervous system. The HIV-associated lymphomas are usually of B-cell origin and of high-grade histology.

Bacteria

Helicobacter pylori infection has been implicated in the pathogenesis of gastric mucosa B-cell (MALT) lymphoma (p. 212).

Protozoa

Endemic Burkitt's lymphoma occurs in the tropics, particularly in malarial areas. It is thought that malaria may alter host immunity and predispose to tumour formation as a result of EBV infection.

The genetics of haemopoietic malignancy

Malignant transformation occurs as a result of the accumulation of genetic mutations in cellular genes. The genes that are involved in the development of

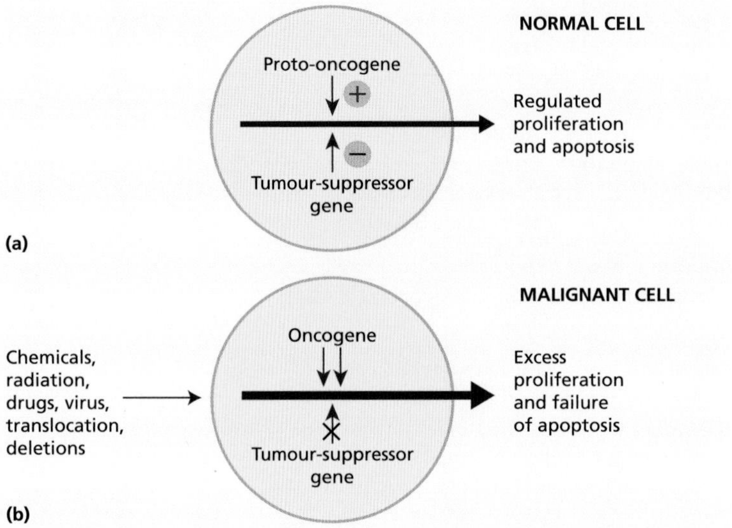

Fig. 10.3 Proliferation of normal cells depends on a balance between the action of proto-oncogenes **(a)** and tumour-suppressor genes **(b)**. In a malignant cell this balance is disturbed leading to uncontrolled cell division.

cancer can be divided broadly into two groups: ***oncogenes*** and ***tumour-suppressor genes***.

Oncogenes

Oncogenes arise because of gain-of-function mutations in normal cellular genes called ***proto-oncogenes*** (Fig. 10.3). Proto-oncogenes are involved in a variety of important cellular processes, often in the pathway by which external signals are transduced to the cell nucleus to activate genes. Oncogenic versions are generated when the activity of proto-oncogenes is increased or they acquire a novel function. This can occur in a number of ways including translocation, mutation or duplication. One of the striking features of haematological malignancies (in contrast to most solid tumours) is their high frequency of chromosomal translocations. A subset of proto-oncogenes are involved in control of apoptosis (e.g. *BCL-2* which is overexpressed in follicular lymphoma) (p. 209).

Tumour-suppressor genes

Tumour-suppressor genes may acquire loss-of-function mutations, usually by point mutation or deletion, which lead to malignant transformation (Fig. 10.3). Tumour-suppressor genes commonly act as components of control mechanisms which regulate entry of the cell from the G_1 phase of the cell cycle into the S phase or passage through the S phase to G_2 and mitosis (Fig. 1.8). Examples of oncogenes and tumour-suppressor genes involved in haemopoietic malignancies are shown in Table 10.2. The most significant tumour-suppressor gene in human cancer is p53 which is mutated or inactivated in over 50% of cases of malignant disease, including many haemopoietic tumours.

Clonal progression

Malignant cells appear to arise as a multistep process with acquisition of mutations in different intracellular pathways (Fig. 10.4). Another feature of malignancy is clonal progression. In many cases the disease develops new characteristics during its clinical course and this may be accompanied by new chromosome changes. Selection of subclones may occur during treatment or reflect disease acceleration. Drug resistance can arise through a variety of molecular mechanisms. In one example the cells express a protein that actively pumps a number of different drugs to the outside of the cells (multidrug resistance, MDR).

Table 10.2 Some of the more frequent genetic abnormalities in leukaemia, lymphoma and myeloproliferative diseases.

Disease	Genetic abnormality*	Oncogene(s) involved
Myeloid		
AML M_2	t(8; 21)	*ETO* and *CBF*α (*AML1*)
	t(6; 9)	*DEK, CAN*
AML M_3	t(15; 17)	*RAR*α*, PML*
AML M_4	inv(16), del(16q)	*CBF*β*, MYH11*
AML M_5	del(11q); t(9; 11); t(11; 19)	*MLL*
AML (all types)	Nucleotide insertion	Nucleophosmin
	Mutation, ITD	*Flt3*
MDS	–5/del(5q)	Unclear
	–7/del(7q)	
	Point mutation	*N-RAS*
Secondary myeloid leukaemia	11q23 translocations	*MLL* gene
CML	t(9; 22)	*ABL, BCR*
Myeloproliferative disease	Point mutation	*JAK2*
	20q–	
Chronic eosinophilic syndrome	4q12 del	*FIP1L1-PDGFRA* fusion
Lymphoid		
Precursor B lineage ALL	t(12; 21)	*TEL, AML1*
	t(4; 11)	*AF4, MLL* (*ALL1, HRX*)
	t(9; 22)	*ABL, BCR*
	t(1; 19)	*PBX-1, E2A*
	Hyperdiploidy	
	Hypodiploidy	
Burkitt's lymphoma, B-ALL	t(8; 14)†	*MYC* to *IgH* locus
	t(2; 8)	*MYC* to *IgK* locus
	t(8; 22)	*MYC* to *Ig*λ locus
T-ALL	t(1; 14)	*TAL-1* to *TCR*δ locus
	t(8; 14)†	*MYC*
	t(11; 14)	*RBTN-1* or *RBTN-2*
	t(7; 9)	*TAL-2* to *TCR*β locus
Follicular lymphoma	t(14; 18)	*BCL-2* to *IgH*
Anaplastic lymphoma	t(2; 5)	*ALK* to *NPM*
Mantle cell lymphoma	t(11; 14)†	*BCL-1* (cyclin D1) to *IgH*
	Mutation	p53 and *ATM*
CLL	Trisomy 12	Unknown
	13q14 deletion	Unknown
	11q22–23 deletion or mutation	*ATM*
	17p deletion or mutation	*p53*
	6q21 deletion	Unknown
MALT B-cell lymphoma	t(1; 14)	*BCL10* to *IgH* locus
T-PLL	inv(14q) or t(14q)	
	Mutations	*ATM*

ALL, acute lymphoblastic leukaemia; AML, acute myeloid leukaemia; CLL, chronic lymphocytic leukaemia; CML, chronic myeloid leukaemia; ITD, internal tandem duplication; MALT, mucosa-associated lymphoid tissue; MDS, myelodysplasia; PLL, prolymphocytic leukaemia.

* Several chromosomal abnormalities may occur in patients with many of the conditions listed (e.g. *Flt-3* mutation occurs in 30% of AML cases with or without chromosome translocations).

† The breakpoints on chromosome 14 are in different positions in T-ALL, B-ALL, mantle cell lymphoma and Burkitt's lymphoma.

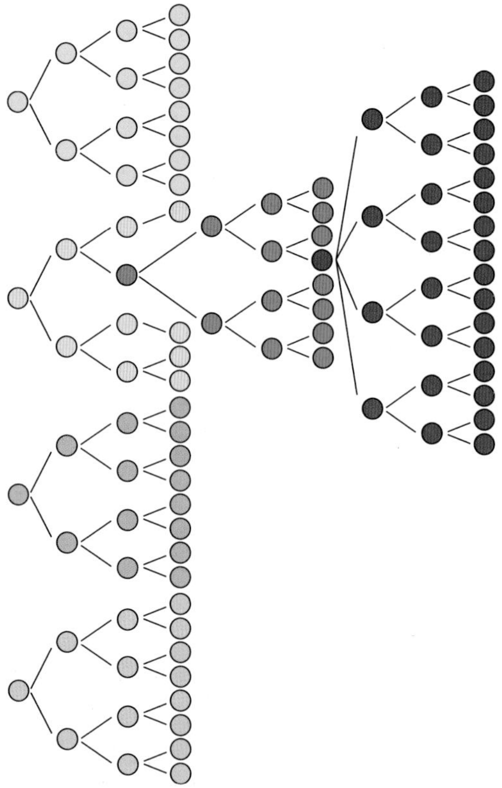

Fig. 10.4 Multistep origin of a malignant tumour. Successive mutations lead to a growth advantage of one subclone.

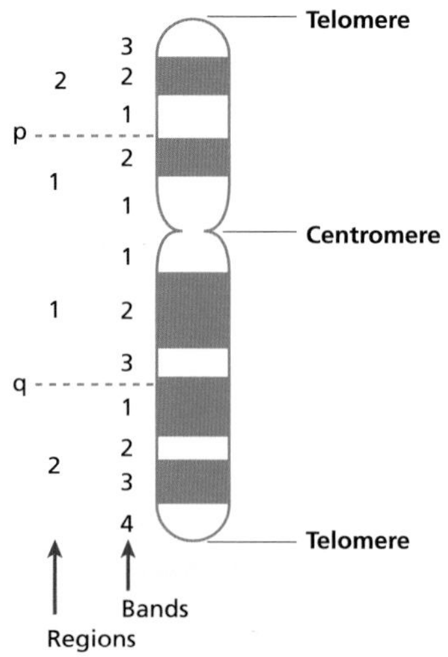

Fig. 10.5 A schematic representation of a chromosome. The bands may be divided into subbands according to staining pattern.

Chromosome nomenclature

The normal somatic cell has 46 chromosomes and is called *diploid*; ova or sperm have 23 chromosomes and are called *haploid*. The chromosomes occur in pairs and are numbered 1–22 in decreasing size order; there are two sex chromosomes, XX in females, XY in males. *Karyotype* is the term used to describe the chromosomes derived from a mitotic cell which have been set out in numerical order (see Fig. 13.1d). A somatic cell with more or less than 46 chromosomes is termed *aneuploid*; more than 46 is *hyperdiploid*, less than 46 *hypodiploid*; 46 but with chromosome rearrangements, *pseudodiploid*.

Each chromosome has two arms, the shorter called 'p', the longer called 'q'. These meet at the *centromere* and the ends of the chromosomes are called *telomeres*. On staining each arm divides into regions numbered outwards from the centromere and each region divides into bands (Fig. 10.5).

When a whole chromosome is lost or gained, a – or + is put in front of the chromosome number. If part of the chromosome is lost it is prefixed with del for deletion. If there is extra material replacing part of a chromosome the prefix add for additional material is used. Chromosome translocations are denoted by t, the chromosomes involved placed in brackets with the lower numbered chromosome first. The prefix inv describes an inversion where part of the chromosome has been inverted to run in the opposite direction. An *isochromosome*, denoted by i, describes a chromosome with identical chromosome arms at each end; for example, i(17q) would consist of two copies of 17q joined at the centromere.

Telomeres

Telomeres are repetitive sequences at the ends of chromosomes. They decrease by approximately 200 base pairs of DNA with every round of replication. When they decrease to a critical length, the cell exits from cell cycle. Germ cells and stem cells, which need to self-renew and maintain a high proliferative potential, contain the enzyme *telomerase* which can add extensions to the telomeric repeats and compensate for loss at replication and so enable the cells to continue proliferation. Telomerase is also often expressed in malignant cells but this is probably a consequence of the malignant transformation rather than an initiating factor.

Genetic abnormalities associated with haematological malignancies

Some of the genetic abnormalities commonly associated with different types of leukaemia and lymphoma are listed in Table 10.2. The types of gene abnormality include the following (Fig. 10.6).

Point mutation

This is best illustrated by the Val617Phe mutation in the *JAK2* gene which leads to constitutive activation of the JAK2 protein in most cases of myeloproliferative disease (Chapter 19). Mutations within the *RAS* oncogenes or p53 tumour-suppressor gene are common in many haemopoietic malignancies. The point mutation may involve several base pairs. In 35% of cases of AML the *nucleophosmin* gene shows an insertion of 4 base pairs resulting in a frameshift change. Internal tandem duplication or point mutations occur in the *Flt-3* gene in 30% of cases of AML.

Translocations

These are a characteristic feature of haematological malignancies and there are two main mechanisms whereby they may contribute to malignant change (Fig. 10.7).

1 Fusion of parts of two genes to generate a chimeric fusion gene that encodes a novel ***'fusion protein'***, e.g. *BCR-ABL* in t(9; 22) in chronic myeloid leukaemia (CML) (see Fig. 13.1), *RARα-PML* in t(15; 17) in AML M_3 (Fig. 10.8) or *TEL-AML1* in t(12; 21) in precursor B-ALL (Fig. 10.9).

2 Overexpression of a normal cellular gene; for example, overexpression of *BCL-2* in the t(14; 18) translocation of follicular lymphoma or of *MYC* in Burkitt's lymphoma (Fig. 10.10). Interestingly, this class of translocation nearly always involves a *TCR* or immunoglobulin gene locus, presumably as a result of aberrant activity of the recombinase enzyme which is involved in immunoglobulin or *TCR* gene rearrangement in immature B or T cells.

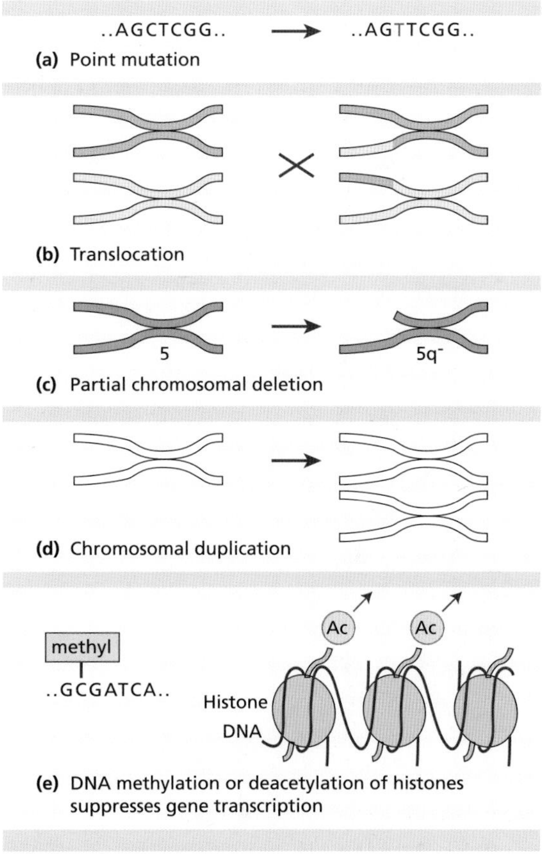

Fig. 10.6 Types of genetic abnormality which may lead to haemopoietic malignancy. **(a)** Point mutation; **(b)** chromosomal translocation; **(c)** chromosomal deletion or loss; **(d)** chromosomal duplication; **(e)** DNA methylation or deacetylation of histone tails suppresses gene transcription.

Deletions

Chromosomal deletions may involve a small part of a chromosome, the short or long arm (e.g. 5q–) (Fig. 10.12b) or the entire chromosome (e.g. monosomy 7). Losses most commonly affect chromosomes 5, 6, 7, 11, 20 and Y. The critical event is probably loss of a tumoursuppressor gene or of a microRNA as in the 13q14 deletion in CLL (see below).

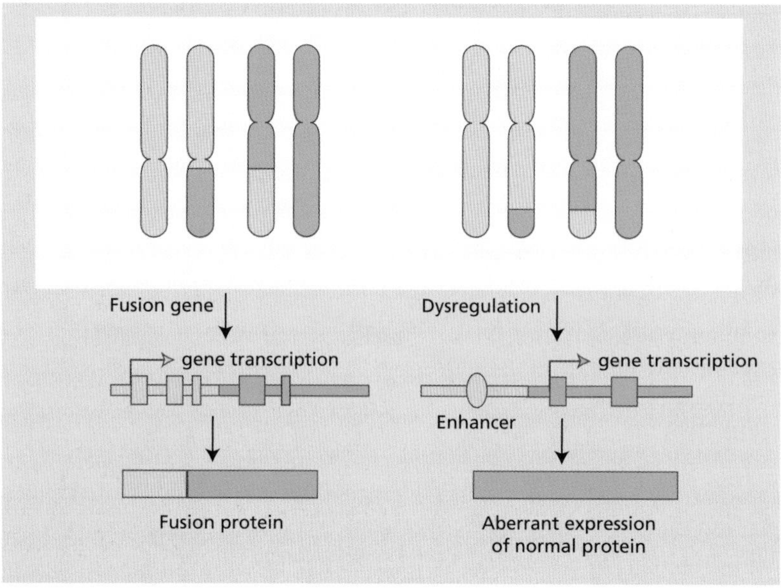

Fig. 10.7 The two possible mechanisms by which chromosomal translocations can lead to expression of an oncogene.

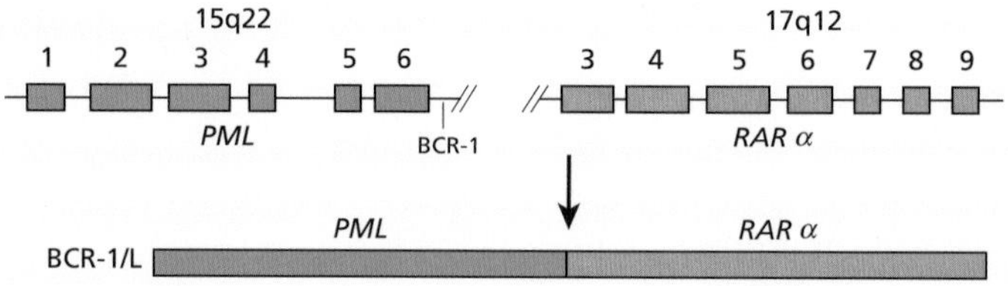

Fig. 10.8 Generation of the t(15; 17) translocation. The *PML* gene at 15q22 may break at one of three different breakpoint cluster regions (BCR-1, -2 and -3) and joins with exons 3–9 of the *RARα* gene at 17q12. Three different fusion mRNAs are generated (termed long (L), variable (V) or short (S)) and these give rise to fusion proteins of different size. In this diagram only the long version resulting from a break at BCR-1 is shown.

Duplication or amplification

In chromosomal duplication (e.g. trisomy 12 in CLL) or gene amplification, gains are common in chromosomes 8, 12, 19, 21 and Y. Gene amplification is not a common feature in haemopoietic malignancy but has been described involving the *MLL* gene.

Epigenetic alterations

Gene expression may be dysregulated in cancer, not only by structural changes to the genes themselves but also by alterations in the mechanism by which genes are transcribed. These changes are called ***epigenetic*** and are stably inherited with each cell division so they are passed on as the malignant cell divides. The most important mechanisms are methylation of cytosine residues in DNA and enzymatic alterations, such as acetylation or methylation, of the histone proteins that package DNA within the cell (Fig. 10.6e). Demethylating agents such as azacytidine increase gene transcription and are finding a role in the management of haemopoietic malignant disease.

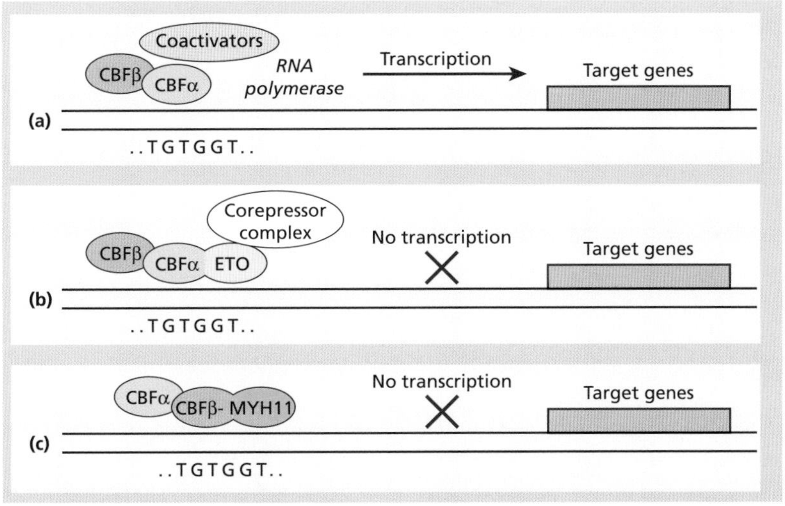

Fig. 10.9 Mechanism of action of the core binding factor (CBF) transcription factor and its disruption in acute myeloid leukaemia. CBF consists of two subunits, *CBFβ* and *CBFα* (or *AML1*), which together form a heterodimer **(a)**. This complex binds to the DNA sequence TGTGGT in the regulatory region of certain target genes. This binding allows recruitment of coactivators which lead to transcription from these genes. **(b)** The t(8; 21) translocation leads to a fusion protein of CBFα with ETO. Although the CBF subunits can still form heterodimers, their binding to DNA leads to recruitment of a co-repressor complex which blocks transcription. **(c)** In the inv(16) mutation, a CBFα-MYH10 fusion protein is generated which again can form CBF heterodimers but these do not gain access to DNA.

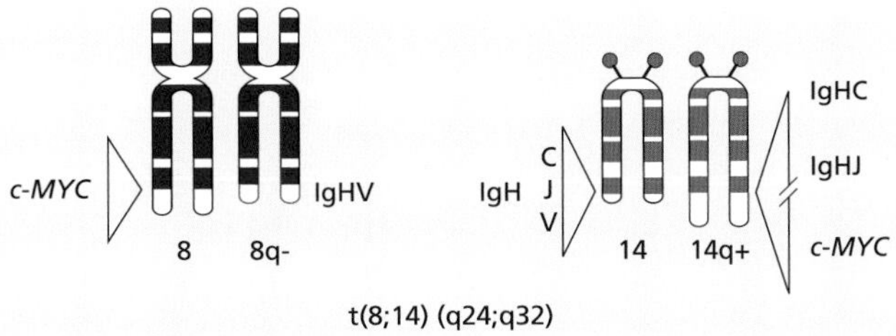

Fig. 10.10 The genetic events in one of the three translocations found in Burkitt's lymphoma and B-cell acute lymphoblastic leukaemia. The oncogene *c-MYC* is normally located on the long arm (q) of chromosome 8. In the (8; 14) translocation, *c-MYC* is translocated into close proximity to the immunoglobulin heavy-chain gene on the long arm of chromosome 14. Part of the heavy-chain gene (the V region) is reciprocally translocated to chromosome 8. C, constant region; IgH, immunoglobulin heavy-chain gene; J, joining region; V, variable region.

MicroRNAs

Chromosomal abnormalities, both deletions and amplifications, can result in loss or gain of short (micro) RNA sequences. These are normally transcribed but not translated. MicroRNAs (miRNAs) control expression of adjacent or distally located genes. Deletion of the miR15a/miR16-1 locus may be relevant to CLL development with the common 13q deletion.

Specific examples of translocations associated with haematological malignancy

Philadelphia (Ph) chromosome

The translocation t(9; 22) which underlies Philadelphia chromosome positive chronic myeloid leukaemia (CML) and some cases of ALL is discussed in detail in Chapter 13.

Retinoic acid receptor

In the t(15; 17) translocation associated with AML M_3 (p. 158), the promyelocytic leukaemia gene *PML* on chromosome 15 is fused to the retinoic acid receptor α gene, *RARα*, on chromosome 17 (Fig. 10.8). The resultant PML-RARα fusion protein functions as a transcriptional repressor whereas normal (wild-type) *RARα* is an activator. Normally, the PML protein forms homodimers with itself whereas the RARα protein forms heterodimers with the retinoid X receptor protein, RXR. The PML-RARα fusion protein binds to PML and RXR, preventing them from linking with their natural partners. This results in the cellular phenotype of arrested differentiation. Cases of AML M_3 associated with the t(15; 17) translocation respond to treatment with high doses of all-*trans* retinoic acid (ATRA) which causes differentiation of the abnormal promyelocytes and results in improved prognosis (p. 170). Interestingly, in rare variants of AML M_3, *RARα* is fused to other genes and in these cases ATRA treatment is not successful.

Translocations involving the core binding factor genes

Core binding factor (CBF) is a heterodimeric transcription factor and is important in regulating expression of a number of genes such as *IL-3* and *GM-CSF*. Genes encoding the two components of CBF, *CBFα* and *CBFβ*, are involved in a number of chromosomal translocations associated with leukaemia (Fig. 10.9). These include t(8; 21) in which the *CBFα* gene, also known as *AML1*, is translocated to the *ETO* gene on chromosome 8. Another common rearrangement in AML is inv(16) in which the *CBFβ* gene is fused to the *SMMHC* (*MYH11*) gene. In the t(12; 21) translocation associated with pre-B-ALL the *TEL* gene is fused to the *CBFα* gene to generate a novel fusion protein. All three translocations appear to act as dominant inhibitors of normal wild-type CBF activity. They are all associated with a relatively good prognosis.

Translocation of *MYC*

In Burkitt's lymphoma and B-ALL one of three translocations is normally found. All of these bring the *MYC* oncogene into close proximity with one of the immunoglobulin genes (Fig. 10.10); the most frequent is translocation to the heavy-chain locus, t(8; 14). As a result, expression of the *MYC* gene is deregulated and the gene is expressed in parts of the cell cycle during which it should normally be switched off.

Translocation of the *BCL-2* gene

This oncogene is translocated from chromosome 18 to chromosome 14 in the (14; 18) translocation found in approximately 85% of cases of follicular lymphoma and in some cases of diffuse large cell lymphoma. The translocation leads to constitutive expression of the *BCL-2* gene with increased survival of cells because of reduced apoptosis.

Diagnostic methods used to study malignant cells

Karyotype analysis

Karyotype analysis involves direct morphological analysis of chromosomes from tumour cells under the microscope (Fig. 10.11; see Fig. 13.1). This requires tumour cells to be in metaphase and so cells are cultured to encourage cell division prior to chromosomal preparation.

Fluorescent *in situ* hybridization analysis

Fluorescent *in situ* hybridization (FISH) analysis involves the use of fluorescent-labelled genetic probes which hybridize to specific parts of the genome. It is possible to label each chromosome with a different

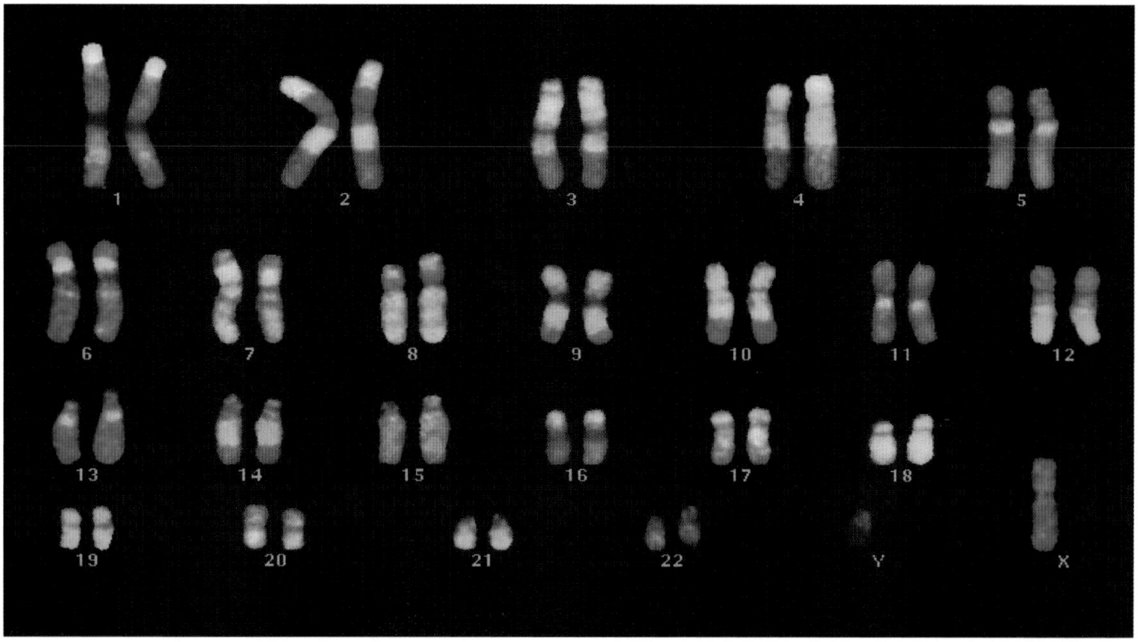

Fig. 10.11 A colour-banded karyotype from a normal male. Each chromosome pair shows an individual colour-banding pattern. This involves a cross-species multiple colour chromosome banding technique. Probe sets developed from the chromosomes of gibbons are combinatorially labelled and hybridized to human chromosomes. The success of cross-species colour banding depends on a close homology between host and human conserved DNA, divergence of repetitive DNA and a high degree of chromosomal rearrangement in the host relative to the human karyotype. (Courtesy of Dr C.J. Harrison)

combination of fluorescent labels (Fig. 10.12a). This is a sensitive technique that can detect extra copies of genetic material in both metaphase and interphase (non-dividing) cells (e.g. trisomy 12 in CLL) or, by using two different probes, reveal chromosomal translocations (Fig. 10.12c); for example, t(9;22) in CML (Fig. 13.1e) or reduced chromosome numbers or segments (e.g. monosomy 7 or 5 in myelodysplasia) (Fig. 10.12b).

Southern blot analysis

Southern blot analysis involves the extraction of DNA from leukaemic cells followed by restriction enzyme digestion, gel electrophoresis and transfer by 'blotting' to a suitable membrane. The DNA is then hybridized to a probe complementary to the gene of interest. When the probe recognizes a segment within the boundaries of a single restriction fragment one band is identified but if the gene has been translocated to a new area in the genome a novel band of different electrophoretic mobility is seen. Although time consuming and relatively insensitive, this remains a powerful technique.

Polymerase chain reaction

Polymerase chain reaction (PCR) (see Fig. 6.23) can be performed on blood or bone marrow for a number of specific translocations such as t(9;22) and t(15;17) (Fig. 10.13). It can also be used to detect 'clonal' cells of B- or T-cell lineage by immunoglobulin or T-cell receptor (TCR) gene rearrangement analysis. As it is relatively straightforward and extremely sensitive (detecting one abnormal cell in 10^5–10^6 normal cells), it has become of great value in the diagnosis and monitoring of minimal residual disease (p. 144).

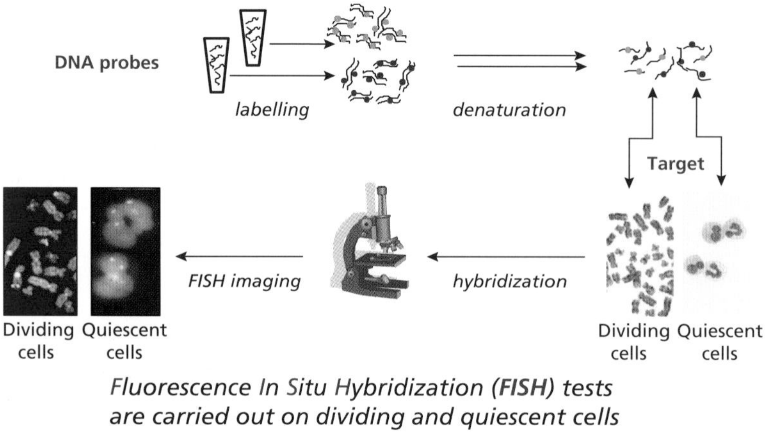

(a)

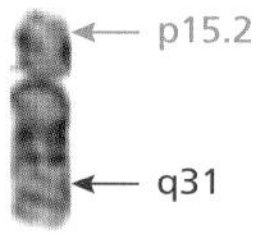

DNA probes from the short arm (control, in green) and the long arm (commonly deleted region in patients with leukemia, in red) of chromosome 5 are used for FISH analysis

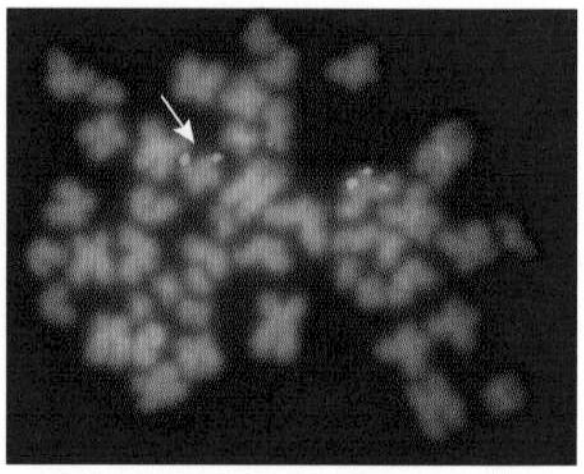

Missing red FISH signal (arrow) shows deletion of the long arm of chromosome 5, while the normal homologue 5 is marked by red & green signals

(b)

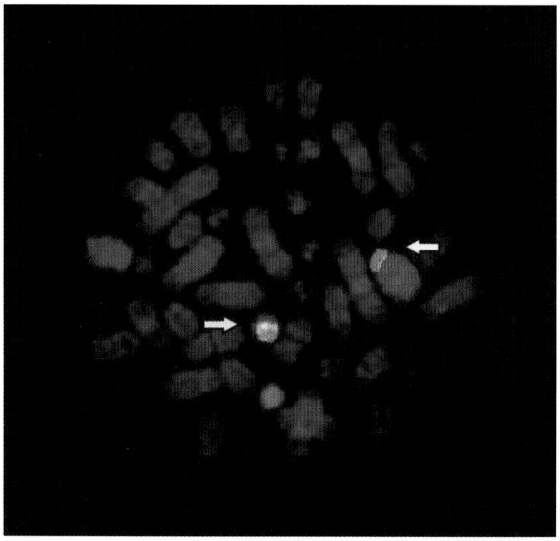

(c)

Fig. 10.12 **(a)** The principles of fluorescent *in situ* hybridization (FISH). A particular strength is that it may be performed on both dividing and non-dividing (quiescent) cells. **(b)** Deletion of long arm (q) of chromosome 5. (Courtesy of Dr Ellie Nacheva) **(c)** An example of FISH analysis showing the t(12;21) translocation. The green probe hybridizes to the region of the *TEL* gene on chromosome 12 and the red probe hybridizes to the region of the *AML1* gene on chromosome 21. The arrows point to the two derived chromosomes resulting from the reciprocal translocation. (Courtesy of Dr C.J. Harrison)

DNA microarray platforms

DNA microarrays allow a rapid and comprehensive analysis of cellular transcription by hybridizing labelled cellular mRNA to DNA probes which are immobilized on a solid support (Fig. 10.14a). Oligonucleotides or complementary DNA (cDNA) arrays may be immobilized on the array and RNA from the tissue of interest is used to generate fluorescent cDNA or RNA which is then annealed to the nucleic acid matrix. This approach can rapidly determine mRNA expression from a large number

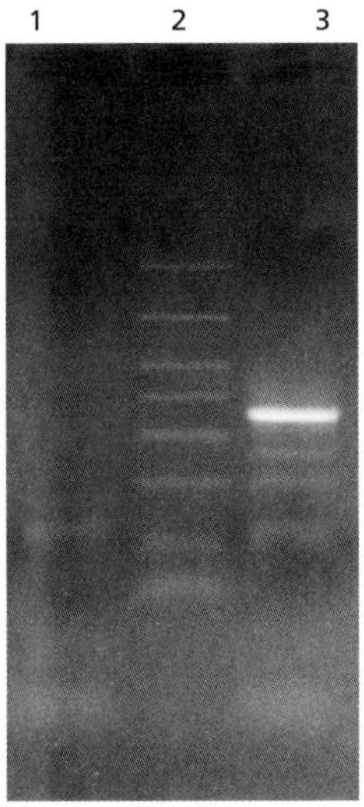

Fig. 10.13 Reverse transcription polymerase chain reaction (PCR) analysis of bone marrow from a patient with AML M_3 (acute promyelocytic leukaemia) at diagnosis. The PML-RARα fusion product (cDNA) formed by the t(15; 17) translocation has been amplified by PCR using oligonucleotide primers from the *PML* and *RARα* genes. Lane 1, water control; lane 2, low molecular weight DNA marker; lane 3, patient sample. A single 355 base pair fusion message has been amplified showing the presence of the fusion gene.

of genes and may be used to determine the mRNA expression pattern of different leukaemia or lymphoma subtypes (Fig. 10.14b). The technique cannot be used to detect (minimal) residual disease and is not yet in routine diagnostic use but it is clear that it can give valuable information for subclassfication of large cell non-Hodgkin's lymphoma diffuse (Fig. 17.5), or AML without cytogenetic changes.

Flow cytometry

In this technique, antibodies labelled with different fluorochromes recognize the pattern and intensity of expression of different antigens on the surface of normal and leukaemic cells (see Appendix 1). Normal cells each have a characteristic profile but malignant cells often express an aberrant phenotype that can be useful in allowing their detection. In the case of B cell malignances (e.g. CLL), expression of only one light chain, κ or λ, by the tumour cells distinguishes them from a normal polyclonal population which express both κ and λ chains, usually in a κ : λ ratio of 2 : 1 (Fig. 10.15).

Immunohistology

Antibodies can also be used to stain tissue sections with fluorescent markers and this is known as ***immunohistology*** or ***immunohistochemistry***. The presence and architecture of tumour cells can be identified by visualization of stained tissue sections under the microscope. The clonal nature of B-cell malignancies can be shown in tissue sections by staining for κ or λ chains. A malignant clonal population (e.g. in B-cell NHL) will express one or other light chain but not both (Fig. 17.4).

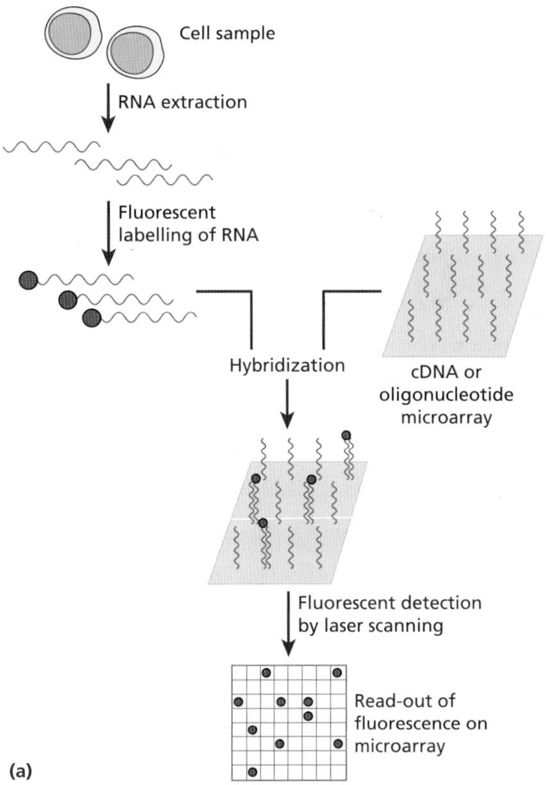

Fig. 10.14 **(a)** Principle of transcriptional profiling of RNA expression in leukaemia samples using DNA microarrays. *(Continued)*

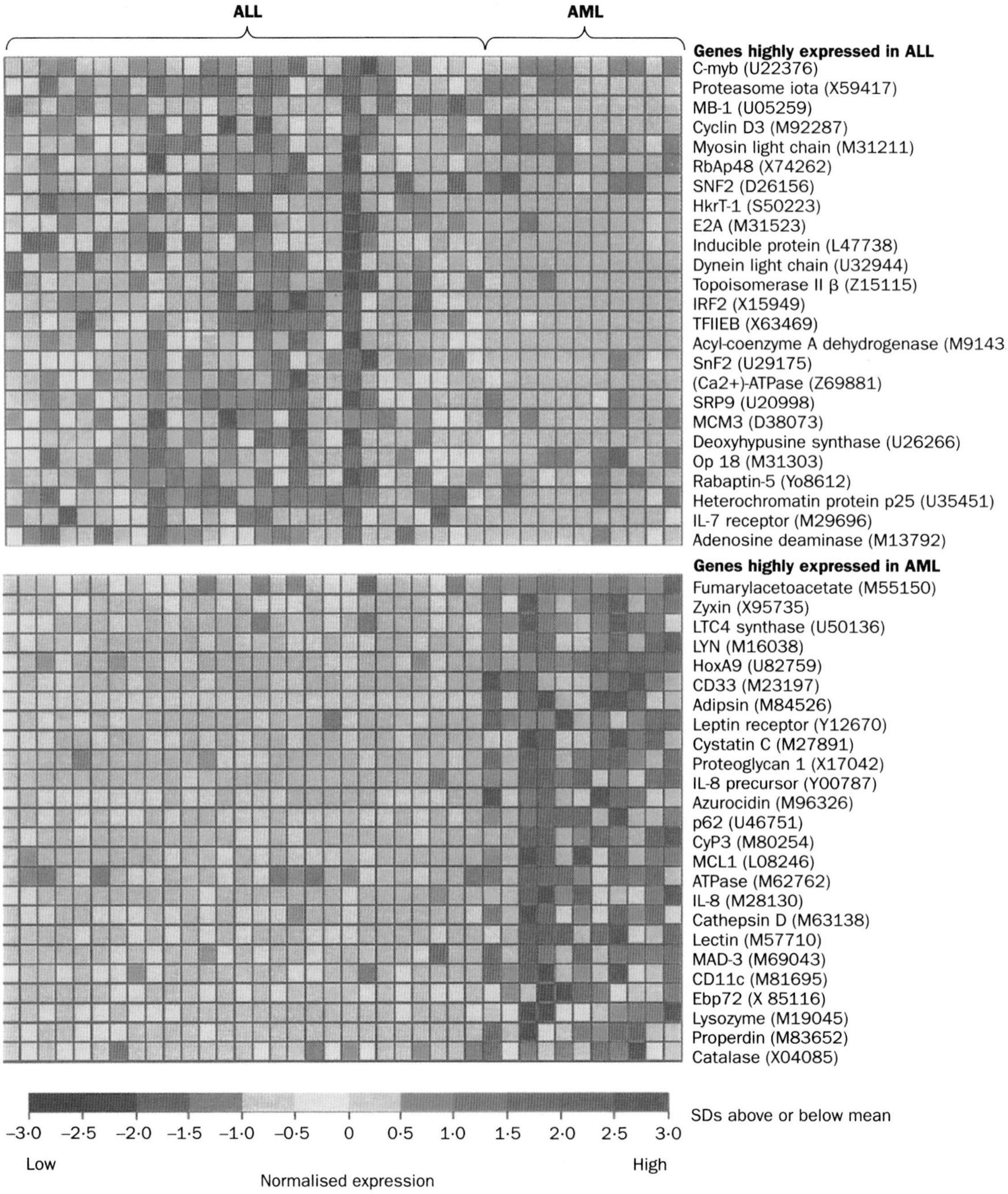

(b)

Fig. 10.14 (*Continued*) **(b)** Microarray analysis of genes distinguishing acute lymphoblastic leukaemia (ALL) from acute myeloid leukaemia (AML). The 50 genes most highly correlated on gene-expression microarrays with each of these leukaemias are shown. Each row corresponds to a gene; each column corresponds to the expression value in a particular sample. Expression for each gene is normalized across the samples such that the mean is 0 and the SD is 1. Expression greater than the mean is shaded in red, and that below the mean is shaded in blue. Although the genes as a group appear correlated with the type of leukaemia under study, no single gene is uniformly expressed across the class, illustrating the value of a multigene prediction method. (Reproduced courtesy of Golub and colleagues)

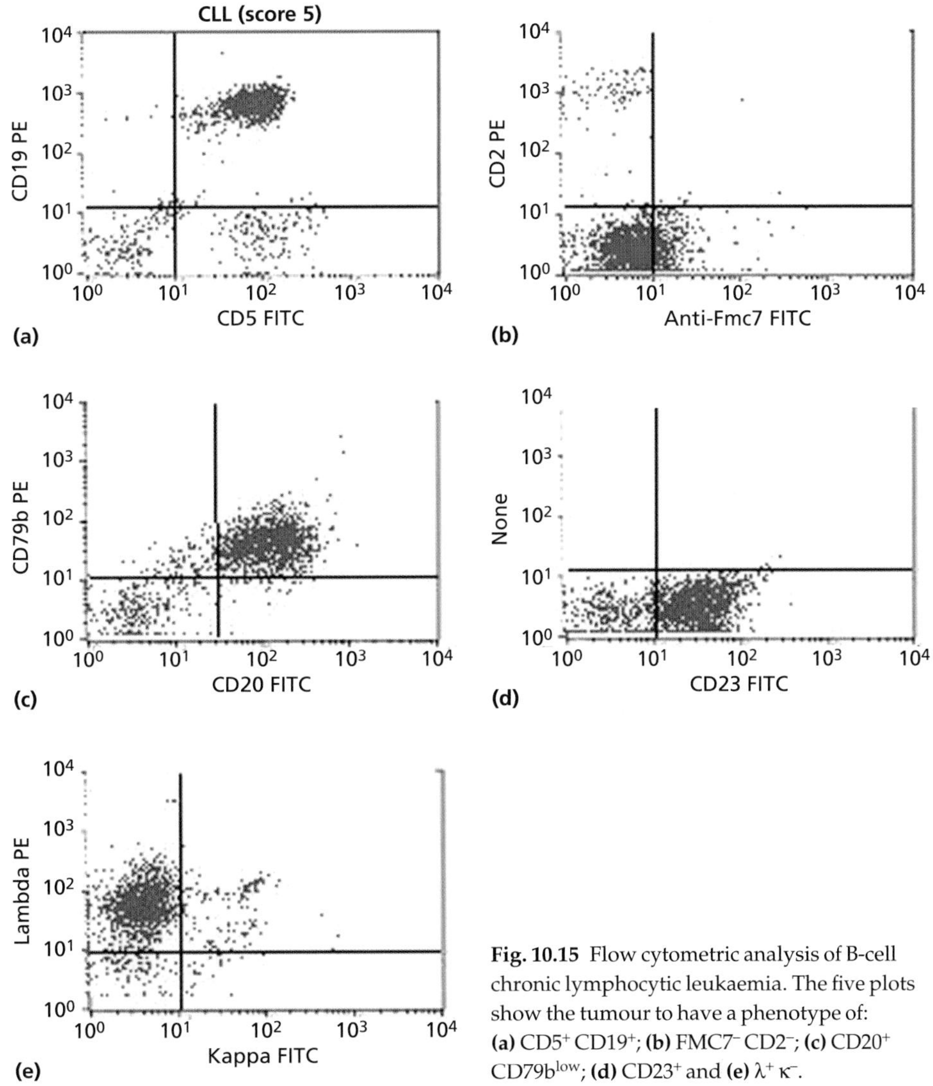

Fig. 10.15 Flow cytometric analysis of B-cell chronic lymphocytic leukaemia. The five plots show the tumour to have a phenotype of: **(a)** $CD5^+$ $CD19^+$; **(b)** $FMC7^-$ $CD2^-$; **(c)** $CD20^+$ $CD79b^{low}$; **(d)** $CD23^+$ and **(e)** λ^+ κ^-.

Value of genetic markers in management of haematological malignancy

The detection of genetic abnormalities may be important in several aspects of the management of patients with leukaemia or lymphoma.

Initial diagnosis

Many genetic abnormalities are so specific for a particular disease that their presence determines that diagnosis. An example is the t(15; 17) translocation which classifies an AML as promyelocytic leukaemia. Clonal immunoglobulin or TCR gene rearrangements are useful in establishing clonality and determining the lineage of a lymphoid malignancy.

For establishing a treatment protocol

Each major type of haematological malignancy can be further subdivided on the basis of detailed genetic information. For instance, AML is a diverse group of disorders with characteristic genotypes. Individual subtypes respond differently to standard treatment.

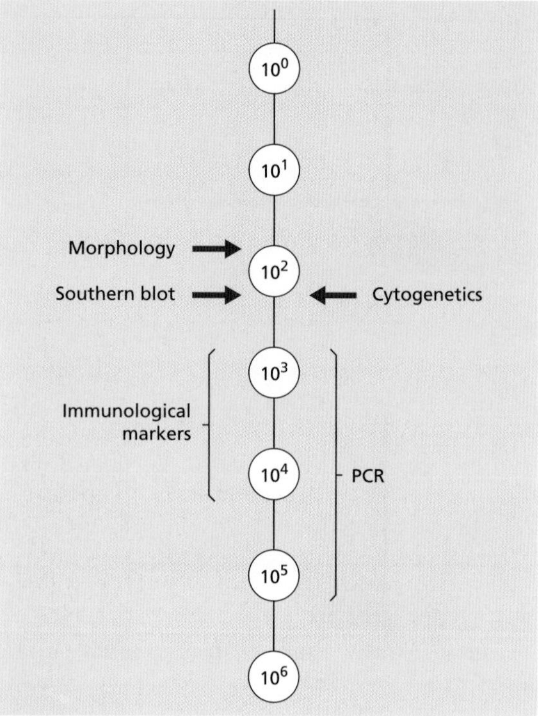

Fig. 10.16 Sensitivity of detection of leukaemic cells using five different techniques. 10^1 to 10^6 = 1 cell in 10 to 1 cell in 10^6 detected.

The t(15; 17), inv(16) and t(8; 21) subgroups do well, whereas monosomy 7 carries a poor prognosis. Treatment strategies are now tailored for the individual and in some instances knowledge of the underlying genetic abnormality can lead to more rational treatment. The best examples are the use of retinoic acid in the treatment of acute promyelocytic leukaemia associated with the t(15; 17) translocation and the use of imatinib for treatment of Ph+ CML. Genetic information is also valuable for giving a prognosis. For instance, Ph+ ALL has a particularly poor prognosis, whereas hyperdiploidy in ALL is a favourable finding. DNA microarrays are valuable for prognosis (e.g. in diffuse large B-cell lymphoma) which can be divided into good and bad prognostic groups according to the pattern of gene expression (Fig. 17.5).

Monitoring the response to therapy

The detection of minimal residual disease (MRD) (disease that cannot be seen by conventional microscopy of the blood or bone marrow) in AML, ALL or CML when the patient is in remission after chemotherapy or stem cell transplantation is possible using the following techniques (in increasing order of sensitivity; Fig. 10.16).

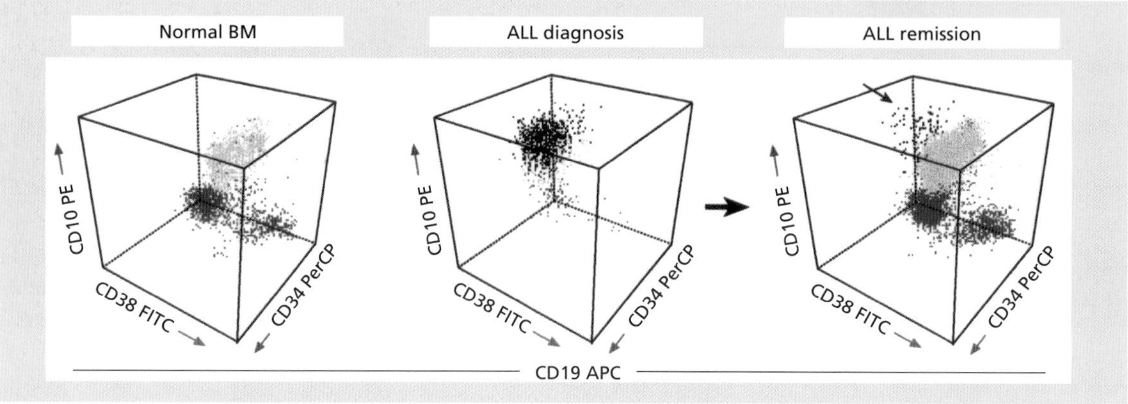

Fig. 10.17 Detection of minimal residual disease (MRD) by four-colour flow cytometry in: normal bone marrow mononuclear cells (BM), BM from a patient with B lineage ALL at diagnosis and in remission 6 weeks after diagnosis. The cells were detected with four different antibodies (anti-CD10, anti-CD19, anti-CD34, anti-CD38) attached to fluorescent labels abbreviated as PE, APC, PerCP and FITC, respectively. The tridimensional plot shows the immunophenotype of $CD19^+$ lymphoid cells in the three samples. MRD of 0.03% of cells expressing the leukaemia-associated phenotype ($CD10^+$, $CD34^+$, $CD38^-$) were detected at 6 weeks, confirmed by PCR analysis. (From D. Campana and E. Coustan-Smith (1999). Cytometry. *Commun Clin Cytometry* **38**,139–52, with permission)

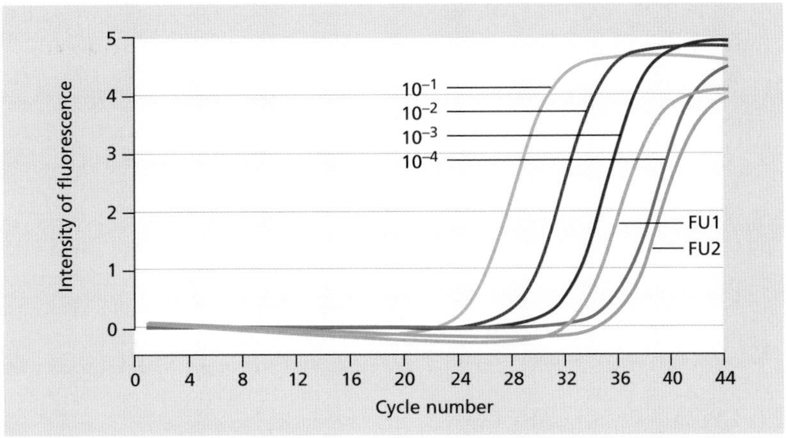

Fig. 10.18 Real-time quantitative PCR in acute B-lineage lymphoblastic leukaemia for minimal residual disease using the immunoglobulin heavy chain as target. Primers are designed based on DNA from sequence analysis of the presenting leukaemic clone. Bone marrow samples taken in clinical remission are amplified by PCR using these primers and fluorescent labelled using Sybergreen. The intensity of the signal measures the total DNA molecules amplified in successive cycles. In this example, the intensities of amplification of DNA from two follow-up bone marrow samples (FU1 and FU2) are compared with serial deletions of (10^{-1} to 10^{-4}) of the DNA from the presentation bone marrow. FU1 shows a level of residual disease approximately 1 in 5000 (0.02%) and FU2 of 1 in 12 000 (0.008%). (Courtesy of Dr L. Foroni)

1 Cytogenetic analysis.
2 Southern blot analysis to look for a tumour-specific DNA rearrangement.
3 Fluorescence-activated cell sorting (FACS) to detect tumour cells using immunological markers that detect 'leukaemia-specific' combinations of antigens (Fig. 10.17).
4 PCR to amplify tumour-specific translocations or immunoglobulin/TCR sequences specific to the original clone (Fig. 10.18).

These approaches are being evaluated but they already have an important role in determining the treatment of individual patients (e.g. persistence of MRD in childhood ALL after the initial 1–3 months of therapy predicts probable relapse; Fig. 10.19) while persistence of the *BCR-ABL* fusion gene after

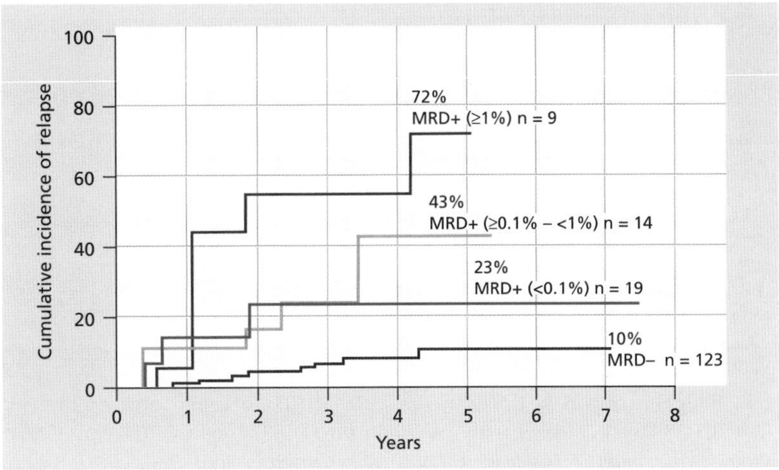

Fig. 10.19 Cumulative incidence of relapse according to minimal residual disease (MRD) levels at the end of remission induction in children with acute lymphoblastic leukaemia (ALL) treated at St Jude Children's Research Hospital. (Courtesy of Dr D. Campana)

allogeneic stem cell transplantation for CML suggests the need for early treatment with donor leucocytes (p. 262).

Bibliography

Abramson J.S. and Shipp M.A. (2005) Advances in the biology and therapy of diffuse large B-cell lymphoma: moving toward a molecularly targeted approach. *Blood* **106**,1164–74.

Bullinger L. (2006) Gene expression profiling in acute myeloid leukemia. *Haematologica* **91**,733–8.

Chou W.C., Tang J.L., Lin L.I. *et al.* (2006) Nucleophosmin mutations in *de novo* acute myeloid leukemia: the age-dependent incidences and the stability during disease evolution. *Cancer Res* **66**,3310–6.

Foroni, L., Gameiro, P.M., Hoffbrand, A.V. (2005) Minimal residual disease in acute leukaemia. In: Hoffbrand A.V., Catovsky D., Tuddenham E.G.D. (eds) *Postgraduate Haematology*, 5th edn. Blackwell Science, Oxford: pp. 561–74.

Gilliland D.G. and Griffin J.D. (2002) The roles of FLT3 in hematopoiesis and leukemia. *Blood* **100**,1532–42.

Haferlach T., Kohlmann A., Schnittger S. *et al.* (2005) General approach to the diagnosis of leukemia using gene expression profiling. *Blood* **106**,1189–98.

Hubank M. (2004) Gene expression profiling and its application in studies of haematological malignancy. *Br J Haematol* **124**,577–94.

Kottaridis P.D., Gale R.F. and Linch D.C. (2003) FLT3 mutations and leukaemia. *Br J Haematol* **122**,523–38.

Krause D.S. and Van Etten R.A. (2005) Mechanisms of disease: tyrosine kinases as targets for cancer therapy. *N Engl J Med* **353**,172–87.

Lossos I.S., Czerwinski D.K., Alizadeh A.A. *et al.* (2004) Prediction of survival in diffuse large-B-cell lymphoma based on the expression of six genes. *N Engl J Med* **350**,1828–37.

Lotem J. and Sachs L. (2006) Epigenetics and the plasticity of differentiation in normal and stem cancer cells. *Oncogene*: advanced on line publication, doi:10.1038/sj.onc.1209816.

Speck N.A. and Gilliland D.G. (2002) Core-binding factors in haematopoiesis and leukaemia. *Nat Rev Cancer* **2**,502–13.

Staudt L.M. and Dave S. (2005) The biology of human lymphoid malignancies revealed by gene expression profiling. *Adv Immunol* **87**,163–208.

Wiemels J.L., Ford A.M., Van Wering E.R., Postma A. and Greaves M. (1999) Protracted latency of acute lymphoblastic leukaemia after *TEL-AML* gene fusion *in utero*. *Blood* **94**,1057–62.

CHAPTER 11

11 Management of haematological malignancy

The treatment of haematological malignancy has improved greatly over the last 40 years. This has resulted from developments in ***support therapy*** and in ***specific treatment***. Details of specific treatment are discussed in relation to individual diseases in the appropriate chapter. Support care and general aspects of the agents used in the treatment of haematological malignancy are described here.

General support therapy

Patients with haematological malignancies often present with medical problems related to suppression of normal haemopoiesis and this problem is compounded by the treatments that are given to eradicate the tumour. General supportive therapy for bone marrow failure includes the following.

1 ***Insertion of a central venous catheter*** A central venous catheter is usually inserted prior to intensive treatment via a skin tunnel from the chest into the superior vena cava (Fig. 11.1). This gives ease of access for administering chemotherapy, blood products, antibiotics and intravenous feeding. In addition, blood may be taken for laboratory tests.

2 ***Blood product support*** (Chapter 27). Red cell and platelet transfusions are used to treat anaemia and thrombocytopenia. A number of particular issues apply to the support of patients with haematological malignancy:

(i) The threshold haemoglobin for transfusion will depend on clinical factors such as symptoms and speed of onset of anaemia but most units give red cell support for a Hb <8 g/dL, with a higher threshold in older patients. In patients needing both red cells and platelets, platelets are given first to reduce the risk of a further fall in the platelet count.

(ii) The trigger for platelet transfusion is typically a platelet count $<10 \times 10^9$/L but this should be doubled in the presence of active bleeding or infection.

(iii) Fresh frozen plasma (FFP) may be needed to reverse coagulation defects.

(iv) Cytomegalovirus (CMV) negative blood should be given to all patients until it has been shown that they are either CMV seropositive or that they will never be candidates for stem cell transplantation. This is to prevent transmission of CMV to uninfected patients as the virus is a significant problem in stem cell transplant recipients (p. 258).

(v) Red cell transfusions should be avoided if at all possible in patients with a very high white cell count ($>100 \times 10^9$/L) because of the hyperviscosity and the risk of precipitating thrombotic episodes as a result of white cell stasis.

(vi) Large volume transfusions, such as 3 units of blood or more, can precipitate pulmonary oedema in older patients and should be given slowly and with clinical monitoring. Diuretics such as frusemide (furosemide) are often given.

(vii) Febrile reactions with blood products are not uncommon and should be managed by slowing the infusion and administration of drugs such as

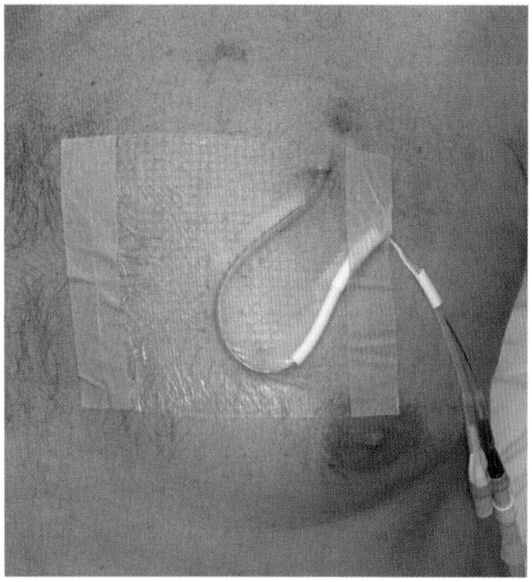

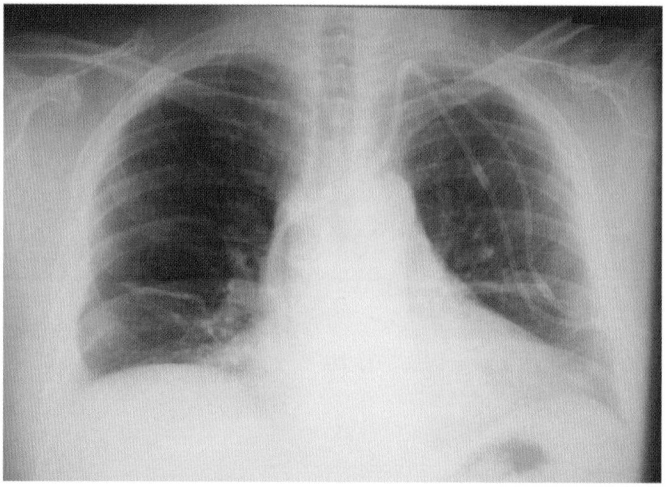

(a) (b)

Fig. 11.1 (a) A central venous line in a patient undergoing intensive chemotherapy. **(b)** Chest X-ray showing correct placement of a central venous line. (Courtesy of Dr D. Tattersall)

antihistamines, pethidine or hydrocortisone. The dosage of steroids should be limited because of concerns with immunosuppression.

(viii) Blood products given to highly immunosuppressed patients (e.g. from chemotherapy, such as fludarabine, or with aplastic anaemia or Hodgkin's disease) should be irradiated prior to administration to prevent graft-versus-host disease (p. 256).

(ix) The use of recombinant erythropoietin to reduce the need for blood transfusion and improve patient well being (e.g. in myeloma or myelodysplasia) is discussed on p. 14.

3 *Haemostasic support* A coagulation screen should be performed regularly on patients undergoing intensive chemotherapy and support with vitamin K or FFP may be required. Cryoprecipitate may be needed for fibrinogen deficiency (e.g. precipitated by asparaginase in the management of acute lymphoblastic leukaemia (ALL)). Antiplatelet drugs such as aspirin or clopidogrel are usually discontinued in patients undergoing intensive chemotherapy and patients on long-term warfarin can be switched to low molecular weight heparin, which can then itself be stopped if the platelet count falls below 50×10^9/L. Progesterones are given to premenopausal women undergoing intensive chemotherapy to prevent menstruation. Tranexamic acid can be given to reduce haemorrhage in patients with chronic low-grade blood loss.

4 *Antiemetic therapy* Nausea and vomiting are common side-effects of chemotherapy. A key objective is to try to prevent nausea occurring early in the treatment as it is more difficult to control once problems have arisen. The 5-HT_3 (serotonin) receptor antagonists such as ondansetron or granisetron can control nausea from intensive chemotherapy in over 60% of cases and the addition of dexamethasone can increase this by approximately 20%. Metoclopramide, prochlorperazine or cyclizine, benzodiazepines (e.g. lorazepam), domperidone or cannabinoids (e.g. nabilone) can all have a role.

5 *Tumour lysis syndrome* Chemotherapy may trigger an acute rise in plasma uric acid, potassium and phosphate and cause hypocalcaemia because of rapid lysis of tumour cells. This syndrome is seen most commonly with rapidly dividing tumours such as lymphoblastic lymphoma or acute leukaemia and can cause acute renal failure. Allopurinol, intravenous fluids and electrolyte replacement are the mainstay of prevention and alkalinization of the urine is sometimes used. Rasburicase, the oxidation of uric acid to allantoin, is highly effective in controlling hyperuricaemia.

6 ***Psychological support*** Patients with a diagnosis of malignant disease commonly feel concerns about such issues as the discomfort of treatment, finance, sexuality and fear of mortality. Even when patients achieve a clinical remission there is understandable concern about the chance of disease relapse. Psychological support should be an integral part of the relationship between physician and patient, and patients should be allowed to express their fears and concerns at the earliest opportunity. Most patients value the opportunity to read more about their disorder and many excellent booklets or websites are now available. Teamwork is also crucial and the nursing staff and trained counsellors have a vital role in offering support and information during inpatient and outpatient care. Many units have specialist input from clinical psychologists and psychiatric help may occasionally be required. Inadequate communication is perhaps the most common failing of medical teams. The immediate family should be kept informed of the patient's progress whenever possible and appropriate.

7 ***Reproductive issues*** Men who are to receive cytotoxic drugs should be offered sperm storage, ideally before treatment commences or, if impossible, within a short period of time thereafter. Ethical issues relating to storage or potential usage of tissue in the event of treatment failure will need to be addressed. Permanent infertility in women is less common after chemotherapy although premature menopause may occur. Storage of fertilized ova is usually impractical and storage of unfertilized ova is currently very difficult and, despite some recent progress, is not offered as a routine service.

8 ***Nutritional support*** Some degree of weight loss is virtually inevitable in patients undergoing inpatient chemotherapy because of the combination of a poor nutritional intake, malabsorption caused by drugs and a catabolic disease state. If a weight loss of >10% occurs, support with total nutrition is often given, either enterally via a nasogastric tube or parenterally through a central venous catheter.

9 ***Pain*** is rarely a major problem in haematological malignancies except myeloma although bone pain can be a presenting feature. The mucositis that follows intensive chemotherapy can cause severe discomfort and continuous infusions of opiate analgesia are often required. Pain is often a considerable issue in patients with multiple myeloma and can be managed by a combination of analgesia and chemotherapy/radiotherapy. Advice from palliative care teams or specialist pain management practitioners should be sought when required.

10 ***Prophylaxis and treatment of infection*** Patients with haematological malignancy are at great risk of infection which remains the major cause of morbidity and mortality. Immunosuppression may result from neutropenia, hypogammglobulinaemia and impaired cellular function. These can be secondary to the primary disease or its treatment. Neutropenia is a particular concern and in many patients neutrophils are totally absent from the blood for periods of 2 weeks or more. The use of granulocyte colony-stimulating factor (G-CSF) to reduce periods of neutropenia is discussed on p. 97. The likely sequence of infection following stem cell transplantation is illustrated in Fig. 11.2.

Bacterial infection

This is the most common problem and usually arises from the patient's own commensal bacterial flora. Gram-positive skin organisms (e.g. *Staphylococcus* and *Streptococcus*) commonly colonize central venous lines, whereas Gram-negative gut bacteria (e.g. *Pseudomonas aeruginosa, Escherichia coli, Proteus, Klebsiella* and anaerobes) can cause overwhelming septicaemia. Even organisms not normally considered pathogenic, such as *Staphyloccus epidermidis*, may cause life-threatening infection. In the absence of neutrophils, local superficial lesions can rapidly cause severe septicaemia.

Prophylaxis of bacterial infection

Protocols used to limit bacterial infection vary from unit to unit and may include the use of a prophylactic antibiotic such as ciprofloxacin. During periods of neutropenia, topical antiseptics for bathing and chlorhexidine mouthwashes and a 'clean diet' are recommended. The patient is nursed in a reverse-barrier room. The severity and length of mucositis may be reduced by treatment with recombinant human keratinocyte growth factor (Palifermin) which reduces the severity of oral mucositis. Oral non-absorbed antimicrobial agents such as neomycin and colistin reduce gut commensal flora but

- Fever 38°C or higher twice within 1 hour
- Fever 38°C or higher and circulatory/respiratory impairment
- Afebrile but suspicion of sepsis, e.g. hypotension in patient on high dose steroids

↓

Investigations

- Culture : Blood – peripheral vein
  - central venous cannulae

  Urine

  Swab at potential site of sepsis
- FBC/Biochem/CRP
- Consider CXR

↓

Treatment

Broad spectrum antibiotic, e.g. meropenem/tazocin
± vancomycin (esp. if central line in place)
Circulatory support if appropriate, e.g. fluids

↓

Resolution of fever
Continue treatment
for 5–10 days after
fever settles

↓

Fever persists 48–72 hours

↓

- Additional antibiotic?
  e.g. teicoplanin/vancomycin
- Consider use of anti-fungal agents
- Change antibiotics?

Fig. 11.2 A protocol for the management of fever in the neutropenic patient. CRP, C-reactive protein; CXR, chest X-ray.

their value is unclear. Regular surveillance cultures are taken to document the patient's bacterial flora and its sensitivity.

Treatment of bacterial infection

Fever is the main indication that infection is present because if neutropenia is present pus will not be formed and infections are often not localized. Fever may be caused by blood products or drugs, but infection is the most common cause and fever of over 38°C in neutropenic patients should be investigated and treated within hours. Cultures should be taken from any likely focus of infection including blood from central venous lines and peripheral veins, from urine and mouth swabs. The mouth and throat, intravenous catheter site, and perineal and perianal areas are particularly likely foci. A chest X-ray is indicated as chest infections are frequent.

Antibiotic therapy must be started immediately after blood and other cultures have been taken; in many febrile episodes no organisms are isolated.

There are many different antibiotic regimes in use and a close link with the microbiology team is essential. A typical regimen might be based on a single agent such as a broad-spectrum penicillin (e.g. Tazocin), meropenem or a broad-spectrum cephalosporin. An aminoglycoside such as gentamicin or vancomycin is often added. *Staphylococcus epidermidis* is a common source of fever in patients with intravenous lines and an agent such as teicoplanin, vancomycin or linezolid may be needed. If an infective agent and its antibiotic sensitivities become known, appropriate changes in the regimen are made. If no response occurs within 48–72 h, changing the antibiotics or treating a fungal or viral infection are considered.

Viral infection

Prophylaxis and treatment of viral infection

Herpes viruses, such as herpes simplex, varicella zoster, CMV and Epstein–Barr virus (EBV), undergo latency following primary infection and are never eradicated from the host. Most patients with haematological malignancy have already been infected with these agents and viral reactivation is therefore the most common problem. Aciclovir is frequently given prophylactically. Herpes simplex is a common cause of oral ulcers but is usually controlled easily by aciclovir. Varicella zoster frequently reactivates in patients with lymphoproliferative diseases to cause shingles which requires treatment with high doses of aciclovir or valaciclovir. Primary infection, usually in children, can be very serious and immunoglobulin can be used to prevent infection following recent exposure. Reactivation of CMV infection is particularly important following stem cell transplantation (Chapter 21) but may occur following intensive chemotherapy. Failure of immune control of EBV following allogeneic transplantation can lead to outgrowth of a B-cell tumour known as post-transplant lymphoproliferative disease (PTLD).

Fungal infection

Prophylaxis and treatment of fungal infection

Because of the intensity of current chemotherapy, fungal infections are a major cause of morbidity and mortality. The two major subtypes are yeasts such as *Candida species* and moulds of which *Aspergillus fumigatus* is the most common.

Invasive aspergillosis is now the most common cause of infectious death in intensively immunocompromised patients. Infection occurs through inhalation of *Aspergillus* spores (conidia) (Fig. 11.3) and air filtration systems are used in many haematology wards. The diagnosis of invasive aspergillosis can be difficult. Definitive diagnosis requires demonstration of invasive growth on a biopsy specimen but such evidence is rarely available. Polymerase chain reaction (PCR) for fungal DNA or enzyme-linked immunosorbent assay (ELISA) for *Aspergillus* galactomannan are often used and the detection of β1–3 D-glucan is also showing promise. High resolution computed tomography (HRCT) scan is a valuable tool and early features are nodular lesions with a 'ground glass' appearance. Later on, wedge lesions, the halo sign and the air crescent sign are seen (Fig. 11.4). A high index of suspicion for fungal infection should be maintained and treatment is often started empirically for a fever that has failed to resolve after 3–4 days of antibiotic treatment.

Treatment of established *Aspergillus* infection is

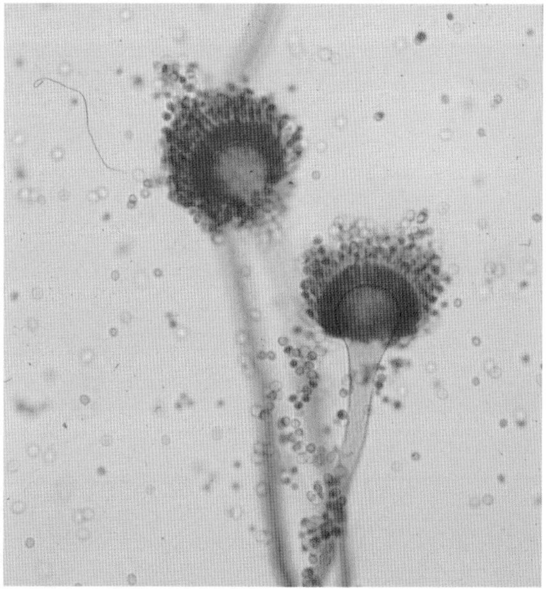

Fig. 11.3 Sporing heads of *Aspergillus fumigatus*. (Courtesy of Dr Elizabeth Johnson)

with amphotericin (usually liposomal), voriconazole or caspofungin. Surgery to remove lung lesions may be needed.

Candida species are a common hospital pathogen and frequently cause oral infection. *Candida* can be significant when isolated from normally sterile body fluids such as blood or urine. Prophylaxis or treatment is usually with fluconazole or itraconazole.

Pneumocystis carinii (also known as *Pneumocystis jiroveci*) is an important cause of pneumonitis. Prophylaxis with co-trimoxazole or nebulized pentamidine is highly effective and is given to those who have received intensive (combination) chemotherapy. Treatment is with high dose co-trimoxazole.

Specific therapies for haematological malignancy

Specific therapy is aimed at reducing the tumour cell burden by the use of drugs or radiotherapy. The hope in some diseases is to eradicate the tumour completely and cure rates for haematological malignancy are gradually improving. However, cure is often not achievable so palliation can also be an important aim.

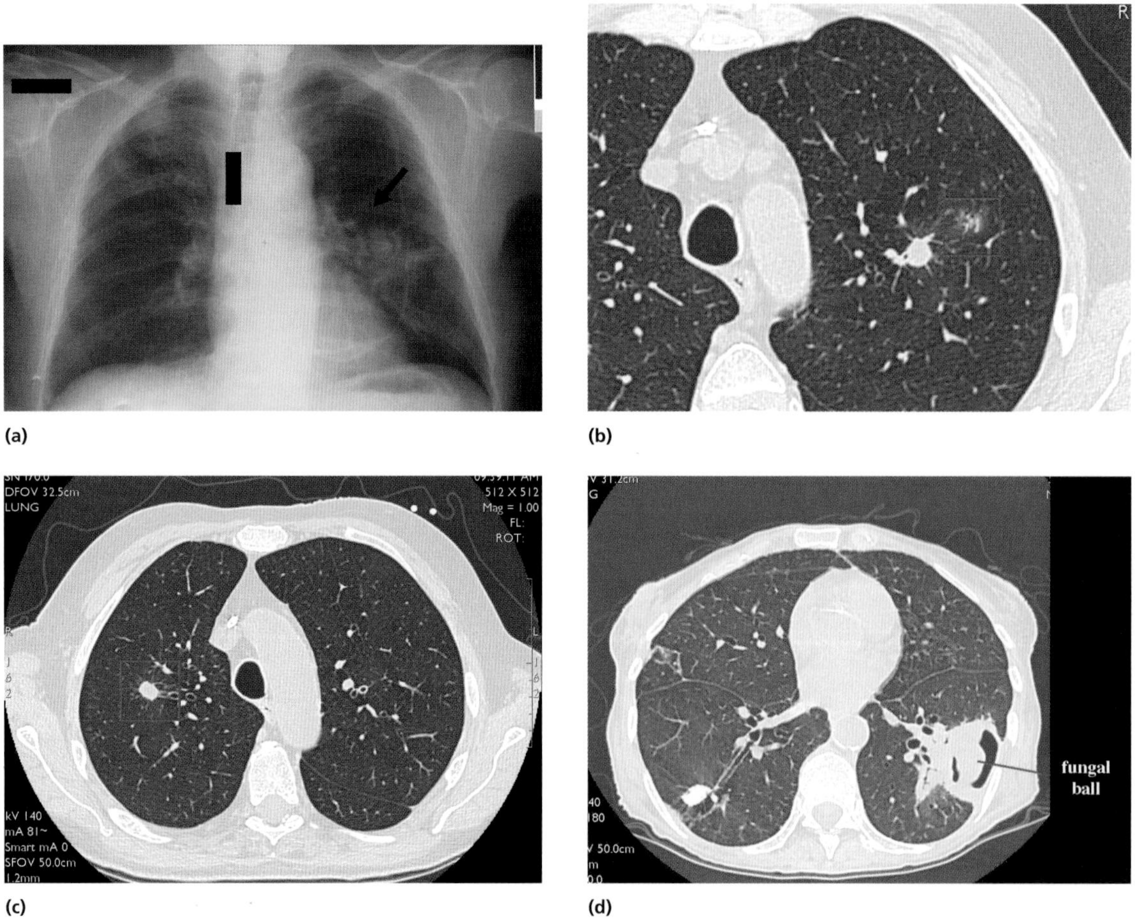

Fig. 11.4 **(a)** Chest X-ray of patient with pulmonary aspergillosis which shows an area of cavitation containing a central fungal ball (arrow) leading to the typical 'air-crescent' sign. Hazy ground-glass shadowing with bronchiolar dilatation **(b)** and **(c)** nodules are seen in early aspergillosis, whereas a fungal ball with surrounding air is typical of more advanced disease **(d)**.

A wide variety of drugs are used in the management of haemopoietic malignancies and several drugs are often combined together in regimens that minimize the potential for resistance to occur against a single agent. Many act specifically on dividing cells and their selectivity is dependent on the high proliferation rate within the tumour. Not all tumour cells will be killed by a single course of treatment and it is usual to give several courses of treatment which gradually eradicate the tumour burden. This 'log kill' hypothesis also gives the residual normal haemopoietic cells the opportunity to recover between treatment courses.

Drugs used in the treatment of haemopoietic malignancies

Cytotoxic drugs (Table 11.1)

Alkylating agents such as chlorambucil, cyclophosphamide and melphalan are activated to expose reactive alkyl groups which make covalent bonds to molecules within the cell. These have a particular affinity for purines and are thus able to cross-link DNA strands and impair DNA replication, resulting in a block at G_2 (Fig. 1.8) and death of the cell by apoptosis (Fig. 1.11).

Table 11.1 Drugs used in the treatment of leukaemia and lymphoma.

	Mechanism of action	Particular side-effects*
Alkylating agents		
Cyclophosphamide	Cross-link DNA, impede RNA formation	Haemorrhagic cystitis, cardiomyopathy, loss of hair
Chlorambucil		Marrow aplasia, hepatic toxicity, dermatitis
Busulfan		Marrow aplasia, pulmonary fibrosis, hyperpigmentation
Melphalan		Marrow aplasia
Nitrosoureas BCNU, CCNU		Renal and pulmonary toxicity
Cisplatin	Intrastrand DNA linkage	Renal dysfunction, neurotoxicity, ototoxicity
Antimetabolites		
Methotrexate	Inhibit pyrimidine or purine synthesis or incorporation into DNA	Mouth ulcers, gut toxicity
6-Mercaptopurine†		Jaundice
6-Tioguanine†		Gut toxicity
Cytosine arabinoside		CNS especially cerebellar toxicity and conjunctivitis at high doses
Cytotoxic antibiotics		
Anthracyclines (e.g. daunorubicin)	Bind to DNA and interfere with mitosis	Cardiac toxicity, hair loss
Hydroxodaunorubicin (Adriamycin)		
Mitoxantrone		
Idarubicin		
Bleomycin	DNA breaks	Pulmonary fibrosis, skin pigmentation
Plant derivatives		
Vincristine (Oncovin)	Spindle damage	Neuropathy (peripheral or bladder or gut)
Vinblastine		
Vindesine		
Epipodophyllotoxin (etoposide, VP-16)	Mitotic inhibitor	Hair loss, oral ulceration
Purine analogues		
Fludarabine	Inhibits adenosine deaminase or other purine pathways	Immunosuppression (low CD4 counts); renal and neurotoxicity (at high doses)
2-Chlorodeoxyadenosine		
Deoxycoformycin		
Miscellaneous		
Hydroxyurea	Inhibits ribonucleotide reductase	Pigmentation, nail dystrophy, skin ulceration
Signal transduction inhibitors (imatinib)	Inhibits tyrosine kinase activity	Myelosuppression, fluid retention
Corticosteroids	Lymphoblast lysis	Peptic ulcer, obesity, diabetes, osteoporosis, psychosis, hypertension
Trans-retinoic acid	Induces differentiation	Liver dysfunction, skin hyperkeratosis, leucocytosis and hyperviscosity, pleural or pericardial effusion

(Continued on p. 154)

Table 11.1 (*Continued*) Drugs used in the treatment of leukaemia and lymphoma.

	Mechanism of action	Particular side-effects*
Arsenic	Induces differentiation or apoptosis	Hyperleucocytosis, cardiac
α-Interferon	Activation of RNAase and natural killer activity	Flu-like symptoms, thrombocytopenia, leucopenia, weight loss
Monoclonal antibodies		
Rituximab (anti-CD20)	Induction of apoptosis	Infusion reactions, immunosuppression
Campath (anti-CD52)	Lysis of target cell by complement fixation	
Ibritumomab (Zevalin) (anti-CD20+ ^{90}Y)	Toxicity to bound cell	Myelosuppression, nausea
Tositumomab (Bexxar) (anti-CD20+ ^{131}I)	Toxicity to bound cell	Myelosuppression
L-Asparaginase	Deprive cells of asparagine	Hypersensitivity, low albumin and coagulation factors, pancreatitis

* Most of the drugs cause nausea, vomiting, mucositis and bone marrow toxicity, and in large doses infertility. Tissue necrosis is a problem if the drugs are extravasated during infusion.
† Allopurinol potentiates the action and side-effects of 6-mercaptopurine.

Antimetabolites block metabolic pathways used in DNA synthesis. There are three major groups:

1 ***Folate antagonists***, such as methotrexate (Fig. 4.5). Methotrexate is widely used alone or in combination with cytosine arabinoside as intrathecal prophylaxis of CNS disease in patients with ALL, AML or high grade non-Hodgkin lymphomas. High systemic closes may also prenetrate the CNS. Folinic acid (formyl THF) is able to overcome the activity of methotrexate and is sometimes administered to 'rescue' normal cells after high-dose methotrexate therapy.

2 ***Pyrimidine analogues*** include cytosine arabinoside (cytarabine; ara-C) which is an analogue of 2′-deoxycytidine and is incorporated into DNA where it inhibits DNA polymerase and blocks replication.

3 ***Purine analogues*** include fludarabine (which inhibits DNA synthesis in a manner similar to ara-C), mercaptopurine, azathioprine and deoxycoformycin.

Cytotoxic antibiotic drugs include the anthracyclines such as doxorubicin, hydroxodaunorubicin, epirubicin and mitozantrone. These are able to intercalate into DNA and then bind strongly to enzymes called topoisomerases. These enzymes are critical for relieving torsional stress in replicating DNA by nicking and resealing DNA strands. If their activity is blocked, DNA replication cannot take place.

Bleomycin is a metal chelating antibiotic that generates superoxide radicals within cells that degrade preformed DNA. It is active on non-cycling cells.

Plant derivatives include the vinca alkaloids such as vincristine which is derived from the periwinkle plant. It binds to tubulin and prevents its polymerization to microtubules. This blocks cell division in metaphase (Fig. 1.8). Etoposide inhibits topisomerase action.

Other agents

Hydroxyurea (hydroxycarbamide) is used widely in the treatment of myeloproliferative disorders. It inhibits the enzyme ribonucleotide reductase which converts ribonucleotides to deoxyribonucleotides. It is not thought to damage DNA and is used in non-malignant disorders such as sickle cell anaemia (p. 89).

Imatinib is a new class of drug that binds to the bcr-abl fusion protein generated from the Philadelphia chromosome translocation in chronic

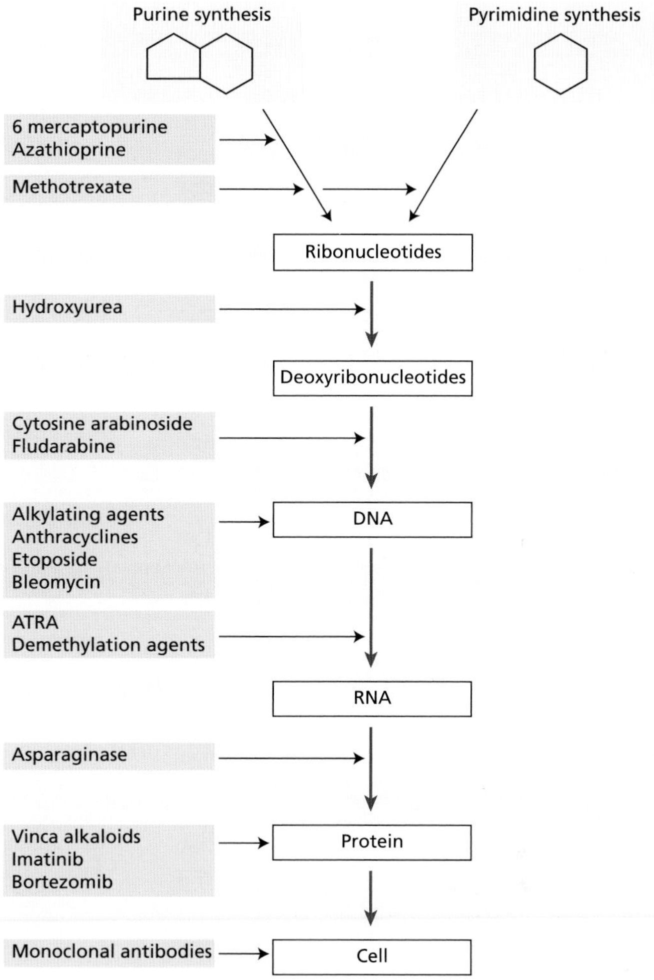

Fig. 11.5 The site of action of drugs used in the management of haemopoietic malignancies. ATRA, all-trans retinoic acid.

myeloid leukaemia (CML; p. 177). It blocks binding of adenosine triphosphate (ATP) and thus prevents phosphorylation of substrate proteins leading to apoptosis of the cell (Fig. 13.4).

Corticosteroids have a potent lymphocytotoxic activity and have an important role in many chemotherapeutic regimens used in the treatment of lymphoid malignancy and myeloma.

All-trans retinoic acid (ATRA) is a vitamin A derivative that acts as a differentiation agent in acute promyelocytic leukaemia (APML). Tumour cells in APML are arrested at the promyelocyte stage as a result of transcriptional repression resulting from the PML-RARA fusion protein (p. 136). ATRA relieves this block and may lead to a brisk neutrophila within a few days of treatment with other side-effects known as the 'ATRA syndrome' (p. 170).

Demethylation agents (e.g. azacytidine) act to increase transcription by reducing methylation on cytosine resides within DNA.

Interferon-α is an antiviral and antimitotic substance produced in response to viral infection and inflammation. It has proven useful in CML, myeloma and myeloproliferative diseases.

Monoclonal antibodies are highly effective against B-cell malignancies. Rituximab binds to CD20 on B cells and appears to mediate cell death, primarily through direct induction of apoptosis and opsonization (p. 212). Alemtuzumab (Campath) binds to CD52 and is highly efficient at fixing complement which lyzes the target B and T cells. Antibodies may also carry attached toxins (e.g. Mylotarg) (anti-CD33) or radioactive isotopes (e.g. Zevalin or Bexaar).

Asparaginase is an enzyme derived from bacteria which breaks down the amino acid asparagine within the circulation. ALL cells lack asparagine synthase and thus need a supply of exogenous asparagine for protein synthesis. Intramuscular asparaginase is an important agent in the treatment of ALL, although hypersensitivity reactions are not uncommon and blood clotting may be disturbed.

Platinum derivatives (e.g. cisplatin) are used in combinations for treating lymphoma.

Arsenic is useful in treatment of relapsed AML M_3. It induces differentiation and apoptosis.

Bibliography

Cairo M.S. and Bishop M. (2004) Tumour lysis syndrome: new therapeutic strategies and classification. *Br J Haematol* **127**,3–11.

Donnelly J.P. (2001) Prophylaxis of infections. In: Rolston K.V.I. and Rubenstein E.B. (eds) *Textbook of Febrile Neutropenia*. Martin Dunitz, London: pp. 215–43.

Furno P., Bucaneve G., Del Favero A. (2002) Monotherapy or aminoglycoside-containing combinations for empirical antibiotic treatment of febrile neutropenic patients: a meta-analysis. *Lancet Infect Dis* **2**,231–42.

Glasmacher A., Prentice A., Gorschluter M. *et al.* (2003) Itraconazole prevents invasive fungal infections in neutropenic patients treated for hematologic malignancies: evidence from a meta-analysis of 3597 patients. *J Clin Oncol* **21**,4615–26.

Prentice A.G. and Donnelly J.P. (2005) Supportive care in the management of leukaemia. In: Hoffbrand A.V., Catovsky D., Tuddenham E.G.D. (eds) *Postgraduate Haematology*, 5th edn. Blackwell Publishing, Oxford: pp. 586–602.

Rebulla P., Finazza G., Marangoni F. *et al.* (1997) The threshold for prophylactic platelet transfusions in adults with acute myeloid leukemia. The Gruppo Italiano Malattie Ematologiche Maligne dell'Adulto. *N Engl J Med* **337**,1870–5.

Shoham S. and Levitz S.M. (2005) The immune response to fungal infections. *Br J Haematol* **129**,569–82.

Spielberger R., Stiff P., Bensinger W. *et al.* (2004) Palifermin for oral mucositis after intensive therapy for hematologic cancers. *N Engl J Med* **351**,2590–8.

Stewart A.F. (2005) Hypercalcemia associated with cancer. *N Engl J Med* **352**,373–9.

Swanton C. (2004) Cell-cycle targeted therapies. *Lancet Oncol* **5**,27–34.

Walsh T.J., Teppler H., Donowitz G.R. *et al.* (2004) Caspofungin versus liposomal amphotericin B for empirical antifungal therapy in patients with persistent fever and neutropenia. *N Engl J Med* **351**,1391–402.

CHAPTER 12

12 Acute leukaemias

The leukaemias are a group of disorders characterized by the accumulation of malignant white cells in the bone marrow and blood. These abnormal cells cause symptoms because of: (i) bone marrow failure (i.e. anaemia, neutropenia, thrombocytopenia) and (ii) infiltration of organs (e.g. liver, spleen, lymph nodes, meninges, brain, skin or testes).

Classification of leukaemia

The main classification is into four types: acute and chronic leukaemias, which are further subdivided into lymphoid or myeloid (Table 12.1).

Classification and pathogenesis of acute leukaemia

Acute leukaemias are usually aggressive diseases in which malignant transformation occurs in the haemopoietic stem cell or early progenitors. Genetic damage is believed to involve several key biochemical steps resulting in: (i) an increased rate of proliferation; (ii) reduced apoptosis and (iii) a block in cellular differentiation. Together these events cause accumulation of the early bone marrow haemopoietic cells which are known as ***blast cells***. The dominant clinical feature of these diseases is usually bone marrow failure caused by accumulation of blast cells although organ infiltration also occurs. If untreated these diseases are usually rapidly fatal but, paradoxically, they are also easier to cure than chronic leukaemias.

Acute leukaemia is defined as the presence of over 20% of blast cells in the blood or bone marrow at clinical presentation. It can be diagnosed with even less than 20% blasts if specific leukaemia-associated cytogenetic or molecular genetic abnormalities are present. It is further subdivided into acute myeloid leukaemia (AML) and acute lymphoblastic leukaemia (ALL) on the basis of whether the blasts are shown to be myeloblasts or lymphoblasts (Table 12.2).

Table 12.1 Classification of leukaemias.

Acute (see Table 12.2)
Acute myeloid leukaemia: M_0–M_7
Acute lymphoblastic leukaemia: L_1–L_3
Chronic (see Tables 13.1 and 15.1)
Chronic myeloid leukaemias
Chronic lymphoid leukaemias

Differentiation of ALL from AML

In most cases the clinical features and morphology on routine staining distinguish ALL from AML. In ALL the blasts show no differentiation (with the exception of B-cell ALL (B-ALL)) whereas in AML some evidence of differentiation to granulocytes or monocytes is usually seen in the blasts or their progeny. Specialized tests are needed to confirm the diagnosis of AML or ALL and to subdivide

Table 12.2 Classification of acute myeloid (AML) and acute lymphoblastic (ALL) leukaemia according to the French–American–British (FAB) groups. For more detailed WHO classification, see page 366.

AML	Cytogenetic abnormality
M_0 undifferentiated	
M_1 without maturation	
M_2 with granulocytic maturation	t(8; 21)
M_3 acute promyelocytic	t(15; 17)
M_4 granulocytic and monocytic maturation	inv (16)
M_5 monoblastic (M_{5a}) or monocytic (M_{5b})	
M_6 erythroleukaemia	
M_7 megakaryoblastic	
ALL	
L_1 blast cells small, uniform high nuclear to cytoplasmic ratio	
L_2 blast cells larger, heterogeneous, lower nuclear to cytoplasmic ratio	
L_3 vacuolated blasts, basophilic cytoplasm (usually B-ALL)*	

* In WHO classification, L_3 cases with mature immunophenotype and Burkitt's lymphoma translocations are not classified as ALL (p. 367).

cases of AML or ALL into their different subtypes (Tables 12.3 and 12.4).

In a minority of cases of acute leukaemia the blast cells show features of both AML and ALL. These features may be on the same cell (biphenotypic) or on separate populations (bilineal) and they include inappropriate expression of immunological markers or inappropriate gene rearrangements. This is termed hybrid acute leukaemia and treatment is usually given on the basis of the dominant pattern.

Acute lymphoblastic leukaemia

This is caused by an accumulation of lymphoblasts in the bone marrow and is the most common malignancy of childhood.

Incidence and pathogenesis

ALL is the most common form of leukaemia in children; its incidence is highest at 3–7 years, falling off by 10 years with a secondary rise after the age of 40 years. The common ($CD10^+$) precursor B type which is most usual in children has an equal sex incidence; there is a male predominance for T-cell ALL (T-ALL).

The pathogenesis is varied. In a proportion of cases the first event occurs in the fetus *in utero*, with a secondary event possibly precipitated by infection in childhood. This is discussed further on p. 130. In other cases, the disease seems to arise as a postnatal mutation in an early lymphoid progenitor cell.

Table 12.3 Specialized tests for acute lymphoblastic leukaemia (ALL) and acute myeloid leukaemia (AML).

	ALL	AML
Cytochemistry		
Myeloperoxidase	–	+ (including Auer rods)
Sudan black	–	+ (including Auer rods)
Non-specific esterase	–	+ in M_4, M_5
Periodic acid–Schiff	+ (coarse block positivity in ALL)	+ (fine blocks in M_6)
Acid phosphatase	+ in T-ALL (Golgi staining)	+ in M_6 (diffuse)
Immunoglobulin and TCR genes	Precursor B-ALL: clonal rearrangement of immunoglobulin genes T-ALL: clonal rearrangement of TCR genes	Germline configuration of immunoglobulin and TCR genes
Chromosomes and genetic analysis (see Table 10.2)		
Immunological markers (flow cytometry) (Table 12.4)		

B-ALL, B-cell acute lymphoblastic leukaemia; T-ALL, T-cell acute lymphoblastic leukaemia; TCR, T-cell receptor.

Table 12.4 Immunological markers for classification of acute myeloid (AML) and acute lymphoblastic (ALL) leukaemia.

		ALL	
Marker	**AML**	**Precursor B***	**T**
Myeloid			
CD13	+	–	–
CD33	+	–	–
CD117	+	–	–
Glycophorin	+ (M_6)	–	–
Platelet antigens (e.g. CD41)	+ (M_7)	–	–
Myeloperoxidase	+ (M_0)		
B lineage			
CD19	–	+	–
cCD22	–	+	–
cCD79a	–	+	–
CD10	–	+ or –	–
cIg	–	+ (pre-B)	–
SIg	–	– (early pre-B)	–
TdT	–	+	+
T lineage			
CD7	–	–	+
cCD3	–	–	+
CD2	–	–	+
TdT	–	+	+

c, Cytoplasmic; S, surface.
* B-ALL resembles precursor B-ALL immunologically but has surface immunoglobulin (Ig) and is terminal deoxynucleotidyl transferase negative (TdT^-).

Classification

This may be on the basis of morphology or immunological markers.

Morphology The French–American–British (FAB) group subclassifies ALL into three subtypes (Table 12.2 and Fig. 12.1):

1 The L_1 type show uniform, small blast cells with scanty cytoplasm;

2 The L_2 type comprise larger blast cells with more prominent nucleoli and cytoplasm and with more heterogeneity; and

3 The L_3 blasts are large with prominent nucleoli, strongly basophilic cytoplasm and cytoplasmic vacuoles.

Immunophenotype Immunological markers can be used to divide ALL cases into early pre-B, pre-B, B- and T-cell subtypes (Table 12.4).

Clinical features

Clinical features are a result of the following.

1 ***Bone marrow failure*** Anaemia (pallor, lethargy and dyspnoea); neutropenia (fever, malaise, features of mouth, throat, skin, respiratory, perianal or other infections; Fig. 12.3); and thrombocytopenia (spontaneous bruises, purpura, bleeding gums and menorrhagia; Fig. 12.4).

2 ***Organ infiltration*** Tender bones, lymphadenopathy (Fig. 12.5a), moderate splenomegaly, hepatomegaly and meningeal syndrome (headache, nausea and vomiting, blurring of vision and diplopia). Fundal examination may reveal papilloedema and sometimes haemorrhage. Many patients have a fever which usually resolves after starting chemotherapy. Less common manifestations include testicular swelling (Fig. 12.5b) or signs of mediastinal compression in T-ALL (Fig. 12.6).

Investigations

Haematological investigations may reveal a normochromic, normocytic anaemia with thrombocytopenia in most cases. The total white cell count may be decreased, normal or increased to 200×10^9/L or more. Blood film examination typically shows a variable numbers of blast cells. The bone marrow is hypercellular with >20% leukaemic blasts. The blast cells are characterized by morphology, immunological tests and cytogenetic analysis. Identification of the immunoglobulin/T-cell receptor (TCR) gene rearrangement, (aberrant) immunophenotype and molecular genetics of the tumour cells is important to determine treatment and to detect minimal residual disease during follow-up.

Lumbar puncture for cerebrospinal fluid examination should be performed and may show that the spinal fluid has an increased pressure and contains leukaemic cells. Biochemical tests may reveal a raised serum uric acid, serum lactate dehydrogenase or, less commonly, hypercalcaemia. Liver and renal function tests are performed as a baseline before treatment begins. Radiography may reveal

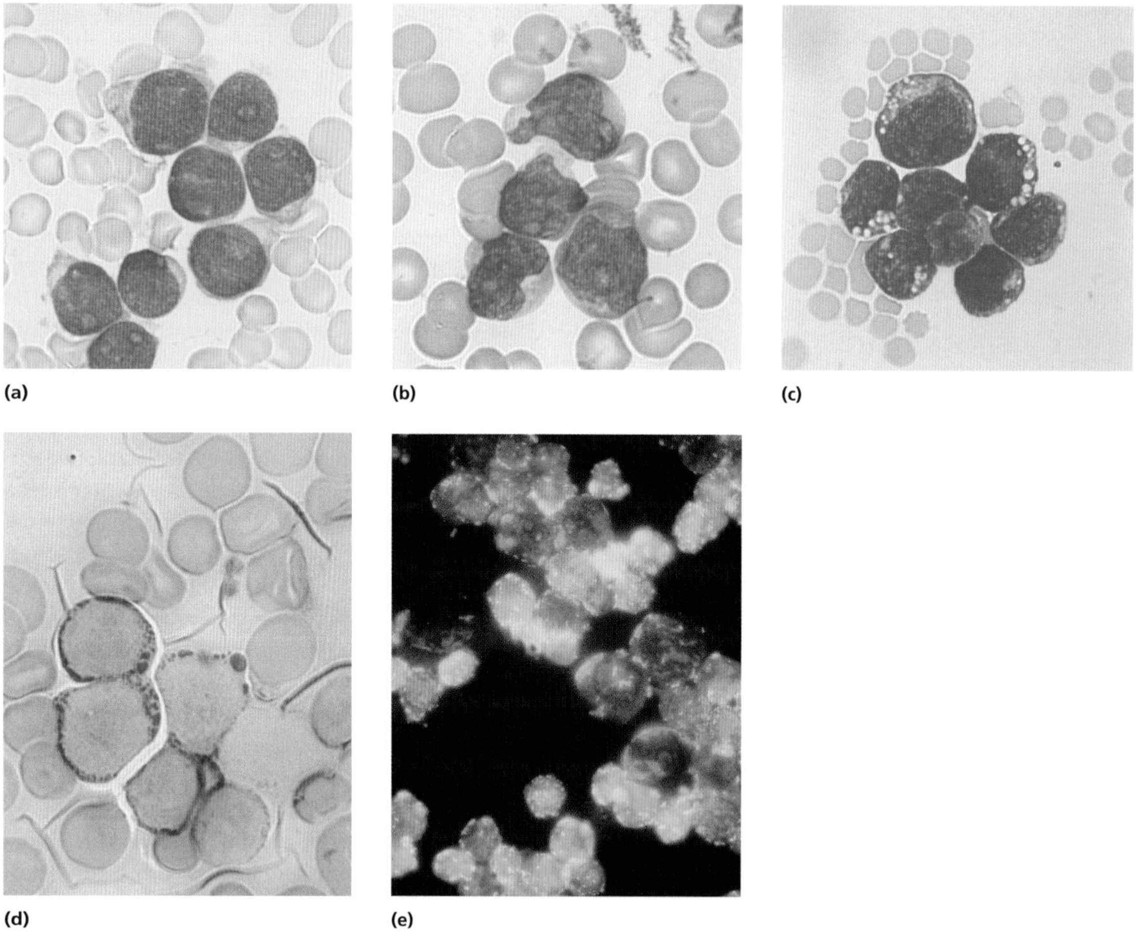

Fig. 12.1 Acute lymphoblastic leukaemia. **(a)** L_1 subtype—blasts show scanty cytoplasm without granules. **(b)** L_2 subtype—blasts are larger and heterogeneous with more abundant cytoplasm. **(c)** L_3 subtype—blasts are deeply basophilic with cytoplasmic vacuolation. **(d)** Periodic acid–Schiff (PAS) staining reveals coarse granules. **(e)** Indirect immunofluorescence reveals nuclear terminal deoxynucleotidyl transferase (TdT) (green) and membrane CD10 (orange). (Courtesy of Professor G. Janossy)

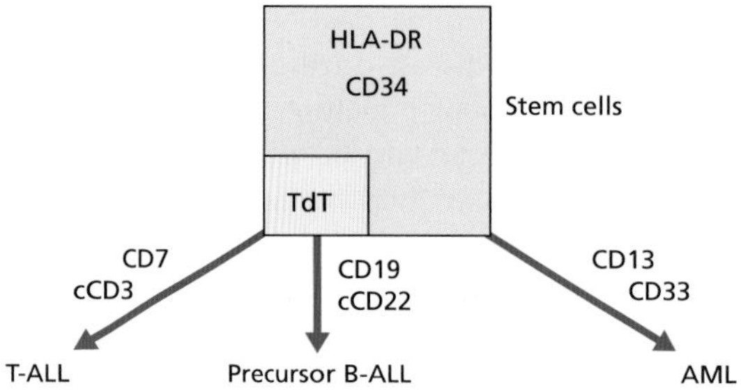

Fig. 12.2 Development of three cell lineages from pluripotential stem cells giving rise to the three main immunological subclasses of acute leukaemia. The immunological characterization using pairs of markers is shown, as well as the three markers characterizing the early 'stem' cells. ALL, acute lymphoblastic leukaemia; AML, acute myeloid leukaemia; c, cytoplasmic.

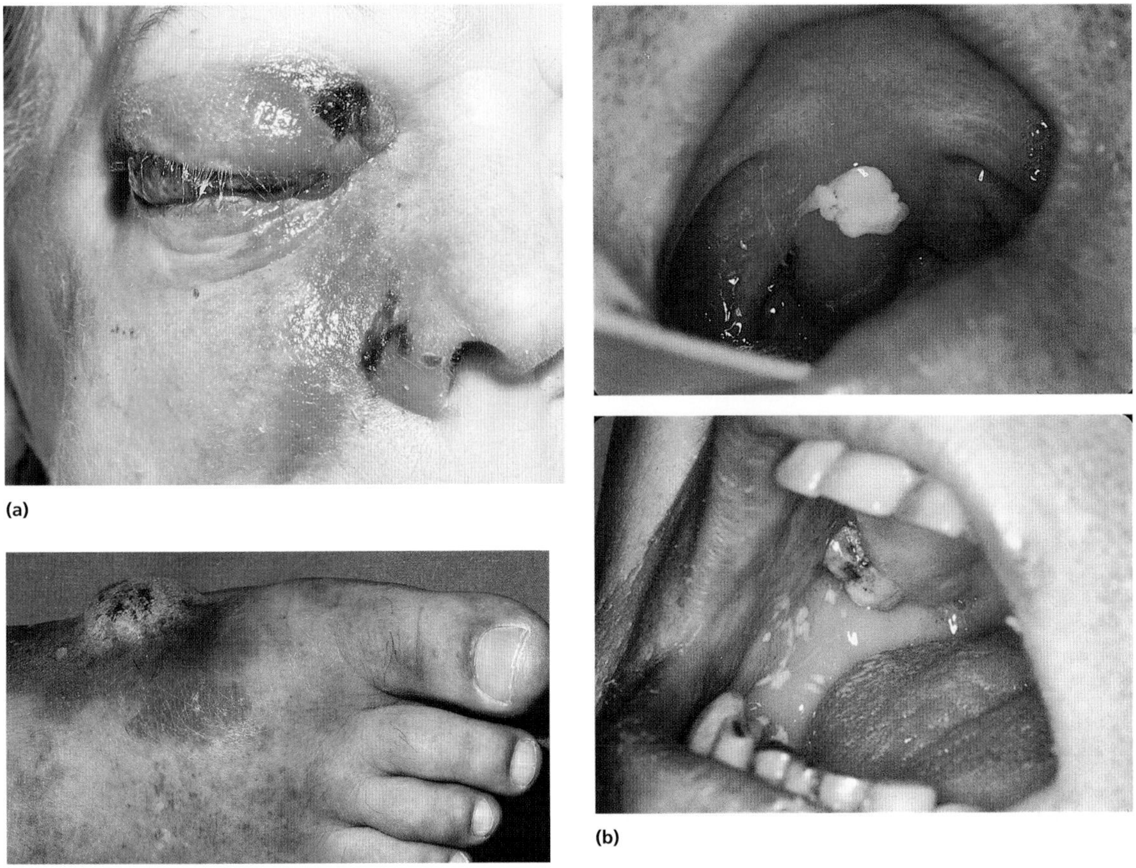

(a) (b) (c)

Fig. 12.3 **(a)** An orbital infection in a female patient (aged 68 years) with acute myeloid leukaemia and severe neutropenia (haemoglobin 8.3 g/dL, white cells 15.3 × 10^9/L, blasts 96%, neutrophils 1%, platelets 30 × 10^9/L). **(b)** Acute myeloid leukaemia: top plaque *Candida albicans* on soft palate; lower: plaque *Candida albicans* in the mouth, with lesion of herpes simplex on the upper lip. **(c)** Skin infection (*Pseudomonas aeruginosa*) in a female patient (aged 33 years) with acute lymphoblastic leukaemia receiving chemotherapy and with severe neutropenia (haemoglobin 10.1 g/dL, white cells 0.7 × 10^9/L, neutrophils <0.1 × 10^9/L, lymphocytes 0.6 × 10^9/L, platelets 20 × 10^9/L).

lytic bone lesions and a mediastinal mass caused by enlargement of the thymus and/or mediastinal lymph nodes characteristic of T-ALL (Fig. 12.6).

The differential diagnosis includes AML, aplastic anaemia (with which ALL sometimes presents), marrow infiltration by other malignancies (e.g. rhabdomyosarcoma, neuroblastoma and Ewing's sarcoma), infections such as infectious mononucleosis and pertussis, juvenile rheumatoid arthritis and immune thrombocytopenic purpura.

Cytogenetics and molecular genetics

Cytogenetic analysis shows differing patterns in infants, children and adults which partly explains the different prognoses of these groups (Fig. 12.7). Cases are stratified according to the number of chromosomes in the tumour cell (***ploidy***) or by specific molecular abnormalities. Hyperdiploid cells have >50 chromosomes and generally have a good prognosis whereas hypodiploid cases carry a poor

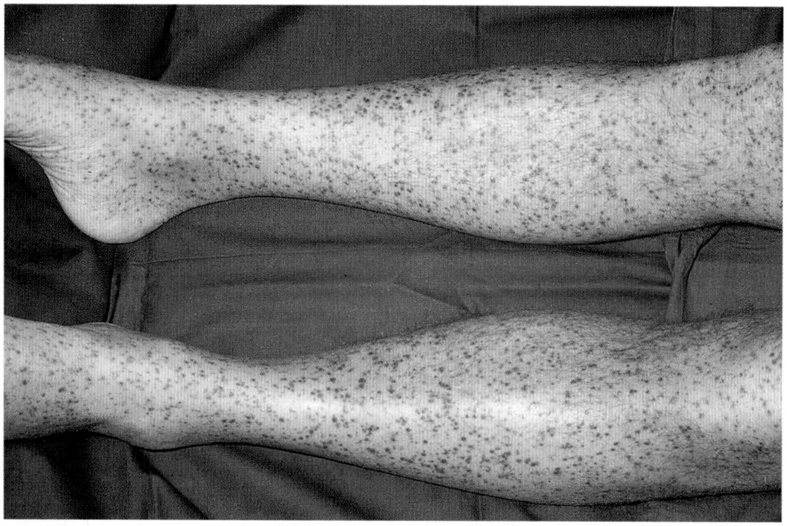

Fig. 12.4 Purpura over the lower limbs in a male patient (aged 53 years) with acute leukaemia.

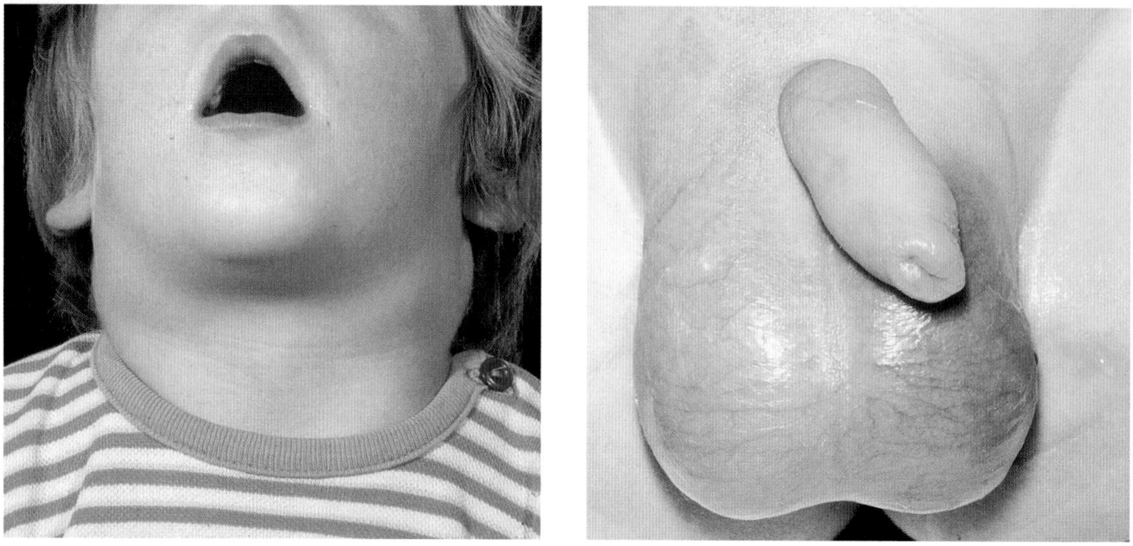

(a) (b)

Fig. 12.5 Acute lymphoblastic leukaemia. **(a)** Marked cervical lymphadenopathy in a boy. **(b)** Testicular swelling and erythema on the left-hand side of the scrotum caused by testicular infiltration. (Courtesy of Professor J.M. Chessels)

prognosis. The most common specific abnormality in childhood ALL is the t(12; 21)(p13; q22) *TEL-AML1* translocation (p. 133). The AML1 protein plays an important part in transcriptional control of haemopoiesis and this is repressed by the TEL-AML1 fusion protein. The frequency of the Philadelphia chromosome translocation t(9; 22) increases with age and carries a poor prognosis. Translocations of chromosome 11q23 involve the *MLL* gene and are seen particularly in cases of infant leukaemia. Using more sensitive molecular genetic tests, as well as fluorescence *in situ* hydridization (FISH) analysis, some cases normal by conventional cytogenetic testing are found to have fusion genes or other genetic abnormalities. These molecular genetic changes carry prognostic significance whether or not the corresponding chromosomal change is present.

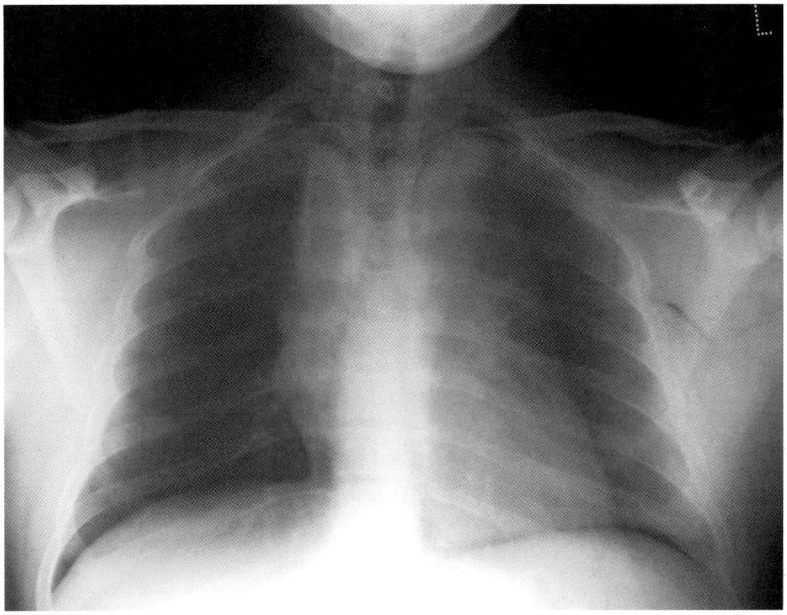

(a)

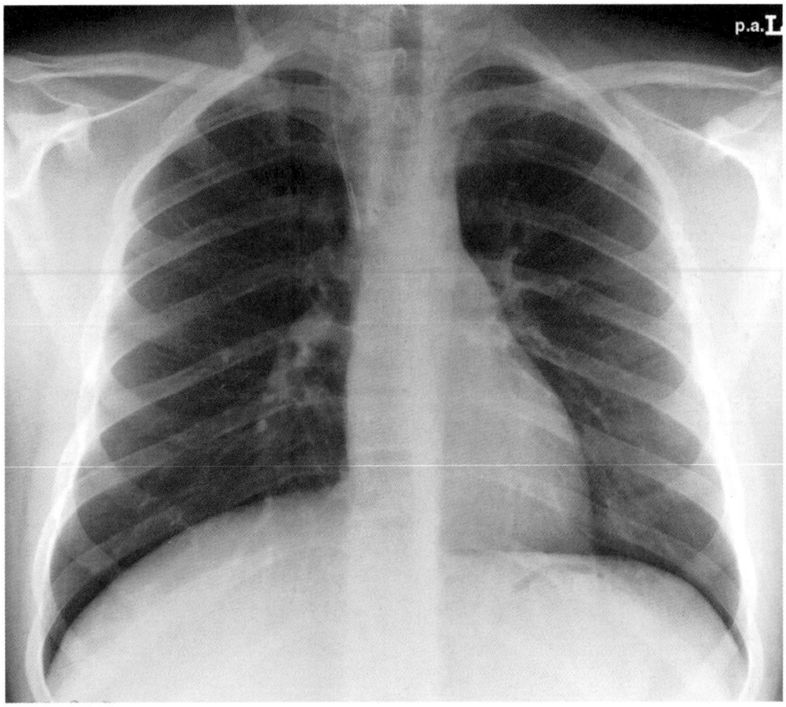

(b)

Fig. 12.6 Chest X-ray of a boy aged 16 years with acute lymphoblastic leukaemia (T-ALL). **(a)** There is a large mediastinal mass caused by thymic enlargement at presentation. **(b)** After 1 week of therapy with prednisolone, vincristine and daunorubicin the mass has resolved.

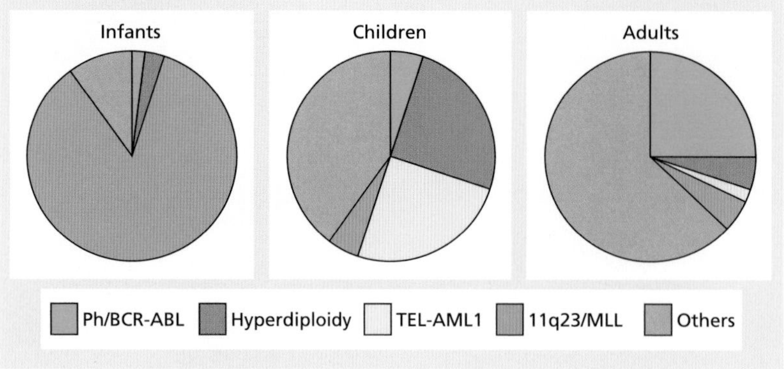

Fig. 12.7 Cytogenetic subsets of acute lymphoblastic leukaemia (ALL). The incidence of different cytogenic abnormalities in infants, children and adults.

Treatment

This may be conveniently divided into supportive and specific treatments.

General supportive therapy

General supportive therapy for bone marrow failure is described in Chapter 11 and includes the insertion of a central venous cannula, blood product support and prevention of tumour lysis syndrome. Any episode of fever must be treated promptly.

Specific therapy

Specific therapy of ALL is with chemotherapy and sometimes radiotherapy (Fig. 12.8). These are used in various phases in a treatment course which usually has four components (Fig. 12.9). The protocols differ in infants, children and adults and are also ***risk adjusted*** to reduce the treatment given to patients with good prognosis. The rare B-ALL is treated by a different protocol involving short and intensive courses of drugs.

Remission induction

At presentation, the patient with acute leukaemia has a very high tumour burden and is at great risk from the complications of bone marrow failure and leukaemic infiltration. The aim of ***remission induction*** is to rapidly kill most of the tumour cells and get the patient into remission. This is defined as less than 5% blasts in the bone marrow, normal peripheral blood count and no other symptoms or signs of the disease. Prednisolone or dexamethasone (in children), vincristine and asparaginase are the drugs usually used and they are very effective—achieving remission in over 90% of children and in 80–90% of adults (in whom daunorubicin is also usually added). However, it should be remembered that remission is not the same as cure. In remission a patient may still be harbouring large numbers of tumour cells and without further chemotherapy virtually all patients will relapse. Nevertheless, achievement of remission is a valuable first step in the treatment course. Patients who fail to achieve remission have a poor prognosis.

Intensification (consolidation)

These courses use high doses of multidrug chemotherapy in order to completely reduce or eliminate the tumour burden to very low levels. The doses of chemotherapy are near the limit of patient tolerability and during intensification blocks patients may need a great deal of support. Typical protocols involves the use of vincristine, cyclophosphamide, cytosine arabinoside, daunorubicin, etoposide, thioguanine or mercaptopurine given as blocks in different combinations. The optimal number of intensification blocks is under trial but two or three is typical in children, with more blocks given in adults.

Central nervous system directed therapy

Few of the drugs given systemically reach the cerebrospinal fluid (CSF) and specific treatment is required to prevent or treat central nervous system (CNS) disease. Options are high-dose methotrexate given intravenously, intrathecal methotrexate or cytosine arabinoside or cranial irradiation. Cranial irradiation is now avoided as far as possible in

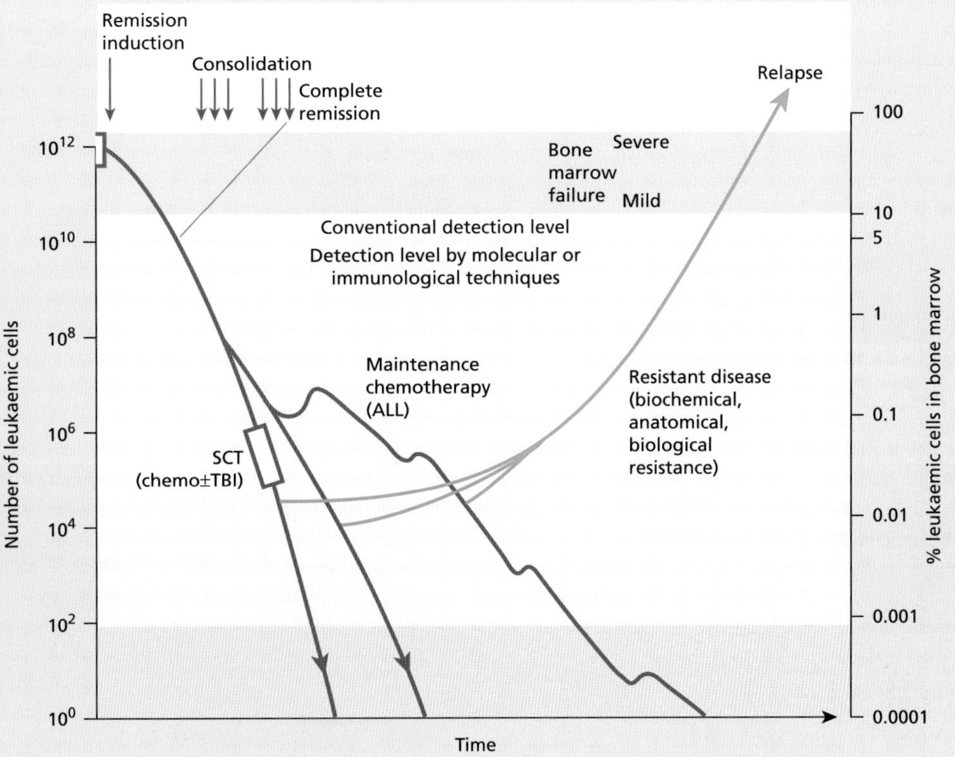

Fig. 12.8 Acute leukaemia: principles of therapy. ALL, acute lymphoblastic leukaemia; chemo ± TBI, chemotherapy ± total-body irradiation; SCT, stem cell transplantation.

children because of substantial side-effects. CNS relapses still occur and present with headache, vomiting, papilloedema and blast cells in the CSF. Treatment is with intrathecal methotrexate, cytosine arabinoside and hydrocortisone, with or without cranial irradiation and systemic reinduction because bone marrow disease is usually also present.

Maintenance

This is given for 2 years in girls and adults and for 3 years in boys, with daily oral mercaptopurine and once-weekly oral methotrexate. Intravenous vincristine with a short course (5 days) of oral corticosteroids is added at monthly or 3-monthly (in adults) intervals. The value of tests for minimal residual disease (MRD) at the end of induction or during consolidation is being explored in trials in which the intensity of consolidation or maintenance therapy is reduced in those who rapidly become MRD negative, whereas more intensified therapy, or even stem cell transplantion, is given to those with persistent MRD. There is a high risk of varicella or measles during maintenance therapy in children who lack immunity to these viruses. If exposure to these infections occurs, prophylactic immunoglobulin should be given. In addition, oral co-trimoxazole is given to reduce the risk of *Pneumocystis carinii*.

Other treatments

Allogeneic stem cell transplantation is indicated for patients with Ph (BCR-ABL) positive ALL, for primary refractory disease or for early relapsed disease. Imatinib mesylate is included into treatment protocols for patients with BCR-ABL positive ALL.

Prognosis

There is a great variation in the chance of individual

Induction
e.g. vincristine, asparginase,
dexamethasone (or prednisolone) ± daunorubicin

↓

Consolidation
e.g. daunorubicin, cytosine arabinoside, vincristine,
etoposide, thioguanine or mercaptopurine,
cyclophosphamide in one to four courses

↓ ⇨ Possible stem cell transplantation

Cranial prophylaxis
e.g. high dose systemic methotrexate
+ multiple intrathecal methotrexate
(or cytosine arabinoside)
or multiple intrathecal methotrexate
cranial irradiation (1800-2400 rad)
+ intrathecal methotrexate

↓

Maintenance therapy
e.g. mercaptopurine, methotrexate, vincristine,
dexamethasone (or prednisolone)

↓

Late intensification (as consolidation)

↓

Maintenance therapy as above (2–3 years)

(a)

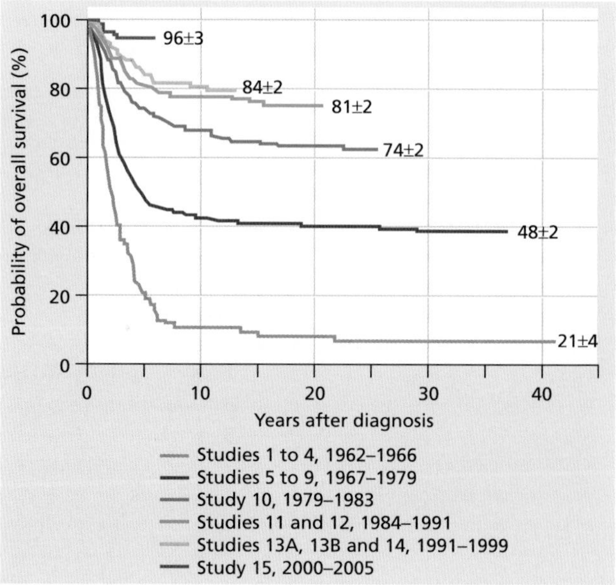

(b)

Fig. 12.9 Acute lymphoblastic leukaemia (ALL). **(a)** Flow chart illustrating typical treatment regimen. **(b)** Kaplan-Meier analyses of overall survival in 2628 children with newly diagnosed ALL. (From Pui CH and Evans WE (2006) Treatment of acute lymphoblastic leukaemia. *New Engl J Med* **354**,169)

Table 12.5 Prognosis in acute lymphoblastic leukaemia (ALL).

	Good	Poor
WBC	Low	High (e.g. >50 × 10^9/L)
Sex	Girls	Boys
Immunophenotype	B-ALL	T-ALL (in children)
Age	Child	Adult (or infant <2 years)
Cytogenetics	Normal or hyperdiploidy (>50) TEL rearrangement	Ph+, 11q23 rearrangements
Time to clear blasts from blood	<1 week	>1 week
Time to remission	<4 weeks	>4 weeks
CNS disease at presentation	Absent	Present
Minimal residual disease	Negative at 1–3 months	Still positive at 3–6 months

CNS, central nervous system; Ph+, Philadelphia chromosome positive; WBC, white blood cell count.

patients achieving a long-term cure based on a number of biological variables (Table 12.5). Approximately 90% of children can expect to be cured, whereas in adults this drops significantly to less than 5% over the age of 70 years. When treatment fails, death usually occurs because of resistant disease or from infections or other complications during treatment.

Table 12.6 Prognosis in acute myeloid leukaemia (AML).*

	Favourable	Unfavourable
Cytogenetics	t(15; 17) t(8; 21) inv(16) NPM mutation	Deletions of chromosome 5 or 7 *Flt-3* mutation 11q23 t(6; 9) abn(3q) Complex rearrangements
Bone marrow response to remission induction	<5% blasts after first course	>20% blasts after first course
Age	<60 years	>60 years
Onset	Primary	Secondary

* Detection of the relevant molecular abnormality, for example by fluorescence *in situ* hybridization (FISH) analysis, carries the same prognostic significance whether or not the corresponding chromosomal abnormality is present.

Treatment of relapse

The treatment of this is unsatisfactory at present. If it occurs during or soon after initial chemotherapy the outlook is very poor. Novel drugs such as clofarabine may help. Chemotherapy is usually followed, where possible, by allogeneic stem cell transplantation.

Acute myeloid leukaemia

Incidence and pathogenesis

AML occurs in all age groups. It is the common form of acute leukaemia in adults and is increasingly common with age. AML forms only a minor fraction (10–15%) of the leukaemias in childhood. An important distinction is between ***primary AML*** which appears to arise *de novo* and ***secondary AML*** which can develop from myelodysplasia and other haematological diseases such as the myeloproliferative diseases or follow previous treatment with chemotherapy. The two types are associated with distinct genetic markers and have different prognoses (Table 12.6). In addition, cytogenetic abnormalities and response to initial treatment have a major influence on prognosis (Table 12.6).

The most common genetic abnormality is the presence of internal tandem repeats of the *FLT-3* gene whose expression is normally tightly regulated in healthy $CD34^+$ cells. Some cases of primary AML demonstrate the chromosomal translocations inv(16) and t(8; 21) which generate fusion proteins involving the cord binding factor (CBF) genes (p. 138). These, together with the t(15; 17) variant (p. 138) exhibit a good prognosis. Many cases of AML with an apparently normal karyotype carry mutations in the nucleophosmin (NPM) gene and these also carry a favourable prognosis. This mutation leads to dysregulated cytoplasmic expression of NPM protein which normally acts as a nucleocytoplasmic shuttling protein and regulates the p53 pathway (Fig. 1.8). On the other hand, other chromosome abnormalities carry an unfavourable prognosis (Table 12.6). Those with normal karyotype may also be subdivided into favourable or poor prognosis on the basis of DNA microarray analysis.

Classification

Classification is usually based on the morphological criteria of the FAB (French–American–British) scheme (modified by the World Health Organization, WHO) in which at least 20% blast cells in the blood or bone marrow are required and which divides AML into eight variants (Table 12.2; Fig. 12.10). These FAB subtypes are associated with characteristic patterns of cytochemical stains (Fig. 12.11), immunophenotype and chromosomal changes (Chapter 10; Table 12.4). The typical 'myeloid immunophenotype' is $CD13^+$, $CD33^+$ and TdT^- (Table 12.4; Fig. 12.2) and special antibodies are helpful in the diagnosis of AML M_0 (a rare undifferentiated form), M_6 or M_7 (Table 12.4).

Although the distinct AML subtypes are in fact different genetic diseases, their grouping together is

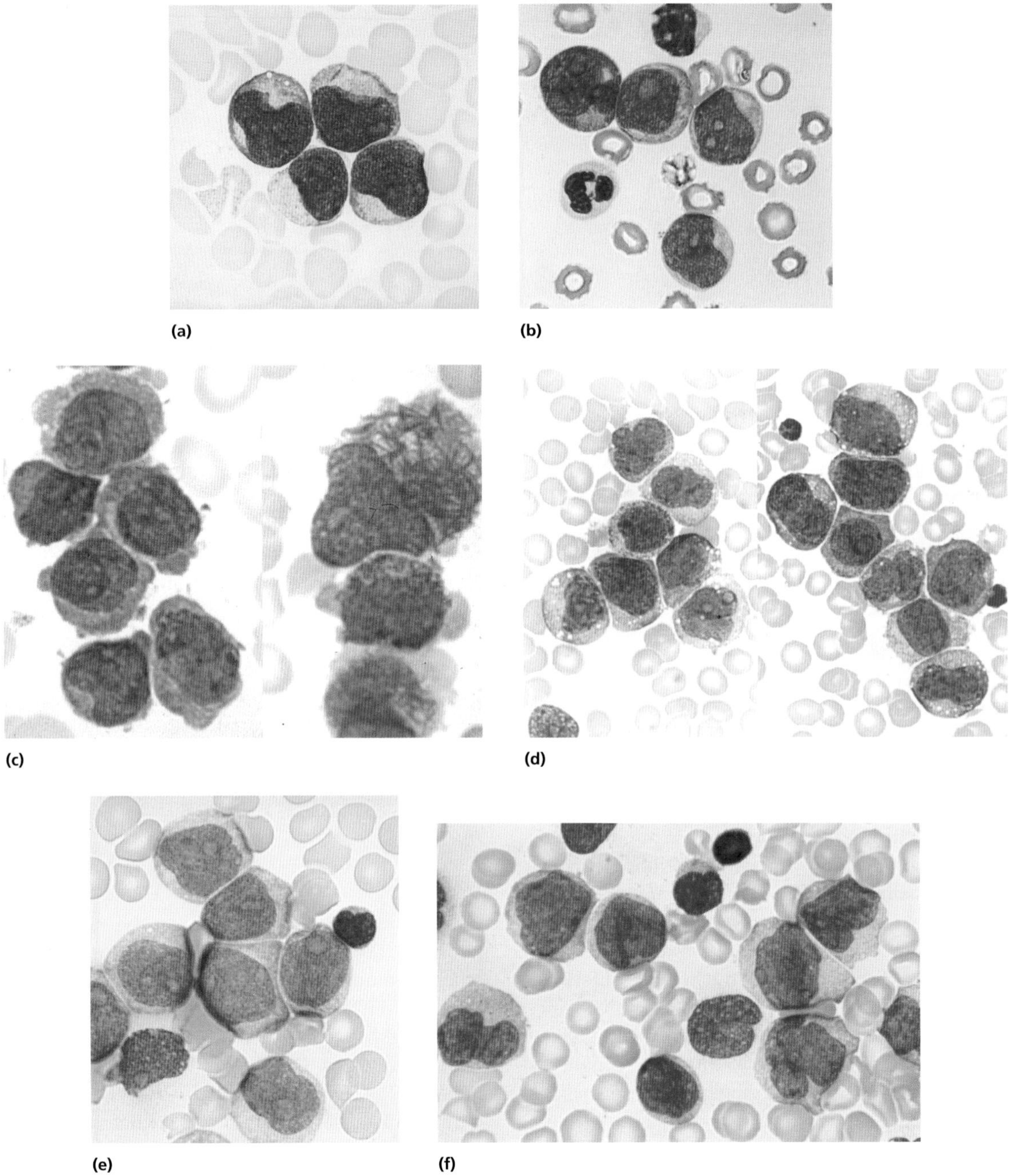

Fig. 12.10 The French–American–British (FAB) classification of acute myeloid leukaemia. **(a)** M_1 blast cells show few granules but may show Auer rods, as in this case; **(b)** M_2 cells show multiple cytoplasmic granules; **(c)** M_3 blast cells contain prominent granules or multiple Auer rods; **(d)** M_4 blasts have some monocytoid differentiation; **(e)** M_{5a}—monoblastic leukaemia in which >80% of blasts are monoblasts; **(f)** M_{5b}—monocytic but <80% of blasts are monoblasts.

(Continued)

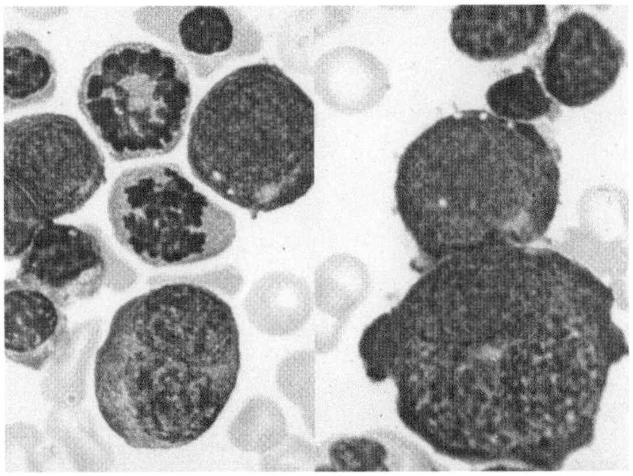

(g)

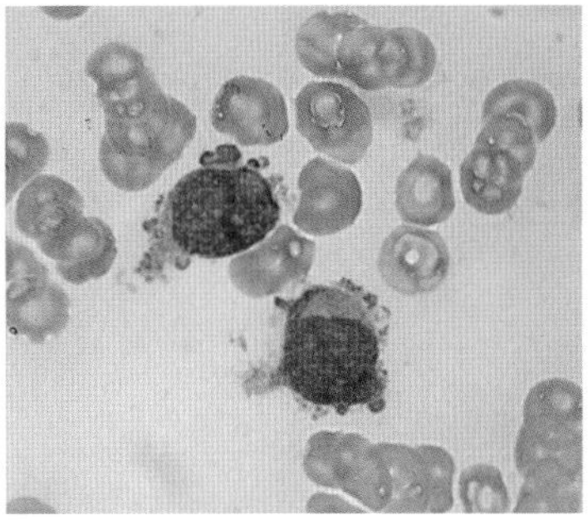

(h)

Fig. 12.10 (*Continued*) **(g)** M_6 showing preponderance of erythroblasts; **(h)** M_7—megakaryoblastic leukaemia showing cytoplasmic blebs on blasts.

Fig. 12.11 Cytochemical staining in acute myeloid leukaemia. **(a)** Sudan black B shows black staining in the cytoplasm. **(b)** M_4 (myelomonocytic): non-specific esterase/chloracetate staining shows orange-staining monoblast cytoplasm and blue-staining (myeloblast) cytoplasm.

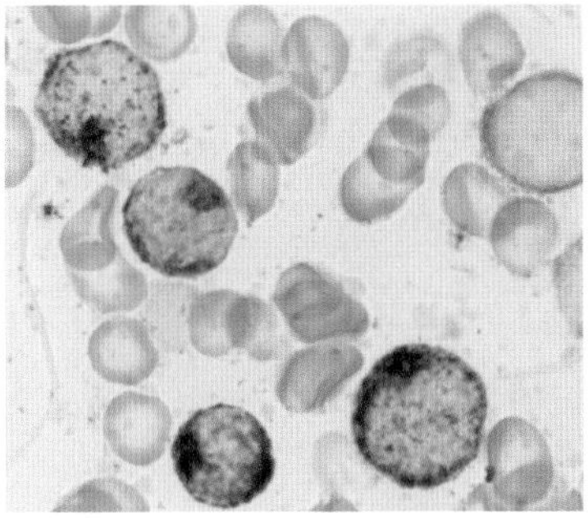

(a)

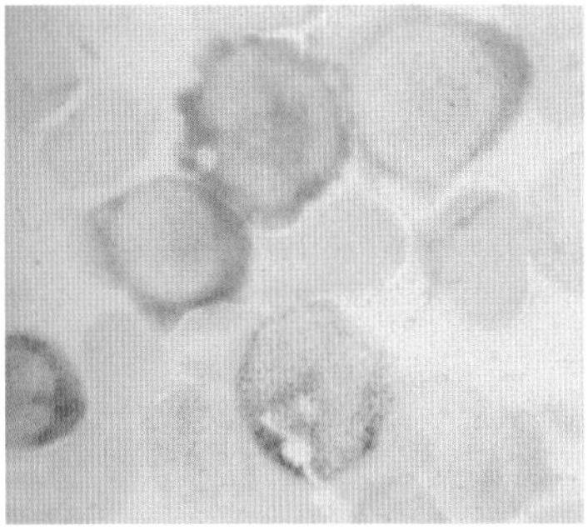

(b)

valid as generally their treatment and prognosis are similar. However, differences in treatment according to subtype are being introduced.

Clinical features

Clinical features resemble those of ALL. Anaemia and thrombocytopenia are often profound. A bleeding tendency caused by thrombocytopenia and disseminated intravascular coagulation (DIC) is characteristic of the M_3 variant of AML. Tumour cells can infiltrate a variety of tissues. Gum hypertrophy and infiltration (Fig. 12.12), skin involvement and CNS disease are characteristic of the myelomonocytic (M_4) and monocytic (M_5) types. An isolated mass of leukaemic blasts is usually referred to as a granulocytic sarcoma.

Investigations

The general haematological and biochemical findings are similar to those seen in ALL. Tests for DIC are often positive in patients with the promyelocytic (M_3) variant of AML. As explained earlier, cytogeneic and molecular analysis is critical for determining the prognosis and developing a treatment plan (Table 12.6).

Treatment

Management is both supportive and specific.

1 Supportive treatment is based on the same principles as that for ALL. Problems unique to AML include the haemorrhagic syndrome associated with the AML M_3 variant. The disease may present

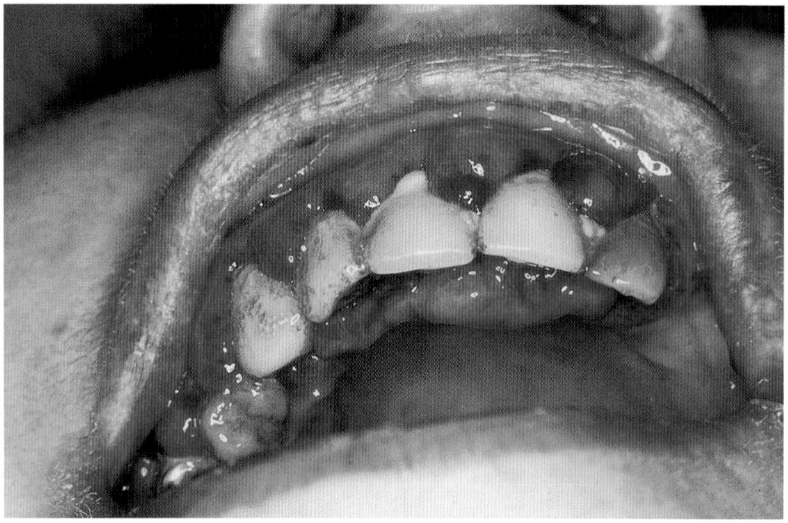

Fig. 12.12 Acute myeloid leukaemia FAB type M_5 (monocytic): the gums are swollen and haemorrhagic because of infiltration by leukaemic cells.

with catastrophic haemorrhage or this may develop in the first few days of treatment. It is treated as for DIC with multiple platelet transfusions and replacement of clotting factors with fresh frozen plasma (p. 349). In addition all-*trans* retinoic acid (ATRA) therapy is given in conjunction with chemotherapy for the M_3 disease.

ATRA syndrome is a specific complication that may arise after treatment of AML-M_3 with ATRA. Clinical problems, which are thought to result from the neutrophilia that follows differentiation of promyelocytes from the bone marrow (p. 138), include fever, hypoxia with pulmonary infiltrates and fluid overload. Treatment is with dexamethasone 10 mg intravenously twice daily and ATRA is only discontinued in very severe cases.

2 Specific therapy of AML is primarily with the use of intensive chemotherapy. This is usually given in four blocks each of approximately 1 week and the most commonly used drugs include cytosine arabinoside (in conventional or high doses), daunorubicin, idarubicin, mitoxantrone and etoposide (Fig. 12.13). All the AML subtypes (FAB M_0–M_7) are treated similarly except for the promyelocytic (M_3) variant associated with the t(15; 17) translocation in which ATRA is added to the initial chemotherapy. A typical good response in AML to cytotoxics is shown in Fig. 12.14. The drugs are myelotoxic with limited selectivity between leukaemic and normal marrow cells and so marrow failure resulting from the chemotherapy is severe, and prolonged and intensive supportive care is required. Maintenance therapy is of no value except in AML M_3 and CNS prophylaxis is not usually given in AML.

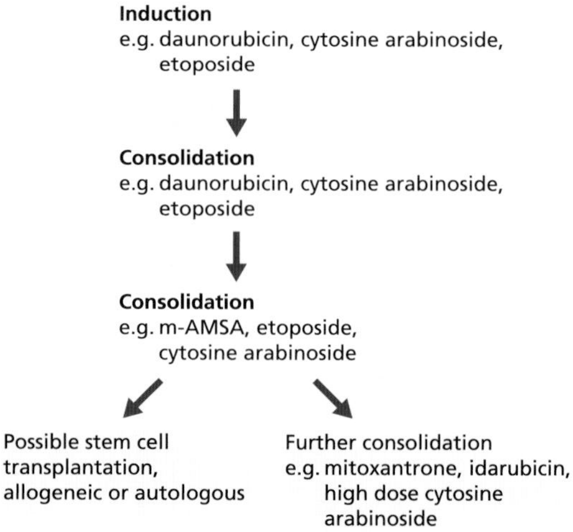

Fig. 12.13 Acute myeloid leukaemia: flow chart illustrating typical treatment regimen.

An important concept developing in AML therapy is that of basing the treatment schedule of individual patients on their risk group. Favourable cytogenetics and remission after one course of chemotherapy both predict for a better prognosis. In contrast, monosomy 5 or 7 abnormalities, blast cells

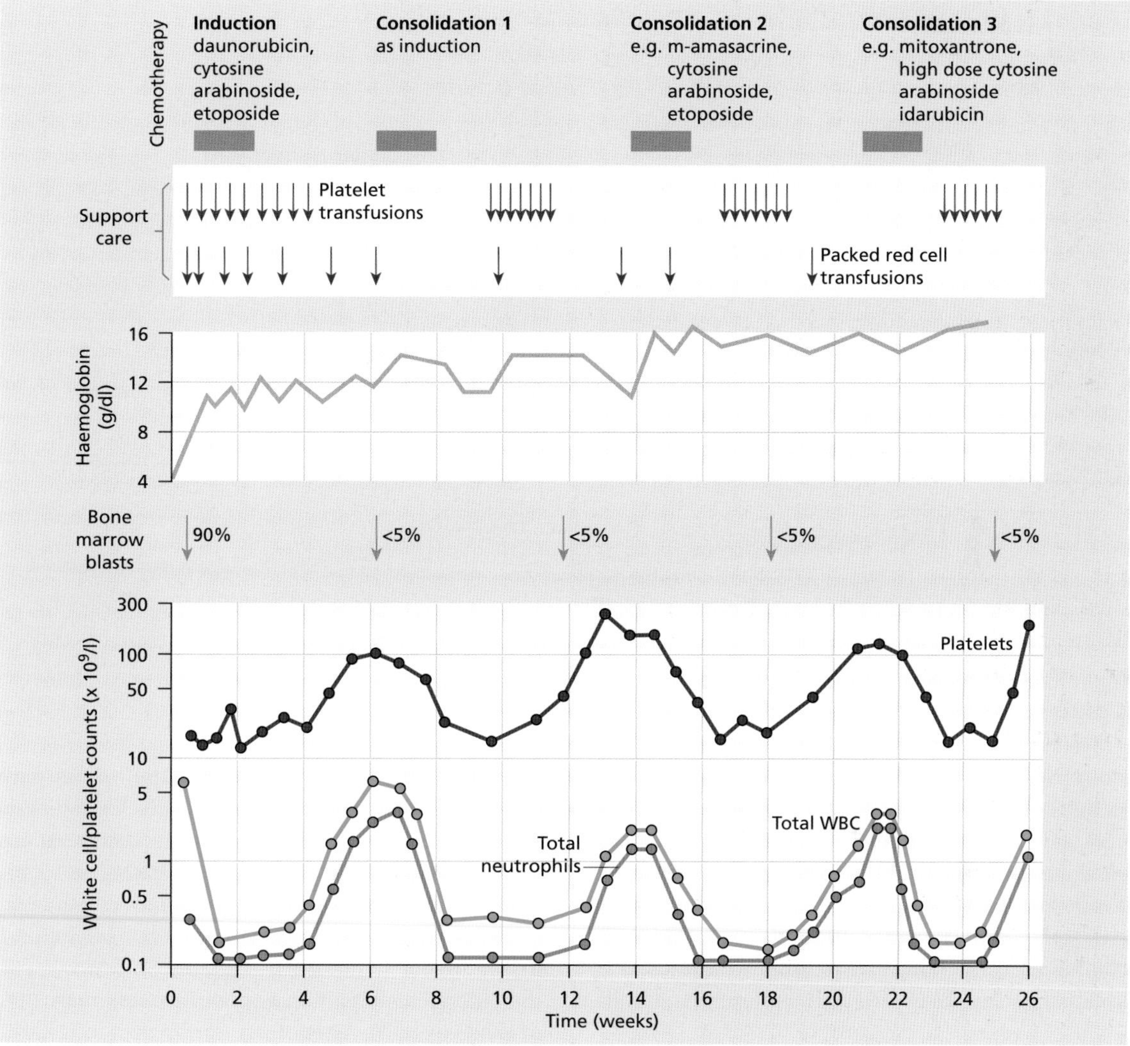

Fig. 12.14 Typical flow chart for the management with chemotherapy of acute myeloid leukaemia.

with *Flt-3* mutations or poorly responsive disease places patients into poor risk groups which may need more intensive treatments (Table 12.6). Monoclonal immunoconjugates targeted against CD33 (e.g. Mylotarg) or CD45 provide an additional therapeutic option for AML therapy.

Stem cell transplantation

Autologous transplantation reduces the rate of relapse but adds further toxicity to the treatment regime and is of no overall benefit. Allogeneic stem cell transplantation (SCT) is used in some centres in patients under 65 years old with a human leucocyte antigen (HLA) matching sibling donor with standard or poor risk AML in first remission, although other groups save it as an option for relapsed disease. Patients with t(8; 21), t(15; 17) and inv16 who go into remission after the first course do not have SCT unless they subsequently relapse.

Patients over 70 years of age

Results of AML therapy in the elderly are poor because of primary disease resistance and poor tolerability of intensive treatment protocols. Death

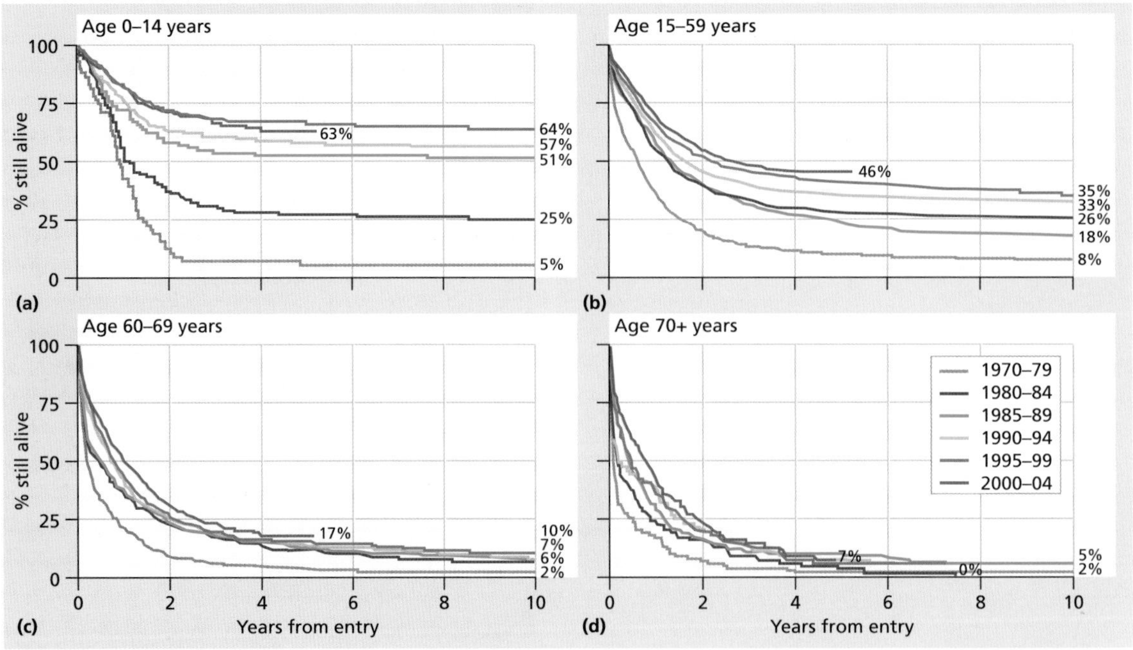

Fig. 12.15 Survival in children and adults with acute myeloid leukaemia (Medical Research Council trials). **(a)** Children 0–14 years; **(b)** patients 15–59 years; **(c)** age 60–69 years; **(d)** 70+ years. (Courtesy of Professor A.K. Burnett)

from haemorrhage, infection or failure of the heart, kidneys or other organs is more frequent than in younger patients. In elderly patients with serious disease of other organs, the decision may be made to use supportive care with or without gentle single-drug chemotherapy. However, in those otherwise well, combination chemotherapy similar to that used in younger patients may produce long-term remissions.

Treatment of relapse

Most patients suffer relapse of their disease and the outlook will depend on age, the duration of the first remission and the cytogenetic risk group. In addition to further chemotherapy, allogeneic SCT is usually performed in those patients who can tolerate the procedure and who have a suitable HLA matching related or unrelated donor. Arsenic trioxide is useful in management of relapsed M_3 variant.

Prognosis

The prognosis for patients with AML has been improving steadily, particularly for younger patients and most recently for the 60–70-year-old group. Fifty per cent of children and young adults may expect a long-term cure (Fig. 12.15). Cytogenetic abnormalities and initial response to treatment are major predictors of prognosis. Tracking of minimal residual disease using molecular cytogenetic markers or aberrant phenotypes may be helpful in predicting long-term remission or relapse. For the elderly the situation is poor and less than 10% of those over 70 years of age can expect long-term remission.

Bibliography

Bullinger L., Dohner K., Bair E. *et al.* (2004) Use of gene-expression profiling to identify prognostic subclasses in adult acute myeloid leukemia. *N Engl J Med* **350**,1605–16.

Burnett A.K. (2002) Current controversies: which patients with acute myeloid leukaemia should receive a bone marrow transplantation? An adult treater's view. *Br J Haematol* **118**,357–64.

Döhner K., Schlenk R.F., Habdank M. *et al.* (2005) Mutant nucleophosmin (NPM1) predicts favorable prognosis in younger adults with acute myeloid leukemia and normal cytogenetics: interaction with other gene mutations. *Blood* **106**,3740–6.

Falini B., Mecucci C., Tiacci E. *et al.* (2005) Cytoplasmic nucleophosmin in acute myelogenous leukemia with a normal karyotype. *N Engl J Med* **352**,254–66.

Fröhling S., Scholl C., Gilliland D.G., Levine R.L. (2005) Genetics of myeloid malignancies: pathogenetic and clinical implications. *J Clin Oncol* **23**,6285–95.

Gilham C., Peto J., Simpson J. *et al.* (2005) UKCCS Investigators. Day care in infancy and risk of childhood acute lymphoblastic leukaemia: findings from UK case–control study. *BMJ* **330**,1294.

Gokbuget N., Kneba M., Raff T. *et al.* (2002) Related articles, links risk-adapted treatment according to minimal residual disease in adult ALL. *Best Pract Res Clin Haematol* **15**,639–52.

Ottmann O., Druker B.J., Sawyers C.L. *et al.* (2002) A phase 2 study of imatinib in patients with relapsed or refractory Philadelphia chromosome-positive acute lymphoid leukemias. *Blood* **100**,1965–71.

Pui C.-H. (ed.) (2006) *Childhood Leukemias*, 2nd edn. Cambridge University Press, New York.

Pui C.-H. and Evans W.E. (2006) Treatment of acute lymphoblastic leukemia. *N Engl J Med* **354**,166–78.

Pui C.-H., Relling M.V., Downing J.R. (2004) Mechanisms of disease: acute lymphoblastic leukemia. *N Engl J Med* **350**,1535–48.

Rowe J.M., Buck G., Burnett A.K. *et al.* (2005) Induction therapy for adults with acute lymphoblastic leukemia: results of more than 1500 patients from the international ALL trial: MRC UKALL XII/ECOG E2993. *Blood* **106**,3760–7.

Tallman M.S., Gilliland D.G., Rowe J.M. (2005) Drug therapy for acute myeloid leukemia. *Blood* **106**,1154–63.

Valk P.J.M., Verhaak R.G.W., Beijen M.A. *et al.* (2004) Prognostically useful gene-expression profiles in acute myeloid leukemia. *N Engl J Med* **350**,1617–28.

CHAPTER 13

13 Chronic myeloid leukaemia

The chronic leukaemias are distinguished from acute leukaemias by their slower progression. Paradoxically, they are also more difficult to cure. Chronic leukaemias can be broadly subdivided into myeloid (Table 13.1) and lymphoid groups (Chapter 15).

Chronic myeloid leukaemia

Chronic myeloid leukaemia (CML) is a clonal disorder of a pluripotent stem cell. The disease accounts for around 15% of leukaemias and may occur at any age. The diagnosis of CML is rarely difficult and is assisted by the characteristic presence of the Ph chromosome (Fig. 13.1d). This results from the t(9; 22) (q34; q11) translocation between chromosomes 9 and 22 as a result of which part of the proto-oncogene c-*ABL* is moved to the *BCR* gene on chromosome 22 (Fig. 13.1a) and part of chromosome 22 moves to chromosome 9. The abnormal chromosome 22 is the Ph chromosome (Fig. 13.1d). In the Ph translocation 5′ exons of *BCR* are fused to the 3′ exons of *ABL* (Fig. 13.1b,c). The resulting chimeric *BCR-ABL* gene codes for a fusion protein of size 210 kDa (p210). This has tyrosine kinase activity in excess of the normal 145-kDa ABL product. The Ph translocation is also seen in a minority of cases of acute lymphoblastic leukaemia (ALL) and in some of these the breakpoint in *BCR* occurs in the same region as in CML. However, in other cases the breakpoint in *BCR* is further upstream, in the intron between the first and second exons, leaving only the first *BCR* exon intact. This chimeric *BCR-ABL* gene is expressed as a p190 protein which, like p210, has enhanced tyrosine kinase activity. In a minority of patients, the Ph abnormality cannot be seen by microscopic karyotypic analysis but the same molecular rearrangement is detectable by more sensitive techniques; for example, fluorescence *in situ* hybridization (FISH) (Fig. 13.1e) or polymerase chain reaction (PCR) (see p. 90). This Ph-negative *BCR-ABL*-positive CML behaves clinically like Ph-positive CML. As the Ph chromosome is an acquired abnormality of haemopoietic stem cells it is found in cells of both the myeloid (granulocytic, erythroid and megakaryocytic) and lymphoid (B and T cell) lineages.

A great increase in total body myeloid cell mass is responsible for most of the clinical feaures. In at least 70% of patients who do not respond well to imatinib there is a terminal metamorphosis to acute leukaemia, often preceded by an accelerated phase.

Table 13.1 Classification of chronic myeloid leukaemias (CML).

Chronic myeloid leukaemia, Ph positive (CML, Ph+) (chronic granulocytic leukaemia, CGL)
Chronic myeloid leukaemia, Ph negative (CML, Ph–) (atypical)
Juvenile chronic myeloid leukaemia
Chronic neutrophilic leukaemia
Eosinophilic leukaemia
Chronic myelomonocytic leukaemia (CMML) (see myelodysplasia, p. 186)

Clinical features

This disease occurs in either sex (male : female ratio of 1.4 : 1), most frequently between the ages of 40 and 60 years. However, it may occur in children and neonates, and in the very old. In most cases there are no predisposing factors but the incidence was increased in survivors of the atom bomb exposures in Japan. Its clinical features include the following:

1 Symptoms related to hypermetabolism (e.g. weight loss, lassitude, anorexia or night sweats).
2 Splenomegaly is nearly always present and is frequently massive. In some patients, splenic enlargement is associated with considerable discomfort, pain or indigestion.
3 Features of anaemia may include pallor, dyspnoea and tachycardia.
4 Bruising, epistaxis, menorrhagia or haemorrhage from other sites because of abnormal platelet function.
5 Gout or renal impairment caused by hyperuricaemia from excessive purine breakdown may be a problem.
6 Rare symptoms include visual disturbances and priapism.
7 In up to 50% of cases the diagnosis is made incidentally from a routine blood count.

Laboratory findings

1 Leucocytosis is usually $>50 \times 10^9/L$ and sometimes $>500 \times 10^9/L$ (Fig. 13.2). A complete spectrum of myeloid cells is seen in the peripheral blood. The levels of neutrophils and myelocytes exceed those of blast cells and promyelocytes (Fig. 13.3).
2 Increased circulating basophils.
3 Normochromic, normocytic anaemia is usual.
4 Platelet count may be increased (most frequently), normal or decreased.
5 Neutrophil alkaline phosphatase score is invariably low. It is raised in the myeloproliferative diseases and infections.

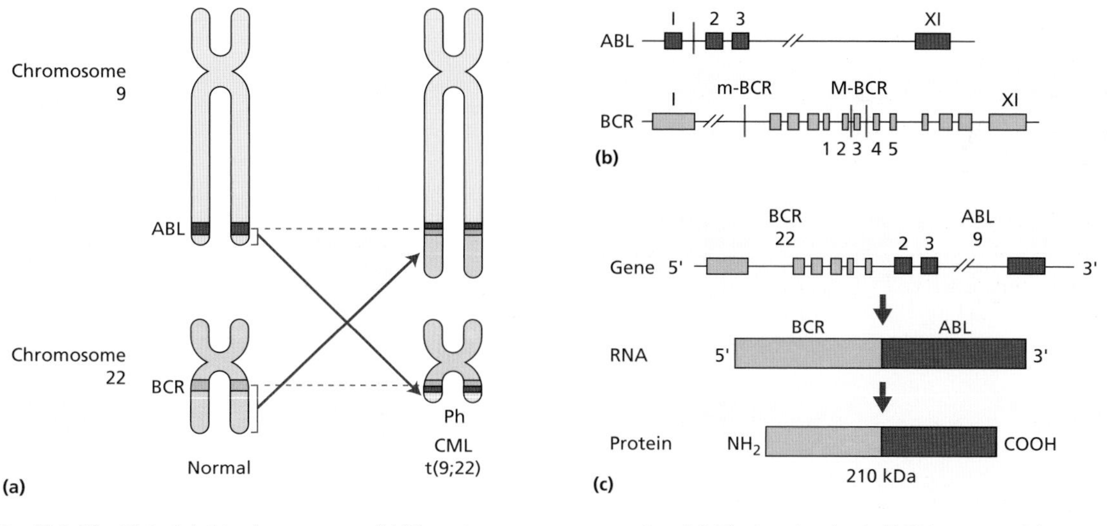

Fig. 13.1 The Philadelphia chromosome. **(a)** There is translocation of part of the long arm of chromosome 22 to the long arm of chromosome 9 and reciprocal translocation of part of the long arm of chromosome 9 to chromosome 22 (the Philadelphia chromosome). This reciprocal translocation brings most of the *ABL* gene into the *BCR* region on chromosome 22 (and part of the *BCR* gene into juxtaposition with the remaining portion of *ABL* on chromosome 9). **(b)** The breakpoint in *ABL* is between exons 1 and 2. The breakpoint in *BCR* is at one of the two points in the major breakpoint cluster region (M-BCR) in chronic myeloid leukaemia (CML) or in some cases of Ph+ acute lymphoblastic leukaemia (ALL). **(c)** This results in a 210-kDa fusion protein product derived from the *BCR-ABL* fusion gene. In other cases of Ph+ ALL, the breakpoint in *BCR* is at a minor breakpoint cluster region (m-BCR) resulting in a smaller *BCR-ABL* fusion gene and a 190-kDa protein. *(Continued)*

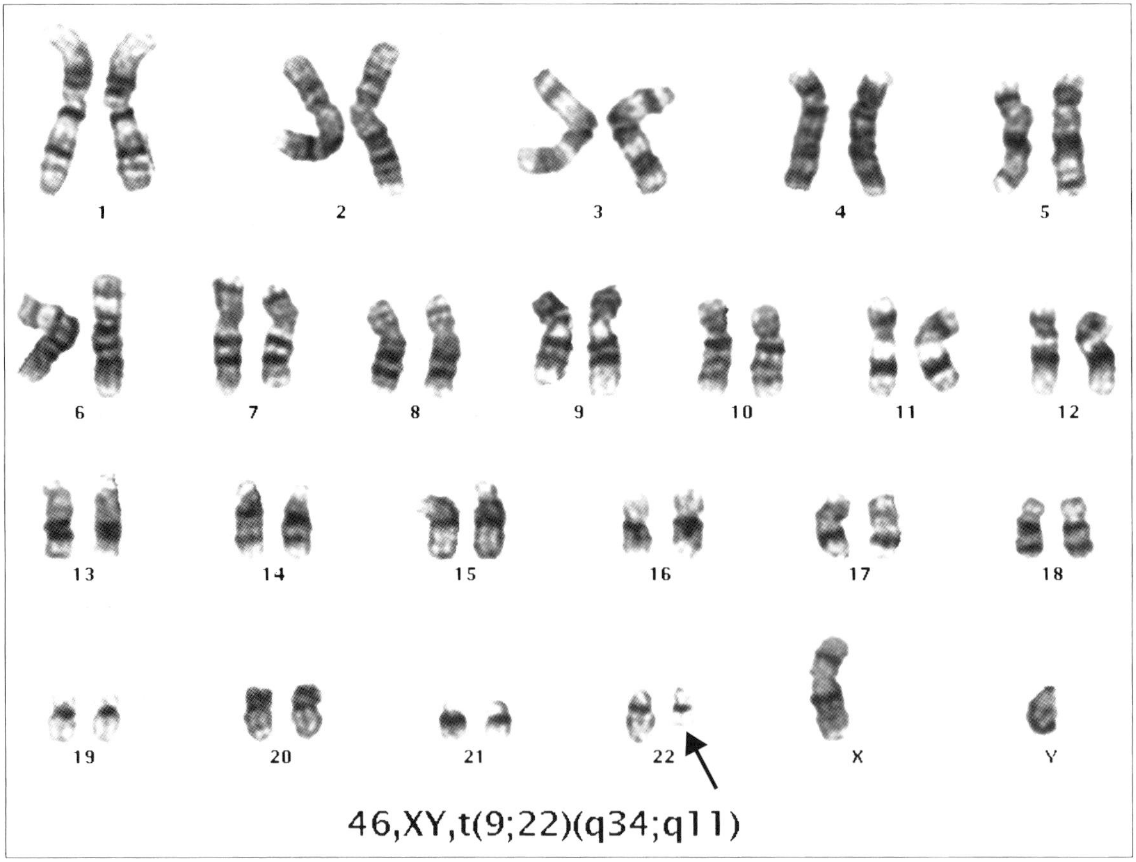

(d)

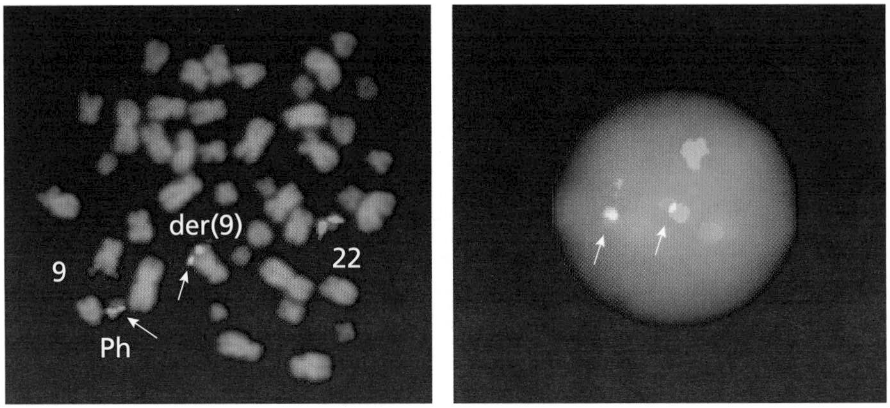

(i) (ii)

(e)

Fig. 13.1 (*Continued*) **(d)** Karyotype showing the t(9; 22) (q34; q11) translocation. The Ph chromosome is arrowed. **(e)** Visualization of the Philadelphia chromosome on: (i) dividing (metaphase); and (ii) quiescent (interphase) cells by fluorescence *in situ* hybridization (FISH) analysis (ABL probe in red and BCR probe in green) with fusion signals (red / green) on the Ph and der(9) chromosomes. (Courtesy of Dr Ellie Nacheva)

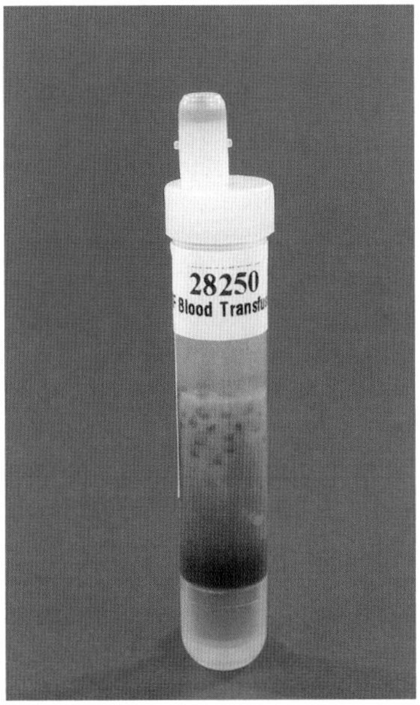

Fig. 13.2 Chronic myeloid leukaemia: peripheral blood showing a vast increase in buffy coat. The white cell count was $532 \times 10^9/L$.

6 Bone marrow is hypercellular with granulopoietic predominance.
7 Ph chromosome on cytogenetic analysis (conventional or FISH) of blood or bone marrow (Fig. 13.1).
8 Serum uric acid is usually raised.

Treatment

Treatment of chronic phase

Tyrosine kinase inhibitors Imatinib (Glivec) was designed as a specific inhibitor of the BCR-ABL fusion protein and blocks tyrosine kinase activity by competing with adenosine triphosphate (ATP) binding (Fig. 13.4). It is the first-line drug in the management of chronic phase disease. At a dose of 400 mg/day it is able to produce a complete haematological response in virtually all patients (Fig. 13.5). Side-effects include skin rash, fluid retention, muscle pains and nausea. Neutropenia and thrombocytopenia may occur and although neutropenia may be managed by granulocyte colony-stimulating factor (G-CSF) in some cases, dose reduction or cessation may be required. Imatinib is highly effective in reducing the number of tumour cells in the bone marrow and this may be monitored by karyotypic analysis of the bone marrow together with PCR analysis for BCR-ABL transcripts in marrow or blood. A complete cytogenetic response is defined as the absence of Ph-positive metaphases on cytogenetic analysis of the bone marrow. The aim is to achieve complete cytogenetic response in all patients as this is associated with improved survival. In the first year after starting treatment, blood should be studied every 3 months and the marrow

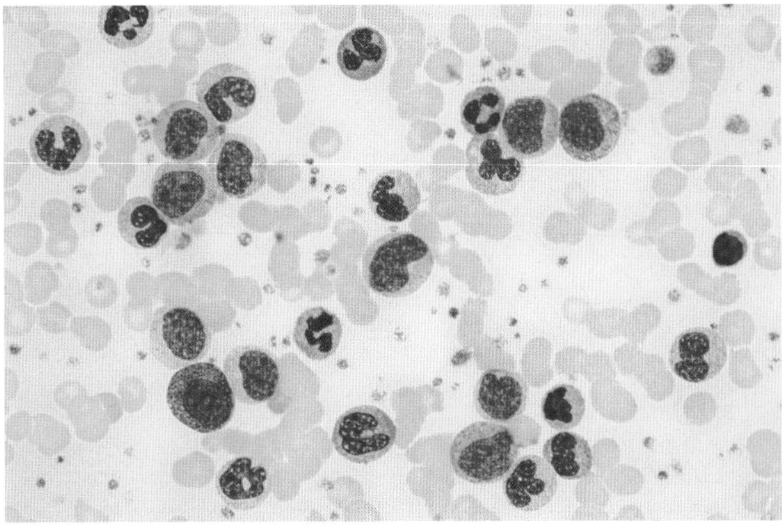

Fig. 13.3 Chronic myeloid leukaemia: peripheral blood film showing various stages of granulopoiesis including promyelocytes, myelocytes, metamyelocytes and band and segmented neutrophils.

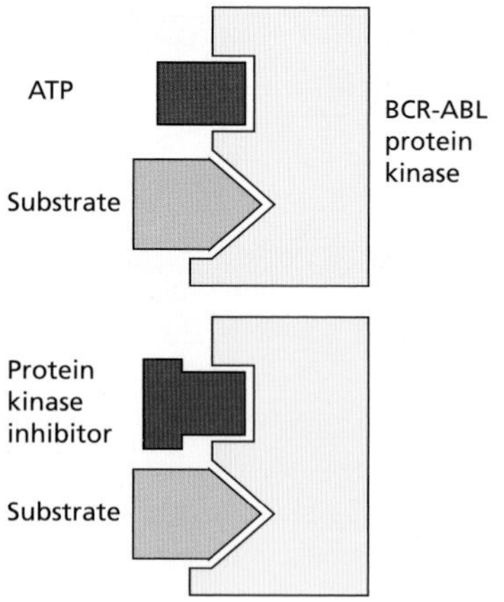

Fig. 13.4 Mode of action of the tyrosine kinase inhibitor STI-571. It blocks the adenosine triphosphate (ATP) binding site.

at 6 monthly intervals. Patients with suboptimal response can be identified as those who:

1 Fail to achieve a complete haematological response after 3 months;

2 Fail to achieve any significant cytogenetic response in bone marrow after 6 months; or

3 Fail to achieve a major cytogenetic response in bone marrow – <25% Ph+ metaphases by cytogenetic analysis after 1 year.

It is unclear how patients who have a suboptimal response should be treated. Potential options are an increase in the dose of imatinib to 600 or 800 mg/day, substitution or addition of second generation tyrosine kinase inhibitors dasatinib or nilotinib which can overcome resistance to imatinib or early allogeneic stem cell transplantation. These questions, as well as combination of imatinib with other drugs (e.g. interferon or cytosine arabinoside), are being assessed in trials. Molecular screening for mutations in the *BCR-ABL* fusion gene can be predictive for

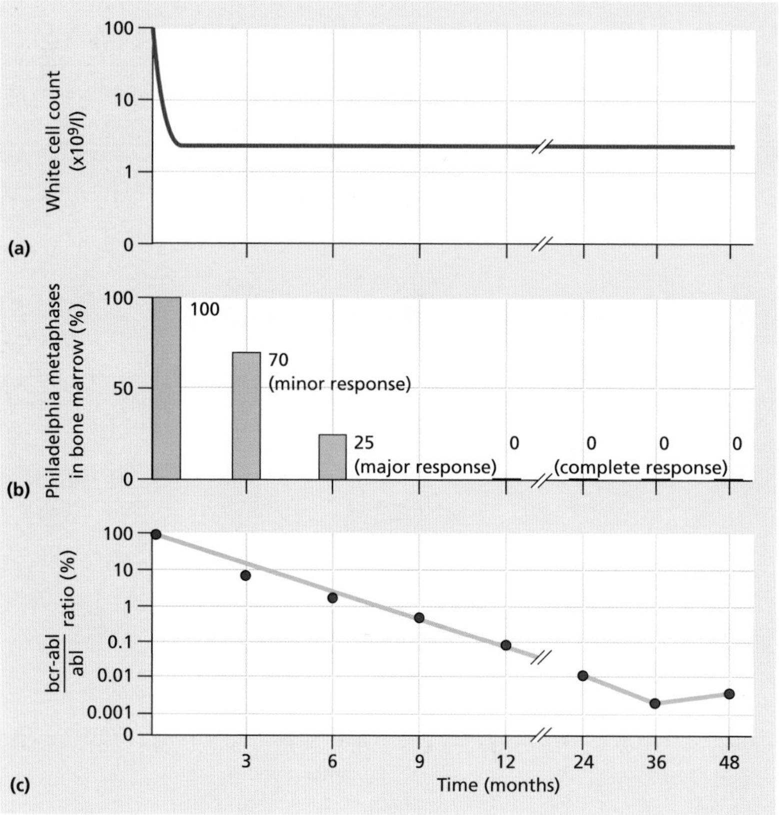

Fig. 13.5 Example of the haematological and cytogenetic response in a patient with chronic myeloid leukaemia who achieves complete remission with imatinib therapy. **(a)** The white cell count returns to normal within days. **(b)** Karyotypic examination of the bone marrow reveals a gradual reduction in the number of Philadelphia chromosomes over the first year. **(c)** Polymerase chain reaction (PCR) analysis of the bone marrow or blood shows a reduction in the number of bcr-abl transcripts in comparision with the normal abl transcript. Bcr-abl transcripts continue to be detected at a very low level but can become negative in some patients. In this case analysis was performed on bone marrow for the first 12 months and on peripheral blood thereafter.

acquired resistance to imatinib in patients in whom there is an increase in bcr-abl transcripts.

It is not yet known if patients may stop imatinib if they become negative for *BRC-ABL* transcripts by PCR analysis. It is possible that imatinib, and similar drugs in development, may prove to be a cure for some patients with CML but this will need much longer clinical follow-up than is available at the present time.

Allopurinol is used in the initial phase of treatment to prevent hyperuricaemia and gout.

Second-line drugs for patients unable to take imatinib or have a poor response to it are discussed below.

Chemotherapy Hydroxyurea treatment can control and maintain the white cell count in the chronic phase but usually needs to be given indefinitely. A typical regimen would be to start with 1.0–2.0 g/day and then to reduce this in weekly increments to a maintenance dosage of 0.5–1.5 g/day. The alkylating agent busulfan is also effective in controlling the disease but has considerable long-term side-effects and is now reserved for patients who are intolerant of hydroxyurea. Imatinib has now largely replaced both drugs.

α-Interferon This was often used after the white cell count had been controlled by hydroxyurea but has now been superceded by imatinib. A typical regimen would be from 3 (to 9) megaunits between three to seven times each week given as a subcutaneous injection. The aim is to keep the white cell count low (around 4×10^9/L). Almost all patients have symptoms of a 'flu-like' illness in the first few days of treatment which responds to paracetamol and gradually wears off. More serious complications include anorexia, depression and cytopenias (see Table 11.1). A minority (approximately 15%) of patients may achieve long-term remission with loss of the Ph chromosome on cytogenetic analysis although the *BCR-ABL* fusion gene can still be detected by PCR. Interferon produces an overall prolongation of the chronic phase with increased life expectancy. Combinations of interferon with pulses of cytosine arabinoside may be more effective than interferon alone.

Stem cell transplantation Allogeneic stem cell transplantation (SCT) is the only established curative treatment for CML but, because of the risk, is usually reserved for imatinib failures. The results are better when it is performed in chronic rather than acute or accelerated phases. Only patients below approximately 65 years of age can tolerate SCT (low intensity in the older group) and only 30% of these will have a matched sibling. The 5-year survival is approximately 50–70% although this is reduced by approximately 10% if transplantation is delayed for

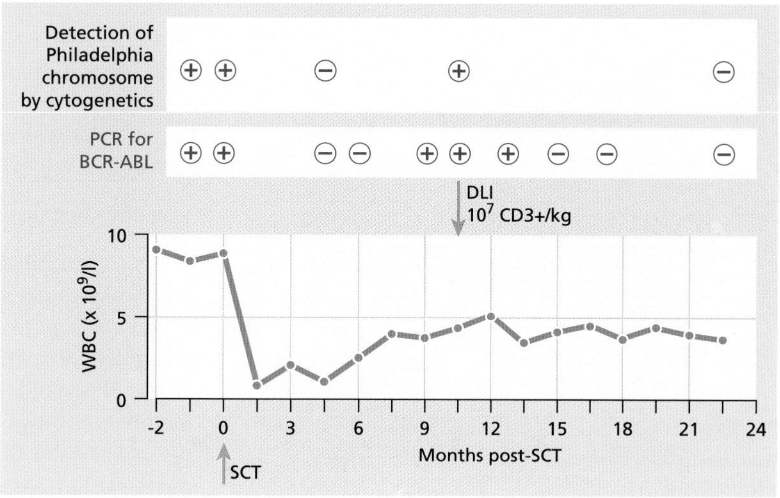

Fig. 13.6 Example of donor leucocyte infusion (DLI) in the treatment of chronic myeloid leukaemia (CML) which relapsed following allogeneic stem cell transplantation (SCT). Polymerase chain reaction (PCR) analysis of the blood for the *BCR-ABL* transcript shows that there was transient loss of the transcript but molecular and cytogenetic relapse occurred at 10 months. One infusion of donor leucocytes led to re-establishment of a durable complete remission.

more than 1 year following diagnosis. Although international bone marrow donor panels are playing an increasingly important part in providing human leucocyte antigen (HLA) matching unrelated donors, allogeneic SCT can only be offered to a minority of patients. Leukaemia relapse post-transplant is a significant problem but donor leucocyte infusions are highly effective in CML (Fig. 13.6 and p. 261), particularly if relapse is diagnosed early by molecular detection of the *BCR-ABL* transcript.

Course and prognosis

CML usually shows an excellent response to imatinib in the chronic phase. Survival is now much prolonged by imatinib. It is possible but not yet established that the best responders to imatinib may never relapse. If death occurs it is usually from terminal acute transformation or from intercurrent haemorrhage or infection. The patients may be divided into prognostic groups according to age, spleen size, platelet count, peripheral blood or bone marrow blast cells on presentation. These are only rough guides to outcome. Ease of response to imatinib is most important.

Accelerated phase disease and blastic transformation

Acute transformation (20% or more blasts in the marrow) may occur rapidly over days or weeks

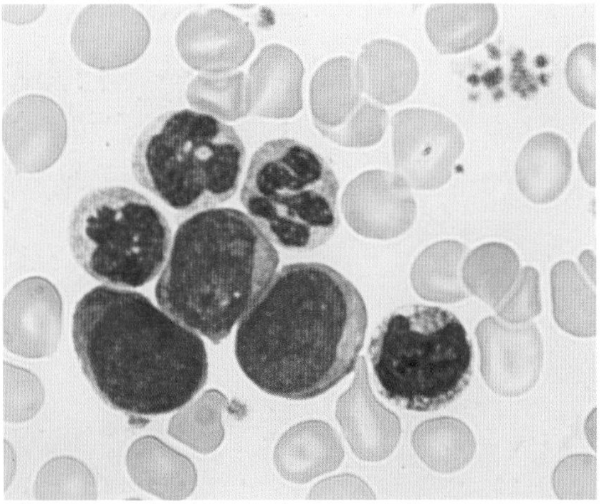

Fig. 13.7 Chronic myeloid leukemia: acute myeloblastic transformation. Peripheral blood showing frequent myeloblasts.

(Fig. 13.7). More commonly, the patient has an accelerated phase with anaemia, thrombocytopenia and an increase in basophils, eosinophils or blast cells in the blood and marrow. The spleen may be enlarged despite control of the blood count and the marrow may become fibrotic. The patient may be in this phase for several months during which the disease is less easy to control than in the chronic phase. In both the accelerated and acute phases, new chromosome abnormalities are often present. In approximately one-fifth of cases, acute transformation is lymphoblastic and patients may be treated in a similar way to ALL with a number of patients returning to the chronic phase for months or even a year or two. In the majority, transformation is into acute myeloid leukaemia (AML) or mixed types. These are more difficult to treat and survival is rare beyond a few months. Imatinib is valuable in the management of blastic transformation but resistance to treatment usually occurs within a few weeks. New tyrosine kinase inhibitors aimed at overcoming resistance to imatinib are in dasatinib and nilotinib (p. 178) trials. SCT is usually offered to younger patients with an HLA matching donor but the results are less good than in chronic phase.

Variants of chronic myeloid leukaemia

Philadelphia-negative chronic myeloid leukaemia

Less than 5% of patients with features suggestive of CML are negative for the Philadelphia chromosome and *BCR-ABL* translocation. These patients usually have some of the haematological features typical of myelodysplasia. The prognosis appears to be worse than for Ph-positive CML.

Juvenile chronic myeloid leukaemia

This rare condition affects young children and has characteristic clinical features including skin rashes, lymphadenopathy, hepatosplenomegaly and recurrent infections. The blood film shows monocytosis. A high haemoglobin F level is a useful diagnostic feature, the neutrophil alkaline phosphatase score is normal and the Ph chromosome test is negative. The prognosis is poor and SCT is the treatment of choice.

Eosinophilic leukaemia and chronic neutrophilic leukaemia

These are rare conditions in which there is a relatively pure proliferation of mature cells. Some patients with idiopathic hypereosinophilia have an interstital deletion of chromosome 4 that results in a *FIP1L1-PDGFRA* fusion gene. These patients are often responsive to low doses of imatinib (p. 104). Patients with chronic neutrophilic leukaemia may have mild splenomegaly and in general the prognosis is good.

Chronic myelomonocytic leukaemia

This is classified with the myelodysplastic syndromes and with the myeloproliferative disorders (p. 186).

Bibliography

Cools J., DeAngelo D.J., Gotlib J. *et al.* (2003) A tyrosine kinase created by fusion of the PDGFRA and FIP1L1 genes as a therapeutic target of imatinib in idiopathic hypereosinophilic syndrome. *N Engl J Med* **348**,1201–14.

Deininger M., Buchdunger E., Druker B.J. (2005) The development of imatinib as a therapeutic agent for chronic myeloid leukemia. *Blood* **105**,2640–53.

Druker B.J., Talpaz M., Resta R.N. *et al.* (2001) Efficacy and safety of a specific inhibitor of the BCR-ABL tyrosine kinase in chronic myeloid leukemia. *N Engl J Med* **344**,1031–7.

Kantarjian H., Giles F., Wunderle L. *et al.* (2006) Nilotinib in imatinib-resistant CML and Philadelphia chromosome positive ALL. *N Engl J Med* **354**,2542–51.

Mauro M.J. and Deininger M.W.N. (2006) Chronic myeloid leukemia in 2006: a perspective. *Haematologica* **91**,152–9.

Melo J.V., Deininger M.W. (2004) Biology of chronic myelogenous leukemia — signaling pathways of initiation and transformation. *Hematol Oncol Clin N Am* **18**,545–68.

Ren R. (2005) Mechanisms of BCR-ABL in the pathogenesis of chronic myelogenous leukaemia. *Nat Rev Cancer* **5**,172–8.

Talpaz M., Shah N.P., Kantarjian *et al.* (2006) Dasatinib in imatinib-resistant Philadelphia chromosome-positive leukemias. *N Engl J Med* **354**,2531–41.

Willis S.G., Lange T., Demehri S. *et al.* (2005) High-sensitivity detection of BCR-ABL kinase domain mutations in imatinib-naive patients: correlation with clonal cytogenetic evolution but not response to therapy. *Blood* **106**,2128–37.

CHAPTER 14

14 Myelodysplasia

Myelodysplasia (myelodysplastic syndromes)

This is a group of clonal disorders of multipotent haemopoietic stem cells which are characterized by increasing bone marrow failure with quantitative and qualitative abnormalities of all three myeloid cell lines. A hallmark of the disease is ineffective haemopoiesis so that cytopenias often accompany a marrow of normal or increased cellularity. There is a tendency to progress to acute myeloid leukaemia (AML), although death often occurs before this develops. In most cases, the disease is *primary* but in a significant proportion of patients the disease is *secondary* to chemotherapy and/or radiotherapy which has been given for treatment of another malignancy.

Pathogenesis

The pathogenesis of myelodysplastic syndromes (MDS) is unclear but is presumed to start following genetic damage to a multipotent haemopoietic progenitor cell. This leads to increased stem cell proliferation but ineffective differentiation and maturation, leading to the paradox of a hypercellular bone marrow but a pancytopenia in peripheral blood. A high rate of apoptosis is present in bone marrow precursors. The immune system may have a role in suppressing bone marrow function; immunosuppression is sometimes used in treatment (see below).

Clinical features

The disease has an incidence of 4 in 100 000 and a slight male predominance. Over half of patients are over 70 years and fewer than 25% are less than 50 years old. The evolution is often slow and the disease may be found by chance when a patient has a blood count for some unrelated reason. The symptoms, if present, are those of anaemia, infections or of easy bruising or bleeding (Fig. 14.1). In some patients transfusion-dependent anaemia dominates the course, while in others recurring infections or spontaneous bruising and bleeding are the major clinical problems. Because the neutrophils, monocytes and platelets are often functionally impaired, spontaneous infections in some cases, or bruising or bleeding in others, may occur out of proportion to the severity of the cytopenia. The spleen is not usually enlarged.

Dysplastic features in bone marrow may be seen in a wide range of conditions such as excess alcohol intake, megaloblastic anaemia, recovery from cytotoxic chemotherapy and response to growth-factor therapy and these must be ruled out before making a diagnosis of MDS.

Laboratory findings

Peripheral blood Pancytopenia is a frequent finding. The red cells are usually macrocytic or dimorphic but occasionally hypochromic; normoblasts may be present. The reticulocyte count is low. Granulocytes

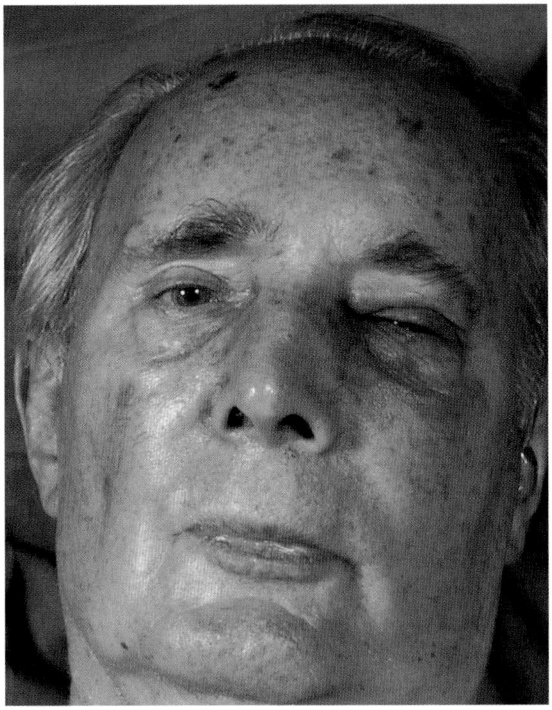

(a)

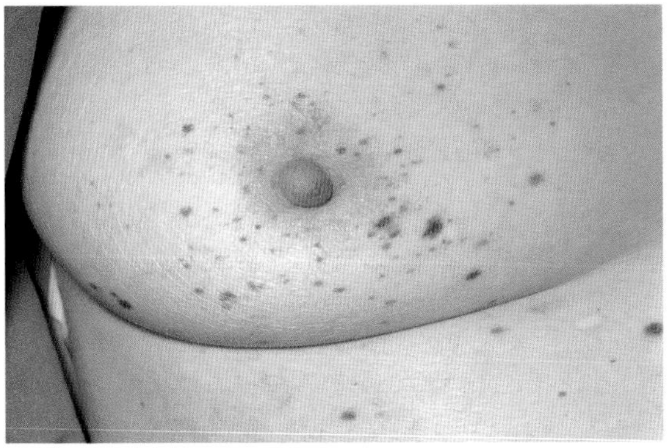

(b)

Fig. 14.1 Myelodysplasia. **(a)** A 78-year-old male patient with refractory anaemia had recurring infections of the face and maxillary sinuses associated with neutropenia (haemoglobin 9.8 g/dL; white cells 1.3×10^9/L; neutrophils 0.3×10^9/L; platelets 38×10^9/L). **(b)** Purpura in a 58-year-old female with refractory anaemia (haemoglobin 10.5 g/dL; white cells 2.3×10^9/L; platelets 8×10^9/L).

are often reduced in number and frequently show lack of granulation (Fig. 14.2). Their chemotactic, phagocytic and adhesive functions are impaired. The Pelger abnormality (single or bilobed nucleus) is often present. The platelets may be unduly large or small and are usually decreased in number but in 10% of cases are elevated. In poor prognosis cases variable numbers of myeloblasts are present in the blood.

Bone marrow The cellularity is usually increased but is decreased in approximately 20% of cases. Multinucleate normoblasts and other dyserythropoietic features are seen (Fig. 14.2). The appearance of ring sideroblasts is caused by iron deposition in the mitochondria of erythroblasts. The granulocyte precursors show defective primary and secondary granulation; cells that are difficult to identify as either agranular myelocytes, monocytes or promonocytes are frequent. Megakaryocytes are abnormal with micronuclear, small binuclear or polynuclear forms. A small number of dysplastic cells may be seen in marrow from normal elderly individuals so at least 10% of the cells in a lineage should be dysplastic in order to consider the diagnosis of MDS. In a minority of cases the marrow is hypocellular and may resemble aplastic anaemia; in others there is fibrosis.

Cytogenetic abnormalities are more frequent in secondary than primary MDS and most commonly constitute partial or total loss of chromosomes 5 or 7 or trisomy 8. The loss of chromosome 5 bands q13 to q33 in elderly females with macrocytic anaemia, normal or raised platelet counts and micromegakaryocytes has been termed the 5q-syndrome and has a good prognosis. *RAS* oncogene (usually *N-RAS*) mutations occur in about 20% of cases and mutations of *FMS* in approximately 15%.

Classification of myelodysplastic syndromes

The myelodysplastic syndromes are classified on the basis of the blood count, their morphological appearance and the number of blast cells in blood or bone marrow (Table 14.1).

Although the classification appears rather complex, the principles are:

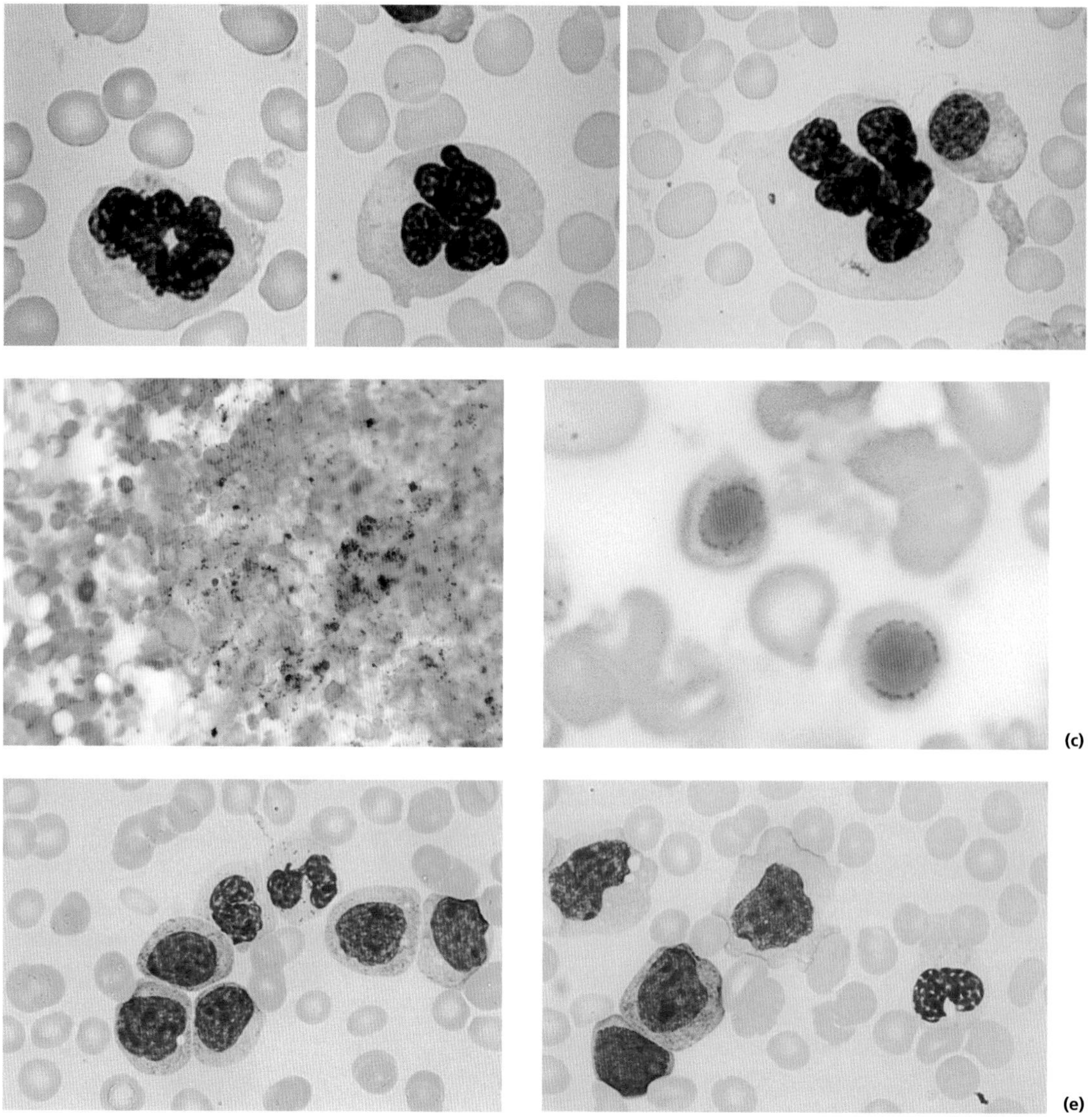

(a) (b) (c) (d) (e)

Fig. 14.2 Myelodysplasia: appearances of the peripheral blood and bone marrow. **(a)** Multinucleate polychromatic erythroblasts. **(b)** Perls' stain showing iron overload in macrophages of a bone marrow fragment. **(c)** Ring sideroblasts. **(d)** White cells showing pseudo-Pelger cells, agranular myelocytes and neutrophils. **(e)** Monocytoid cells and an agranular neutrophil. **(f)** Mononuclear megakaryocyte.

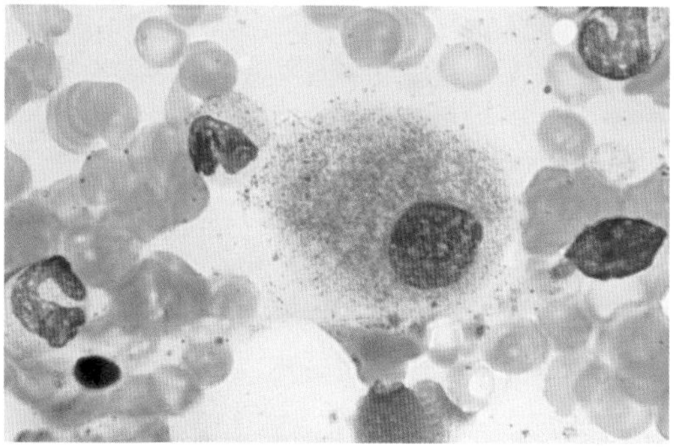

(f)

Table 14.1 The World Health Organization (WHO) classification of myelodysplasia.

Subtype	Blood	Bone marrow
Refractory anaemia (RA)	Anaemia, no blasts	Erythroid dysplasia only, <5% blasts
Refractory anaemia with ringed sideroblasts (RARS)	Anaemia, no blasts	Erythroid dysplasia only and >15% ringed sideroblasts
Refractory cytopenia with multilineage dysplasia (RCMD)	Bi- or pancytopenia or more cell lineages	Dysplasia in >10% of cells in ≥2 myeloid lineages
Refractory cytopenia with multilineage dysplasia (RCMD) and ringed sideroblasts	Bi- or pancytopenia or more cell lineages and	Dysplasia in >10% of cells in ≥2 myeloid lineages >15% ringed sideroblasts
Refractory anaemia with excess blasts-1 (RAEB-1)	Cytopenias; <5% blasts no Auer rods	Uni- or multilineage dysplasia 5–9% blasts
Refractory anaemia with excess blasts-2 (RAEB-2)	Cytopenias or 5–19% blasts or Auer rods	Uni- or multilineage dysplasia 10–19% blasts or Auer rods
Myelodysplasia syndrome unclassified (MDS-U)	Cytopenias no blasts or Auer rods	Myeloid or megakaryocytic dysplasia <5% blasts
MDS associated with isolated del (5q)	Anaemia; normal or increased platelets	Megakaryocytes with hypolobated nuclei <5% blasts

Patients with dysplastic features and over 20% blast cells in the bone marrow are considered to have *acute myeloid leukaemia with multilineage dysplasia* (p. 366).

- Dysplasia may be present solely in red cells (*refractory anaemia*) or present in two or more myeloid lineages (*refractory cytopenia with multilineage dysplasia*, RCMD).
- Both of these subsets can also be associated with *ring sideroblasts* and these subtypes are classified separately.
- If the blast cell count is increased in blood or bone marrow, the diagnosis is made of *refractory anaemia with excess blasts* and these subtypes have a poor prognosis.
- *5q-Syndrome* receives its own classification. It has a particularly good prognosis (Table 14.2).
- Cases with unilineage dysplasia of myeloid or megakaryocytic lineage are termed *unclassified*.

Treatment

This is often extremely difficult because chemotherapy rarely cures the disease and intensive or even low-dose chemotherapy may in some cases make the situation worse rather than better.

Table 14.2 World Health Organization (WHO) classification: clinical and laboratory features.

Subtype	MDS (%)	Cytogenetic abnormalities (%)	Median survival (months)
RA	5–10	25	66
RARS	10	<10	72
RCMD	24	50	33
RCMD-RS	15	50	33
RAEB	40	30–50	10 (RAEB-1)
Isolated del 5q	5	100	116

MDS, myelodysplastic syndromes; RA, refractory anaemia; RAEB, RA with excess blasts; RARS, RA with ringed sideroblasts; RCMD, refractory cytopenia with multilineage dysplasia; RCMD-RS, RCMD with ringed sideroblasts.

Low-risk myelodysplastic syndromes

Patients with less than 5% blasts in the marrow and only one cytopenia and favourable cytogenetics are defined as having low-grade MDS. They are usually managed conservatively with red cell transfusions, platelet transfusions or antibiotics as required. Attempts may be made to improve marrow function with haemopoietic growth factors, either singly or in combination. Erythropoietin (Epo) benefits the anaemia in many cases of refractory anaemia and may obviate the need for transfusions. Granulocyte colony-stimulating factor (G-CSF) shows synergy with Epo and may increase the response rate. Ciclosporin or antilymphocyte globulin (ALG) occasionally improve patients, particularly those with a hypocellular bone marrow. In the long term, iron overload may be a problem after multiple transfusions; iron chelation therapy (p. 83) should be started after 30–50 units have been transfused and if the anaemia and the need for transfusion continues to be the dominant problem. Other agents (e.g. thalidomide or its derivative Lenalidomide) may be of benefit, especially in the 5q-syndrome. In selected patients, standard or low-intensity allogeneic transplantation offers a permanent cure.

High-risk myelodysplastic syndromes

In these patients, with 5% or more blasts in the marrow and often unfavourable cytogenetics and pancytopenia, a variety of treatments have been attempted to improve the overall prognosis with varying degrees of success. These treatments extend from general support alone to intensive chemotherapy.

General support care only This is most suitable in elderly patients with other major medical problems. Transfusions of red cells and platelets, and therapy with antibiotics and antifungals, are given as needed. Fewer patients in the high-risk group with anaemia are helped by recombinant Epo, even with the addition of G-CSF, than in the low-risk group.

Single-agent chemotherapy Hydroxyurea, etoposide, mercaptopurine or low-dose cytosine arabinoside may be given with some benefit to patients with refractory anaemia with excess blasts (RAEB). The demethylating agents 5′ azacytidine or decitabine have been of benefit to approximately 60% of patient trials.

Intensive chemotherapy Chemotherapy as given in AML (p. 169) may be tried in high-risk patients. Although the majority of patients may expect to obtain a remission, relapse is almost inevitable and frequently occurs within a few months. The risks of intensive chemotherapy are great because prolonged pancytopenia may occur in some cases without normal haemopoietic regeneration, presumably because normal stem cells are not present.

Stem cell transplantation SCT offers the prospect of complete cure for MDS and the advent of non-myeloablative conditioning is increasing the age range of patients that may be treated. SCT is usually carried out in MDS without a complete remission being first obtained with chemotherapy, although in high-risk cases initial chemotherapy may be tried to reduce the blast proportion and the risk of recurrence of the MDS. Older age, poor-risk cytogenetics, advanced disease and treatment-related MDS all increase the risk of an unfavourable outcome.

Myelodysplastic/myeloproliferative diseases

These disorders are characterized by the presence of dysplastic features but also increased number of circulating cells in one or more lineages (Table 14.3).

Chronic myelomonocytic leukaemia

This constituted approximately 20% of cases of

Table 14.3 The World Health Organization (WHO) classification of myelodysplastic/myeloproliferative diseases.

Chronic myelomonocytic leukaemia	CMML
Atypical chronic myeloid leukaemia*	aCML
Juvenile myelomonocytic leukaemia	JMML
Myelodysplastic/myeloproliferative disease	Unclassifiable

* This is discussed in Chapter 13.

MDS when it was classified with them. It is defined by a persistent monocytosis of $>1.0 \times 10^9$/L. The total white cell count is usually raised and may exceed 100×10^9/L. Patients may develop skin rashes and around half have splenomegaly. Gum hypertrophy and lymphadenopathy may also be present. Treatment is difficult although hydroxyurea, etoposide or mercaptopurine may be useful. SCT may be tried in younger patients. Median survival is approximately 2 years, with increased marrow blasts a predictor of poor outcome.

Juvenile myelomonocytic leukaemia

This presents in the first 4 years of life and has features of both myelodysplasia and a myeloproliferative disease. There is often a skin rash, hepatosplenomegaly and lymphadenopathy. There is a monocytosis to $>1.0 \times 10^9$/L, clonal cytogenetic changes but not the *BCR-ABL* fusion gene. The only curative treatment is allogeneic SCT. If untreated, death usually occurs within 4 years, often from acute transformation with leukaemic infiltration (e.g. of the lungs).

Bibliography

Bennett J.M. (ed.) (2002) *The Myelodysplastic Syndromes: Pathobiology and Clinical Management*. Marcel Dekker, New York.

Bowen D., Culligan D., Jowitt S. *et al.* (2003) UK MDS Guidelines Group. Guidelines for the diagnosis and therapy of adult myelodysplastic syndromes. *Br J Haematol* **120**,187–200.

Cazzola M. and Malcovati L. (2005) Myelodysplastic syndromes: coping with ineffective hematopoiesis. *N Engl J Med* **352**,536–8.

Deeg, J., Bowen D.T., Gore S.D. *et al.* (eds) (2006) *Hematologic Malrgnancies*. Springer-Verlag, Berlin.

Greenberg P., Cox C., LeBeau M.M. *et al.* (1997) International scoring system for evaluating prognosis in myelodysplastic syndromes. *Blood* **89**,2079–88.

Jaffe E.S., Harris N.L., Stein H., Vardiman J.W. (eds). (2001) *World Health Organization Classification of Tumours: Pathology and Genetics of Tumours of Haematopoietic and Lymphoid Tissues*. IARC Press, Lyon.

List A., Kurtin S., Roe D.J. (2005) Efficacy of lenalidomide in myelodysplastic syndromes. *N Engl J Med* **352**,549–57.

Rowe J.M. (ed.) (2004) Myelodysplastic syndromes: etiology, natural history, current and future therapies. *Clin Haematol* **17**,535–661.

CHAPTER 15

15 The chronic lymphoid leukaemias

Several disorders are included in this group characterized by accumulation in the blood of mature lymphocytes of either B- or T-cell type (Table 15.1). There is considerable overlap with the lymphomas. In many cases of non-Hodgkin's lymphoma, lymphoma cells are found in the blood and the distinction between chronic leukaemia and lymphoma is arbitrary, depending on the relative proportion of the disease in soft tissue masses compared to blood and bone marrow. In general, the diseases are incurable but tend to run a chronic and fluctuating course.

Table 15.1 Classification of the chronic lymphoid leukaemias and leukaemia/lymphoma syndromes.*

B-cell	T-cell
Chronic lymphoid leukaemias	
Chronic lymphocytic leukaemia (CLL)	Large granular lymphocytic leukaemia
Prolymphocytic leukaemia (PLL)	T-cell prolymphocytic leukaemia (T-PLL)
Hairy cell leukaemia (HCL)	
Plasma cell leukaemia	
Leukaemia/lymphoma syndromes	
Splenic lymphoma with villous lymphocytes	Sézary syndrome
Follicular lymphoma	Adult T-cell leukaemia/lymphoma
Mantle cell lymphoma	Large cell lymphoma
Lymphoplasmacytic lymphoma	
Large cell lymphoma	

* WHO classification see page 367.

Diagnosis

This group is characterized by a chronic persistent lymphocytosis. Subtypes are distinguished by morphology, immunophenotype and cytogenetics. DNA analysis may be useful in showing a monoclonal rearrangement of either immunoglobulin or T-cell receptor genes.

B-cell diseases

Chronic lymphocytic leukaemia

Chronic lymphocytic leukaemia (CLL) is by far the most common of the chronic lymphoid leukaemias and has a peak incidence between 60 and 80 years of age. The aetiology is unknown but there are geographical variations in incidence. It is the most common of the leukaemias in the Western world but rare in the Far East. In contrast to other forms of leukaemia there is no higher incidence after previous chemotherapy or radiotherapy. There is a sevenfold increased risk of CLL in the close relatives of patients. The tumour cell appears to be a relatively mature B cell with weak surface expression of immunoglobulin (Ig) M or IgD. The cells accumulate in the blood, bone marrow, liver, spleen and lymph nodes as a result of a prolonged lifespan with impaired apoptosis.

Clinical features

1 The disease occurs in older subjects with only 15%

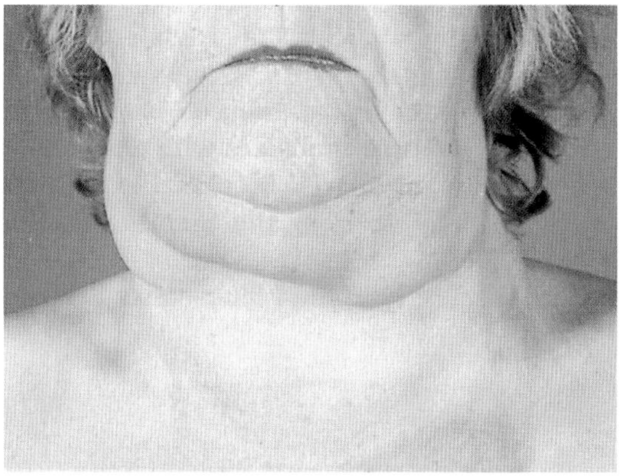

Fig. 15.1 Chronic lymphocytic leukaemia: bilateral cervical lymphadenopathy in a 67-year-old woman. Haemoglobin 12.5 g/dL; white blood count 150×10^9/L (lymphocytes 146×10^9/L); platelets 120×10^9/L.

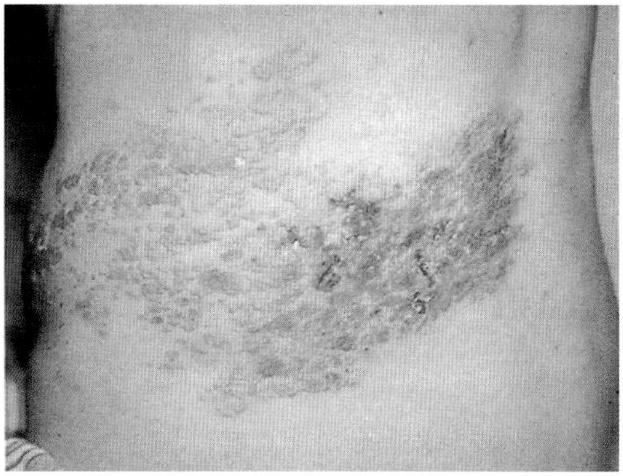

Fig. 15.2 Chronic lymphocytic leukaemia: herpes zoster infection in a 68-year-old female.

of cases before 50 years of age. The male to female ratio is 2 : 1.

2 Most cases are diagnosed when a routine blood test is performed. With increasing routine medical check-ups, this proportion is rising.

3 Symmetrical enlargement of cervical, axillary or inguinal lymph nodes is the most frequent clinical sign (Fig. 15.1). The nodes are usually discrete and non-tender. Tonsillar enlargement may be a feature.

4 Features of anaemia may be present. Patients with thrombocytopenia may show bruising or purpura.

5 Splenomegaly and, less commonly, hepatomegaly are common in later stages.

6 Immunosuppression is a significant problem resulting from hypogammaglobulinaemia and cellular immune dysfunction. Early in the disease course bacterial infections predominate but with advanced disease viral and fungal infections such as herpes zoster are also seen (Fig. 15.2).

Laboratory findings

1 Lymphocytosis. The absolute lymphocyte count is $>5 \times 10^9$/L and may be up to 300×10^9/L or more. Between 70 and 99% of white cells in the blood film appear as small lymphocytes. Smudge or smear cells are also present (Fig. 15.3).

2 Immunophenotyping of the lymphocytes shows them to be B cells (surface $CD19^+$), weakly expressing surface immunoglobulin (IgM or IgD). This is shown to be monoclonal because of expression of only one form of light chain (κ or λ; p. 141). Characteristically, the cells are also surface $CD5^+$ and $CD23^+$ but $CD79b^-$ and $FMC7^-$ (Table 15.2). Similar clones are found in some healthy subjects but with a normal total lymphocyte count.

3 Normocytic normochromic anaemia is present in later stages as a result of marrow infiltration or hypersplenism. Autoimmune haemolysis may also occur (see below). Thrombocytopenia occurs in many patients.

4 Bone marrow aspiration shows lymphocytic replacement of normal marrow elements. Lymphocytes comprise 25–95% of all the cells. Trephine biopsy reveals nodular, diffuse or interstitial involvement by lymphocytes.

5 Reduced concentrations of serum immunoglobulins are found and this becomes more marked with advanced disease. Rarely a paraprotein is present.

6 Autoimmunity directed against cells of the haemopoietic system is common. Autoimmune haemolytic anaemia is most frequent but immune thrombocytopenia (p. 283), neutropenia and red cell aplasia are also seen.

Prognostic markers

Cytogenetics The four most common chromosome abnormalities are deletion of 13q14, trisomy 12, deletions at 11q23 and structural abnormalities of

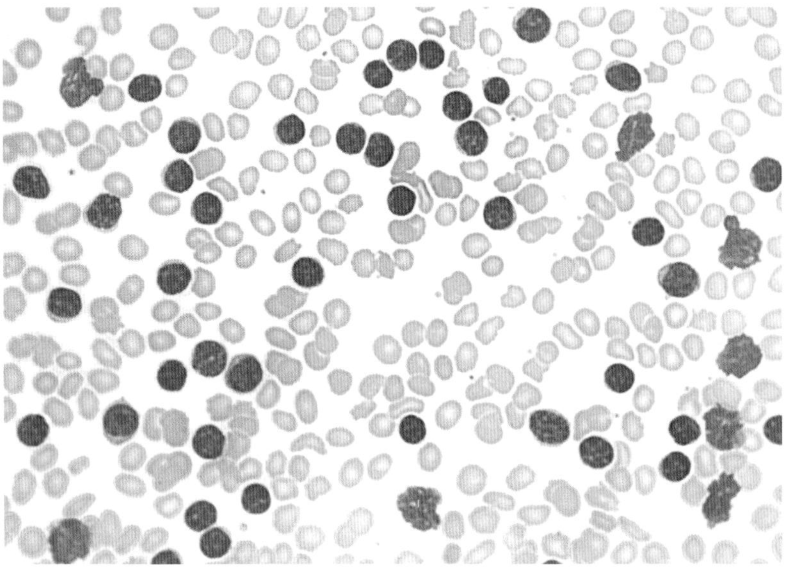

Fig. 15.3 Chronic lymphocytic leukaemia: peripheral blood film showing lymphocytes with thin rims of cytoplasm, coarse condensed nuclear chromatin and rare nucleoli. Typical smudge cells are present.

Table 15.2 Immunophenotype of the chronic B-cell leukaemias/lymphomas (all cases CD19⁺).

	CLL	PLL	HCL	FL	MCL
SIg	Weak	++	++	++	+
CD5	+	–	–	–	+
CD22/FMC7	–	+	+	+	+
CD23	+	–	–	–	–
CD79b	–	++	–/+	++	++
CD103*	–	–	+	–	–

CLL, chronic lymphocytic leukaemia; FL, follicular lymphoma; HCL, hairy cell leukaemia; MCL, mantle cell lymphoma; PLL, prolymphocytic leukaemia.
* CD103 is positive only in HCL.

17p involving the p53 gene. These abnormalities carry prognostic significance (Table 15.3). The 13q14 deletion prevents expression of microRNAs which control expression of proteins relevant to the CLL lifespan (p. 137). Expression of a novel gene CLLU.1 is substantially greater in unmutated than mutated cases.

Somatic hypermutation of the immunoglobulin genes When B cells recognize antigen in the germinal centre of secondary lymphoid tissues they undergo a process called *somatic hypermutation* in which random mutations occur in the immunoglobulin heavy-chain gene (p. 113). In CLL, the *IGVH* gene shows evidence of this hypermutation in approximately 50% of cases whereas in the other cases the *VH* genes are unmutated. CLL with unmutated immunoglobulin genes has an unfavourable prognosis (Table 15.3).

Tumour cell phenotype ZAP-70 is a protein tyrosine kinase that is involved in cell signalling following recognition of antigen by antigen receptors on lymphocytes. Its expression is normally restricted to T cells but is also aberrantly expressed in cases of CLL. Its expression is associated with an unfavourable clinical outcome.

Staging

It is useful to stage patients at presentation both for prognosis and for deciding on therapy. The Rai and Binet staging systems are shown in Table 15.4. Typical survival ranges from 12 years for Rai stage 0 to less than 3 years for stage IV.

Treatment

Cures are rare in CLL and so the approach to therapy is conservative, aiming for symptom control rather than a normal blood count. Indeed, chemotherapy given too early in the disease can

Table 15.3 Prognostic factors in chronic lymphocytic leukaemia.

	Good	Bad
Stage	Binet A (Rai 0–I)	Binet B, C (Rai II–IV)
Sex	Female	Male
Lymphocyte doubling time	Slow	Rapid
Bone marrow biopsy appearance	Nodular	Diffuse
Chromosomes	Deletion 13q14	Trisomy 12; deletion 17p; deletion 11q23
VH immunoglobulin genes	Hypermutated	Unmutated
ZAP expression	Low	High
CD38 expression	Negative	Positive
CLLU.1 expression	Low	High
LDH	Normal	Raised

LDH, lactate dehydrogenase.

Table 15.4 Staging of chronic lymphocytic leukaemia (CLL).
(a) Rai classification

Stage	
0	Absolute lymphocytosis $>15 \times 10^9/L^+$
I	As stage 0 + enlarged lymph nodes (adenopathy)
II	As stage 0 + enlarged liver and/or spleen ± adenopathy
III	As stage 0 + anaemia (Hb <10.0 g/dL)$^+$ ± adenopathy ± organomegaly
IV	As stage 0 + thrombocytopenia (platelets $<100 \times 10^9/L)^+$ ± adenopathy ± organomegaly

(b) International Working Party classification (From J.L. Binet *et al.* 1981)

Stage	Organ enlargement*	Haemoglobin† (g/dL)	Platelets† ($\times 10^9$/L)
A (50–60%)	0, 1 or 2 areas		
B (30%)	3, 4 or 5 areas	≥10	≥100
C (<20%)	Not considered	<10	and/or <100

* One area = lymph nodes >1 cm in neck, axillae, groins or spleen, or liver enlargement.
† Secondary causes of anaemia (e.g. iron deficiency) or autoimmune haemolytic anaemia or autoimmune thrombocytopenia must be treated before staging.

shorten rather than prolong life expectancy. Many patients never receive treatment. Treatment is given for troublesome organomegaly, haemolytic episodes and bone marrow suppression. The lymphocyte count alone is not a good guide to treatment. Usually, patients in Binet stage C will need treatment as will some in stage B.

Chemotherapy

Chlorambucil This oral alkylating agent can be used as a daily treatment (e.g. 4–6 mg/day) or in a monthly cycle (e.g. 10 mg/m^2/day for 7 days) and is effective in reducing disease bulk in the majority of cases. Typically the drug will need to be given for several months after which a remission of variable duration will be obtained. Chlorambucil can be reintroduced when required although resistance may develop.

Purine analogues These drugs are effective in the treatment of chronic lymphoid leukaemias and lymphomas. The most effective agent in CLL appears to be fludarabine. Its place in the overall management of CLL is currently under trial. It is the drug of first choice in younger patients as well as having value in patients resistant to chlorambucil. Myelosuppression and prolonged reduction of CD4 (helper) T lymphocytes lead to an increased infection risk and prophylaxis against *Pneumocystis carinii* infection with co-trimoxazole is given until CD4 counts recover. The combination of fludarabine with cyclophosphamide (FC) is more effective than fludarabine alone and fludarabine, cyclophosphamide and rituximab (FCR) increases further the response rate and duration of response.

Monoclonal antibodies Campath-1H (anti-CD52) is a monoclonal antibody that is effective in killing white cells by complement fixation. It is given intravenously or subcutaneously over several weeks and as well as being valuable in resistant and relapsed disease, it may also find a role earlier in treatment. It is highly immunosuppressive and antibacterial and antiviral prophylaxis is advisable.

CD20 expression on CLL cells is not high; rituximab (p. 217), however, appears to be valuable in combination therapy (e.g. with fludarabine). It also has a role in treating autoimmune haemolytic anaemia, thrombocytopenia and red cell aplasia.

Corticosteroids Patients in bone marrow failure should be treated initially with prednisolone alone until there is significant recovery of the platelet, neutrophil and haemoglobin levels. The peripheral lymphocyte count initially rises as infiltrated organs shrink, but later the count falls. Corticosteroids are also indicated in autoimmune haemolytic anaemia or thrombocytopenia.

Other forms of treatment

Radiotherapy This is valuable in reducing the size of bulky lymph node groups that are unresponsive to chemotherapy. Radiotherapy to the spleen may be valuable in late-stage disease.

Combination chemotherapy Cyclophosphamide, hydroxodaunorubicin, oncovin (vincristine) and prednisolone (CHOP; p. 213) with rituximab is sometimes used in late-stage cases and in patients refractory to chlorambucil.

Ciclosporin Red cell aplasia may respond to ciclosporin.

Splenectomy This is generally reserved for those patients with immune-mediated cytopenias that do not respond to short courses of steroids or those with painful bulky enlargement of the spleen.

Immunoglobulin replacement Immunoglobulin (e.g. 400 mg/kg/month by intravenous infusion) is useful for patients with hypogammaglobulinaemia and recurrent infections.

Stem cell transplantation This is currently an experimental approach in younger patients. Allogeneic stem cell transplantation (SCT) may be curative but has a high mortality rate. Autologous SCT after prior therapy with fludarabine and other drugs is undergoing clinical trials.

Course of disease

Many patients in Binet stage A or Rai stage 0 or I never need therapy and this is particularly likely for those with favourable prognostic markers (Table 15.3). For those who do need treatment a typical pattern is that of a disease that is responsive to several courses of chemotherapy before the gradual onset of extensive bone marrow infiltration, bulky disease and recurrent infection. The disease may transform into a localized high-grade lymphoma (Richter's transformation) or there may be the appearance of an increasing number of prolymphocytes that are resistant to treatment.

Prolymphocytic leukaemia

Although prolymphocytic leukaemia (PLL) may initially appear similar to CLL, the diagnosis is

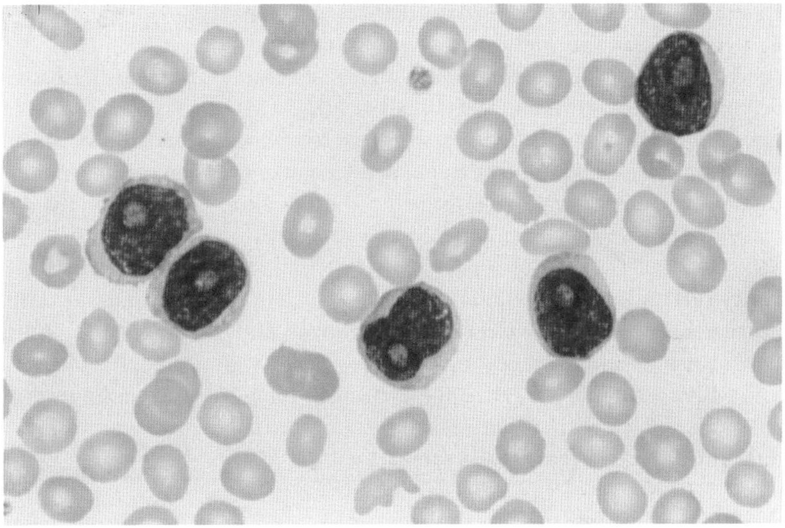

Fig. 15.4 Prolymphocytic leukaemia: blood film showing prolymphocytes that have prominent central nucleoli and an abundance of pale cytoplasm.

made by the appearance of a majority of prolymphocytes in the blood. The prolymphocyte is around twice the size of a CLL lymphocyte and has a large central nucleolus (Fig. 15.4). B-cell PLL is three times more common than T-cell PLL.

PLL and CLL also differ in their clinical features. PLL typically presents with splenomegaly without lymphadenopathy and with a high and rapidly rising lymphocyte count. Anaemia is a poor prognostic feature. Treatment is difficult in PLL. Splenectomy is usually of benefit and purine nucleoside analogues and rituximab may help.

Hairy cell leukaemia

Hairy cell leukaemia (HCL) is an uncommon B-cell lymphoproliferative disease with a male : female ratio of 4 : 1 and a peak incidence at 40–60 years. Patients typically present with infections, anaemia or splenomegaly. Lymphadenopathy is very uncommon. Pancytopenia is usual at presentation and the lymphocyte count is rarely over 20×10^9/L. Monocytopenia is a distinctive feature. The blood film reveals a variable number of unusual large lymphocytes with villous cytoplasmic projections (Fig. 15.5). Immunophenotyping shows CD22, FMC7 and CD103 positivity in most cases (Table 15.2). The hairy cells stain for tartrate-resistant acid phosphatase (TRAP). The bone marrow trephine shows a characteristic appearance of mild fibrosis and a diffuse cellular infiltrate.

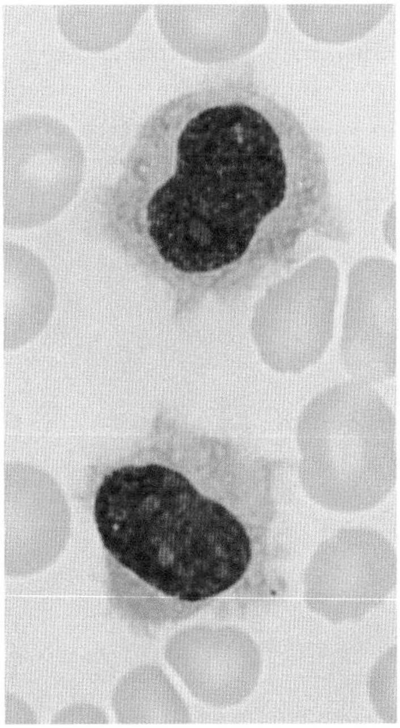

Fig. 15.5 Hairy cell leukaemia: peripheral blood film showing typical 'hairy' cells with oval nuclei and finely mottled pale grey/blue cytoplasm with an irregular edge.

There are several effective treatments for HCL and a patient can expect a long-term remission. The treatment of choice is 2-chlorodeoxyadenosine or deoxycoformycin and both agents achieve responses in over 90% of cases. In two-thirds of cases no relapse occurs, even after 5–10 years. HCL was one of the first diseases in which α-interferon was shown to be effective and it remains an excellent treatment. These drugs have largely replaced the need for splenectomy or combination chemotherapy.

Hairy cell leukaemia variant

Some cases of HCL have clear differences from the typical disease and warrant a separate classification. The white cell count is higher, the hairy cells have a prominent nucleolus and response to purine analogues and interferon is less satisfactory.

Splenic lymphoma with villous lymphocytes

This is now classified within the World Health Organization (WHO) as splenic marginal zone lymphoma (p. 367). It is characterized by massive splenomegaly and circulating monoclonal B cells with a villous appearance. It is a disease of the elderly with a benign clinical course. Although many patients will not need treatment, splenectomy is valuable and purine nucleoside analogues are also effective. The outlook is good.

Plasma cell leukaemia

This rare disease is characterized by a high number of circulating plasma cells. The clinical features tend to be a combination of those found in acute leukaemia (pancytopenia and organomegaly) with features of myeloma (hypercalcaemia, renal involvement and bone disease; Chapter 18). Treatment is with supportive care and systemic chemotherapy; for example, with CHOP, cyclophosphamide-VAD (vincristine, Adriamycin and dexamethasone) or cyclophosphamide, dexamethasone and thalidomide as for multiple myeloma (Chapter 18).

Lymphoma/leukaemia syndromes

Circulating malignant lymphoid cells occur in a variety of syndromes in association with otherwise typical cases of non-Hodgkin's lymphoma. This syndrome is most frequently seen in B-cell tumours of the follicle centre cell type (with circulating indented or cleaved nuclei; Fig. 15.6) and the course is that of the non-Hodgkin's lymphoma (p. 209). Mantle zone lymphoma is often associated with circulating B cells (Fig. 15.6) and, because these are $CD5^+$, mantle zone lymphoma may be confused with CLL. Other types of lymphoma may also show

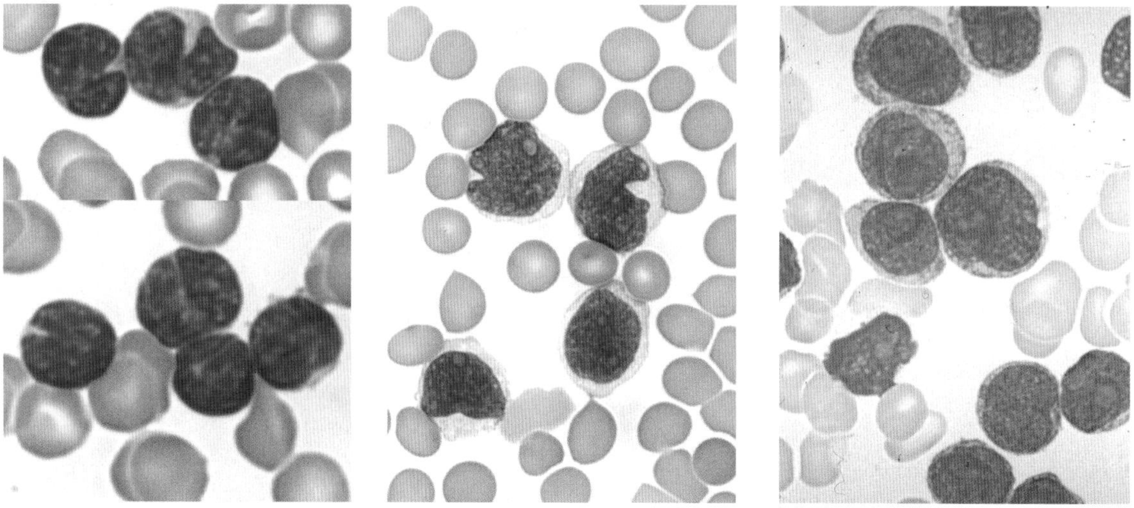

(a) (b) (c)

Fig. 15.6 Blood involvement by malignant lymphoma: **(a)** small cleaved lymphoid cells in follicle centre cell lymphoma; **(b)** mantle cell lymphoma; **(c)** large B-cell lymphoma.

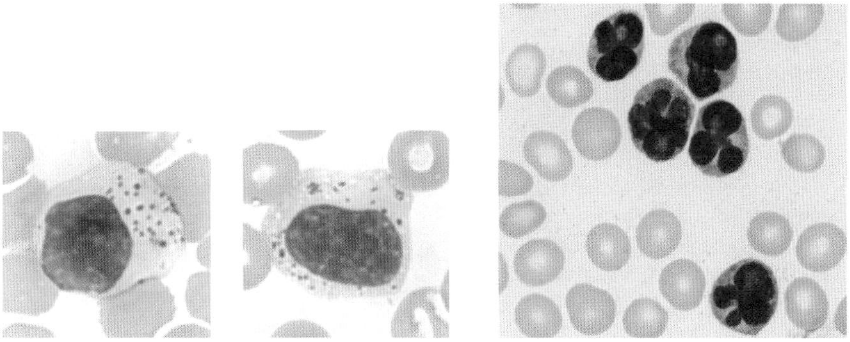

(a) (b)

Fig. 15.7 (a) Large granular lymphocytes in the peripheral blood. **(b)** Adult T-cell leukaemia/lymphoma. Typical convoluted lymphoid cells in peripheral blood.

tumour cells in the peripheral blood and bone marrow and in some cases it is difficult to define the disease as either lymphoma (with mainly soft tissue masses) or leukaemia.

T-cell diseases

Large granular lymphocytic leukaemia

Large granular lymphocytic leukaemia (LGL-L) is characterized by the presence of circulating lymphocytes with abundant cytoplasm and large azurophilic granules (Fig. 15.7a). Such cells may be either T or natural killer (NK) cells and show variable expression of CD16, CD56 and CD57. Cytopenia, especially neutropenia, is the main clinical problem although anaemia, splenomegaly and arthropathy with positive serology for rheumatoid arthritis are also common. The mean age is 50 years. Treatment may not be needed but, if required, steroids, cyclophosphamide, ciclosporin or methotrexate may relieve the cytopenia. Granulocyte colony-stimulating factor (G-CSF) or granulocyte–macrophage colony-stimulating factor (GM-CSF) have been used in cases associated with neutropenia.

Adult T-cell leukaemia/lymphoma

Adult T-cell leukaemia/lymphoma (ATLL) was the first malignancy to be associated with a human retrovirus, human T-cell leukaemia/lymphoma virus type 1 (HTLV-1). The virus is endemic in parts of Japan and the Caribbean but the disease is very rare in people who have not lived in these areas. ATLL lymphocytes have a bizarre morphology with a convoluted 'clover-leaf' nucleus and a consistent $CD4^+$ phenotype (Fig. 15.7b).

Most subjects infected with the virus do not develop the disease. The clinical presentation is often acute and dominated by hypercalcaemia, skin lesions, hepatosplenomegaly and lymphadenopathy. Diagnosis is by morphology and serology and although combination chemotherapy may be tried the prognosis is poor. Antiretroviral drugs may prove to have a valuable role.

Sézary syndrome

Patients with Sézary syndrome present with skin disease, usually a pruritic exfoliative erythroderma affecting the palms, soles and face ('red man syndrome'). Biopsy of the skin reveals lymphocytic infiltration and Sézary cells in peripheral blood have a characteristic morphology with deep nuclear clefting, similar to ATLL cells. A variety of treatments are available including chemotherapy, radiotherapy and a photoactivable drug (psoralens) combined with ultraviolet A light (PUVA).

Bibliography

Binet J.L., Auquier A., Dighiero G. *et al.* (1981) A new prognostic classification of chronic lymphocytic leukemia derived from a multivariate survival analysis. *Cancer* **48**,198–206.

Buhl A.M., Jurlander J., Jørgensen F.S. *et al.* (2006) Identification of a gene on chromosome 12q22 uniquely overexpressed in chronic lymphocytic leukemia. *Blood* **107**,2904–11.

Calin G.A., Ferracin M., Cimmino A. *et al.* (2005) A microRNA signature associated with prognosis and progression in chronic lymphocytic leukemia. *N Engl J Med* **353**,1793–801.

Chiorazzi N., Rai K.R., Ferrarini M. (2005) Chronic lymphocytic leukemia. *N Engl J Med* **352**,804–15.

Crespo M., Bosch F., Villamor N. *et al.* (2003) ZAP-70 expression as a surrogate for immunoglobulin-variable-region mutations in chronic lymphocytic leukemia. *N Engl J Med* **348**,1764–75.

Montserrat E., Moreno C., Esteve J. *et al.* (2006) How I treat refractory CLL. *Blood* **107**,1276–83.

Oscier D., Fegan C., Hillmen P. *et al.* (2004) Guidelines Working Group of the UK CLL Forum. British Committee for Standards in Haematology. Guidelines on the diagnosis and management of chronic lymphocytic leukaemia. *Br J Haematol* **125**,294–317.

Paneesha S. and Milligan D.W. (2005) Stem cell transplantation for chronic lymphocytic leukaemia. *Br J Haematol* **128**,145–52.

Rai K.R., Sawitsky A., Cronkite E.P. *et al.* (1975) Clinical staging of chronic lymphocytic leukemia. *Blood* **46**,219–34.

Rawstron A.C., Yuille M.R., Fuller J. *et al.* (2002) Inherited predisposition to CLL is detectable as subclinical monoclonal B-lymphocyte expansion. *Blood* **100**,2289–90.

Stevenson F.K. and Caligaris-Cappio F. (2004) Chronic lymphocytic leukemia: revelations from the B-cell receptor. *Blood* **103**,4389–95.

Wiestner A., Rosenwald A., Barry T.S. *et al.* (2003) ZAP-70 expression identifies a chronic lymphocytic leukemia subtype with unmutated immunoglobulin genes, inferior clinical outcome, and distinct gene expression profile. *Blood* **101**,4944–51.

CHAPTER 16

16 Hodgkin's lymphoma

Lymphomas are a group of diseases caused by malignant lymphocytes that accumulate in lymph nodes and cause the characteristic clinical features of lymphadenopathy. Occasionally, they may spill over into blood ('leukaemic phase') or infiltrate organs outside the lymphoid tissue.

The major subdivision of lymphomas is into Hodgkin's lymphoma and non-Hodgkin's lymphoma and this is based on the histological presence of Reed–Sternberg (RS) cells in Hodgkin's lymphoma.

Pathogenesis

Hodgkin's disease is a lymphoma in which RS cells are found in the disease tissue. The characteristic RS cells, and the associated abnormal mononuclear cells, are neoplastic whereas the infiltrating inflammatory cells are reactive. Immunoglobulin gene rearrangement studies suggest that the RS cell is of B-lymphoid lineage and that it is often derived from a B cell with a 'crippled' immunoglobulin gene caused by the acquisition of mutations that prevent synthesis of full-length immunoglobulin. The Epstein–Barr virus (EBV) genome has been detected in 50% or more of cases in Hodgkin tissue but its role in the pathogenesis is unclear.

Clinical features

The disease can present at any age but is rare in children and has a peak incidence in young adults. There is an almost 2 : 1 male predominance. The following symptoms are common.

1 Most patients present with painless, non-tender, asymmetrical, firm, discrete and rubbery enlargement of superficial lymph nodes (Fig. 16.1). The cervical nodes are involved in 60–70% of patients, axillary nodes in approximately 10–15% and inguinal nodes in 6–12%. In some cases the size of the nodes decreases and increases spontaneously. They may

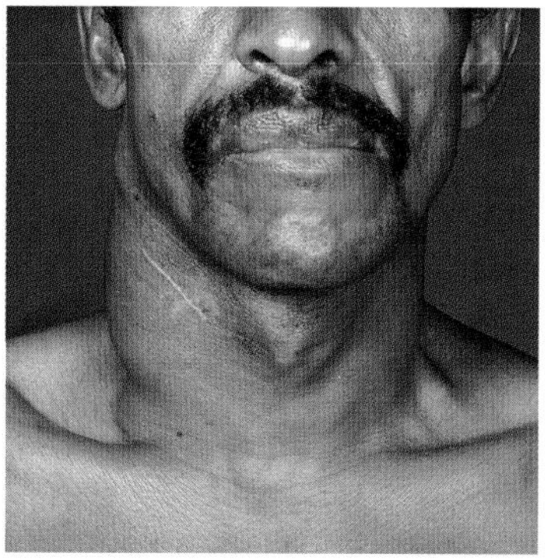

Fig. 16.1 Cervical lymphadenopathy in a patient with Hodgkin's lymphoma.

become matted. Typically the disease is localized initially to a single peripheral lymph node region and its subsequent progression is by contiguity within the lymphatic system. Retroperitoneal nodes are also often involved but usually only diagnosed by computed tomography (CT) scan.

2 Clinical splenomegaly occurs during the course of the disease in 50% of patients. The splenic enlargement is seldom massive. The liver may also be enlarged because of liver involvement.

3 Mediastinal involvement is found in 6–11% of patients at presentation. This is a feature of the nodular sclerosing type, particularly in young women. There may be associated pleural effusions or superior vena cava obstruction.

4 Cutaneous Hodgkin's disease occurs as a late complication in approximately 10% of patients. Other organs (e.g. bone marrow, gastrointestinal tract, bone, lung, spinal cord or brain) may also be involved, even at presentation, but this is unusual.

5 Constitutional symptoms are prominent in patients with widespread disease. The following may be seen:

(a) fever occurs in approximately 30% of patients and is continuous or cyclic;

(b) pruritus, which is often severe, occurs in approximately 25% of cases;

(c) alcohol-induced pain in the areas where disease is present occurs in some patients;

(d) other constitutional symptoms include weight loss, profuse sweating (especially at night), weakness, fatigue, anorexia and cachexia. Haematological and infectious complications are discussed below.

Haematological and biochemical findings

1 Normochromic, normocytic anaemia is most common. Bone marrow involvement is unusual in early disease but if it occurs bone marrow failure may develop with a leucoerythroblastic anaemia.

2 One-third of patients have a neutrophilia; eosinophilia is frequent.

3 Advanced disease is associated with lymphopenia and loss of cell-mediated immunity.

4 The platelet count is normal or increased during early disease, and reduced in later stages.

5 The erythrocyte sedimentation rate (ESR) and C-reactive protein are usually raised and are useful in monitoring disease progress.

6 Serum lactate dehydrogenase (LDH) is raised initially in 30–40% of cases.

Diagnosis and histological classification

The diagnosis is made by histological examination of an excised lymph node. The distinctive multinucleate polyploid RS cell is central to the diagnosis of the four classic types (Figs 16.2 and 16.3) and mononuclear Hodgkin cells are also part of the malignant clone. These cells stain with CD30 and CD15 but are usually negative for B-cell antigen expression. Inflammatory components consist of lymphocytes, neutrophils, eosinophils, plasma cells and variable fibrosis.

Histological classification is into five types (Table 16.1), each of which implies a different prognosis. Nodular sclerosis and mixed cellularity are most frequent. Patients with lymphocyte predominant histology have the most favourable prognosis. Nodular lymphocyte predominant does not show RS cells and has many features of non-Hodgkin's lymphoma and may be treated as such.

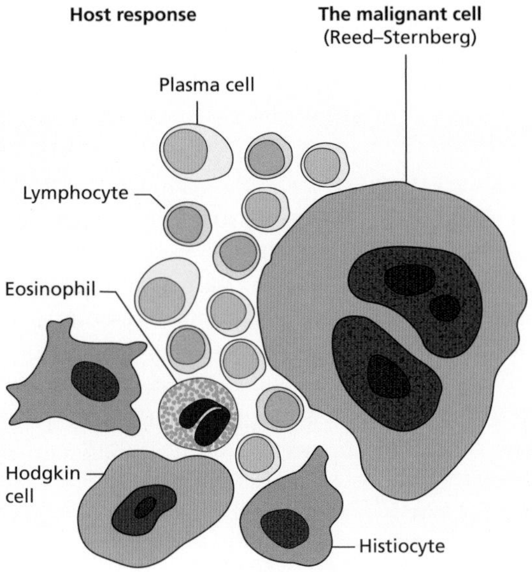

Fig. 16.2 Diagrammatic representation of the different cells seen histologically in Hodgkin's lymphoma.

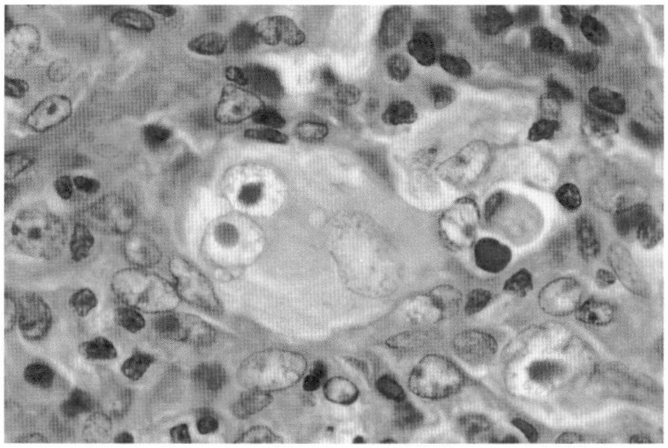

(a)

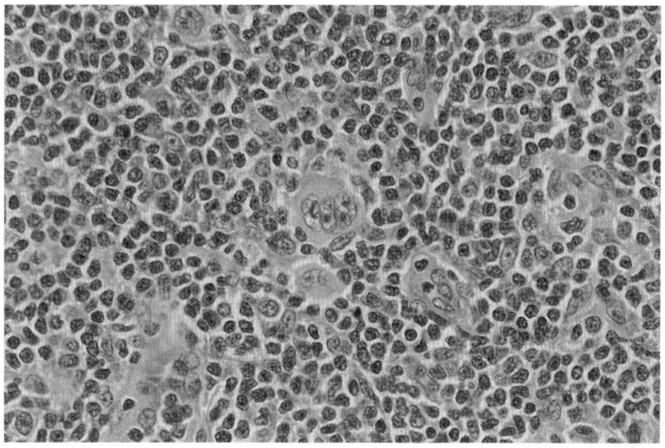

(b)

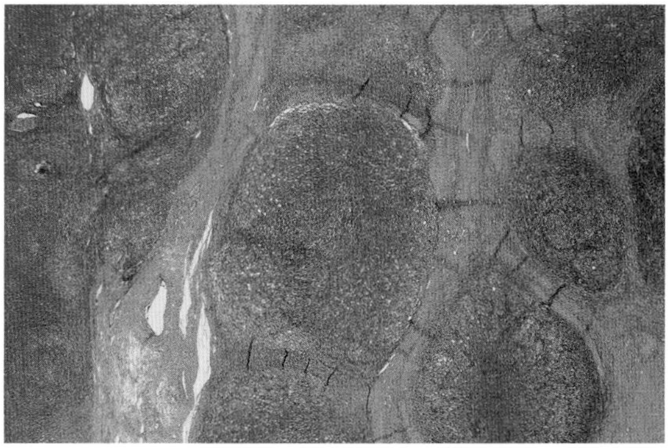

(c)

Fig. 16.3 Hodgkin's disease: **(a)** high power view of a lymph node biopsy showing two typical multinucleate Reed–Sternberg cells, one with a characteristic owl eye appearance, surrounded by lymphocytes, histiocytes and an eosinophil; **(b)** mixed cellularity; and **(c)** nodular sclerosing Hodgkin's lymphoma.

Table 16.1 Histology of Hodgkin's lymphoma (WHO classification).

Classic Hodgkin's lymphoma	
Nodular sclerosis	Collagen bands extend from the node capsule to encircle nodules of abnormal tissue. A characteristic lacunar cell variant of the Reed–Sternberg cell is often found. The cellular infiltrate may be of the lymphocyte-predominant, mixed cellularity or lymphocyte-depleted type; eosinophilia is frequent
Mixed cellularity	The Reed–Sternberg cells are numerous and lymphocyte numbers are intermediate
Lymphocyte depleted	There is either a reticular pattern with dominance of Reed–Sternberg cells and sparse numbers of lymphocytes or a diffuse fibrosis pattern where the lymph node is replaced by disordered connective tissue containing few lymphocytes. Reed–Sternberg cells may also be infrequent in this latter subtype
Lymphocyte rich	Scanty Reed–Sternberg cells; multiple small lymphocytes with few eosinophils and plasma cells; nodular and diffuse types
Nodular lymphocyte-predominant	Reed–Sternberg cells are absent; abnormal polymorphic B cells

WHO, World Health Organization.

Clinical staging

The selection of appropriate treatment depends on accurate staging of the extent of disease (Table 16.2). Figure 16.4 shows the scheme (Ann Arbor) that is now recommended. Staging is performed by thorough clinical examination together with chest X-ray (Fig. 16.5) and CT scan to detect intrathoracic, intra-abdominal or pelvic disease (Fig. 16.6). It is also used to monitor response to therapy. Magnetic resonance imaging (MRI) scanning may be needed for particular sites (Table 16.2). Bone marrow trephine is carried out in some centres and liver biopsy may also be needed in difficult cases. Positron emission tomography (PET) scanning may also be useful in staging and PET scan combined with CT may be used in staging and to detect small foci of residual disease following treatment (Fig. 17.8).

Table 16.2 Techniques for staging of lymphoma.

Laboratory	Full blood count ESR Bone marrow aspirate and trephine (not routine) Liver function LDH C-reactive protein
Radiology	Chest radiograph CT of thorax, abdomen, chest and pelvis
Special tests	MRI Bone scan PET or PET/CT

CT, computed tomography; ESR, erythrocyte sedimentation rate; LDH, lactate dehydrogenase; MRI, magnetic resonance imaging; PET, positron emission tomography.

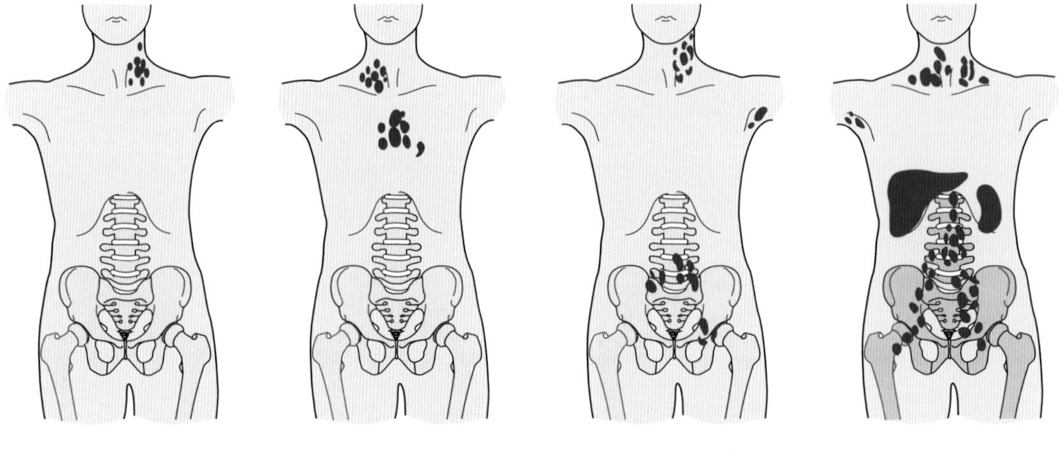

Fig. 16.4 Staging of Hodgkin's lymphoma. Stage I indicates node involvement in one lymph node area. Stage II indicates disease involving two or more lymph nodal areas confined to one side of the diaphragm. Stage III indicates disease involving lymph nodes above and below the diaphragm. Splenic disease is included in stage III but this has special significance (see below). Stage IV indicates involvement outside the lymph node areas and refers to diffuse or disseminated disease in the bone marrow, liver and other extranodal sites. NB. The stage number in all cases is followed by the letter A or B indicating the absence (A) or presence (B) of one or more of the following: unexplained fever above 38°C; night sweats; or loss of more than 10% of body weight within 6 months. Localized extranodal extension from a mass of nodes does not advance the stage but is indicated by the subscript E. Thus, mediastinal disease with contiguous spread to the lung or spinal theca would be classified as I_E. As involvement of the spleen is often a prelude to widespread haematogenous spread of the disease, patients with lymph node and splenic involvement are staged as III_S. Bulky disease (widening of the mediastinum by more than one-third, or the presence of a nodal mass >10 cm in diameter) is relevant to therapy at any stage.

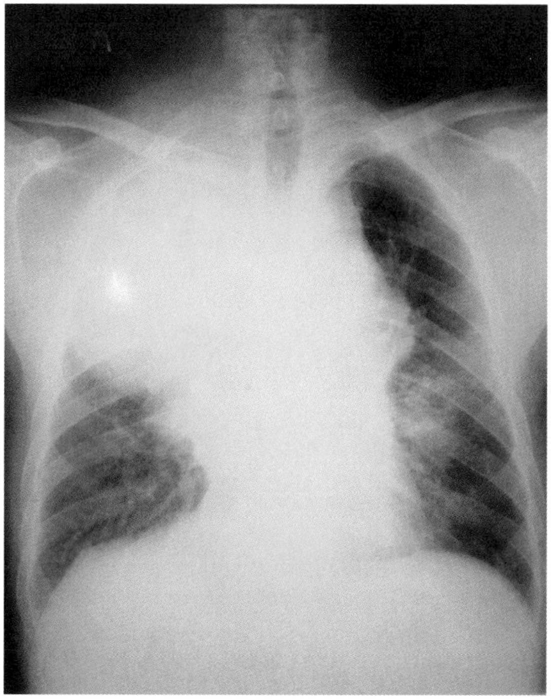

Fig. 16.5 Chest X-ray in Hodgkin's lymphoma showing widespread enlargement of hilar and mediastinal lymph nodes with associated collapse of the right upper lobe and infiltration or possibly pneumonic changes in the mid zone of the left lung.

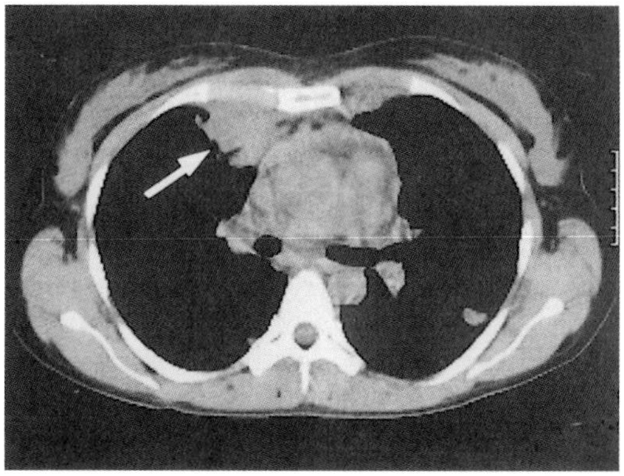

Fig. 16.6 Hodgkin's lymphoma (nodular sclerosing type): CT scan of chest showing anterior mediastinal mass of enlarged lymph nodes (arrowed).

Patients are also classified as A or B according to whether or not constitutional features (fever or weight loss) are present (Fig. 16.4).

Treatment

Treatment is with radiotherapy, chemotherapy or a combination of both. The choice depends primarily on the stage and whether clinically A or B (Fig. 16.4) although histological grading is an additional factor. Semen storage, if appropriate, should be carried out before therapy is begun.

Radiotherapy

Patients with stage I and IIA disease may be cured by radiotherapy alone. A dose of 4000 rad (40 Gy) is able to destroy lymph node Hodgkin's tissue in approximately 80% of these patients. Improved high-voltage radiotherapy techniques allow the treatment of all lymph node areas above or below the diaphragm by single 'upper mantle' or 'inverted Y' blocks. Radiotherapy also has a role in the treatment of bulky tumour masses such as mediastinal tumour that remains after chemotherapy or painful skeletal, nodal or soft tissue deposits.

Combined modality therapy

Concerns over late relapse and the long-term effects of radiotherapy have led to the development of regimens in which chemotherapy and radiotherapy are used together. This combination therapy allows short courses of chemotherapy to be combined with reduced levels of radiotherapy and the most effective combinations are being assessed in clinical trials.

Chemotherapy

Cyclical chemotherapy is used for stage III and IV disease and also in stage I and II patients who have bulky disease, type B symptoms or have relapsed following initial radiotherapy. The combination of Adriamycin, bleomycin, vinblastine and dacarbazine (ABVD) is now most widely used. This has replaced the landmark quadruple therapy with mustine, vincristine (Oncovin), procarbazine and prednisolone (MOPP) which was introduced in the

1970s, but is more likely to cause sterility or secondary leukaemia. Variants of this such as ChlVPP (replacing mustine with chlorambucil or cyclophosphamide) are sometimes used. It is usual to give six cycles of chemotherapy or four following achievement of complete remission.

More intensive chemotherapy regimens such as Stanford V or BEACOPP (bleomycin, etoposide, doxorubicin, cyclophosphamide, vincristine, procarbazine, prednisolone) may be useful for poor-risk disease and trials to compare these with ABVD are underway.

Assessment of response to treatment

Clinical examination and imaging (e.g. CT scan) are used to assess response to treatment. Patients with Hodgkin's lymphoma often show residual masses following treatment which may be because of the large degree of fibrosis present within lymph nodes. It can be difficult to assess whether or not such masses represent residual disease and the label of complete response uncertain (CRu) can be applied in these cases. PET scanning combined with CT (see p. 211) is useful is revealing areas of active disease and further biopsy may also be required.

Relapsed cases

The patient is treated with an alternative combination chemotherapy to the initial regimen and, if necessary, with radiotherapy to sites of bulky disease. If the disease remains chemosensitive, high-dose chemotherapy and autologous stem cell transplantation improve the probability of cure and are recommended for most patients below the age of 65 years. Allogeneic transplantation may also be tried in a minority of patients who fail other therapies.

Prognosis

Approximate 5-year survival rates range from 50% to over 90% depending on age, stage and histology.

The late effects of Hodgkin's lymphoma and its treatment

Long-term follow-up of patients has revealed a considerable burden of late disease following treatment. Secondary cancers such as lung cancer and breast cancer appear to be related to radiotherapy whereas myelodysplasia or acute myeloid leukaemia are more associated with the use of alkylating agents. Non-Hodgkin's lymphomas and other cancers also occur with greater frequency than in controls. Non-malignant complications include sterility, intestinal complications, myocardial infarction and other cardiac or pulmonary complications of the mediastinal radiation and chemotherapy. These features are the main reason why less intensive treatment regimens are now being explored for this disease.

Bibliography

Burton C., Ell P., Linch D. (2004) The role of PET imaging in lymphoma. *Br J Haematol* **126**,772–84.

Cartwright R.A. and Watkins G. (2004) Epidemiology of Hodgkin's disease: a review. *Hematol Oncol* **22**,11–26.

Diehl V., Thomas R.K., Re D. (2004) Part II: Hodgkin's lymphoma — diagnosis and treatment. *Lancet Oncol* **5**,19–26.

Harris N.L., Jaffe E.S., Diebold J. *et al.* (2000) The WHO classification of neoplasms of the hematopoietic and lymphoid tissues. *Hematol J* 1,53–66.

Juweid M.E. and Cheson B.D. (2006) Positron-emission tomography and assessment of cancer therapy. *N Engl J Med* **354**,496–507.

Re D., Thomas R.K., Behringer K., Diehl V. (2005) From Hodgkin disease to Hodgkin lymphoma: biologic insights and therapeutic potential. *Blood* **105**,4553–60.

Thomas R.K., Re D., Wolf J., Diehl V. (2004) Part I. Hodgkin's lymphoma: molecular biology of Hodgkin and Reed–Sternberg cells. *Lancet Oncol* **5**,11–8.

Zekri J.M., Mouncey P., Hancock B.W. (2004) Trials in advanced Hodgkin's disease: more than 30 years experience of the British National Lymphoma Investigation. *Clin Lymphoma* **5**,174–83.

CHAPTER 17

17 Non-Hodgkin's lymphoma

Non-Hodgkin's lymphomas

These are a large group of lymphoid tumours, most commonly of B-cell origin, whose clinical presentation and natural history are more variable than in Hodgkin's lymphoma. They are characterized by an irregular pattern of spread and a significant proportion of patients develop extranodal disease. Their frequency has increased markedly over the last 50 years and with an incidence of approximately 17 in 100 000 they now represent the fifth most common malignancy in some developed countries. The aetiology of the majority of cases of non-Hodgkin's lymphomas (NHL) is unknown although infectious agents are an important cause in particular subtypes (Chapter 10).

Classification and histopathology

No area of diagnostic histopathology has been associated with greater confusion than the classification of NHL. A number of classifications have been used over the years with no one scheme receiving unanimous support. In 1994, the Revised American European Lymphoma (REAL) classification was published and gained widespread application. The more recent World Health Organization (WHO) classification, based on REAL, includes all lymphoid malignancies as well as lymphomas and is more clinically based than previous classification schemes (Table 17.1). In general terms, there is a move away from subdividing lymphomas on the basis of subtle histological appearance and more in terms of distinct syndromes each with characteristic morphological, immunophenotypic, genetic and clinical features. It is also useful to think of the likely origin of individual lymphoid malignancies based on their phenotype and immunoglobulin gene rearrangement status (Fig. 17.1). In this chapter we consider each of the common lymphoma subtypes within this classification.

Low- and high-grade non-Hodgkin's lymphomas

The non-Hodgkin's lymphomas are a diverse group of diseases and vary from highly proliferative and rapidly fatal diseases to some of the most indolent and well-tolerated malignancies. For many years clinicians have subdivided lymphomas into low- and high-grade disease, with some falling into an intermediate grade. This approach has been extremely valuable as, in general terms, the low-grade disorders are relatively indolent, respond well to chemotherapy but are very difficult to cure whereas high-grade lymphomas are aggressive and need urgent treatment but are often curable.

Clinical features of non-Hodgkin's lymphomas

1 *Superficial lymphadenopathy* The majority of patients present with asymmetric painless enlargement

Table 17.1 The World Health Organization (WHO) classification of non-Hodgkin's lymphomas. B-cell disorders comprise of 85% of cases. T cell and NK cell together comprise of 15% of cases.

Precursor B-cell neoplasm	*Precursor T-cell neoplasms*
B-lymphoblastic leukaemia/lymphoma (precursor B-cell ALL, B-ALL/LBL)	T-cell lymphoblastic lymphoma/leukaemia (T-ALL/LBL)
Mature B-cell neoplasms	*Mature T-cell and NK cell neoplasms*
B-cell chronic lymphocytic leukaemia/small lymphocytic lymphoma	T-cell prolymphocytic leukaemia
B-cell prolymphocytic leukaemia	T-cell granular lymphocytic leukaemia
Lymphoplasmacytic lymphoma	Aggressive NK-cell leukaemia
Splenic marginal zone B-cell lymphoma (±villous lymphocytes)	Adult T-cell lymphoma/leukaemia (HTLV-1+)
Hairy cell leukaemia	Extranodal NK/T-cell lymphoma, nasal type
Plasma cell myeloma/plasmacytoma	Enteropathy-type T-cell lymphoma
	Mycosis fungoides/Sézary syndrome
Extranodal marginal zone B-cell lymphoma of MALT type	Anaplastic large cell lymphoma, primary cutaneous type
	Peripheral T-cell lymphoma, unspecified
	Angioimmunoblastic T-cell lymphoma
Mantle cell lymphoma	Anaplastic large cell lymphoma, primary systemic type
Follicular lymphoma	
Nodal marginal zone B-cell lymphoma	
Diffuse large B-cell lymphoma	
Burkitt's lymphoma/Burkitt's cell leukaemia	
Primary effusion lymphoma	
Mediastinal large B-cell lymphoma	

ALL, acute lymphoblastic leukaemia; HTLV, human T-cell leukaemia/lymphoma virus; LBL, lymphoblastic lymphoma; MALT, mucosa-associated lymphoid tissue; NK, natural killer.

of lymph nodes in one or more peripheral lymph node regions.

2 *Constitutional symptoms* Fever, night sweats and weight loss occur less frequently than in Hodgkin's disease and their presence is usually associated with disseminated disease.

3 *Oropharyngeal involvement* In 5–10% of patients there is disease of the oropharyngeal lymphoid structures (Waldeyer's ring) which may cause complaints of a 'sore throat' or noisy or obstructed breathing.

4 *Presenting features* Anaemia, neutropenia with infections or thrombocytopenia with purpura may be presenting features in patients with diffuse bone marrow disease. Cytopenias may also be autoimmune in origin. Infections may occur as a result of neutropenia or reduced cell immunity (e.g. herpes zoster).

5 *Abdominal disease* The liver and spleen are often enlarged and involvement of retroperitoneal or mesenteric nodes is frequent. The gastrointestinal tract is the most commonly involved extranodal site after the bone marrow, and patients may present with acute abdominal symptoms.

6 *Other organs* Skin, brain, testis or thyroid involvement is not infrequent. The skin is also primarily involved in two unusual, closely related T-cell lymphomas: mycosis fungoides and Sézary syndrome.

Investigations

Histology

Lymph node biopsy is the definitive investigation (Figs 17.2 and 17.3) and morphological examination is assisted by immunophenotypic and genetic analysis. For B-cell lymphomas, expression of either κ or λ light chains confirms clonality and distinquishes the disease from a reactive node (Fig. 17.4; Chapter 10).

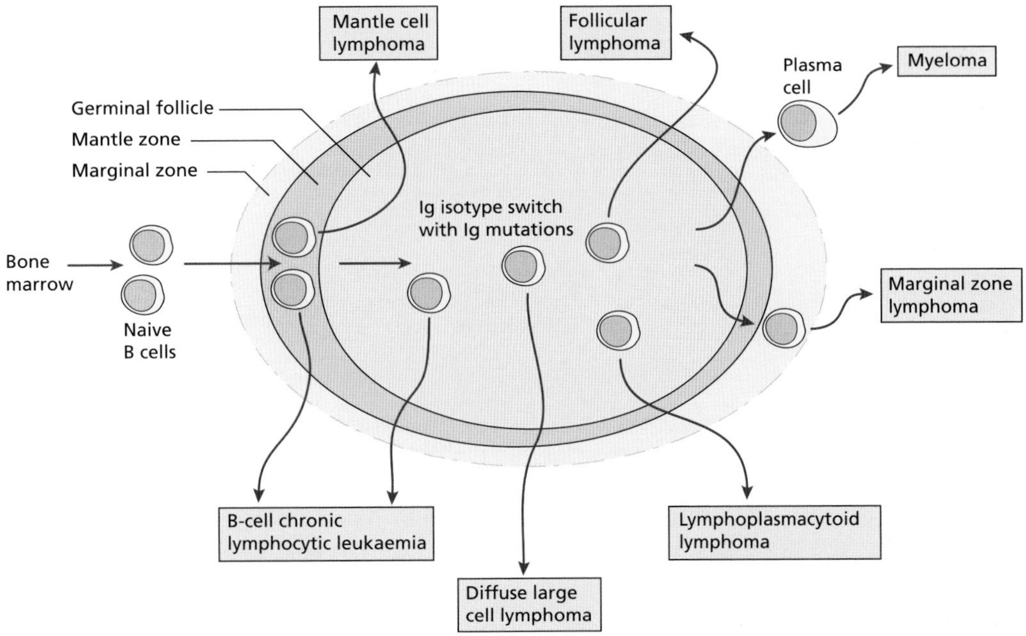

Fig. 17.1 Proposed cellular origin of B-lymphoid malignancies. Normal B cells migrate from the bone marrow and enter secondary lymphoid tissue. When they encounter antigen a germinal centre is formed and B cells undergo somatic hypermutation of the immunoglobulin genes. Finally, B cells exit the lymph node as memory B cells or plasma cells. The cellular origin of the different lymphoid malignancies can be inferred from immunoglobulin gene rearrangement status and membrane phenotype. Mantle cell lymphoma and a proportion of B-CLL cases have unmutated immunoglobulin genes whereas marginal zone lymphoma, diffuse large cell lymphoma, follicle cell lymphoma, lymphoplasmacytoid lymphoma and some B-CLL cases have mutated immunoglobulin genes.

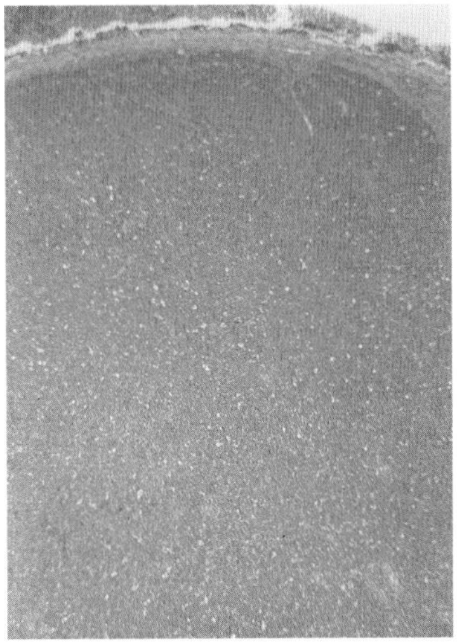

(a)

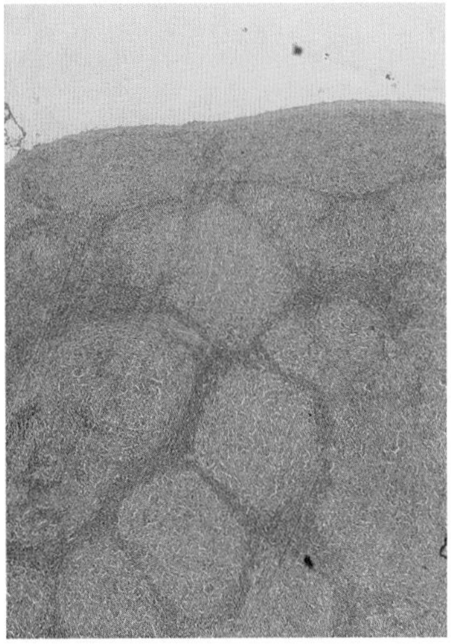

(b)

Fig. 17.2 Non-Hodgkin's lymphoma: histological sections of lymph nodes showing: **(a)** a diffuse pattern of involvement in lymphocytic lymphoma with the normal architecture totally replaced by neoplastic lymphocytic cells; **(b)** a follicular or nodular pattern in follicular lymphoma—the 'follicles' or 'nodules' of neoplastic cells compress surrounding tissue and lack a mantle of small lymphocytes.

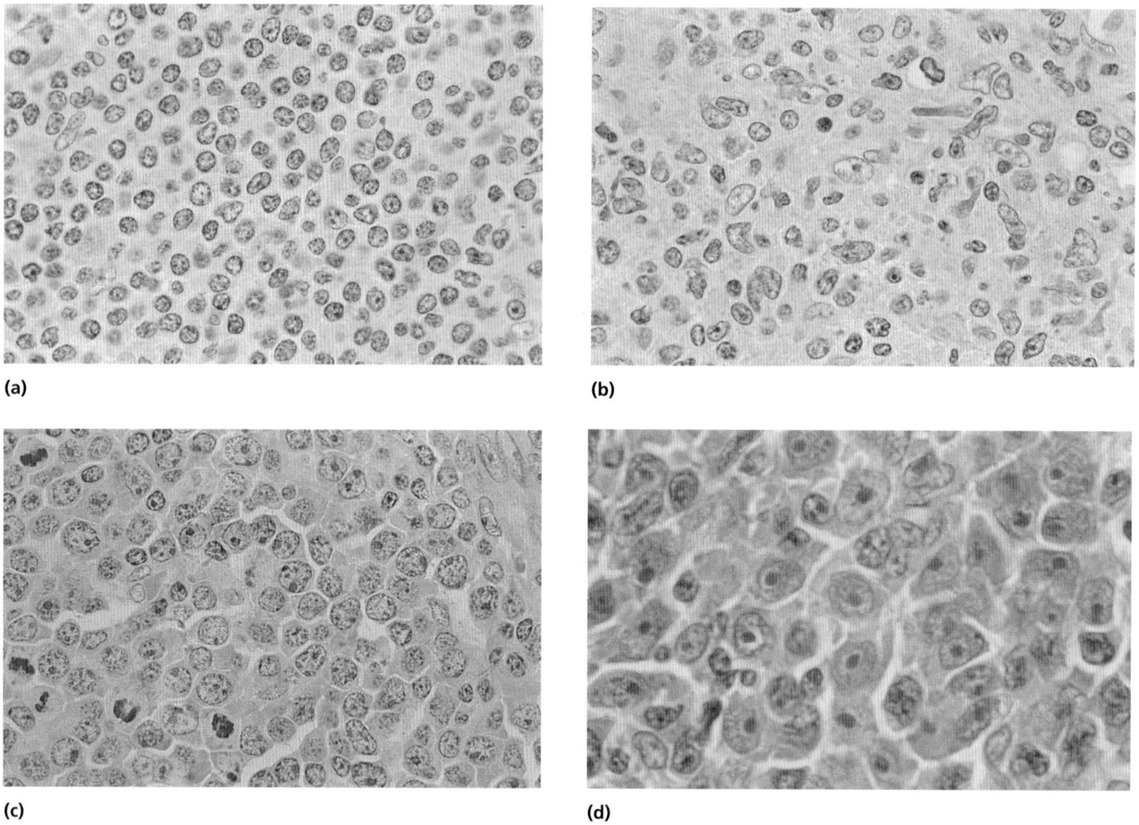

Fig. 17.3 Non-Hodgkin's lymphoma: high power view of lymph node biopsies showing **(a)** lymphocytic lymphoma showing predominantly small lymphocytes with round nuclei containing densely clumped heterochromatin. **(b)** Mantle cell lymphoma: showing characteristic deformed pattern of small lymphocytes with angular nuclei ('centrocytes'). **(c)** Diffuse large B-cell lymphoma: the neoplastic cells are much larger than normal lymphocytes and have a round nucleus with prominent nucleoli, many of which are adjacent to the nuclear membrane ('centroblasts'). A number of mitotic figures are seen. **(d)** Diffuse large B-cell lymphoma showing large neoplastic cells with a single prominent nucleolus and abundant dark-staining cytoplasm (previously termed immunoblasts).

The repertoire of CD antigens expressed on the tumour cell surface is also useful in the classification of malignant lymphoma (Table 17.2; see Appendix 1). Trephine biopsy of the marrow and immunoglobulin or T-cell receptor gene rearrangement studies may also be valuable.

Haematological and biochemical findings

1 A normochromic, normocytic anaemia is usual but autoimmune haemolytic anaemia may also occur.

2 In advanced disease with marrow involvement there may be neutropenia, thrombocytopenia (especially if the spleen is enlarged) or leucoerythroblastic features.

3 Lymphoma cells (e.g. mantle zone cells, 'cleaved follicular lymphoma' or 'blast' cells) with variable nuclear abnormalities may be found in the peripheral blood in some patients (Fig. 15.7).

4 Trephine biopsy of marrow is valuable (Fig. 17.6). Paradoxically, bone marrow involvement is found more frequently in low-grade malignant lymphomas.

5 The serum lactate dehydrogenase (LDH) level is

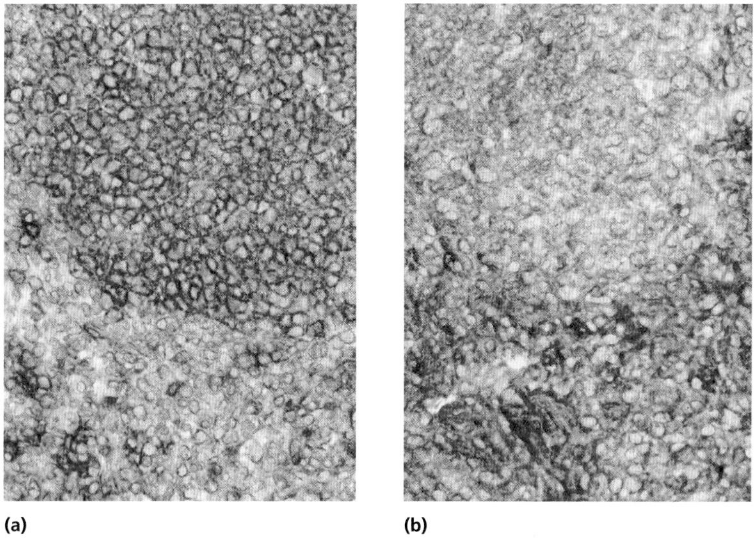

Fig. 17.4 Non-Hodgkin's lymphoma: lymph node stained by immunoperoxidase shows **(a)** brown ring staining for κ in the malignant lymphoid nodule, and **(b)** no labelling for λ confirming the monoclonal origin of the lymphoma.

Table 17.2 Characteristic immunophenotype and cytogenetics of B-cell lymphomas.

Lymphoma	Surface immunoglobulin	CD5	CD10	CD20	CD23	CD43	Cyclin D_1	Typical cytogenetics
CLL/lymphocytic lymphoma	Weak	+	–	+	+	+	–	13q14, 17p or 11q deletions; trisomy 12
Follicular lymphoma	+	–	+	+	+/–	–	–	t(14; 18)
Mantle cell lymphoma	+	+	–	+	–	+	+	t(11; 14)
Diffuse large cell lymphoma	+/–	–	+/–	+	–	+/–	–	various
Burkitt's lymphoma	+	–	+	+	–	–	–	t(8; 14)
MALT lymphoma	+	–	–	+	+/–	+/–	–	t(1; 14)

CLL, chronic lymphocytic leukaemia; MALT, mucosa-associated lymphoid tissue.
More detailed cytogenetics are given in Table 10.2.

raised in more rapidly proliferating and extensive disease and may be used as a prognostic marker (Table 17.3). Elevation of serum uric acid may occur.
6 Immunoglobulin electrophoresis may reveal a paraprotein.

Cytogenetics

The various subtypes of NHL are associated with characteristic chromosomal translocations which are of diagnostic and prognostic value (see Tables 10.2; 17.2). Particularly characteristic translocations are

Table 17.3 International prognostic index for high-grade lymphoma.

	Good	Bad
Age	<60 years	>60 years
Performance status	0 or 1	>2
Stage (p. 200)	I or II	III or IV
Number of extranodal sites	0 or 1	>2
Serum LDH	Normal	Raised

LDH, lactate dehydrogenase.

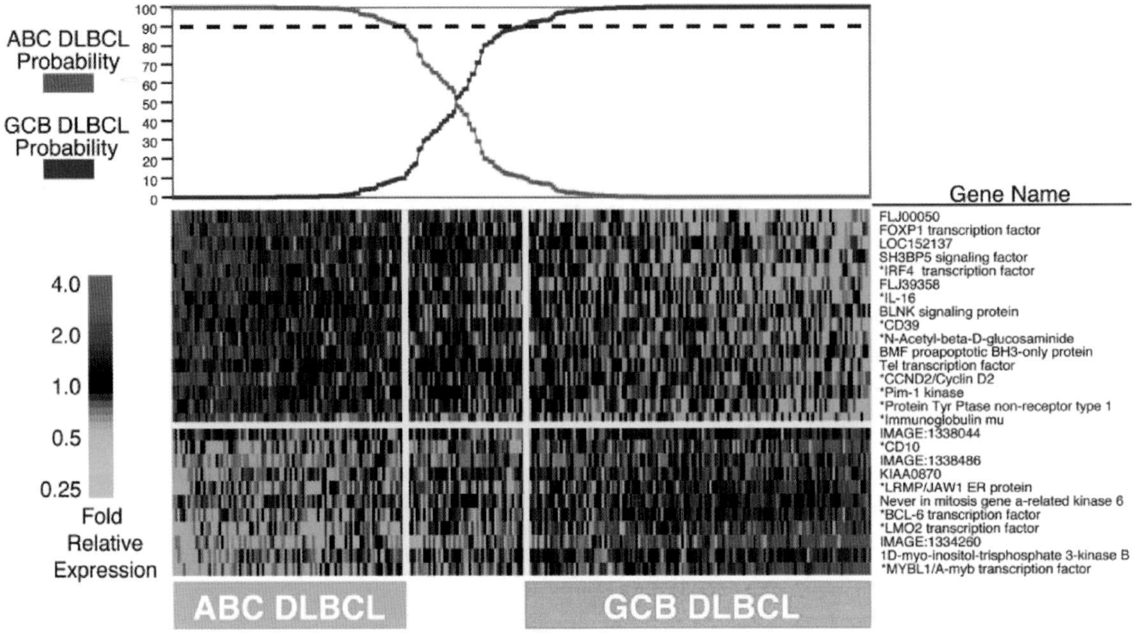

(a)

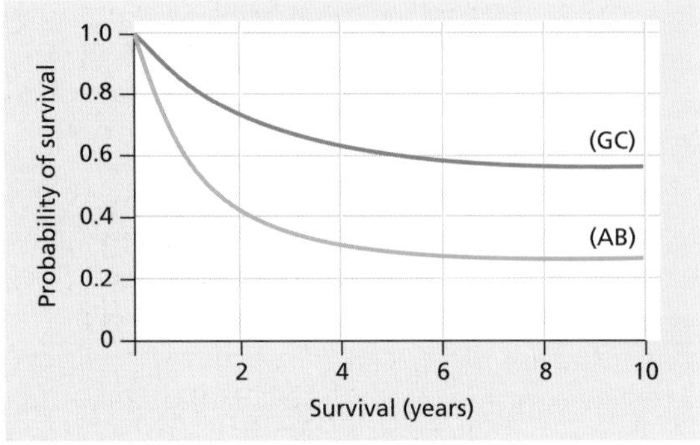

(b)

Fig. 17.5 **(a)** DNA microarray of diffuse large B-cell lymphoma (DLCL) which uses expression analysis of 27 genes to divide cases into those with a typical activated B cell (ABC) or germinal centre B cell (GCB) pattern (Wright *et al.*, 2003). **(b)** Survival of patients with DLCL grouped according to an activated B cell (ABC) or germinal centre B cell (GCB) microarray expression pattern. (After Wright *et al.* 2003)

t(8; 14) in Burkitt's lymphoma, t(14; 18) in follicular lymphoma, t(11; 14) in mantle cell lymphoma and t(2; 5) in anaplastic large cell lymphoma.

In B-cell lymphomas the immunoglobulin genes are clonally rearranged whereas in T-cell lymphomas there is clonal rearrangement of the T-cell receptor genes (Chapter 10). DNA microarray patterns of gene expression have been shown to give valuable diagnostic and prognostic information (Fig. 17.5) but are not yet widely available.

Staging

The staging system is the same as that described for Hodgkin's disease but is less clearly related to prognosis than histological type. Staging procedures usually include chest X-ray, computed tomography (CT) scanning or magnetic resonance imaging (MRI) (Fig. 17.7) and bone marrow aspiration and trephine (Fig. 17.6). Positron-emission tomography (PET) may detect disease not seen on

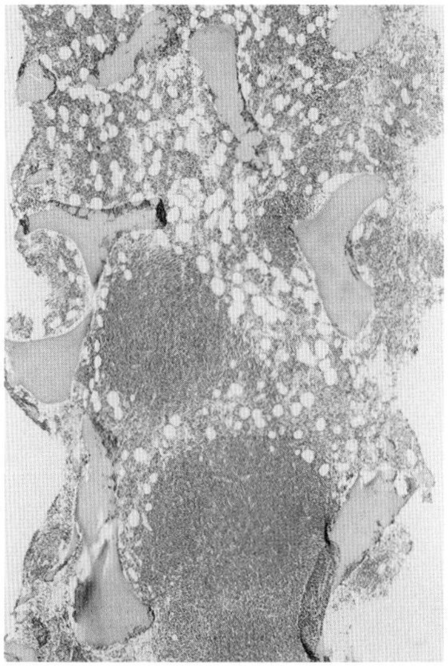

Fig. 17.6 Iliac crest trephine biopsy in lymphocytic lymphoma. Prominent nodules of lymphoid tissue are seen in the intertrabecular space and paratrabecular areas.

CT scan and is useful for following treatment response (Fig. 17.7). Combined PET-CT is now commonly used in initial staging and for detection of residual disease (Fig. 17.8).

Specific subtypes of non-Hodgkin's lymphoma

Low-grade non-Hodgkin's lymphoma

Follicular lymphoma

This is the most common form of NHL and is associated with the t(14; 18) translocation and constitutive BCL-2 expression in the great majority of cases (Fig. 17.9). Patients are likely to be middle-aged or elderly and their disease is often characterized by a benign course for many years. The median survival from diagnosis is approximately 10 years.

Presentation is usually with painless lymphadenopathy, often widespread, and the majority of patients will have stage III or IV disease. However, sudden transformation may occur to aggressive diffuse tumours which are sometimes associated with a leukaemic phase.

Patients with localized disease may achieve cure with radiotherapy alone. Treatment options for disseminated (stage II–IV) disease range from simple observation through oral chemotherapy to experimental high-dose treatment with stem cell support. When used as initial treatment, chlorambucil or cyclophosphamide, vincristine and prednisolone

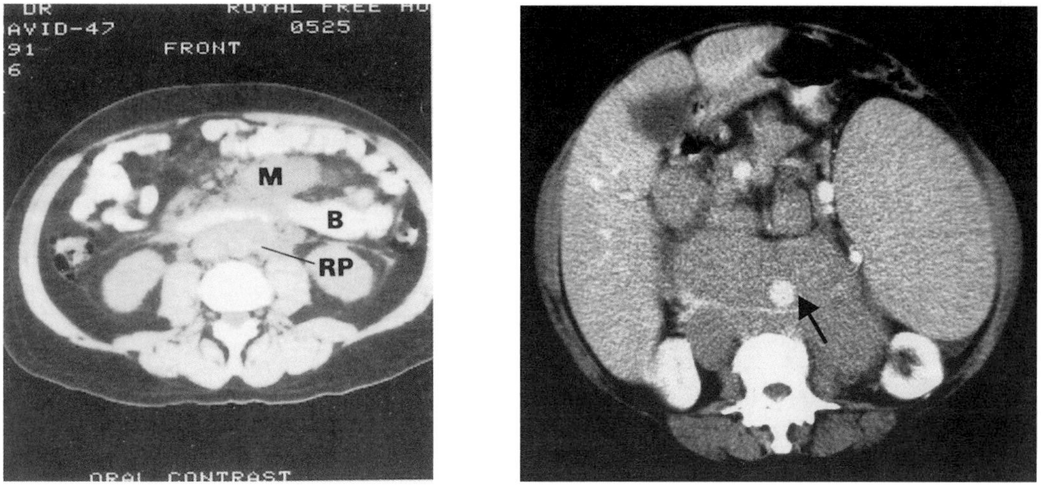

(a) (b)

Fig. 17.7 Non-Hodgkin's lymphoma. **(a)** Computed tomography (CT) scan of the abdomen showing enlarged mesenteric (M) and retroperitoneal (RP; para-aortic) lymph nodes; B, bowel. (Courtesy of Dr L. Berger) **(b)** CT scan of the abdomen: enlarged retroperitoneal and mesenteric nodes from a man causing the 'floating aorta' (arrowed) appearance. (Courtesy of Professor A. Dixon and Dr R.E. Marcus)

(Continued)

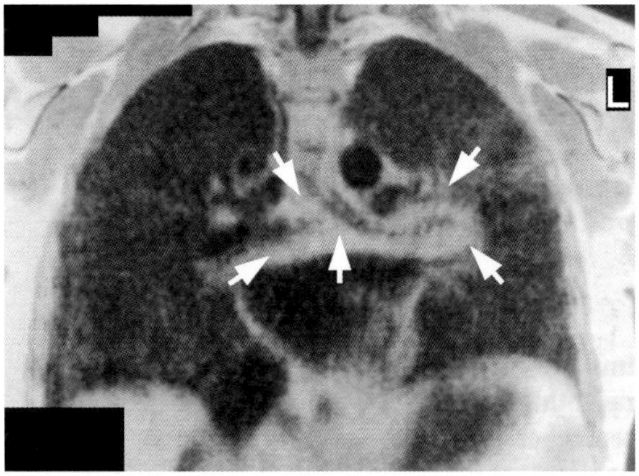

(c)

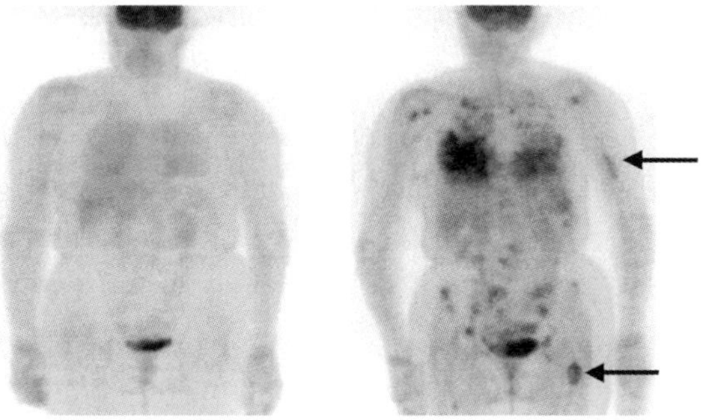

(i) (ii)

(e)

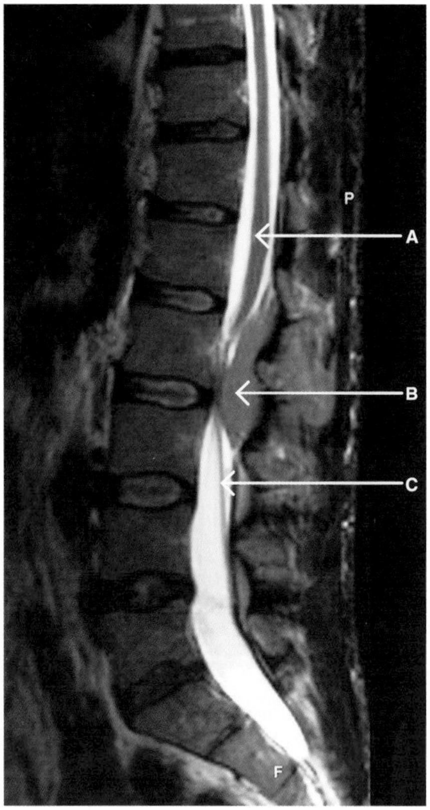

(d)

Fig. 17.7 (*Continued*) **(c)** Magnetic resonance imaging (MRI) scan of the chest showing large mediastinal lymph nodes (white and arrowed) adjacent to the great vessels (black). **(d)** MRI T_2-weighted midline saggital image of a lumbosacral spine showing compression of the dural sac by an extradural mass. A, spinal cord; B, extradural mass; C, roots of corda equina. (Courtesy of Dr A. Valentine) **(e)** Positron emission tomography (PET) body scan of a 59-year-old woman with high-grade non-Hodgkin's lymphoma. (i) The first scan showed no evidence of disease prior to allogeneic transplant. Normal physiological uptake is seen in the brain and bladder. Two months post-transplant the patient relapsed clinically with a mass on the anterior chest wall. (ii) The PET scan showed evidence of widespread relapse in nodal (para-aortic and iliac nodes) and extranodal sites including the lung and bone. The uptake in bone is clearly demonstated in the left humerus and femur (arrowed). This scan illustrates how well PET can detect both nodal and extranodal disease and allows whole body assessment at a single scanning session. (Courtesy of Dr S.F. Barrington)

(CVP) achieve a response in up to 90% of patients with a median duration of approximately 2 years. Fludarabine alone or in combination with cyclophosphamide or mitozantrone and dexamethasone (FMD) is another option. Rituximab, a humanized monoclonal antibody to CD20, is also effective and may be used alone or combined with chemotherapy (e.g. R-CVP; Fig. 17.10). Early studies suggest it is also valuable in maintenance.

Disease relapse is initially treated with similar chemotherapy regimens but the disease becomes increasingly difficult to control and more intensive chemotherapy and radiolabelled antibody therapy may be considered. Autologous stem cell transplantation (SCT) may be valuable in patients with a history of at least one relapse and allogeneic SCT offers the prospect of cure for younger patients.

Lymphocytic lymphomas

Lymphocytic lymphomas are closely related to

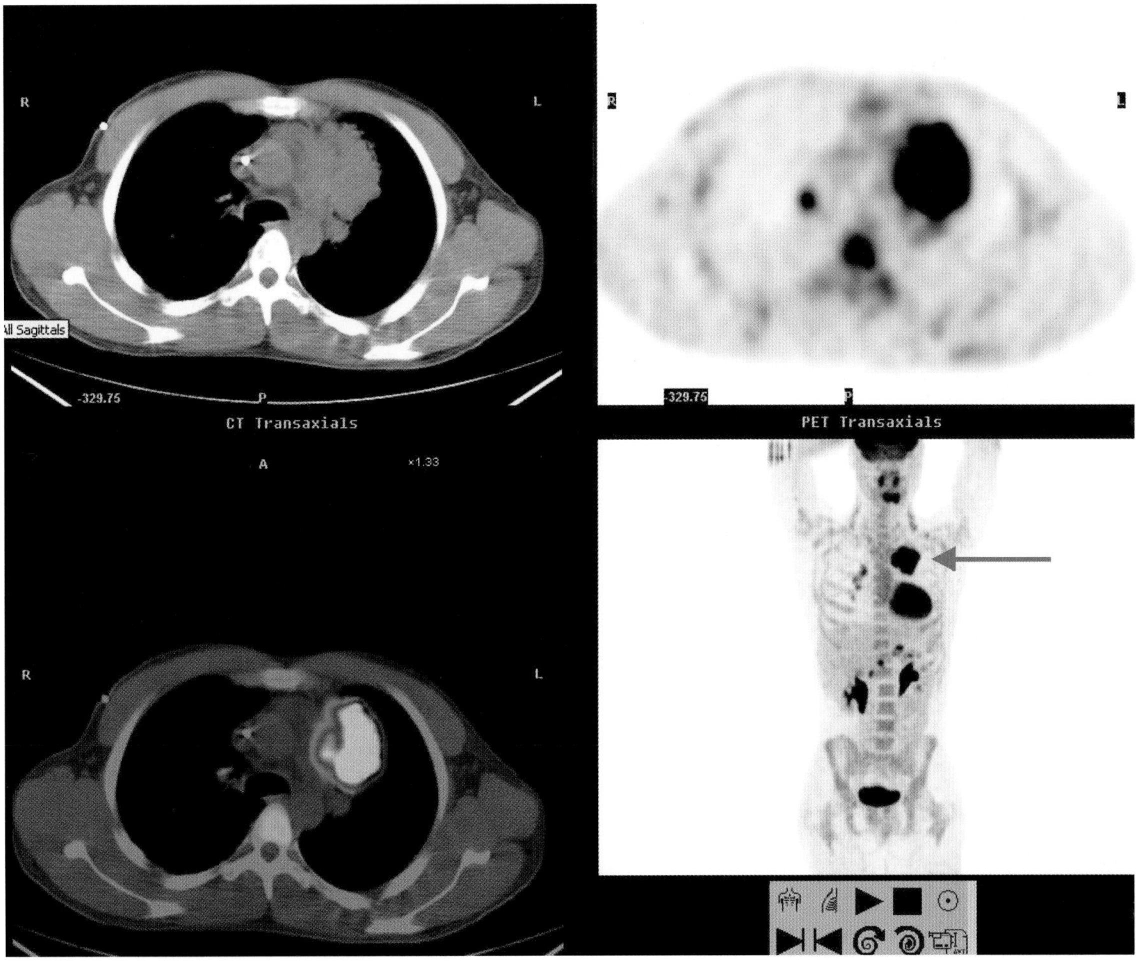

Fig. 17.8 Non-Hodgkin's lymphoma. PET/CT scan of male aged 26 years. Red arrow shows the level at which transaxial section is performed. Upper right-hand panel showing FDG uptake in anterior mediastinal mass and right hilar node. Upper left-hand panel shows corresponding CT section, bottom left-hand panel shows the CT and PET fused image of the corresponding section. Bottom right-hand panel, coronal section showing FDG uptake in mediastinal mass and right hilar node. There is also FDG uptake in the thyroid, heart, bowel, kidneys and bladder. (Courtesy of the Department of Nuclear Medicine, University College, London)

chronic lymphocytic leukaemia (CLL) and this lymphoma appears to be a tissue phase of CLL (Figs 17.2 and 17.3). Many patients with this condition are elderly with slowly progressive disease and may not require treatment for extended periods. Treatment is based on that used for CLL (p. 190).

Lymphoplasmacytoid lymphomas

Lymphoplasmacytoid lymphomas are often associated with the production of monoclonal immunoglobulin M (IgM), in which case they tend to be termed Waldenström's macroglobulinaemia (p. 223). Complications are anaemia and hyperviscosity syndrome. Treatment is with oral chlorambucil, fludarabine or monoclonal antibodies (e.g. rituximab). Plasma exchanges may be needed to reduce hyperviscosity.

Mantle cell lymphoma

Mantle cell lymphoma is derived from pre-germinal centre cells localized in the primary follicles or in the mantle region of secondary follicles. It has a

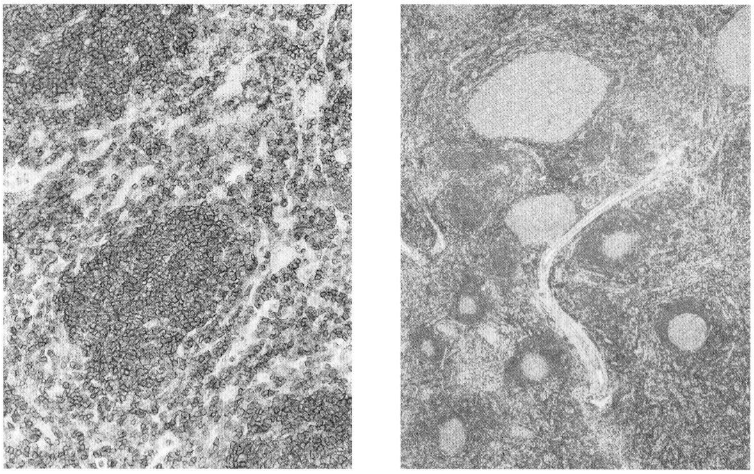

(a) (b)

Fig. 17.9 Follicular lymphoma: immunohistological detection of BCL-2 protein. **(a)** Follicular lymphoma positive because the BCL-2 is activated by the (14; 18) translocation; **(b)** reactive node shows germinal centres unstained for BCL-2 surrounded by positive mantle zone B and T cells. Immunoalkaline phosphatase (APAPP) stain. (Courtesy of Professors K.C. Gatter and D.Y. Mason)

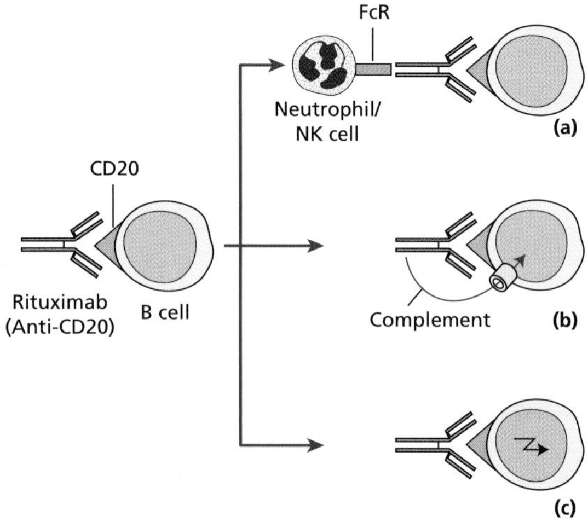

Fig. 17.10 The potential mechanisms of action of rituximab. Rituximab binds to CD20 on the surface of B cells. It can elicit a number of effector mechanisms including: **(a)** antibody dependent cell-mediated cytotoxicity; **(b)** complement mediated lysis of tumour cells; and **(c)** direct apoptosis of the target cell.

characteristic phenotype of $CD19^+$ and $CD5^+$ (like CLL) but in contrast is $CD22^+$, $CD23^-$. A specific t(11; 14) (q13; q32) translocation is seen which leads to deregulation of the cyclin D_1 (*BCL-1*) gene by juxtaposing it with the immunoglobulin heavy-chain gene. Clinical presentation is typically with lymphadenopathy and often there is bone marrow infiltration and tumour cells in the blood. The cells have characteristically angular nuclei in histological sections (Fig. 17.3b) and may circulate in the blood (see Fig. 15.6). Despite its low-grade status, mantle cell lymphoma is characterized by a poor prognosis. Current treatment regimens such as CVP, cyclophosphamide, hydroxodaunorubicin, oncovin (vincristine) and prednisolone (CHOP) or fludarabine, each with rituximab, are used. The role of bortezomid (see p. 223) or autologous stem cell transplantation is being investigated. The prognosis is poor and the median survival is approximately 3 years.

Marginal zone lymphomas

Marginal zone lymphomas are typically extranodal and are usually localized. Mucosa-associated lymphoid tissue (MALT) lymphomas come into this category and usually arise as a consequence of a pre-existing inflammatory or autoimmune disorder at sites such as the stomach or thyroid. Gastric MALT lymphoma is the most common form and is preceded by *Helicobacter (H.) pylori* infection. In the early stages it may respond to antibiotic therapy aimed at eliminating *H. pylori*. Chemotherapy and/ or radiotherapy combined with rituximab as for other low-grade lymphoma may be needed.

Splenic marginal zone lymphoma usually presents as splenomegaly and may be associated with circulating 'villous' lymphocytes (p. 194). Splenectomy is useful for symptomatic patients.

High-grade non-Hodgkin's lymphoma

Diffuse large B-cell lymphomas

Diffuse large B-cell lymphomas (DLCL) are a heterogeneous group of disorders representing the classical 'high-grade' lymphomas. As such they typically present with rapidly progressive lymphadenopathy associated with a fast rate of cellular proliferation. Progressive infiltration may affect the bone marrow, gastrointestinal tract, the spinal cord, the kidneys or other organs.

A variety of clinical and laboratory findings are relevant to the outcome of therapy. According to the international prognostic index these include age, performance status, stage, number of extranodal sites and serum LDH (Table 17.3). Bulky disease (major mass >5 cm in diameter) and prior history of low-grade disease or AIDS are also associated with a poorer prognosis. The cell of origin of DLCL has recently been suggested to be of prognostic significance. If this is germinal centre the outlook has been found to be more favourable than if the origin is from an activated peripheral B cell. Cases associated with 3q27 translocation also have a relatively good prognosis. DNA microarray analysis can give prognostic information (Fig. 17.5).

The CHOP regimen has been the mainstay of treatment of DLCL for many years and consists of cyclophosphomide, hyroxodaunorubicin, vincristine (Oncovin) and prednisolone given in 2-, 3- or 4-weekly cycles, typically for six to eight courses. The addition of anti-CD20 (rituximab) improves the cure rate and so R-CHOP is now the initial treatment. Cycles given at 14-day intervals with G-CSF support are under trial in younger patients. For localized disease, combined radiotherapy and chemotherapy (e.g. three courses of R-CHOP) may be optimal. Prophylactic therapy to prevent central nervous system (CNS) disease such as intrathecal or high-dose systemic methotrexate should be considered for patients with high-risk disease, particularly those with bone marrow involvement.

For patients who relapse and have chemotherapy-sensitive disease, high-dose chemotherapy with ifosfamide, epirubicin and etoposide (IVE) or etoposide, cytosine arabinoside, methylprednisolone and cisplatin (ESHAP), followed by autologous SCT can be effective. For those with primary refractory or chemoresistant disease the outlook is poor. Bortezomib, a proteasome inhibitor is undergoing trials. Alemtuzumab directed against CD52 may be used in both B- and T-cell NHL. Anti-CD20 radioactively linked to yttrium-90 or iodine-131 is currently reserved for relapsed cases. Overall long-term survival is approximately 65%.

Burkitt's lymphoma

Burkitt's lymphoma is the lymphomatous correlate of L_3 acute lymphoblastic leukaemia (p. 159) and occurs in endemic or sporadic forms. Endemic (African) Burkitt's lymphoma is seen in areas with chronic malaria exposure and is associated with Epstein–Barr virus (EBV) infection. In virtually all cases the *C-MYC* oncogene is overexpressed because it is translocated to an immunoglobulin gene, usually the heavy-chain locus t(8; 14). Typically, the patient, usually a child, presents with massive lymphadenopathy of the jaw (Fig. 17.11) which is initially very responsive to chemotherapy although long-term cure is uncommon. Sporadic Burkitt's lymphoma may occur anywhere in the world and is not associated with EBV infection. The histological picture of Burkitt's lymphoma is distinctive (Fig. 17.12). The prognosis for such patients was poor until the introduction of chemotherapy

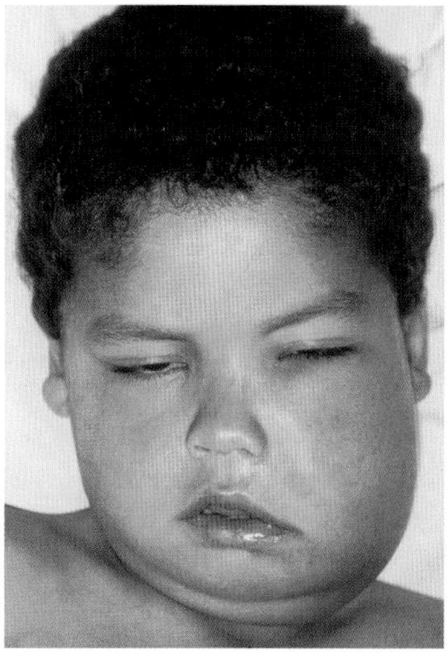

Fig. 17.11 Burkitt's lymphoma: characteristic facial swelling caused by extensive tumour involvement of the mandible and surrounding soft tissues.

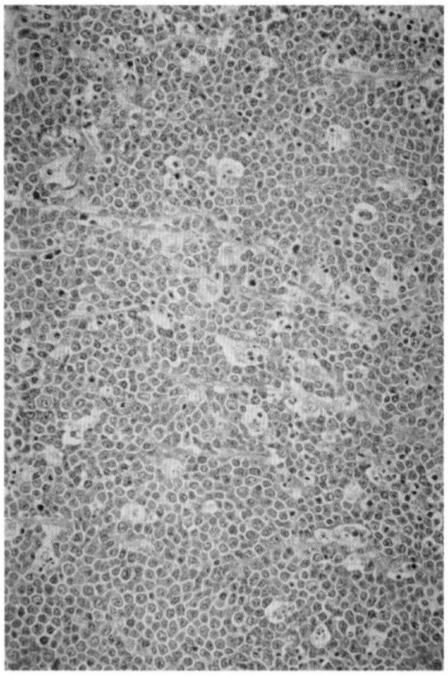

Fig. 17.12 Burkitt's lymphoma: histological section of lymph node showing sheets of lymphoblasts and 'starry sky' tingible body macrophages.

regimes which include high-dose methotrexate and cyclophosphamide. These have transformed the outlook and now the majority of patients are cured. B-ALL is treated with the same regimes.

Lymphoblastic lymphomas

Lymphoblastic lymphomas occur mainly in children and young adults and these conditions merge clinically and morphologically with acute lymphoblastic leukaemia (ALL). They are treated in a similar way.

T-cell lymphomas

Peripheral T-cell lymphomas that present with lymphadenopathy rather than extranodal disease are a heterogeneous group of rare tumours and are usually of $CD4^+$ phenotype. Several variants of T-cell lymphomas are recognized.

Peripheral T-cell non-Hodgkin's lymphoma, unspecified. These derive from post-thymic T cells at various stages of differentiation. They are treated with combined chemotherapy (e.g. CHOP). The prognosis is poor.

Angioimmunoblastic lymphadenopathy usually occurs in elderly patients with lymphadenopathy, hepatosplenomegaly, skin rashes and a polyclonal increase in serum IgG.

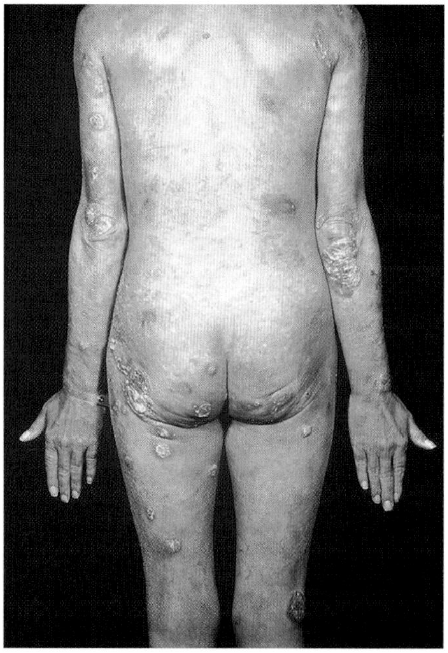

Fig. 17.13 Mycosis fungoides.

Mycosis fungoides is a chronic cutaneous T-cell lymphoma that presents with severe pruritus and psoriasis-like lesions (Fig. 17.13). Ultimately, deeper organs are affected, particularly lymph nodes, spleen, liver and bone marrow.

In **Sézary syndrome** there is dermatitis, erythroderma, generalized lymphadenopathy and circulating T-lymphoma cells. The cells are usually $CD4^+$ and have a folded or cerebriform nuclear chromatin. Initial treatment of these conditions is by local irradiation, topical chemotherapy or photochemotherapy with psoralen and ultraviolet light (PUVA). Chemotherapy (e.g. CHOP) may be needed.

Adult T-cell leukaemia/lymphoma is associated with human T-cell leukaemia/lymphoma virus type 1 (HTLV-1) infection and presents with lymphadenopathy, hepatic and splenic enlargement, cutaneous infiltrations and hypercalcaemia.

Angiocentric lymphomas typically involve the nasal sinuses whereas T-cell intestinal lymphoma is associated with gluten-induced enteropathy in many cases.

Anaplastic large cell lymphoma is particularly common in children and is of T-cell or null cell phenotype. The disease is $CD30^+$ and associated with the t(2; 5) (p23; q35) translocation. It has an aggressive course characterized by systemic symptoms and extranodal involvement.

Bibliography

Abramson J.S. and Shipp M.A. (2005) Advances in the biology and therapy of diffuse large B-cell lymphoma: moving toward a molecularly targeted approach. *Blood* **106**,1164–74.

Barosi G., Carella A., Lazzarino M. *et al.* (2005) Management of nodal indolent (non marginal-zone) non-Hodgkin's lymphomas: practice guidelines from the Italian Society of Hematology, Italian Society of Experimental Hematology and Italian Group for Bone Marrow Transplantation. *Haematologica* **90**,1236–57.

Coiffier B. (2005) Current strategies for the treatment of diffuse large B cell lymphoma. *Curr Opin Hematol* **12**,259–65.

Fisher S.G. and Fisher R.I. (2004) The epidemiology of non-Hodgkin's lymphoma. *Oncogene* **23**,6524–34.

Gandhi M.K. and Marcus R.E. (2005) Follicular lymphoma: time for a re-think? *Blood Rev* **19**,165–78.

Hennessy B.T., Hanrahan E.O., Daly P.A. (2004) Non-Hodgkin lymphoma: an update. *Lancet Oncol* **6**,341–53.

Lossos I.S., Czerwinski D.K., Alizadeh A.A. *et al.* (2004) Prediction of survival in diffuse large-B-cell lymphoma based on the expression of six genes. *N Engl J Med* **350**,1828–37.

Mauch P.M., Armitage J.O., Coiffier B., Dalla-Favera R., Harris N.L. (eds) (2004) *Non-Hodgkin's Lymphomas*. Lippincott Williams and Wilkins, Philadelphia.

Monti S., Savage K.J., Kutok J.L. *et al.* (2005) Molecular profiling of diffuse large B-cell lymphoma identifies robust subtypes including one characterized by host inflammatory response. *Blood* **105**,1851–61.

Peggs K.S., Mackinnon S., Linch D.C. (2005) The role of allogeneic transplantation in non-Hodgkin's lymphoma. *Br J Haematol* **128**,153–68.

Rastetter W., Molina A., White C.A. (2004) Rituximab: expanding role in therapy for lymphomas and autoimmune diseases. *Annu Rev Med* **55**,477–503.

Reichert J.M., Rosensweig C.J., Faden L.B., Dewitz M.C. (2005) Monoclonal antibody successes in the clinic. *Nat Biotechnol* **23**,1073–8.

Rizvi M.A., Evens A.M., Tallman M.S., Nelson B.P., Rosen S.T. (2006) T-cell non-Hodgkin lymphoma. *Blood* **107**,1255–64.

Seyfarth B., Josting A., Dreyling M., Schmitz N. (2006) Relapse in common lymphoma subtypes: salvage treatment options for follicular lymphoma and Hodgkin's disease. *Br J Haematol* **133**,3–18.

Wright G., Tan B., Rosenwald A. *et al.* (2003) A gene-expression-based method to diagnose clinically distinct subgroups of diffuse large B-cell lymphoma. *Proc Natl Acad Sci USA* **100**,9991–6.

CHAPTER 18

18 Multiple myeloma and related disorders

Paraproteinaemia

This term refers to the presence of a monoclonal immunoglobulin band in the serum. Normally, serum immunoglobulins are polyclonal and represent the combined output from millions of different plasma cells. A monoclonal band (M-protein), or ***paraprotein***, reflects the synthesis of immunoglobulin from a single clone of plasma cells. There are several situations in which this may occur (Table 18.1) and not all require treatment.

Table 18.1 Diseases associated with M-proteins.

Malignant or uncontrolled production
Multiple myeloma
Waldenström's macroglobulinaemia
Malignant lymphoma
Chronic lymphocytic leukaemia
Primary amyloidosis
Plasma cell leukaemia
Heavy chain disease
Benign or stable production
Benign monoclonal gammopathy
Solitary plasmacytoma
Chronic cold haemagglutinin disease
Transient (e.g. with infections)
Acquired immune deficiency syndrome (AIDS)
Gaucher's disease
Rarely with carcinoma and other conditions

Multiple myeloma

Multiple myeloma (myelomatosis) is a neoplastic proliferation characterized by plasma cell accumulation in the bone marrow, the presence of monoclonal protein in the serum and/or urine and related tissue damage. Ninety-eight per cent of cases occur over the age of 40 years with a peak incidence in the seventh decade.

The myeloma cell is a post-germinal centre plasma cell that has undergone immunoglobulin class switching and somatic hypermutation and secretes the paraprotein that is present in serum. Plasma cells naturally home to the bone marrow and this characteristic is retained by the tumour cell. The aetiology of the disease is unknown but it is more common in certain racial groups such as those of Afro-Caribbean origin. Tumour cells have very complex genetic changes but dysregulated or increased expression of cyclin D (p. 9) is believed to be an early unifying event. Approximately half of the tumours have an increased number of chromosomes (*hyperdiploid*) whereas non-hyperdiploid cases have a high incidence of translocations involving the immunoglobulin heavy-chain gene (*IGH*). Monoallelic loss of 13q is frequent in both categories and all these genetic abnormalities are also seen in monoclonal gammopathy of undetermined significance (MGUS; p. 224). The characteristic immunophenotype of malignant plasma cells is CD38^{high},

Table 18.2 Features of benign and malignant paraproteinaemia.

	Benign	Malignant
Bence-Jones proteinuria	Absent	May be present
Serum paraprotein concentration	Usually <20 g/L and stationary	Usually >20 g/L and rising
Serum free light chain ratio	Normal	Abnormal
Immuneparesis (hypogammaglobinaemia)	Absent	Present
Underlying lymphoproliferative disease or myeloma	Absent	Present
Bone lesions	Absent	Present
Plasma cells in marrow	<10%	>10%

$CD138^{high}$ and $CD45^{low}$. Interleukin 6 is a potent growth factor for myeloma cells and is often active by an autocrine mechanism.

Diagnosis

This depends on three principal findings (Table 18.2):

1 Monoclonal protein in serum and/or urine (Fig. 18.1).

2 Increased plasma cells in the bone marrow (Fig. 18.2).

3 Related organ or tissue impairment such as bone disease, renal impairment, anaemia, hypercalaemia, hyperviscosity, amyloidosis or recurrent infection.

If the bone marrow plasma cell count is >10% but there is **no** evidence of tissue damage the disease is termed ***asymptomatic*** or ***smouldering myeloma***.

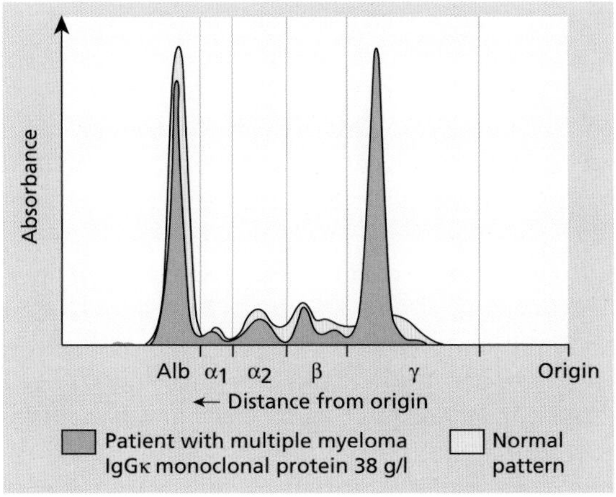

Fig. 18.1 Serum protein electrophoresis in multiple myeloma showing an abnormal paraprotein in the γ-globulin region with reduced levels of background β- and γ-globulins.

Clinical features

1 Bone pain (especially backache) resulting from vertebral collapse and pathological fractures (Fig. 18.3a,b).

2 Features of anaemia: e.g. lethargy, weakness, dyspnoea, pallor, tachycardia.

3 Recurrent infections: related to deficient antibody production, abnormal cell-mediated immunity and neutropenia.

4 Features of renal failure and/or hypercalcaemia: polydipsia, polyuria, anorexia, vomiting, constipation and mental disturbance.

5 Abnormal bleeding tendency: myeloma protein may interfere with platelet function and coagulation factors; thrombocytopenia occurs in advanced disease.

6 Amyloidosis occurs in 5% with features such as macroglossia, carpal tunnel syndrome and diarrhoea.

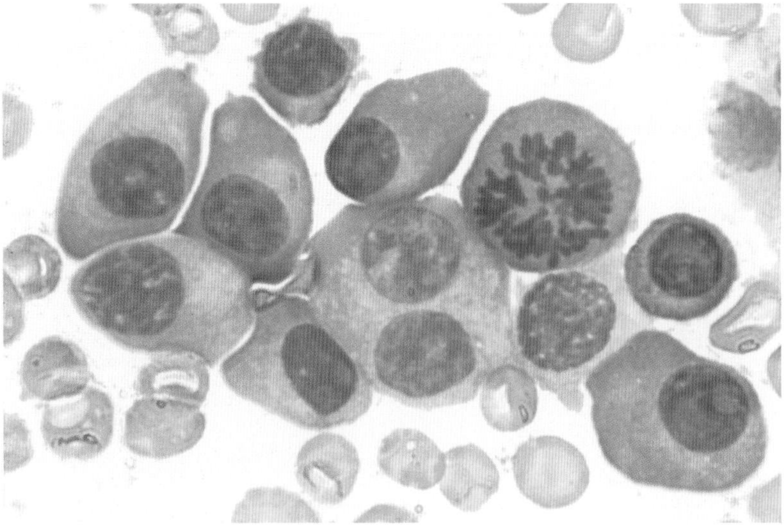

Fig. 18.2 The bone marrow in multiple myeloma showing large numbers of plasma cells, with many abnormal forms.

7 In approximately 2% of cases there is a hyperviscosity syndrome (Fig. 22.6) with purpura, haemorrhages, visual failure, central nervous system (CNS) symptoms, neuropathies and heart failure.

Laboratory findings include the following:

1 ***Presence of a paraprotein*** Serum and urine should be screened by immunoglobulin electrophoresis. The paraprotein is immunoglobulin G (IgG) in 60% of cases, IgA in 20% and light chain only in almost all the rest. Less than 1% have IgD or IgE paraprotein. Free light chains are filtered from the serum into the kidney and are therefore often not detectable in serum using electrophoresis. However, the level of free light chain in serum can be measured with a specific antibody. As free light chains are produced by almost all malignant plasma cells the ***serum free light chain*** assay is useful in diagnosis and monitoring of myeloma and other forms of paraproteinaemia. In myeloma the normal $\kappa : \lambda$ free light chain ratio of 2 : 1 is skewed with an excess of κ or λ chains.

Normal serum immunoglobulin levels (IgG, IgA and IgM) are reduced, a feature known as ***immune paresis***. The urine contains free light chains, known as ***Bence-Jones protein***, in two-thirds of cases. Rare cases of myeloma are non-secretory and therefore not associated with a paraprotein or Bence-Jones proteinuria although some will still show a disturbed free light chain ratio in the serum.

2 There is usually a normochromic normocytic or macrocytic anaemia. Rouleaux formation is marked in most cases (Fig. 18.4). Neutropenia and thrombocytopenia occur in advanced disease. Abnormal plasma cells appear in the blood film in 15% of patients and can be detected by sensitive flow cytometry in over 50%.

3 High erythrocyte sedimentation rate (ESR) and C-reactive protein (CRP).

4 Increased plasma cells in the bone marrow (usually >20%) often with abnormal forms (Fig. 18.2).

5 Radiological investigation of the skeleton reveals bone lesions such as osteolytic areas without evidence of surrounding osteoblastic reaction or sclerosis in 60% of patients (Fig. 18.5) or generalized osteoporosis in 20% (Fig. 18.3). Twenty per cent have no bone lesions. In addition, pathological fractures or vertebral collapse (Fig. 18.3b) are common. The osteolytic lesions are caused by osteoclast activation resulting from high serum levels of RANKL (receptor activator of nuclear factor-κB (NF-κB) ligand), produced by plasma cells and bone marrow stroma, which binds to activatory RANK receptors on the osteoclast surface.

6 Serum calcium elevation occurs in 45% of patients. Typically, the serum alkaline phosphatase is normal (except following pathological fractures).

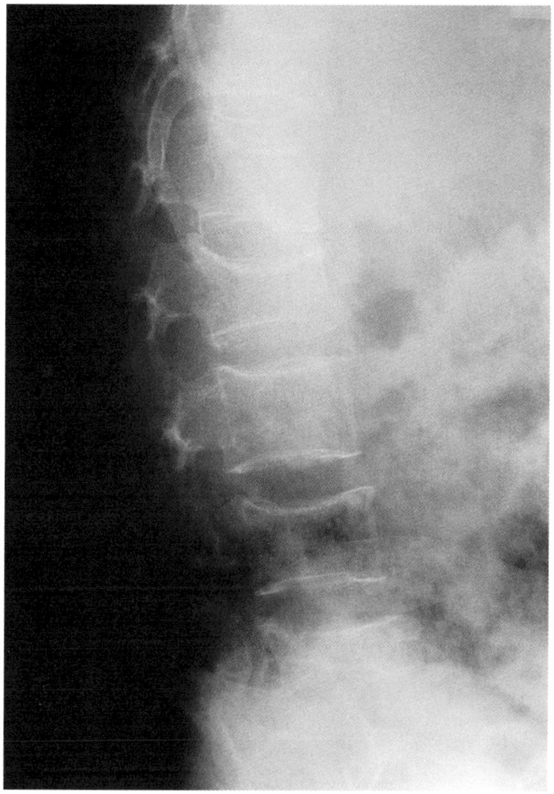

(a)

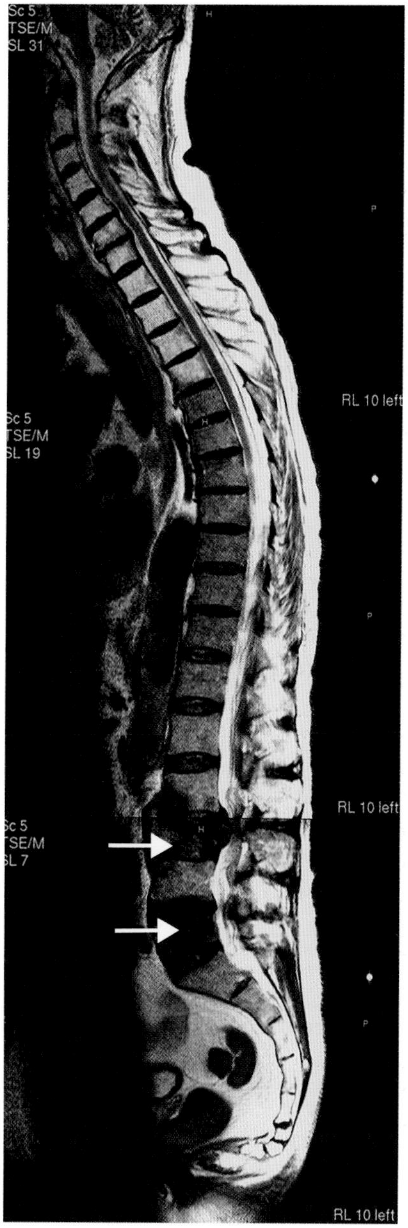

(b)

Fig. 18.3 **(a)** Multiple myeloma: X-ray of lumbar spine showing severe demineralization with partial collapse of L_3. **(b)** Magnetic resonance imaging (MRI) of spine: T_2-weighted study. There is infiltration and destruction of L_3 and L_5 with bulging of the posterior part of the body of L_3 into the spinal canal compressing the corda equina (arrowed). Radiotherapy has caused a marrow signal change in vertebrae C_2–D_4 because of replacement of normal red marrow by fat (bright white signal). (Courtesy of Dr A. Platts)

7 The serum creatinine is raised in 20% of cases. Proteinaceous deposits from heavy Bence-Jones proteinuria, hypercalcaemia, uric acid, amyloid and pyelonephritis may all contribute to renal failure (Fig. 18.6).

8 A low serum albumin occurs with advanced disease.

9 Serum β_2-microglobulin is often raised and is a useful indicator of prognosis. Levels less than 4 mg/L imply a relatively good prognosis.

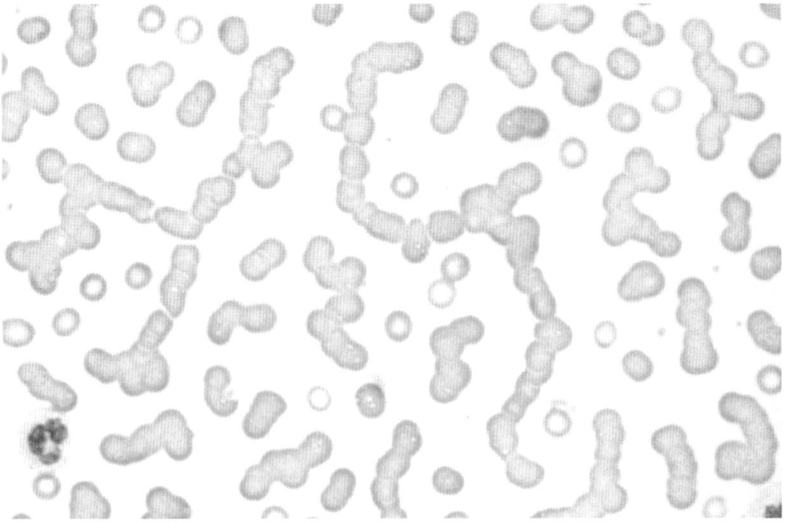

Fig. 18.4 The peripheral blood film in multiple myeloma showing rouleaux formations.

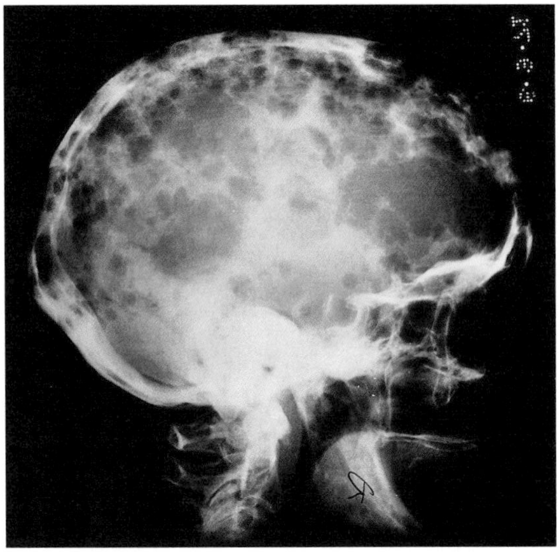

Fig. 18.5 Skull X-ray in multiple myeloma showing many 'punched-out' lesions.

Treatment

This may be divided into specific and supportive (Fig. 18.7).

Specific

At the current time the disease remains incurable except for those very few, mostly younger, patients who may be cured by allogeneic stem cell transplantation (SCT). For all other patients the major treatment decision is between the use of ***intensive therapy*** (mostly for patients aged less than 65–70 years) and ***non-intensive therapy*** for older patients.

Intensive therapy involves the combination of several courses of chemotherapy to reduce the tumour burden followed by stem cell collection and autologous SCT after high-dose chemotherapy. Repeated intravenous or oral chemotherapy cycles such as cyclophosphamide, dexamethasone and thalidomide (CDT), cyclophosphamide, vincristine, adriamycin (hydroxodaunorubicin) and dexamethasone (CVAD) or idarubicin with dexamethasone (IDEX) may be used. Peripheral blood stem cells are collected after mobilization using a combination of chemotherapy and granulocyte colony-stimulating factor (G-CSF). High-dose melphalan, with or without radiotherapy, is the typical conditioning regime for autologous SCT. Two consecutive SCT procedures are used in some centres.

Although allogeneic transplantation may cure the disease it carries a high procedure-related mortality and patients frequently relapse after the procedure.

Non-intensive therapy In elderly patients monthly courses of the oral alkylating agent melphalan, sometimes in combination with prednisolone, are usually effective in reducing the tumour burden. Many centres now also use thalidomide (see below).

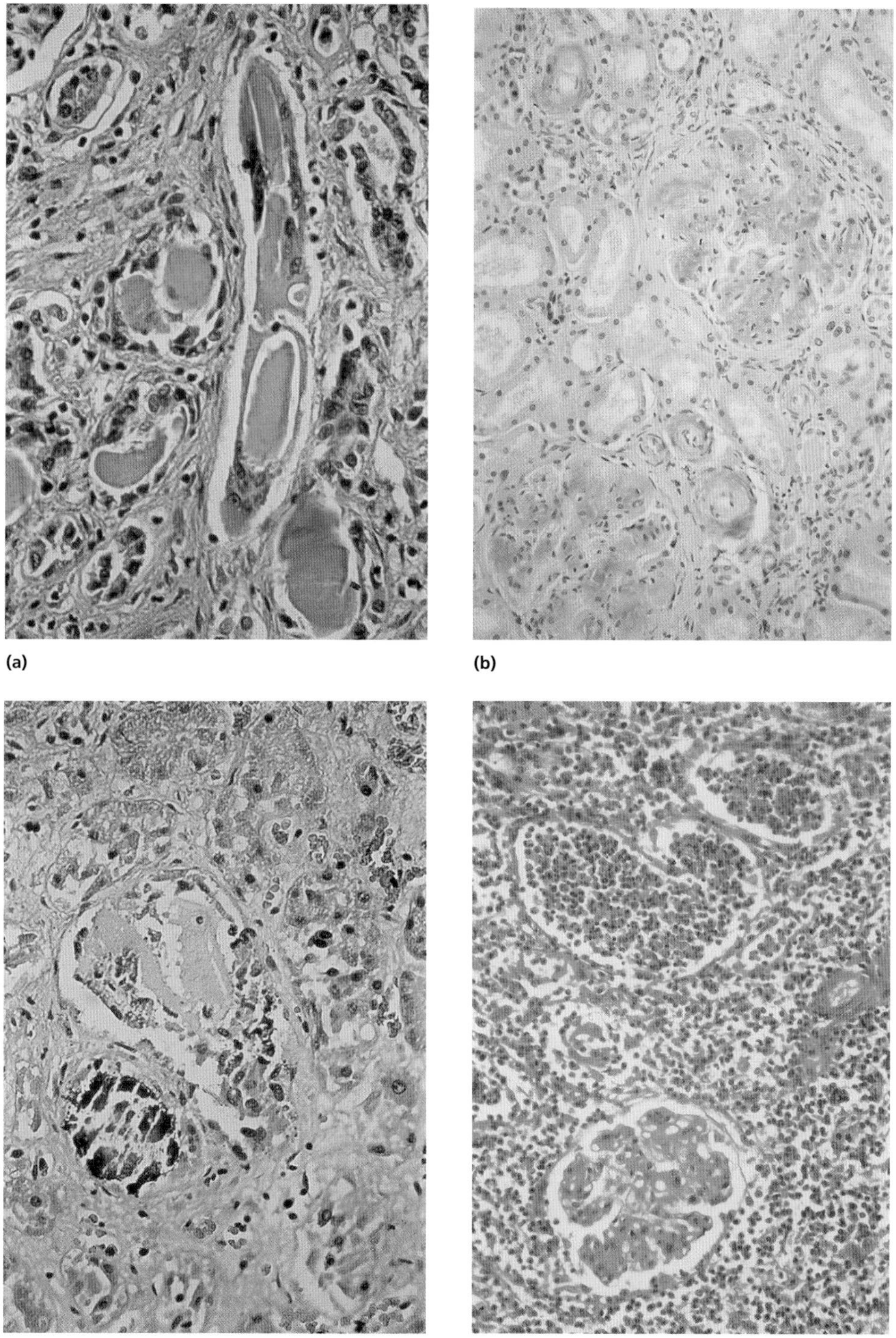

(a) (b) (c) (d)

Fig. 18.6 The kidney in multiple myeloma. **(a)** Myeloma kidney: the renal tubules are distended with hyaline protein (precipitated light chains or Bence-Jones protein). Giant cells are prominent in the surrounding cellular reaction. **(b)** Amyloid deposition: both glomeruli and several of the small blood vessels contain an amorphous pink-staining deposit characteristic of amyloid (Congo red stain). **(c)** Nephrocalcinosis: calcium deposition (dark 'fractured' material) in the renal parenchyma. **(d)** Pyelonephritis: destruction of renal parenchyma and infiltration by acute inflammatory cells.

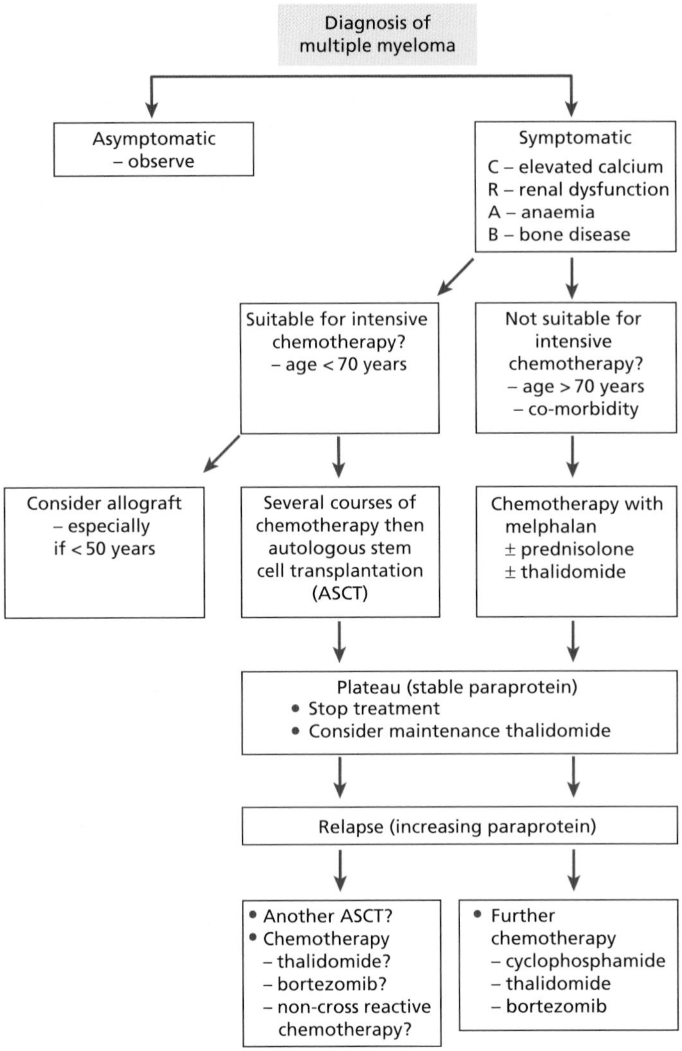

Fig. 18.7 An approach to the management of multiple myeloma.

Typically, paraprotein levels gradually fall, bone lesions show improvement and blood counts may improve. Cyclophosphamide is also effective and simple to use as a single agent. However, after a variable number of courses a 'plateau phase' is reached in which the paraprotein level stops falling. At this point treatment is stopped and the patient is seen at regular intervals in the outpatient clinic. After a variable period of time, often around 18 months, the disease 'escapes' from plateau with rising paraprotein and worsening symptoms. Further chemotherapy may be given although the disease becomes increasingly difficult to control. Trials of drugs designed to overcome multidrug resistance have not proven successful.

Other treatments

Thalidomide is useful in the management of relapsed disease and is being introduced into first-line therapy (e.g. CDT). Its precise mechanism of action is unknown and it has a number of side-effects such as sedation, constipation, neuropathy and thrombosis. The addition of dexamethasone increases the response rate but venous thrombosis becomes a major concern. Prophylactic anticoagulation with warfarin or heparin is needed when thalidomide is used in induction regimes. Analogues of thalidomide which have increased immunomodulatory activity are now showing promise.

Bortezomib (Velcade) is a promising drug which inhibits cellular proteasome and NF-κB activation. Already proven in refractory disease, it is now being assessed in earlier phases of treatment. Its main side-effect is neuropathy.

α-Interferon This may prolong the plateau phase following chemotherapy or transplantation but has little effect on overall survival.

Radiotherapy is highly effective in treating the symptoms of myeloma. It may be used for areas of bone pain or spinal cord compression.

Support care

Renal failure Rehydrate and treat the underlying cause (e.g. hypercalcaemia, hyperuricaemia). Dialysis is generally well tolerated. It is important that all patients with myeloma drink at least 3 L of fluid each day throughout the course of their disease.

Bone disease and hypercalcaemia Bisphosphonates such as pamidronate, clodronate or zoledronic acid are effective in reducing the progression of bone disease and may also improve overall survival. Acute hypercalcaemia is treated with rehydration with isotonic saline, a diuretic and corticosteroids followed by a biphosphonate.

Compression paraplegia Use decompression laminectomy or irradiation; corticosteroid therapy may help.

Anaemia Transfusion or erythropoietin are used.

Bleeding Bleeding caused by paraprotein interference with coagulation and hyperviscosity syndrome may be treated by repeated plasmapheresis.

Infections Rapid treatment of any infection is essential. Prophylactic infusions of immunoglobulin concentrates together with oral broad-spectrum antibiotics and antifungal agents may be needed for recurrent infections.

Prognosis

An international prognostic index has been used based on serum β_2-microglobulin (β_2M) and albumin levels. Patients with serum β_2M >5.5 mg/L and an albumin <35 g/L have a poor survival as do those with frequent circulating plasma cells. Overall, the median survival with non-intensive chemotherapy is 3–4 years and this is improved by approximately 1 year with autologous transplantation.

Other plasma cell tumours

Solitary plasmacytoma

These are isolated plasma cell tumours, usually of bone or soft tissue (e.g. the mucosa of the upper respiratory and gastrointestinal tracts or the skin). The associated paraprotein disappears following radiotherapy to the primary lesion.

Plasma cell leukaemia

This occurs either as a late complication of myeloma or as a primary disease characterized by the presence of 20% or more plasma cells in the blood (Chapter 15). The outlook is poor.

Heavy chain disease

In these rare disorders the neoplastic cells secrete only incomplete immunoglobulin heavy chains (γ, α or μ). The most common form is α-heavy chain disease which occurs mainly in the Mediterranean area and starts as a malabsorption syndrome which may progress to lymphoma.

Waldenström's macroglobulinaemia

This is an uncommon condition, seen most frequently in men over 50 years of age, in which there is a lymphoplasmacytoid lymphoma (Fig. 18.8) which produces a monoclonal IgM paraprotein. The cell of origin appears to be a post-germinal centre B cell with the characteristics of an IgM-bearing memory B cell.

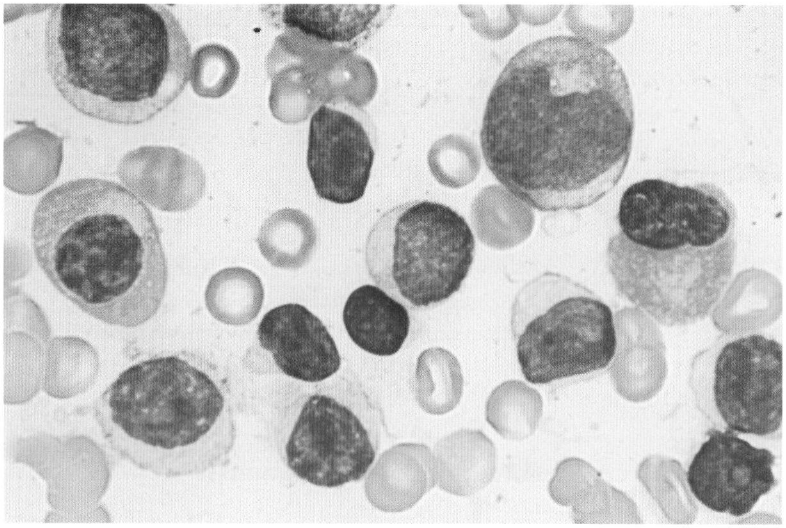

Fig 18.8 Lymphoplasmacytoid lymphoma associated with Waldenström's macroglobulinaemia. Bone marrow shows cells with features of lymphocytes and plasma cells.

Clinical features

These are usually of insidious onset, with fatigue and weight loss. Hyperviscosity syndrome (Fig. 22.6) is common. IgM paraprotein increases blood viscosity more than equivalent concentrations of IgG or IgA, and small increases above 30 g/L in concentration lead to large increases in viscosity. Visual upset is frequent and the retina may show a variety of changes such as engorged veins, haemorrhages, exudates and a blurred disc (Fig. 18.9). If the macroglobulin is a cryoglobulin, features of cryoprecipitation, such as Raynaud's phenomenon, may be present. Anaemia, at least partly caused by an increased plasma volume, is usually a significant problem and a bleeding tendency may result from macroglobulin interference with coagulation factors and platelet function. Neurological symptoms, dyspnoea and heart failure may be presenting symptoms. Moderate lymphadenopathy and enlargement of the liver and spleen are frequently seen.

Diagnosis

This is made by the finding of a monoclonal serum IgM together with bone marrow or lymph node infiltration with lymphoplasmacytoid cells. The ESR is raised and there may be a peripheral blood lymphocytosis.

Treatment

Specific

No therapy is needed for patients without symptoms, significant organomegaly or anaemia. Chlorambucil or cyclophosphamide have been the mainstay of therapy but fludarabine or 2-chlorodeoxyadenosine and rituximab are also useful for initial therapy or for relapsed cases. Combination chemotherapy as for non-Hodgkin's lymphoma is needed in late stages. SCT may be considered for advanced disease.

Support

Acute hyperviscosity syndrome is treated with repeated plasmapheresis. As IgM is mainly intravascular, plasmapheresis is more effective than with IgG or IgA paraproteins when much of the protein is extravascular and so rapidly replenishes the plasma compartment. Erythropoeitin or regular transfusions may be required for chronic anaemia.

Monoclonal gammopathy of undetermined significance

Transient or persistent paraproteins can occur in many other conditions as well as in multiple myeloma (Table 18.1). A serum paraprotein may be sometimes be detected without any evidence of myeloma or other underlying disease and is termed

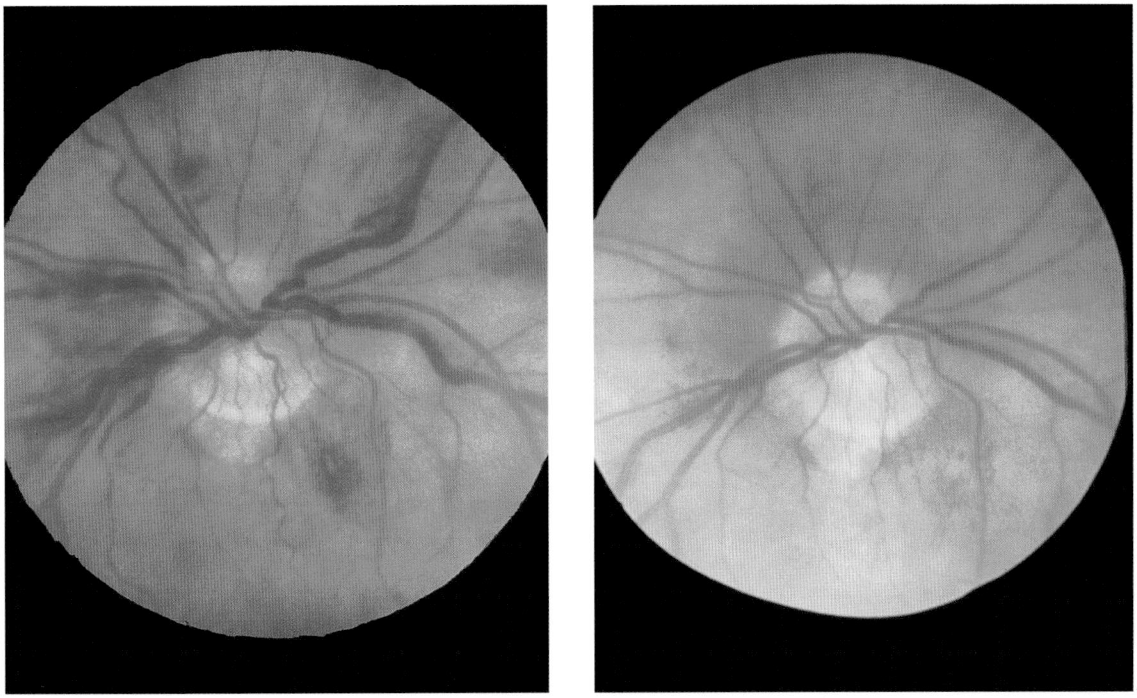

(a) (b)

Fig. 18.9 Waldenström's macroglobulinaemia: hyperviscosity syndrome. **(a)** The retina before plasmapheresis shows distension of retinal vessels, particularly the veins which show bulging and constriction (the 'linked sausage' effect) and areas of haemorrhage; **(b)** following plasmapheresis the vessels have returned to normal and the areas of haemorrhage have cleared.

monoclonal gammopathy of undetermined significance (MGUS). It becomes increasingly common with age, being present in 1% of persons older than 50 years and 3% of those over 70 years. There are no bone lesions, no Bence-Jones proteinuria, and the proportion of plasma cells in the marrow is normal (<4%) or only slightly raised (<10%) (Table 18.2). The concentration of monoclonal immunoglobulin in serum is usually less than 20 g/L and other serum immunoglobulins are not depressed. Serum light chains (either κ or λ) are increased in one-third of patients; the greater the increase, the more the risk of transformation. DNA microarray patterns can distinguish myeloma from MGUS. No treatment is needed but patients with MGUS develop overt myeloma or lymphoma at a rate of approximately 1% each year and so are usually followed up regularly in the outpatient clinic.

Amyloidosis

The amyloidoses are a heterogeneous group of disorders characterized by the extracellular deposition of protein in an abnormal fibrillar form. Amyloidosis may be hereditary or acquired and deposits may be focal, localized or systemic in distribution. The amyloid is made from different amyloid fibril precursor proteins in each type of disease. Except for intracerebral amyloid plaques, all amyloid deposits contain a non-fibrillary glycoprotein amyloid P which is derived from a normal serum precursor structurally related to CRP. The classic diagnostic histological test is red–green birefringence after staining with Congo red and viewing under polarized light (Fig. 18.10).

Amyloidosis is classified in Table 18.3.

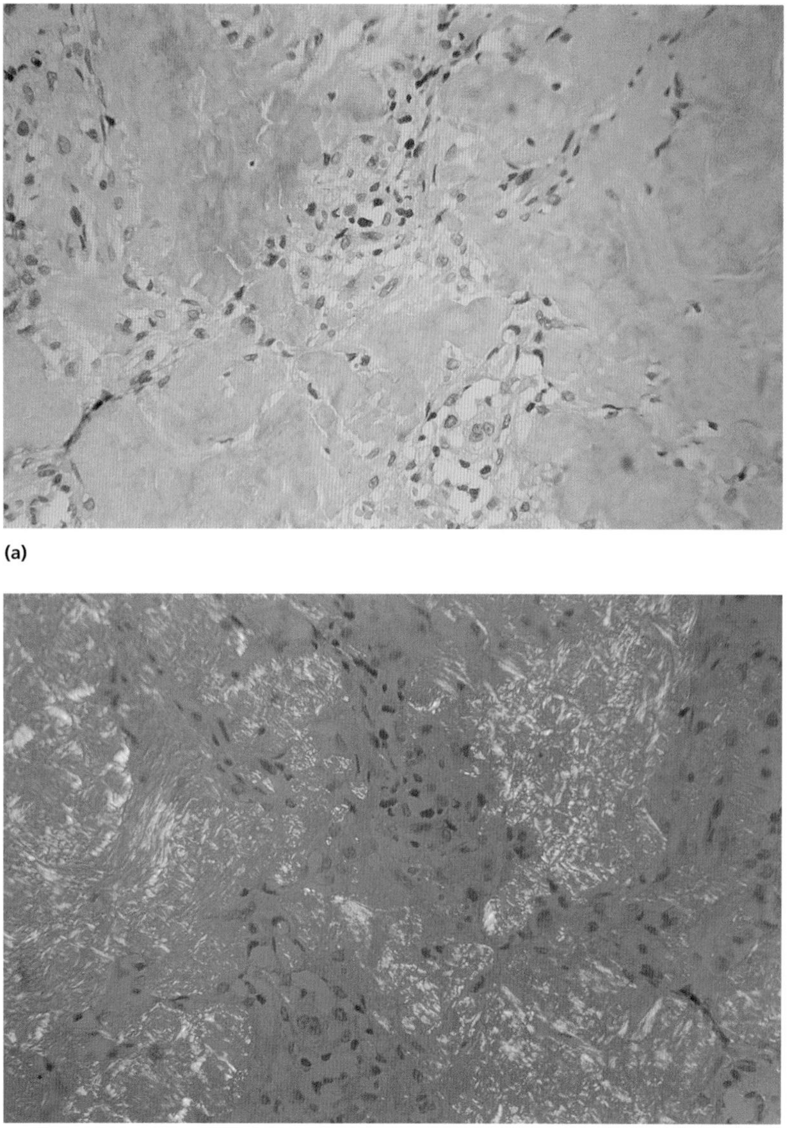

(a)

(b)

Fig. 18.10 Amyloidosis: (a) Congo red staining; and (b) blue–green birefringence under polarized light.

Systemic AL amyloidosis

Systemic amyloid disease is caused by deposition of monoclonal light chains produced from a clonal plasma cell proliferation. The level of paraprotein may be very low and is not always detectable in serum or urine. The clinical features are caused by involvement of the heart, tongue (Fig. 18.11), peripheral nerves and kidneys (Fig. 18.12), and the patient may present with heart failure, macroglossia, peripheral neuropathy, carpal tunnel syndrome or renal failure. Treatment is with chemotherapy similar to that used in myeloma, possibly with autologous SCT, which may improve prognosis.

Hyperviscosity syndrome

The most common cause is polycythaemia (p. 233). Hyperviscosity may also occur in patients with myeloma or Waldenström's macroglobulinaemia

Table 18.3 Classification of amyloidosis: types, structure and organ involvement.

Type	Chemical nature	Organs involved
Systemic AL amyloidosis		
Associated with myeloma, Waldenström's macroglobulinaemia or MGUS	Immunoglobulin light chains (AL)	Tongue
May also occur on its own as primary amyloidosis (associated with an occult plasma cell proliferation)		Skin Heart Nerves Connective tissue
May also occur in localized form with local 'immunocyte' proliferation		Kidneys Liver Spleen
Reactive systemic AA amyloidosis		
Rheumatoid arthritis, tuberculosis, bronchiectasis, chronic osteomyelitis, inflammatory bowel disease	Protein A (AA)	Liver Spleen Kidneys
Hodgkin's lymphoma, carcinomas, familial Mediterranean fever		Bone marrow
Familial amyloidosis	e.g. Transthyretin abnormalities	Nerves Heart Eyes
Localized amyloidosis		
Central nervous system	β-amyloid protein	Alzheimer's disease
Endocrine	Peptic hormones	Endocrine tumours
Senile	Various	Heart, brain, joints, prostate, etc.

AA, AL, these are defined by their chemical nature as in the table; MGUS, monoclonal gammopathy of undetermined significance.

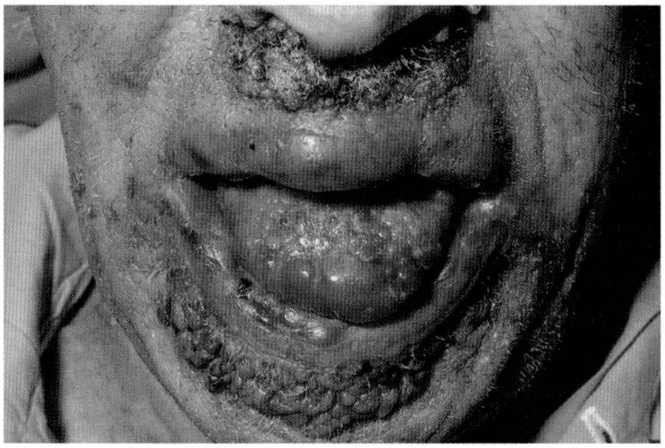

Fig. 18.11 Multiple myeloma: the tongue and lips are enlarged because of nodular and waxy deposits of amyloid.

or in patients with chronic or acute leukaemias associated with very high white cell counts. Rarely, haemophiliac patients with circulating inhibitors, being treated with massive doses of cryoprecipitate, have developed hyperviscosity because of the large volumes of fibrinogen infused.

The clinical features of the hyperviscosity syndrome include visual disturbances, lethargy, confusion, muscle weakness, nervous system symptoms and signs, and congestive heart failure. The retina may show a variety of changes: engorged veins, haemorrhages, exudates and a blurred disc (Fig. 18.9).

Emergency treatment varies with the cause: venesection or isovolaemic exchange with a plasma

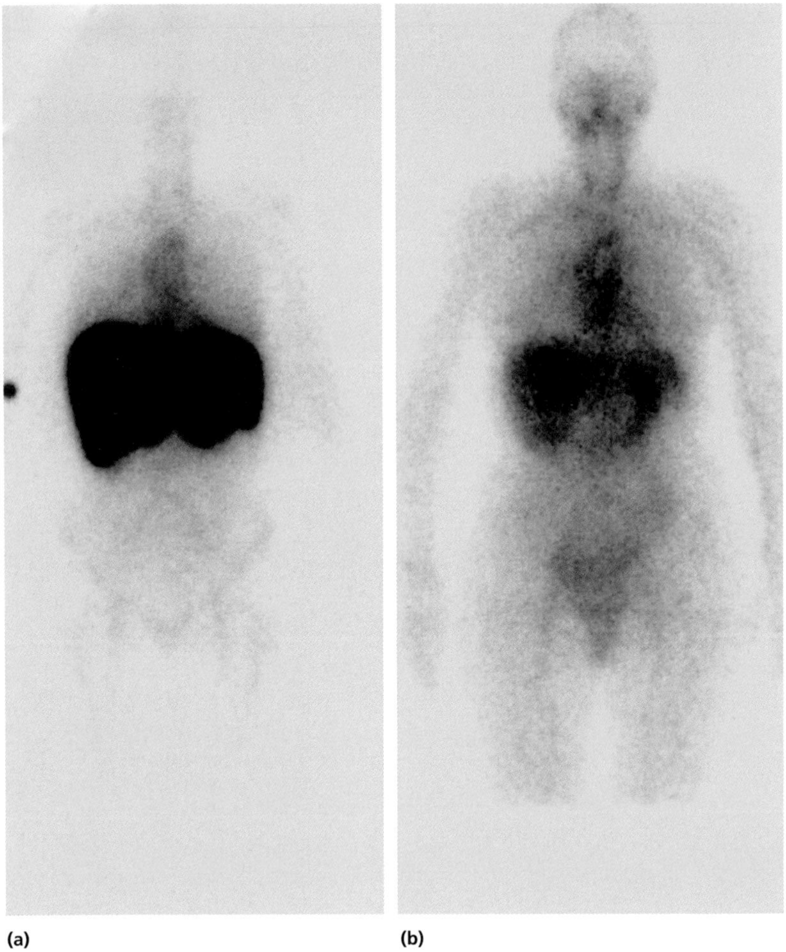

Fig. 18.12 Serial anterior whole body ^{123}I-labelled serum amyloid P component (SAP) scans of a 52-year-old woman who presented with renal failure resulting from systemic AL amyloidosis. **(a)** The initial scan demonstrates a large amyloid load with hepatic, splenic, renal and bone marrow deposits. The underlying plasma cell dyscrasia responded to high-dose melphalan followed by autologous stem cell rescue. **(b)** Follow-up SAP scintigraphy 3 years after chemotherapy showed greatly reduced uptake of tracer indicating substantial regression of her amyloid deposits. (Courtesy of Professor P.N. Hawkins, National Amyloidosis Centre, Royal Free Hospital, London)

substitute for red cells in a polycythaemic patient; plasmapheresis in myeloma, Waldenström's disease or hyperfibrinogenaemia; and leucopheresis or chemotherapy in leukaemias associated with high white counts. The long-term treatment depends on control of the primary disease with specific therapy.

Bibliography

Anderson K.C., Pazdur R., Farrell A.T. (2005) Development of effective new treatments for multiple myeloma. *J Clin Oncol* **23**,7207–11.

Bergsagel P.L. and Kuehl W.M. (2005) Molecular pathogenesis and a consequent classification of multiple myeloma. *J Clin Oncol* **23**,6333–8.

Bergsagel P.L., Kuehl W.M., Zhan F. *et al.* (2005) Cyclin D dysregulation: an early and unifying pathogenic event in multiple myeloma. *Blood* **106**,296–303.

Child J.A., Morgan G.J., Davies F.E. *et al.* (2003) Medical Research Council Adult Leukaemia Working Party. High-dose chemotherapy with hematopoietic stem-cell rescue for multiple myeloma. *N Engl J Med* **348**,1875–83.

Gahrton G., Durie B.G.M., Samson D.M. (2004) *Multiple Myeloma and Related Disorders*. Arnold, London.

Greipp P.R., San Miguel J., Durie B.G. *et al.* (2005) International staging system for multiple myeloma. *J Clin Oncol* **23**,3412–20.

International Myeloma Working Group (2003) Criteria for the classification of monoclonal gammopathies, multiple myeloma and related disorders: a report of the International Myeloma Working Group. *Br J Haematol* **121**,749–57.

Johnson S.A., Birchall J., Luckie C., Oscier D.G., Owen R.G. (2006) Guideline on the management of Waldenström macroglobulinaemia. *Br J Haematol* **132**,683–97.

Kyle R.A. and Rajkumar S.V. (2004) Multiple myeloma. *N Engl J Med* **351**,1860–73.

Kyle R.A., Therneau T.M., Rajkumar S.V. (2006) Prevalence of monoclonal gammopathy of undetermined significance. *N Engl J Med* **354**,362–9.

Kyle R.A., Therneau T.M., Rajkumar S.V. *et al.* (2002) A long-term study of prognosis in monoclonal gammopathy of undetermined significance. *N Engl J Med* **346**,564–9.

Lachmann H.J., Gallimore R., Gillmore J.D. *et al.* (2003) Outcome in systemic AL amyloidosis in relation to changes in concentration of circulating free immunoglobulin light chains following chemotherapy. *Br J Haematol* **122**,78–84.

Nowakowski G.S., Witzig T.E., Dingli D. *et al.* (2005) Circulating plasma cells detected by flow cytometry as a predictor of survival in 302 patients with newly diagnosed multiple myeloma. *Blood* **106**,2276–9.

Palumbo A., Bringhen S., Caravita T. *et al.* (2006) Oral melphelan and prednisone chemotherapy plus thalidomide compared with melphelan and prednisone alone in elderly patients with multiple myeloma: randomised controlled trial. *Lancet* **367**,825–31.

Rajkumar S.V., Kyle R.A., Therneau T.M. *et al.* (2005) Serum free light chain ratio is an independent risk factor for progression in monoclonal gammopathy of undetermined significance. *Blood* **106**,812–7.

Richardson P.G., Barlogie B., Berenson J. *et al.* (2003) A phase 2 study of bortezomib in relapsed, refractory myeloma. *N Engl J Med* **348**,2609–17.

Singal S., Mehta J., Desikan R. (1999) Antitumour activity of thalidomide in refractory myeloma. *N Engl J Med* **341**,1565–71.

Smith A., Wisloff F., Samson D., UK Myeloma Forum; Nordic Myeloma Study Group; British Committee for Standards in Haematology (2006) Guidelines on the diagnosis and management of multiple myeloma. *Br J Haematol* **132**,410–51.

Treon S.P., Gertz M.A., Dimopoulos M. *et al.* (2006) Update on treatment recommendations from the Third International Workshop on Waldenström's macroglobulinemia. *Blood* **107**,3442–6.

CHAPTER 19

19 Myeloproliferative disorders

The term myeloproliferative disorders describes a group of conditions arising from marrow stem cells and characterized by clonal proliferation of one or more haemopoietic components in the bone marrow and, in many cases, the liver and spleen. Three disorders are included in this classification:

1 Polycythaemia rubra vera (PRV).
2 Essential thrombocythaemia (ET).
3 Myelofibrosis.

These disorders are closely related to each other. Indeed, transitional forms occur and in many patients an evolution from one entity into another occurs during the course of the disease (Fig. 19.1). A single acquired mutation of the cytoplasmic tyrosine kinase Janus-associated kinase 2 (JAK2) (Val617Phe) occurs (heterozygous or homozogous) in the marrow and blood of almost all patients with PRV and in approximately 50% of those with ET and myelofibrosis, showing the common aetiology of these three diseases (Fig. 19.2). The mutation occurs in a highly conserved region of the pseudokinase domain, which is believed to negatively regulate JAK2

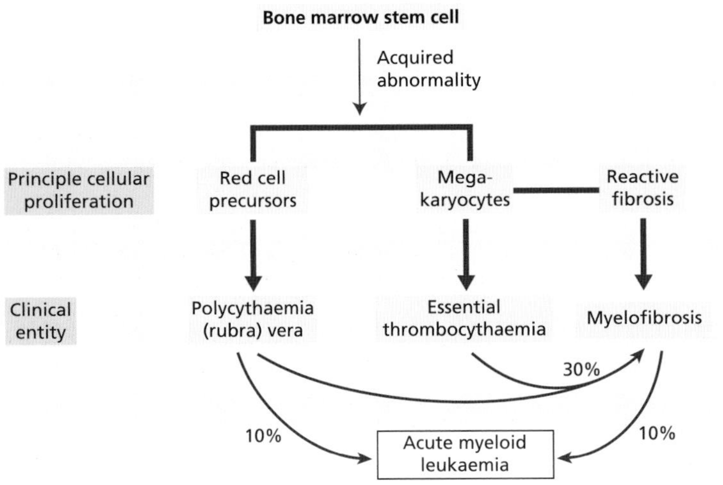

Fig. 19.1 Relationship between the three myeloproliferative diseases. They may all arise by somatic mutation in the pluripotential stem and progenitor cells. Many transitional cases occur showing features of two conditions and, in other cases, the disease transforms during its course from one of these diseases to another or to acute myeloid leukaemia. The three diseases, polycythaemia rubra vera, essential thrombocythaemia and myelofibrosis, are characterised by JAK2 mutation in a varying proportion of cases (see text).

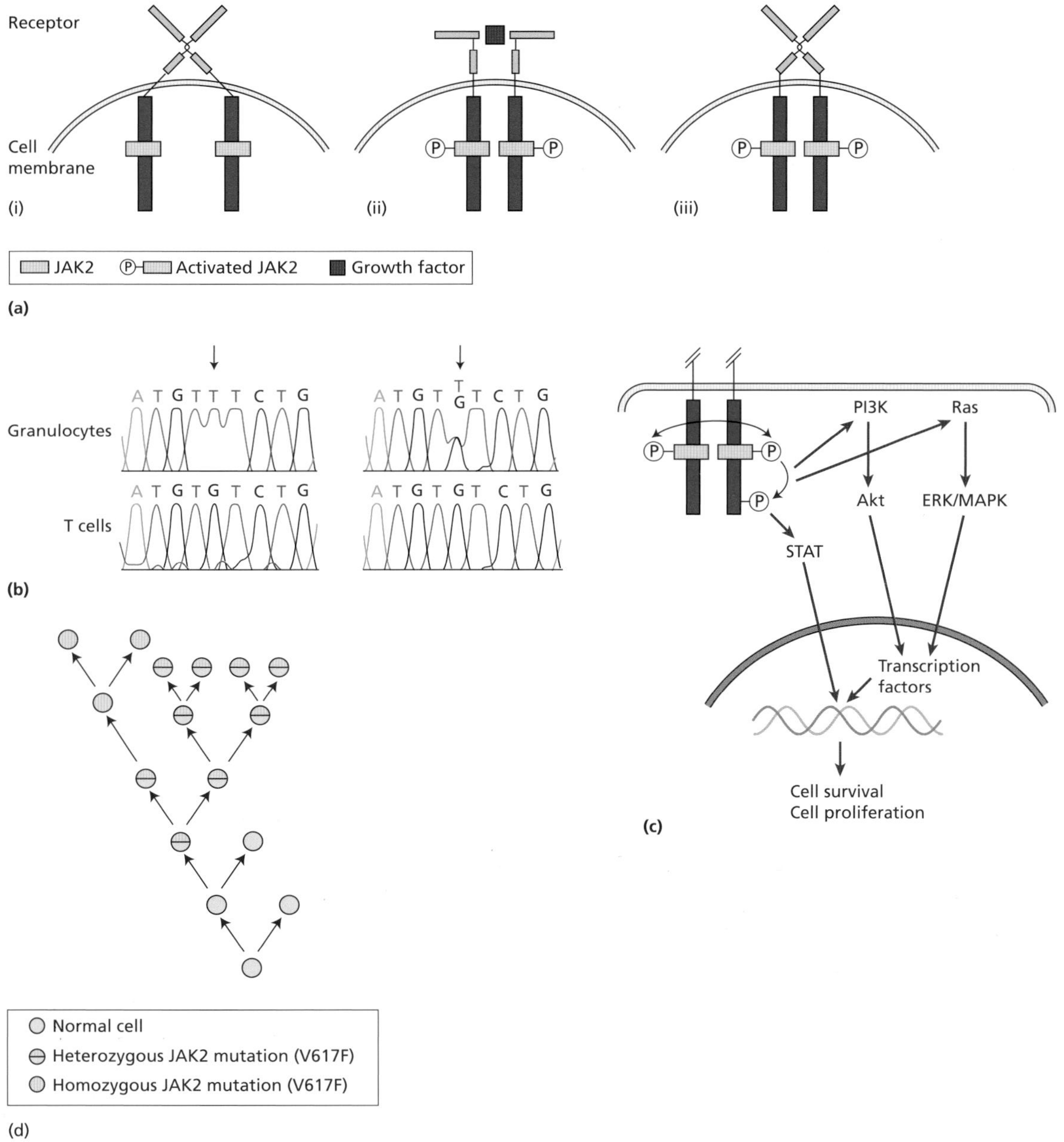

Fig. 19.2 The role of JAK2 mutation in the generation of myeloproliferative diseases. **(a)** (i) Most haemopoietic growth factor receptors do not have intrinsic kinase activity but associate with a protein kinase such as JAK2 in the cytoplasm. (ii) When the receptor binds a growth factor the cytoplasmic domains move closer together and the JAK2 molecules can activate each other by phosphorylation. (iii) The V617F JAK2 mutation allows the JAK protein to become activated even when no growth factor is bound. **(b)** DNA sequencing shows homozygous G → T mutation in JAK2 in granulocytes but not in T lymphocytes (left-hand panel) and heterozygous mutation in right-hand panel. (After Kralovic R. *et al.* (2005) *N Engl J Med* **352**,1779–90) **(c)** JAK2 activation leads to cell survival and proliferation through activation of three major pathways; the STAT transcription factors, the PI3K pathway acting through Akt and Ras activation which subsequently activate ERK and MAPK. The net result is production of a diverse range of proteins that promote cell survival and proliferation. **(d)** A model for the development of myeloproliferative disease following JAK2 mutation. The primary event appears to predispose to an acquired heterozygous mutation of JAK2 (V617F). This leads to a survival advantage. In some patients, a mitotic recombination event leads to a homozygous JAK2 mutation state.

Table 19.1 Radiodilution methods for measuring red cell and plasma volume.

	Normal	Primary or secondary polycythaemia	Relative polycythaemia
Total red cell volume (^{51}Cr)	Men 25–35 mL/kg Women 22–32 mL/kg	Increased	Normal
Total plasma volume (^{125}I-albumin)	40–50 mL/kg	Normal	Decreased

signalling. JAK2 plays a major role in normal myeloid development by transducing signals from diverse cytokines and growth factors including interleukin-3 (IL-3), erythropoietin, granulocyte–macrophage colony-stimulating factor (GM-CSF), granulocyte colony-stimulating factor (G-CSF) and thrombopoietin (Fig. 1.8). Why the same mutation is associated with different myeloproliferative diseases is unclear. The exact cell in which the mutation arises, the genetic background of individual subjects and other factors may be relevant. Chronic myeloid leukaemia, which used to be classified as a myeloproliferative disorder but is now recognized as a separate entity, is discussed in Chapter 13.

Polycythaemia

Polycythaemia (erythrocytosis) is defined as an increase in the haemoglobin concentration above the upper limit of normal for the patient's age and sex.

Classification of polycythaemia

Polycythaemia is classified according to its pathophysiology but the major subdivision is into absolute polycythaemia, in which the red cell mass (volume) is raised, and relative or pseudopolycythaemia in which the red cell volume is normal but the plasma volume is reduced (Table 19.1). Absolute polycythaemia can then be subdivided into primary polycythaemia (PRV) or secondary polycythaemia (Table 19.2).

Table 19.2 Causes of polycythaemia.

Primary
Polycythaemia (rubra) vera
Familial (congenital) polycythaemia

Secondary
Caused by compensatory erythropoietin increase in:
- high altitudes
- pulmonary disease and alveolar hypoventilation (sleep apnoea)
- cardiovascular disease, especially congenital with cyanosis
- increased affinity haemoglobin (familial polycythaemia) (Chapter 19)
- heavy cigarette smoking

Caused by inappropriate erythropoietin increase in:
- renal diseases (e.g. hydronephrosis, vascular impairment, cysts, carcinoma)
- tumours such as uterine leiomyoma, hypernephroma, hepatocellular carcinoma, cerebellar haemangioblastoma

Relative
Stress or pseudopolycythaemia
Cigarette smoking
Dehydration: water deprivation, vomiting
Plasma loss: burns, enteropathy

Polycythaemia (rubra) vera

In PRV, the increase in red cell volume is caused by a clonal malignancy of a marrow stem cell. The disease results from somatic mutation of a single haemopoietic stem cell which gives its progeny a proliferative advantage. The *JAK2* mutation is present in haemopoietic cells in almost 100% of patients. Although the increase in red cells is the diagnostic finding, in many patients there is also an overproduction of granulocytes and platelets.

Chromosome abnormalities (e.g. deletions of 9p or 20q) are found in a minority of subjects.

Diagnosis

Making the diagnosis of PRV in a patient who

Table 19.3 Criteria for diagnosis of polycythaemia (rubra) vera.

Category A
Total red cell mass
male >35 mL/kg
female >32 mL/kg
Arterial oxygen saturation >92%
Splenomegaly
JAK2 mutation
Category B
Platelets $>400 \times 10^9$/L
White cells $>12 \times 10^9$/L
Increased NAP score
Raised serum vitamin B_{12} level

NAP, neutrophil alkaline phosphatase.

presents with polycythaemia can be difficult and the diagnostic criteria of the Polycythaemia Vera Study Group are very valuable (Table 19.3).

Clinical features

This is a disease of older subjects with an equal sex incidence. Clinical features are the result of hyperviscosity, hypervolaemia or hypermetabolism.

1 Headaches, dyspnoea, blurred vision and night sweats. Pruritus, characteristically after a hot bath, can be a severe problem.

2 Plethoric appearance: ruddy cyanosis (Fig. 19.3), conjunctival suffusion and retinal venous engorgement.

3 Splenomegaly in 75% of patients (Fig. 19.4a).

4 Haemorrhage (e.g. gastrointestinal, uterine, cerebral) or thrombosis either arterial (e.g. cardiac, cerebral, peripheral) or venous (e.g. deep or superficial leg veins, cerebral, portal or hepatic veins) are frequent.

5 Hypertension in one-third of patients.

6 Gout (as a result of raised uric acid production; Fig. 19.5a).

7 Peptic ulceration occurs in 5–10% of patients.

Laboratory findings

1 The haemoglobin, haematocrit and red cell count are increased. The total red cell volume (TRCV; Table 19.1) is increased.

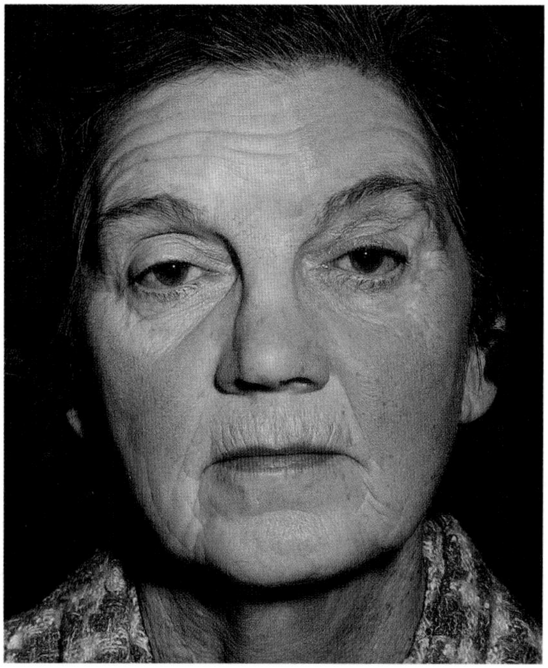

Fig. 19.3 Polycythaemia vera: facial plethora and conjunctival suffusion in a 63-year-old woman. Haemoglobin 18 g/dL; total red cell volume 45 mL/kg.

2 A neutrophil leucocytosis is seen in over half of patients, and some have increased circulating basophils.

3 A raised platelet count is present in about half of patients.

4 The *JAK2* mutation is present in the bone marrow and peripheral blood granulocytes in nearly 100% of patients.

5 The neutrophil alkaline phosphatase (NAP) score is usually increased.

6 Increased serum vitamin B_{12} and vitamin B_{12}-binding capacity because of an increase in haptocorrin.

7 The bone marrow is hypercellular with prominent megakaryocytes, best assessed by a trephine biopsy (Fig. 19.6a).

8 Serum erythropoietin usually low.

9 Expression of PRV-1 (a surface receptor) increased; reduced expression of Mpl (thrombopoietin receptor).

10 Blood viscosity is increased.

11 Plasma urate is often increased; the serum lactate dehydrogenase (LDH) is normal.

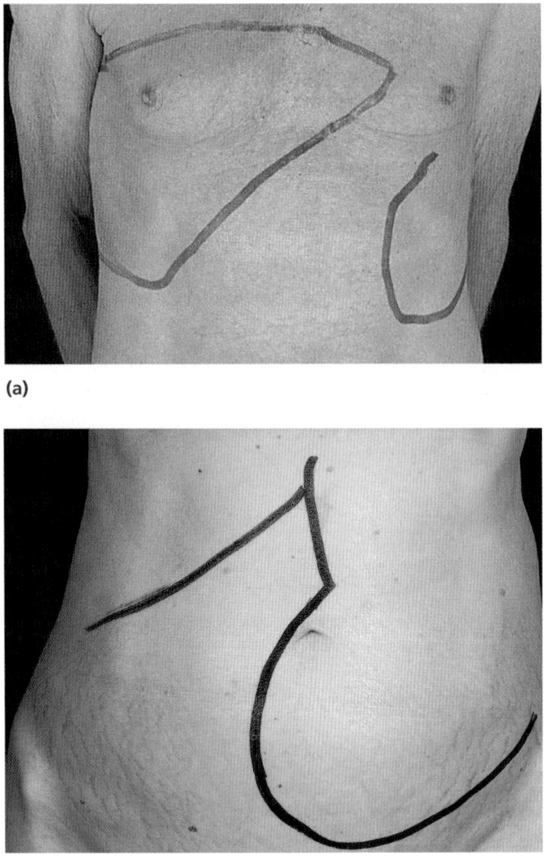

(a)

(b)

Fig. 19.4 Splenomegaly: enlarged spleens in male patients with **(a)** polycythaemia vera and **(b)** myelofibrosis.

12 Circulating erythroid progenitors (erythroid colony-forming unit, CFU_E, and erythroid burst-forming unit, BFU_E; p. 2) are increased compared to normal and grow *in vitro* independently of added erythropoietin (endogenous erythriod colonies).

Treatment

Treatment is aimed at maintaining a normal blood count. The haematocrit should be maintained at about 0.45 and the platelet count below 400×10^9/L.

Venesection

Venesection to reduce the haematocrit to less than 0.45 is particularly useful when a rapid reduction of red cell volume is required (e.g. at the start of therapy). It is especially indicated in younger patients and those with mild disease. The resulting iron deficiency may limit erythropoiesis. Unfortunately, venesection does not control the platelet count.

Cytotoxic myelosuppression

This is considered if there is poor tolerance of venesection, symptomatic or progressive splenomegaly, thrombocytosis, weight loss or night sweats. Daily hydroxycarbamide (hydroxyurea) is valuable in controlling the blood count and may need to be continued for many years (Fig. 19.7). Side-effects of hydroxyurea include myelosuppression, nausea

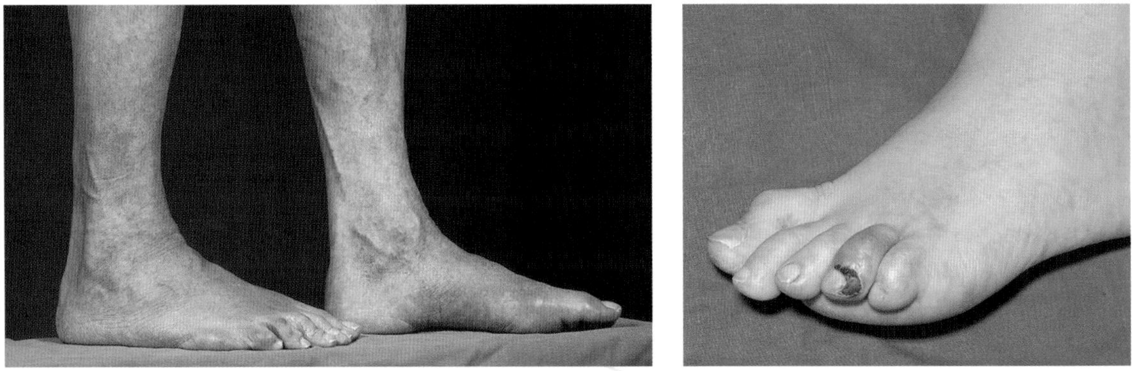

(a) (b)

Fig. 19.5 **(a)** The feet of a 72-year-old man with polycythaemia rubra vera. There is inflammation of the right metatarsophalangeal and other joints caused by uric acid deposits. **(b)** Gangrene of the left fourth toe in essential thrombocythaemia.

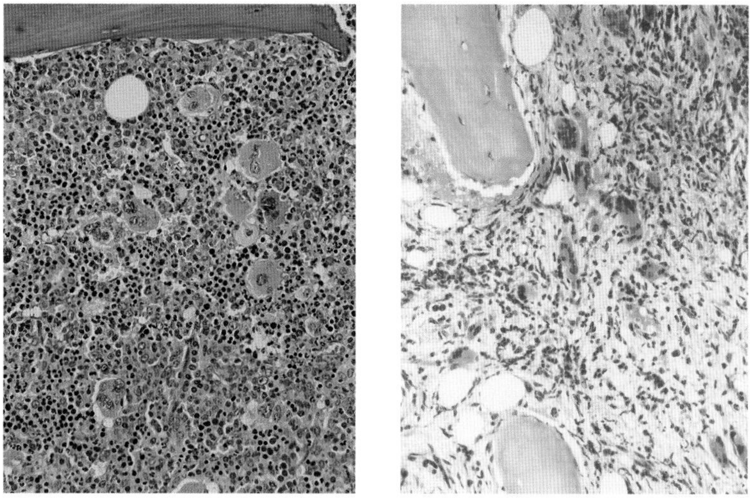

(a) (b)

Fig. 19.6 Iliac crest trephine biopsies. **(a)** Polycythaemia vera: fat spaces are almost completely replaced by hyperplastic haemopoietic tissue. All haemopoietic cell lines are increased with megakaryocytes particularly prominent. **(b)** Myelofibrosis: normal marrow architecture is lost and haemopoietic cells are surrounded by increased fibrous tissue and intercellular substance.

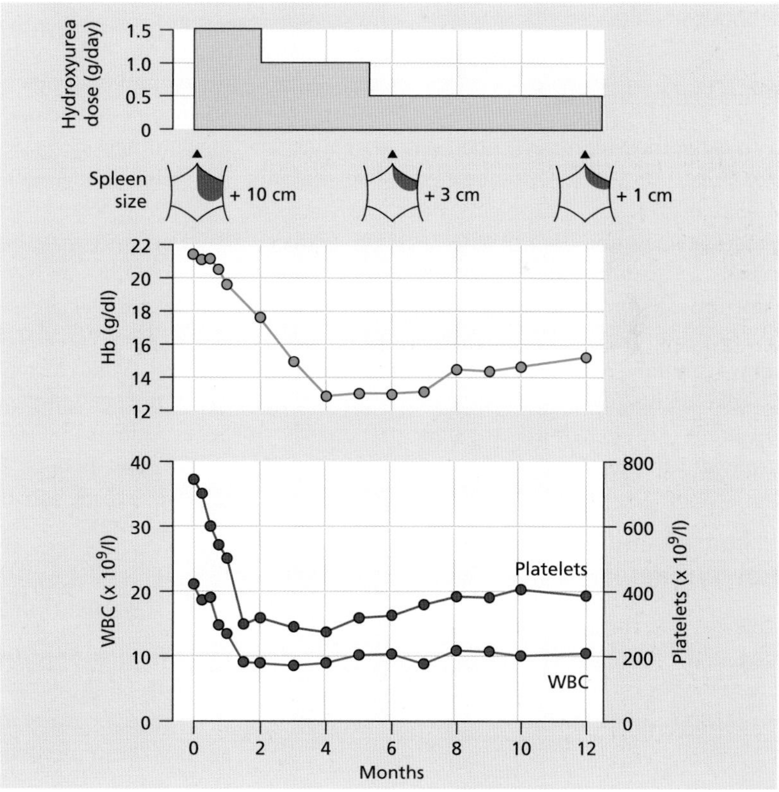

Fig. 19.7 Haematological response to therapy with hydroxyurea in polycythaemia vera. Hb, haemoglobin; WBC, white blood cells.

and skin toxicity. Busulfan, which can be used intermittently, is sometimes used in older patients. Pipobroman is similar to alkyating agents and is used in Europe but not in the UK. The concern with cytotoxic drugs, especially busulfan, is that they may be associated with an increased rate of progression to leukaemia. This risk is low and there may be no increased risk with hydroxyurea.

Phosphorus-32 therapy

This is only used for older patients with severe disease. ^{32}P is a β-emitter, with a half-life of 14.3 days. It is concentrated in bone and is a most effective myelosuppressive agent. The usual remission time after a single dose is 2 years. Concern about late development of leukaemia limits its use.

Interferon

α-Interferon subcutaneously suppresses excess proliferation in the marrow and has produced good haematological responses. It is less convenient than the oral agents and side-effects are frequent. It may be particularly valuable in controlling itching. It is the first-line drug for patients less than 40 years old.

Aspirin

Low-dose aspirin reduces thrombotic complications without an increased risk of major haemorrhage.

Course and prognosis

Typically, the prognosis is good with a median survival of 10–16 years. Thrombosis and haemorrhage are the major clinical problems. Increased viscosity, vascular stasis and high platelet levels may all contribute to thrombosis, whereas defective platelet function may promote haemorrhage.

Transition from PRV to myelofibrosis occurs in approximately 30% of patients and approximately 5% of patients progress to acute leukaemia. ^{32}P and busulfan are generally avoided particularly in younger subjects as they may increase this risk.

Primary familial (congenital) polycythaemia

This is a rare condition. In one type there is a mutation in the von Hippel–Lindau protein gene which creates abnormal oxygen sensing with increased erythropoietin production.

Secondary polycythaemia

The causes of secondary polycythaemia are listed in Table 19.2. Hypoxia caused by chronic obstructive airways disease is one of the most frequent, and measurement of arterial oxygen saturation is a valuable test. Renal and tumour causes of inappropriate erythropoietin secretion are rare. Patients with a high-affinity haemoglobin often have a family history of polycythaemia and present at a young age. Those with cyanotic congenital heart disease should be managed in conjunction with a congenital heart disease unit. Treatment of obesity, hypertension and discontinuation of smoking may lower the haematocrit. These patients are treated by venesection for symptoms such as dizziness, dyspnoea or angina if a raised haematocrit is a contributory factor; also if there has been a previous thrombotic episode. Patients with polycythaemia secondary to hypoxia and pulmonary disease who have symptoms of hyperviscosity or haematocrit of more than 0.56 should have their haematocrit reduced by venesection.

Apparent polycythaemia

Apparent polycythaemia, also known as pseudopolycythaemia, is the result of plasma volume contraction. By definition, the TRCV is normal. The cause is uncertain but it is far more common than PRV. It occurs particularly in young or middle-aged men and may be associated with cardiovascular problems e.g. hypertension (Gaisböck's syndrome) myocardial ischaemia or cerebral transient ischaemic attacks. Diuretic therapy, heavy smoking, obesity and alcohol consumption are frequent associations. Venesection to maintain a haematocrit around 0.45–0.47 is recommended in those with a recent history of thrombosis or with additional risk factors and in all with a haematocrit of more than 0.52.

Differential diagnosis of polycythaemia

A rational approach is needed to evaluate a patient presenting with a high haemoglobin. If PRV is suspected, polymerase chain reaction (PCR) test for the *JAK2* mutation will confirm this in almost all cases. The full blood count, the NAP score, bone marrow aspirate trephine biopsy and ultrasound of the abdomen to assess spleen size and to detect renal abnormalities are the most useful additional tests. Studies with ^{51}Cr-labelled red cells to measure TRCV may be needed if *JAK2* is negative. If absolute polycythaemia is present look for lung or cardiac disease, check arterial Po_2 and consider a check of the oxygen dissociation curve and haemoglobin (Hb) electrophoresis. Finally, look for erythropoietin secreting tumours by ultrasound, computed tomography (CT) or magnetic resonance imaging (MRI). The serum erythropoietin level is also useful in screening for tumours.

Essential thrombocythaemia

In this condition there is a sustained increase in platelet count, because of megakaryocyte proliferation and overproduction of platelets. The haematocrit is normal and the Philadelphia chromosome or *BCR-ABL* rearrangement are absent. The bone marrow shows no collagen fibrosis. A persisting platelet count of >400 × 10^9/L is the central diagnostic feature but other causes of a raised platelet count (particularly iron-deficiency, inflammatory or malignant disorder and myelodysplasia) need to be fully excluded before the diagnosis can be made. Half of patients show the *JAK2* (Val617Phe) mutation and these cases tend to resemble more closely polycythaemia vera with higher haemoglobin and white cell counts and splenomegaly than *JAK2* negative cases. There is endogenous megakaryocyte and possibly erythroid colony growth independent of thrombopoietin or erythropoietin. Rare primary familial cases in children have been associated with mutations on the genes for thrombopoietin or its receptor *c*-Mpl.

Clinical and laboratory findings

The dominant clinical features are thrombosis and haemorrhage. Many cases are symptomless and diagnosed on routine blood counts. Thrombosis may occur in the venous or arterial systems (Fig. 19.5b) whereas haemorrhage, as a result of abnormal platelet function, may cause either chronic or acute bleeding. A characteristic symptom is erythromelalgia, a burning sensation felt in the hands or feet and promptly relieved by aspirin. Up to 40% of patients will have palpable splenomegaly whereas in others there may be splenic atrophy because of infarction. Abnormal large platelets and megakaryocyte fragments may be seen on the blood film (Fig. 19.8). The bone marrow is similar to that in PRV but an excess of abnormal megakaryocytes is typical. Cytogenetics and molecular analysis for the *BCR-ABL* fusion gene are analysed to exclude chronic myeloid leukaemia. The condition must be distinguished from other causes of a raised platelet count (Table 19.4). Platelet function tests (p. 277) are consistently abnormal, failure of aggregation with adrenaline being particularly characteristic.

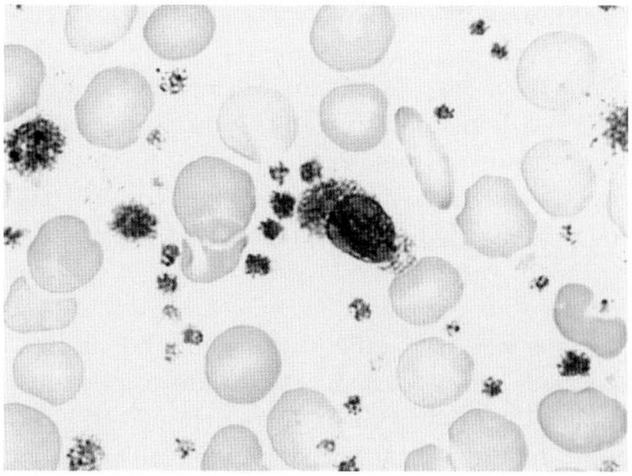

Fig. 19.8 Peripheral blood film in essential thrombocythaemia showing increased numbers of platelets and a nucleated megakaryocytic fragment.

Table 19.4 Causes of a raised platelet count.

Reactive
Haemorrhage, trauma, postoperative
Chronic iron deficiency
Malignancy
Chronic infections
Connective tissue diseases (e.g. rheumatoid arthritis)
Post-splenectomy
Endogenous
Essential thrombocythaemia (*JAK2* mutation + or –)
In some cases of polycythaemia vera, myelofibrosis and chronic myeloid leukaemia

Treatment

The principle is to control the platelet count so as to reduce the risk of thrombosis which is the major clinical problem. The patients most at risk are those over 60 years old, with a platelet count

>1000 × 10^9/L and with previous episodes of thrombosis or haemorrhage. The thrombotic risk depends on other risk factors such as smoking history and hypertension, and the treatment should take account of these risks. In those with a high risk the aim is to keep the platelet count below 600 × 10^9/L. Hydroxyurea is the most widely used treatment. α-Interferon is also valuable in younger patients but has more side-effects. Anagrelide is effective in reducing the platelet count but also has more side-effects, particularly on the cardiovascular system, than hydroxyurea. A possible increased risk of myelofibrosis is also of concern. Busulfan and ^{32}P were used but are not now favoured because of possible long-term complications. Platelet pheresis may be helpful in short-term management. Aspirin is commonly used to reduce thrombotic risk and in patients younger than 60 years with no previous thrombosis or haemorrhage, and platelets <1000 × 10^9/L, it may be the treatment of choice.

Course

Often the disease is stationary for 10–20 years or more. The disease may transform after a number of years to myelofibrosis; the risk of transformation to acute leukaemia is relatively low (<5%). Patients have been stratified as low risk if less than 40 years old, with no previous thrombosis, hypertension or diabetes and platelets <1000–1500 × 10^9/L and are treated with aspirin alone; intermediate risk if less than 60 years with no prior thrombosis, hypertension or diabetes and platelets <1000–1500 × 10^9/L; or high risk if over 60 years or with prior thrombosis or haemorrhage, hypertension or diabetes, platelet count >1000 × 10^9/L. High-risk patients receive hydroxyurea and aspirin. For intermediate risk, trials of aspirin versus hydroxyurea and aspirin are in progress.

Myelofibrosis

Confusingly, the condition has many names: idiopathic myelofibrosis; myelosclerosis; agnogenic myeloid metaplasia; or myelofibrosis with myeloid metaplasia (MMM).

The predominant feature of myelofibrosis is a progressive generalized reactive fibrosis of the bone marrow in association with the development of haemopoiesis in the spleen and liver (known as myeloid metaplasia). Clinically this leads to anaemia and massive hepatosplenomegaly. In some patients there is osteosclerosis. Myelofibrosis is a clonal stem cell disease. The fibrosis of the bone marrow is secondary to hyperplasia of abnormal megakaryocytes. It is thought that fibroblasts are stimulated by platelet-derived growth factor and other cytokines secreted by megakaryocytes and platelets. The *JAK2* mutation occurs in approximately 50% of patients. The absence of the mutation in many patients shows genetic heterogeneity in myelofibrosis as in ET. Non-specific cytogenetic abnormalities may be found in approximately half the patients.

One-third or more of the patients have a previous history of PRV and some patients present with clinical and laboratory features of both disorders.

Clinical features

1 An insidious onset in older people is usual with symptoms of anaemia.
2 Symptoms resulting from massive splenomegaly (e.g. abdominal discomfort, pain or indigestion) are frequent; splenomegaly is the main physical finding (Fig. 19.4b).
3 Hypermetabolic symptoms such as loss of weight, anorexia, fever and night sweats are common.
4 Bleeding problems, bone pain or gout occur in a minority of patients.

Myelofibrosis and chronic myeloid leukaemia are responsible for most cases of massive (>20 cm) splenic enlargement in the UK and North America (see Table 9.1).

Laboratory findings

1 Anaemia is usual but a normal or increased haemoglobin level may be found in some patients.
2 The white cell and platelet counts are frequently high at the time of presentation. Later in the disease leucopenia and thrombocytopenia are common.
3 A leucoerythroblastic blood film is found. The red cells show characteristic 'tear-drop' poikilocytes (Fig. 19.9).
4 Bone marrow is usually unobtainable by aspiration. Trephine biopsy (Fig. 19.6b) shows a fibrotic

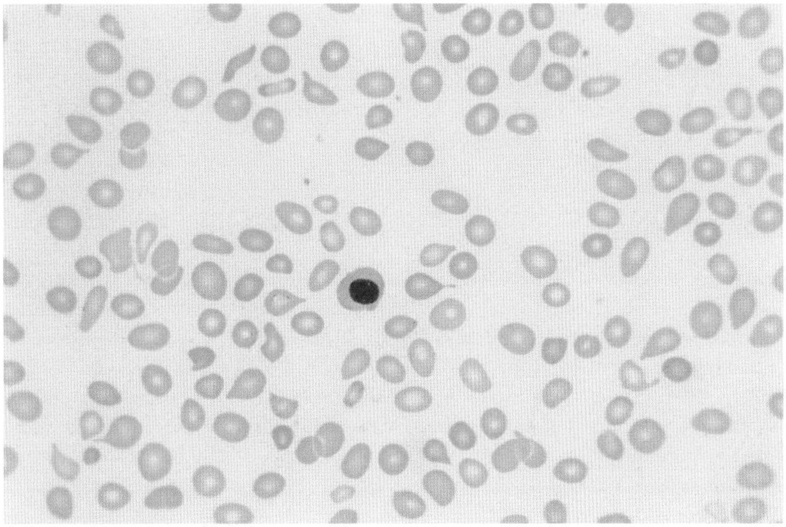

Fig. 19.9 Peripheral blood film in myelofibrosis. Leucoerythroblastic change with 'tear-drop' cells and an erythroblast.

hypercellular marrow. Increased megakaryocytes are frequently seen. In 10% of cases there is increased bone formation with increased bone density on X-ray.

5 *JAK2* kinase is mutated in approximately 50% of cases.

6 NAP score is usually increased.

7 High serum urate and LDH levels reflect the increased but largely ineffective turnover of haemopoietic cells.

8 Transformation to acute myeloid leukaemia occurs in 10–20% of patients.

Treatment

This is usually palliative and aimed at reducing the effects of anaemia and splenomegaly. Blood transfusions and regular folic acid therapy are used in severely anaemic patients. Hydroxyurea may help to reduce splenomegaly and hypermetabolic symptoms. Trials of thalidomide, cyclophosphamide or etanercept (anti-TNFα) are in progress. Danazol, an androgen derivative may improve anaemia in approximately 30% of patients. Erythropoietin may also be tried. Splenectomy is considered for patients with severe symptomatic splenomegaly—mechanical discomfort, thrombocytopenia, portal hypertension, excessive transfusion requirements or hypermetabolic symptoms. Splenic irradiation is an alternative but usually provides relief only for 3–6 months. Allopurinol is indicated in virtually all patients to prevent gout and urate nephropathy from hyperuricaemia. Allogeneic stem cell transplantation may be curative for young patients.

The median survival is approximately 3.5 years and causes of death include heart failure, infection and leukaemic transformation. A haemoglobin level of less than 10 g/dL, a white cell count of less than 4 or greater than 30×10^9/L and the presence of abnormal chromosomes are associated with a worse prognosis.

Systemic mastocytosis

Mast cells are derived from haemopoietic stem cells. Mature cells survive for months or years in vascular tissues and most organs. Systemic mastocytosis is a clonal myeloproliferative disorder involving usually the bone marrow, heart, spleen, lymph nodes and skin.

The somatic *c*-kit mutation Asp816Val is detected in the majority of patients and may be partly responsible for autonomous growth and enhanced survival of the neoplastic mast cells. In many patients this mutation is also detected in other haemopoietic cells.

Symptoms are related to histamine and prostaglandin release and include flushing, pruritus, abdominal pain and bronchospasm. The skin usually shows urticaria pigmentosa.

In many patients the disease runs a chronic indolent course. In others an aggressive course may be associated with acute myeloid leukaemia, mast cell leukaemia or other haemopoietic proliferative or dysplastic conditions (see Appendix 3).

Bibliography

Baxter E.J., Scott L.M., Campbell P.J. *et al.* (2005) Acquired mutation of the tyrosine kinase JAK2 in human myeloproliferative disorders. *Lancet* **365**,1054–61. Erratum in: *Lancet* **366**,122.

Bellané-Chantelot C., Chaumarel I., Labopin M. *et al.* (2006) Genetic and clinical implications of the Val617Phe JAK2 mutation in 72 families with myeloproliferative diseases. *Blood* **108**,346–52.

Cross N.C. and Reiter A. (2002) Tyrosine kinase fusion genes in chronic myeloproliferative diseases. *Leukemia* **16**,1207–12.

Finazzi G., Caruso V., Marchioli R. *et al.* (2005) Acute leukemia in polycythemia vera: an analysis of 1638 patients enrolled in a prospective observational study. *Blood* **105**,2664–70.

Harrison C.N., Campbell P.J., Buck G. *et al.* (2005) Hydroxyurea compared with anagrelide in high-risk essential thrombocythemia. *N Engl J Med* **353**,33–45.

Harrison C.N., Gale R.E., Machin S.J., Linch D.C. (1999) A large proportion of patients with a diagnosis of essential thrombocythemia do not have a clonal disorder and may be at lower risk of thrombotic complications. *Blood* **93**,417–24.

James C., Ugo V., Le Couedic J.P. *et al.* (2005) A unique clonal JAK2 mutation leading to constitutive signalling causes polycythaemia vera. *Nature* **434**,1144–8.

Jones A.V., Kreil S., Zoi K. *et al.* (2005) Widespread occurrence of the JAK2 V617F mutation in chronic myeloproliferative disorders. *Blood* **106**,2162–8.

Kaushansky K. (2005) On the molecular origins of the chronic myeloproliferative disorders: it all makes sense. *Blood* **105**,4187–90.

Kralovics R. and Skoda R.C. (2005) Molecular pathogenesis of Philadelphia chromosome negative myeloproliferative disorders. *Blood Rev* **19**,1–13.

Kralovics R., Passamonti F., Buser A.S. *et al.* (2005) A gain-of-function mutation of JAK2 in myeloproliferative disorders. *N Engl J Med* **352**,1779–90.

Levine R.L., Wadleigh M., Cools J. *et al.* (2005) Activating mutation in the tyrosine kinase JAK2 in polycythemia vera, essential thrombocythemia, and myeloid metaplasia with myelofibrosis. *Cancer Cell* **7**,387–97.

Sandberg E.M., Wallace T.A., Godney M.D., Vonderlinden D., Sayeski P.P. (2004) Jak2 tyrosine kinase: a true jak of all trades? *Cell Biochem Biophys* **41**,207–32.

Schafer A.I. (2006) Molecular basis of the diagnosis and treatment of polycythemia vera and essential thrombocythemia. *Blood* **107**,4214–22.

Tefferi A., Lasho T.L, Wolanskyj A.P., Mesa R.A. (2004) Neutrophil PRV-1 expression across the chronic myeloproliferative disorders and in secondary or spurious polycythemia. *Blood* **103**,3547–8.

Tefferi A., Mesa R.A., Nagorney D.M. *et al.* (2000) Splenectomy in myelofibrosis with myeloid metaplasia: a single institution experience with 223 patients. *Blood* **95**,2226–33.

CHAPTER 20

20 Aplastic anaemia and bone marrow failure

Pancytopenia

Pancytopenia describes a reduction in the blood count of all the major cell lines—red cells, white cells and platelets. It has several causes (Table 20.1) which can be broadly divided into decreased bone marrow production or increased peripheral destruction.

Aplastic anaemia

Aplastic (hypoplastic) anaemia is defined as pancytopenia resulting from aplasia of the bone marrow. It is classified into primary (congenital or acquired) or secondary types (Table 20.2).

Pathogenesis

The underlying defect in all cases appears to be a substantial reduction in the number of haemopoietic pluripotential stem cells, and a fault in the remaining stem cells or an immune reaction against them, which makes them unable to divide and differentiate sufficiently to populate the bone marrow (Fig. 20.1). A primary fault in the marrow microenvironment has also been suggested but the success of stem cell transplantation (SCT) shows this can only be a rare cause because normal donor stem cells are usually able to thrive in the recipient's marrow cavity.

Table 20.1 Causes of pancytopenia.

Decreased bone marrow function
Aplasia
Acute leukaemia, myelodysplasia, myeloma
Infiltration with lymphoma, solid tumours, tuberculosis
Megaloblastic anaemia
Paroxysmal nocturnal haemoglobinuria
Myelofibrosis
Haemophagocytic syndrome
Increased peripheral destruction
Splenomegaly

Congenital

The Fanconi type has an autosomal recessive pattern of inheritance and is often associated with growth retardation and congenital defects of the skeleton (e.g. microcephaly, absent radii or thumbs), of the renal tract (e.g. pelvic or horseshoe kidney) (Fig. 20.2) or skin (areas of hyper- and hypopigmentation); sometimes there is mental retardation. The syndrome is genetically heterogeneous with eight different complementation groups termed A, B, C, D1, D2, E, F and G. The *FAND1* gene is identical to *BRCA2*, the breast cancer susceptibility gene. The encoded proteins cooperate in a common cellular pathway involved in DNA repair. Cells from Fanconi's anaemia (FA) patients show an abnormally high frequency of spontaneous chromosomal breakage and the diagnostic test is elevated breakage after incubation of peripheral blood lymphocytes

Table 20.2 Causes of aplastic anaemia.

Primary	Secondary
Congenital (Fanconi and non-Fanconi types) Idiopathic acquired	**Ionizing radiation**: accidental exposure (radiotherapy, radioactive isotopes, nuclear power stations) **Chemicals**: benzene, organophosphates and other organic solvents, DDT and other pesticides, organochlorines, recreational drugs (ecstasy)
	Drugs Those that regularly cause marrow depression (e.g. busulfan, cyclophosphamide, anthracyclines, nitrosoureas) Those that occasionally or rarely cause marrow depression (e.g. chloramphenicol, sulphonamides, gold, anti-inflammatory, antithyroid, psychotrophic, anticonvulsant/antidepressant drugs)
	Viruses: viral hepatitis (non-A, non-B, non-C, non-G in most cases), EBV

EBV, Epstein–Barr virus.

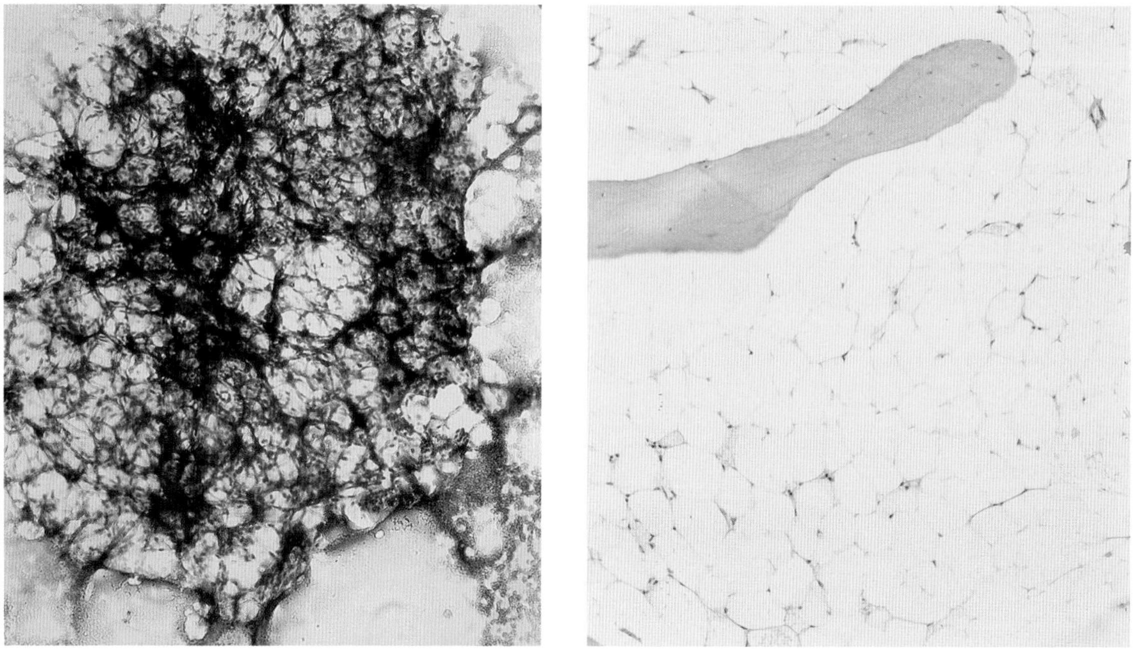

(a) (b)

Fig. 20.1 Aplastic anaemia: low power views of bone marrow show severe reduction of haemopoietic cells with an increase in fat spaces. **(a)** Aspirated fragment. **(b)** Trephine biopsy.

with the DNA cross-linking agent diepoxybutane (DEB test). Dyskeratosis congenita is a rare sex-linked disorder with nail and skin atrophy and is associated with mutations in the *DKC1* (dyskerin) or *TERC* (telomerase reverse transcriptase RNA template) genes which are both involved in the maintenance of telomere length.

The usual age of presentation of FA is 5–10 years.

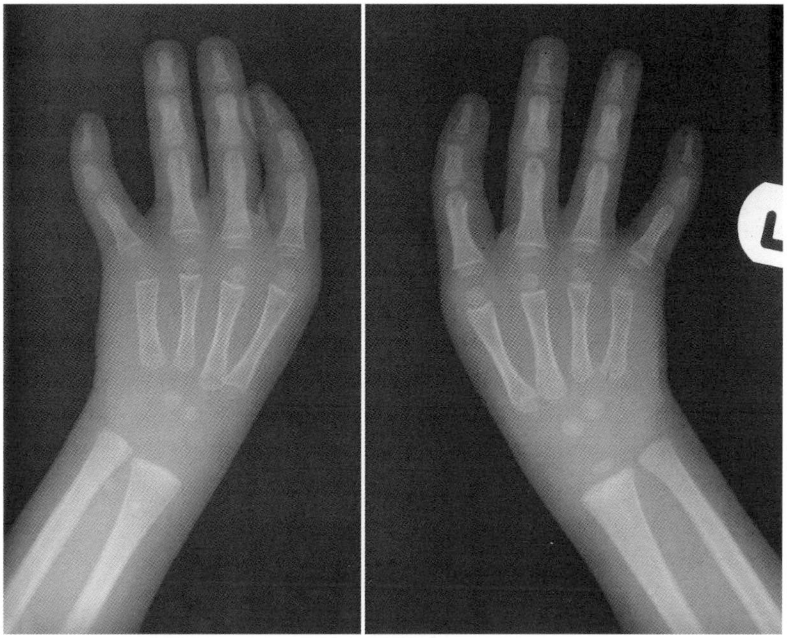

(a)

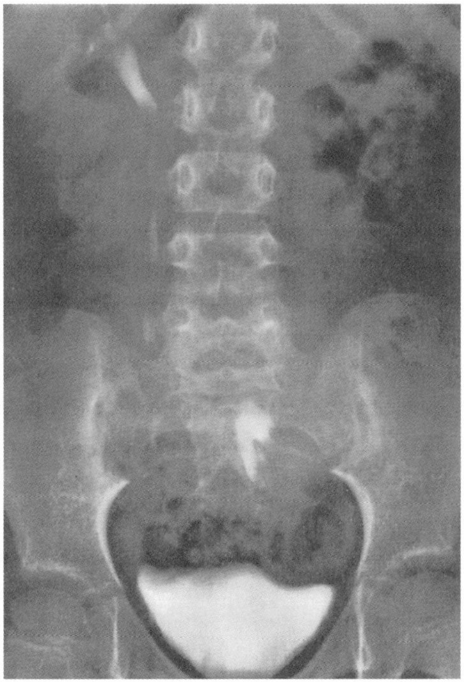

(b)

Fig. 20.2 **(a)** X-rays showing absent thumbs in a patient with Fanconi's anaemia (FA). **(b)** Intravenous pyelogram in a patient with FA showing a normal right kidney but a left kidney abnormally placed in the pelvis.

Approximately 10% of cases develop acute myeloid leukaemia. Treatment is usually with androgens and/or SCT. The blood count usually improves with androgens but side-effects, especially in children, are distressing (virilization and liver abnormalities); remission rarely lasts more than 2 years. SCT may cure the patient. Because of the sensitivity of the patient's cells to DNA damage, conditioning regimes are mild.

Idiopathic acquired

This is the most common type of aplastic anaemia, accounting for at least two-thirds of acquired cases. In most cases haemopoetic tissue is the target of an immune process dominated by oligoclonal expression of cytotoxic T cells which secrete γ-interferon and tumour necrosis factor. In approximately one-third of cases short telomeres are found in leucocytes, especially in those with a prolonged clinical course. Mutations in the telomere repair complex have been described but their relevance is unclear. The favourable responses to antilymphocyte globulin (ALG) and ciclosporin support the concept that autoimmune T-cell mediated damage, possibly against functionally and structurally altered stem cells, is important.

Secondary

This is often caused by direct damage to the haemopoietic marrow by radiation or cytotoxic drugs. The antimetabolite drugs (e.g. methotrexate) and mitotic inhibitors (e.g. daunorubicin) cause only temporary aplasia but the alkylating agents, particularly busulfan, may cause chronic aplasia closely resembling the chronic idiopathic disease. Some individuals develop aplastic anaemia as a rare idiosyncratic side-effect of drugs such as chloramphenicol or gold which are not known to be cytotoxic (Table 20.2). They may also develop the disease during or within a few months of viral hepatitis (rarely hepatitis A, B or C, but more frequently non-A, non-B, non-C). Because the incidence of marrow toxicity is particularly high for chloramphenicol, this drug should be reserved for treatment of those infections that are life-threatening and for which it is the optimum antibiotic (e.g. typhoid). Chemicals such as benzene may be implicated and rarely aplastic anaemia may be the presenting feature of acute lymphoblastic or myeloid leukaemia, especially in childhood. Myelodysplasia (Chapter 14) may also present with a hypoplastic marrow.

Clinical features

The onset is at any age with a peak incidence around 30 years and a slight male predominance; it can be insidious or acute with symptoms and signs resulting from anaemia, neutropenia or thrombocytopenia. Infections, particularly of the mouth and throat, are common and generalized infections are frequently life-threatening; bruising, bleeding gums, epistaxes and menorrhagia are the most frequent haemorrhagic manifestations and the usual presenting features, often with symptoms of anaemia. The lymph nodes, liver and spleen are not enlarged.

Laboratory findings

1 Anaemia is normochromic, normocytic or macrocytic (mean cell volume (MCV) often 95–110 fL). The reticulocyte count is usually extremely low in relation to the degree of anaemia.

2 Leucopenia. There is a selective fall in granulocytes, usually but not always to below 1.5×10^9/L. In severe cases, the lymphocyte count is also low. The neutrophils appear normal.

3 Thrombocytopenia is always present and, in severe cases, is less than 20×10^9/L.

4 There are no abnormal cells in the peripheral blood.

5 The bone marrow shows hypoplasia, with loss of haemopoietic tissue and replacement by fat which comprises over 75% of the marrow. Trephine biopsy is essential and may show patchy cellular areas in a hypocellular background (Fig. 20.1b). The main cells present are lymphocytes and plasma cells; megakaryocytes in particular are severely reduced or absent.

Severe cases show neutrophils $<0.5 \times 10^9$/L (very severe $<0.2 \times 10^9$/L), platelets $<20 \times 10^9$/L, reticulocytes $<20 \times 10^9$/L and marrow cellularity <25%.

Diagnosis

The disease must be distinguished from other causes of pancytopenia (Table 20.1) and this is not usually difficult provided an adequate bone marrow sample is obtained. Cytogenetic analysis should be performed. Paroxysmal nocturnal haemoglobinuria (PNH) must be excluded by flow-cytometry testing of red cells for CD55 and CD59. In older patients, hypoplastic myelodysplasia may show similar appearances. Qualitative abnormalities of the cells and clonal cytogenetic changes suggest myelodysplasia rather than aplastic anaemia. Some patients diagnosed as having aplastic anaemia develop PNH, myelodysplasia or acute myeloid leukaemia in subsequent years. This may occur even in patients who have responded well to immunosuppressive therapy.

Treatment

General

The cause, if known, is removed (e.g. radiation or drug therapy is discontinued). Initial management consists largely of supportive care with blood transfusions, platelet concentrates, and treatment and prevention of infection. All blood products should be filtered to reduce the risk of alloimmunization and irradiated to prevent grafting of live donor lymphocytes. In severely thrombocytopenic (platelet count $<10 \times 10^9$/L) and neutropenic (neutrophils $<0.5 \times 10^9$/L) patients, management is similar to the supportive care of patients receiving intensive chemotherapy with reverse barrier isolation. An antifibrinolytic agent (e.g. tranexamic acid) may be used in patients with severe prolonged thrombocytopenia. Oral antifungal agents and oral antibiotics are used prophylactically in some units to reduce the incidence of infection.

Specific

This must be tailored to the severity of the illness as well as the age of the patient and potential sibling stem cell donors. Severity is assessed by the reticulocyte, neutrophil and platelet counts and degree of marrow hypoplasia. Severe cases have a high mortality in the first 6–12 months unless they respond to specific therapy. Less severe cases may have an acute transient course or a chronic course with ultimate recovery, although the platelet count often remains subnormal for many years. Relapses, sometimes severe and occasionally fatal, may also occur and rarely the disease transforms into myelodysplasia, acute leukaemia or PNH (Chapter 5).

The following 'specific' treatments are used with varying success.

1 ***Antilymphocyte or antithymocyte globulin*** (ALG or ATG) This is prepared in animals (e.g. horse or rabbit) and is of benefit in approximately 50–60% of acquired cases. It is usually given with corticosteroids which also reduce the side-effects of ALG including the serum sickness of fever, rash and joint pains which may occur approximately 7 days after administration. Corticosteroids should not be used alone as they increase the risk of infection. Typically, if there is no response to ALG after 4 months a second course may be tried, prepared from another species. Overall, up to 80% of patients respond to combined ALG, steroids and ciclosporin.

2 ***Ciclosporin*** This is an effective agent which appears particularly valuable in combination with ALG and steroids.

3 ***Androgens*** These are beneficial in some patients with FA and acquired aplastic anaemia although an overall improved survival in acquired aplastic anaemia has not been proven. Oxymetholone is usually tried but side-effects are marked including virilization, salt retention and liver damage with cholestatic jaundice or rarely hepatocellular carcinoma. If there is no response in 4–6 months, androgens should be stopped. If there is a response the drug should be withdrawn gradually.

4 ***Stem cell transplantation*** Allogeneic transplantation offers the chance of permanent cure. For aplastic anaemia conditioning is with cyclophosphamide without irradiation but with ciclosporin which reduces the risks of graft failure and (with methotrexate) of graft-versus-host disease. The relative role of SCT versus immunosuppressive therapy in individual patients with aplastic anaemia is under constant review. In general terms, SCT is favoured in younger patients with severe aplastic anaemia and a human leucocyte antigen (HLA) matching sibling donor. Cure rates of up to 80% are obtained. However, non-myeloablative transplants (p. 262) are used in selected patients over the age of 40 years. SCT using unrelated volunteer donors and mismatched family members is achieving a survival ratio over 50% in patients with severe aplastic anaemia. In older subjects and those with less severe disease, immunosuppression is usually tried first.

5 *Haemopoietic growth factors* Granulocyte colony-stimulating factor (G-CSF) may produce minor responses but does not lead to sustained improvement. Other growth factors have not proved helpful.

Red cell aplasia

Chronic form

This is a rare syndrome characterized by anaemia with normal leucocytes and platelets and grossly reduced or absent erythroblasts in the marrow (Fig. 20.3). The congenital form is known as Diamond–Blackfan syndrome (Table 20.3) and is inherited as a recessive condition. It is associated with a varying number of somatic disorders (e.g. of the face or heart). Mutation of a gene on chromosome 19 that encodes a ribosomal protein underlies some cases. Corticosteriods are the first line of treatment and SCT may be curative. Androgens may also produce improvement but side-effects on growth can be severe.

The acquired chronic form can occur without any obvious associated disease or precipitating factor (idiopathic), or may be seen with autoimmune diseases (especially systemic lupus erythematosus), with a thymoma, lymphoma or chronic lymphocytic leukaemia. Red cell aplasia from anti-erythropoietin antibodies has been rarely described in patients with chronic renal failure receiving recombinant erythropoietin. In some cases, immunosuppression with corticosteroids, ciclosporin, azathioprine or ALG is helpful. Monoclonal antibodies (e.g. Campath (anti-CD52) or rituximab (anti-CD20)) are being increasingly used in treatment of refractory acquired red cell aplasia and other autoimmune cytopenias.

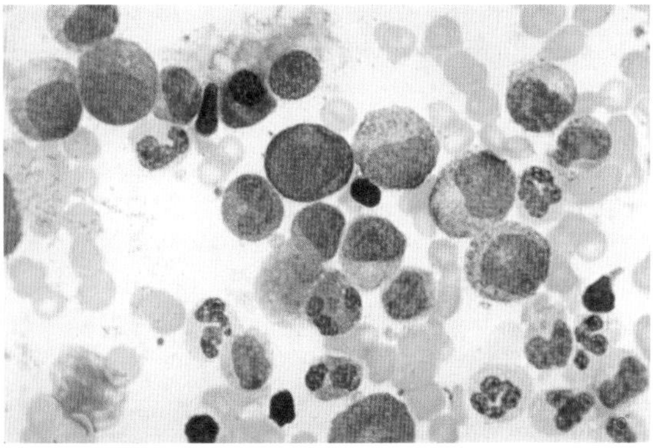

Fig. 20.3 The bone marrow in primary red cell aplasia. There is selective loss of erythropoiesis.

If regular blood transfusions are needed, iron chelation therapy will also be necessary. SCT has been carried out in some severe cases.

Transient form

Parvovirus B19 infects red cell precursors via the P antigen and causes a transient (5–10 days) red cell aplasia with the rapid onset of severe anaemia in patients with pre-existing shortened red cell survival (e.g. sickle cell disease or hereditary spherocytosis; Fig. 20.4). Transient red cell aplasia with anaemia may also occur in association with drug therapy (Table 20.3), and in normal infants or children, often with a history of a viral infection in the preceding 3 months.

Schwachman–Diamond syndrome

This is a rare autosomal recessive syndrome characterized by varying degrees of cytopenia, especially neutropenia with a propensity to transform to myelodysplasia or acute myeloid leukaemia. Exocrine pancreatic dysfunction is an invariable feature while skeletal abnormalities, hepatic impairment and short stature are frequent.

Congenital dyserythropoietic anaemia

Congenital dyserythropoietic anaemias (CDAs) are a group of hereditary refractory anaemias characterized by ineffective erythropoiesis and erythroblast multinuclearity. The patient may be jaundiced with bone marrow expansion. The white cell and platelet counts are normal. The reticulocyte count is low for the degree of anaemia, despite increased marrow cellularity. The anaemia is of variable severity and is usually first noted in infancy or childhood. Iron overload may develop and splenomegaly is common. The CDAs have been classified into four types based on the degree to which megaloblastic changes, giant erythroblasts and dyserythropoietic changes

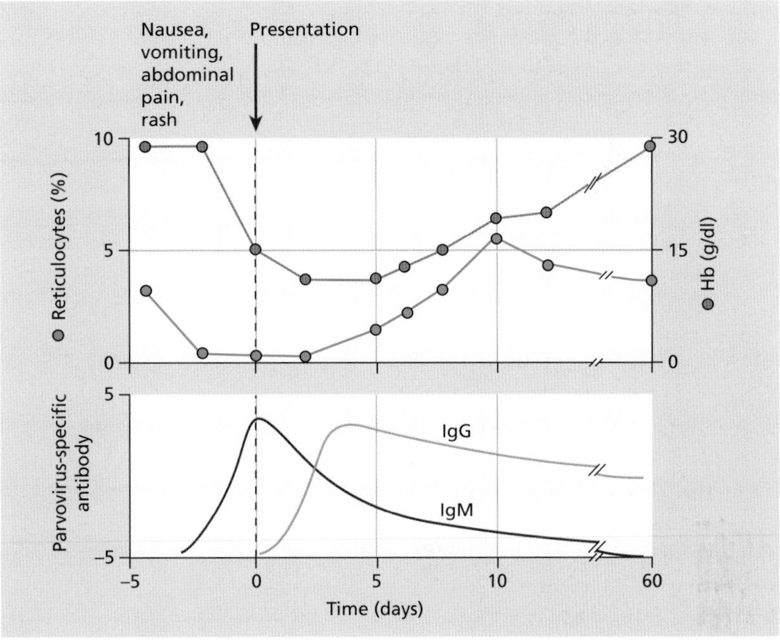

Fig. 20.4 Parvovirus infection: flow chart showing transient fall in haemoglobin and reticulocytes in a patient with hereditary spherocytosis.

Table 20.3 Classification of pure red cell aplasia.

Acute, transient	Chronic Congenital	Chronic Acquired
Parvovirus infection Infancy and childhood Drugs (e.g. azathioprine, co-trimoxazole)	Diamond–Blackfan syndrome	Idiopathic Associated with thymoma, systemic lupus erythematosus, rheumatoid arthritis, lymphoma, chronic lymphocytic leukaemia, T-large granular lymphocytosis, myelodysplasia, viral infection, drugs

are present. Type II is known as HEMPAS (hereditary erythroblast multinuclearity with a positive acidified serum lysis test) with some sera but not the patient's serum. The basic lesion in HEMPAS is a genetic defect in one of two enzymes, *N*-acetylglucosaminyltransferase or α-mannosidase, which are involved in glycosylation of several red cell membrane proteins. α-Interferon has induced remission in some cases.

Bibliography

Dokal I. (2003) Inherited aplastic anaemia. *Hematol J* **4**,3–9.

Dror Y. and Freedman M.H. (2002) Shwachman–Diamond syndrome. *Br J Haematol* **118**,701–13.

Frickhofen N., Heimpel H., Kaltwasser J.P., Schrezenmeier H. for the German Aplastic Anemia Study Group. (2003) Antithymocyte globulin with or without cyclosporin A: 11-year follow-up of a randomized trial comparing treatments of aplastic anemia. *Blood* **101**,1236–42.

Issaragrisil S., Kaufman D.W., Anderson T. *et al*. (2006) The epidemiology of aplastic anemia in Thailand. *Blood* **107**,1299–307.

Joenje H. and Patel K.J. (2001) The emerging genetic and molecular basis of Fanconi anaemia. *Nat Rev Genet* **2**,446–57.

Locasciulli A., Bruno B., Rambaldi A. *et al*. GITMO Prospective Randomized Study Group (2004) Treatment of severe aplastic anemia with antilymphocyte globulin, cyclosporine and two different granulocyte colony-stimulating factor regimens: a GITMO prospective randomized study. *Haematologica* **89**,1054–61.

Marsh J.C. (2005) Management of acquired aplastic anaemia. *Blood Rev* **19**,143–51.

Marsh J.C., Ball S.E., Gordon-Smith E.C. *et al*. for the British

Committee for Standards in Haematology (2003) Guidelines for the diagnosis and management of acquired aplastic anaemia. *Br J Haematol* **123**,782–801.

Muir K.R., Chilvers C.E., Harriss C. *et al.* (2003) The role of occupational and environmental exposures in the aetiology of acquired severe aplastic anaemia: a case–control investigation. *Br J Haematol* **123**,906–14.

Robak T. (2004) Monoclonal antibodies in the treatment of autoimmune cytopenias. *Eur J Haematol* **72**,79–88.

Taniguchi T. and D'Andrea A.D. (2006) Molecular pathogenesis of Fanconi anemia: recent progress. *Blood* **107**,4223–33.

Vulliamy T., Marrone A., Dokal I., Mason P.J. (2002) Association between aplastic anaemia and mutations in telomerase RNA. *Lancet* **359**,2168–70.

Yamaguchi H., Calado R.T., Ly H. *et al.* (2005) Mutations in TERT, the gene for telomerase reverse transcriptase, in aplastic anemia. *N Engl J Med* **352**,1413–24.

Young, N.S. and Brown K.E. (2004) Parvovirus B19. *N Engl J Med* **350**,586–97.

CHAPTER 21

21 Stem cell transplantation

Principles of stem cell transplantation

Stem cell transplantation (SCT) involves eliminating a patient's haemopoietic and immune system by chemotherapy and/or radiotherapy and replacing it with stem cells either from another individual or with a previously harvested portion of the patient's own haemopoietic stem cells (Fig. 21.1). The term encompasses both ***bone marrow transplantation*** (BMT), in which stem cells are collected from bone marrow, and ***peripheral blood stem cell*** (PBSC) ***transplantation*** in which stem cells are collected from peripheral blood.

SCT may be ***syngeneic*** (from an identical twin), ***allogeneic*** (from another person) or ***autologous*** (from the patient's own stem cells) (Table 21.1).

The principal diseases for which SCT is performed are listed in Table 21.2. However, the exact role of SCT in the management of each disease is complex and depends on factors such as disease severity and subtype, remission status, age and, for allogeneic transplantation, availability of donors.

Collection of stem cells

Stem cells can be collected from bone marrow or from peripheral blood.

Bone marrow collection

The donor is given a general anaesthetic and 500–1200 mL of marrow is harvested from the pelvis. The marrow is heparinized and a mononuclear cell count is taken to assess the yield, which should be approximately $2–4 \times 10^8$ nucleated cells/kg body weight of the recipient.

Peripheral blood stem cell collection

PBSCs are taken using a cell-separator machine connected to the patient or donor via peripheral cannulae (Fig. 21.2). Blood is taken through one cannula and pumped around the machine where mononuclear cells are collected by centrifugation before the red cells are returned to the patient. This continuous process may take a few hours before enough mononuclear cells are collected.

Peripheral blood normally contains too few haemopoietic stem cells to allow collection of sufficient numbers for transplantation. Chemotherapy and growth factors can each increase the number by around 100 times. In future it is possible that stem cell populations may also be expanded *in vitro*.

Chemotherapy is used in patients undergoing autologous stem cell collection but not in healthy donors. PBSCs are usually collected during the recovery phase from a cycle of chemotherapy such as 1.5 g/m^2 of cyclophosphamide.

Granulocyte colony-stimulating factor (G-CSF) is given to patients or donors as a course of injections (typically 10 μg/kg/day for 4–6 days) until the white cell count starts to rise. PBSC collections are taken and, depending on the efficiency of stem cell

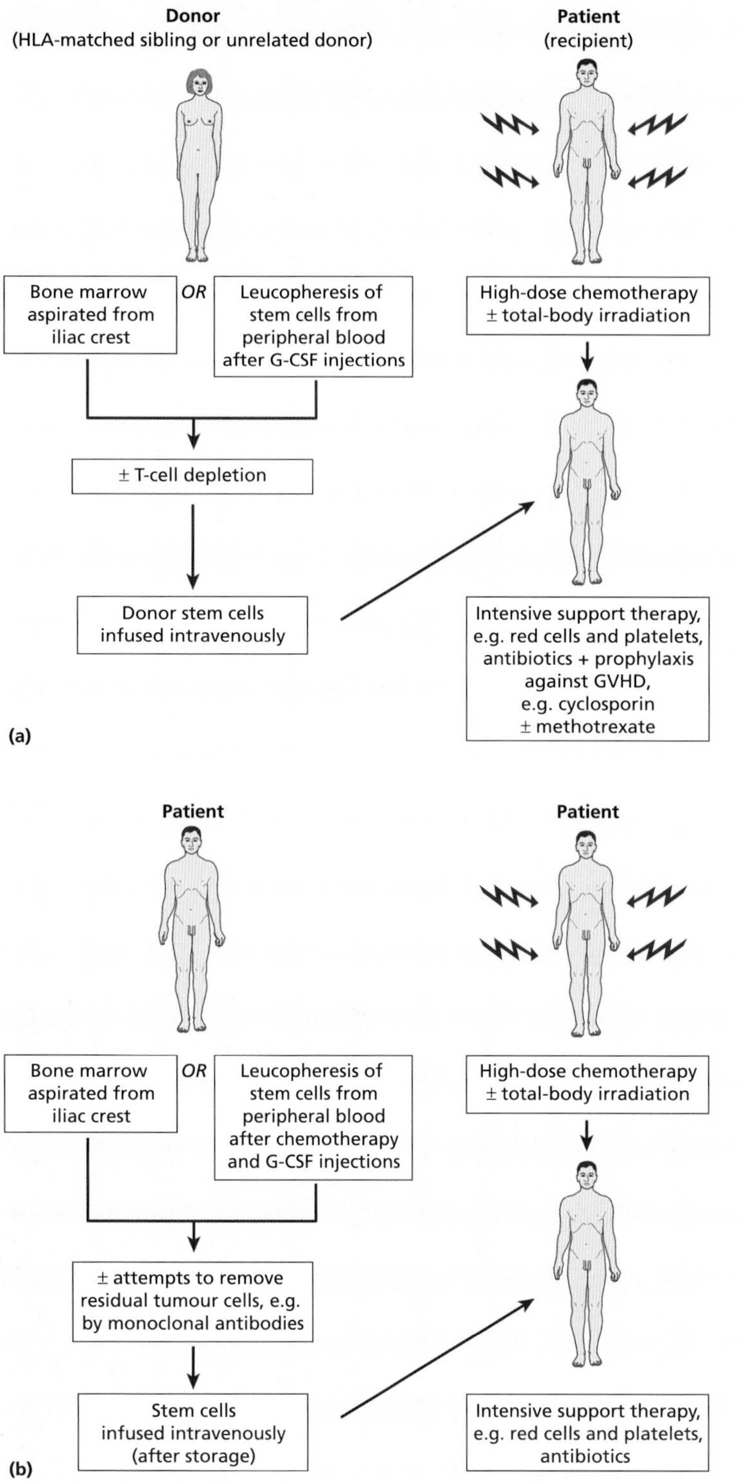

Fig. 21.1 Procedures for **(a)** allogeneic, and **(b)** autologous stem cell transplantation. G-CSF, granulocyte colony-stimulating factor; GVHD, graft-versus-host disease.

Table 21.1 Stem cell transplantation: potential donors.

HLA-matching sibling Unrelated HLA-matching volunteer Umbilical cord blood	Allogeneic
Identical twin	Syngeneic
Self	Autologous

HLA, human leucocyte antigen.

mobilization, repeated collections may be needed for up to 3 days. The adequacy of the collection may be assessed by:

1 $CD34^+$ cell count. Generally $>2.5 \times 10^6$/kg are needed for autologous transplantation.

2 *In vitro* colony assays, particularly granulocyte–macrophage colony-forming unit (CFU-GM) (p. 2), of which $1–5 \times 10^5$/kg would be considered adequate for transplantation.

Table 21.2 Stem cell transplantation: indications.

Allogeneic (or syngeneic)	Autologous
Acute lymphoblastic or myeloid leukaemia	Hodgkin's lymphoma and non-Hodgkin's lymphoma
Chronic myeloid leukaemia	Multiple myeloma
Other malignant disorders of the marrow (e.g. myelodysplasia, multiple myeloma, lymphoma, chronic lymphocytic leukaemia)	Acute and chronic leukaemias
Severe aplastic anaemia including Fanconi's anaemia	Severe autoimmune disease
Inherited disorders: thalassaemia major, sickle cell anaemia, immune deficiencies, inborn errors of metabolism in the haemopoietic and mesenchymal system (e.g. osteopetrosis)	Amyloidosis
Other acquired severe marrow diseases (e.g. paroxysmal nocturnal haemoglobinuria, red cell aplasia, myelofibrosis)	For 'gene therapy' of genetic disease (e.g. adenosine deaminase deficiency)

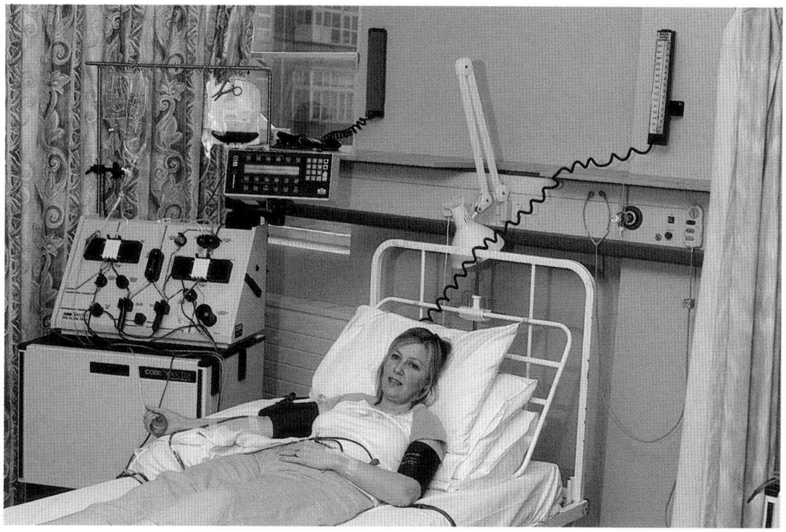

Fig. 21.2 Peripheral blood stem cell (PBSC) collection: a donor undergoing collection of PBSCs on a cell separator.

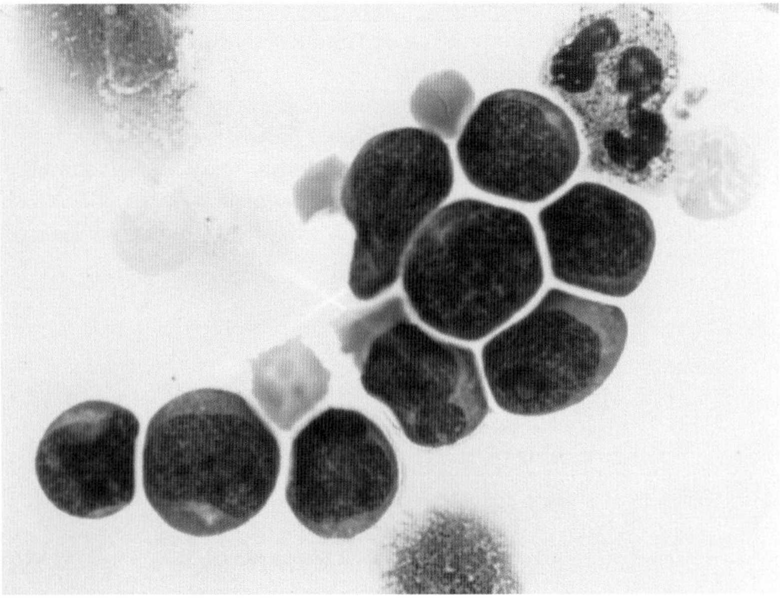

Fig. 21.3 Peripheral blood stem cell collection: enriched $CD34^+$ cells stained by May-Grünwald–Giemsa stain. The cells have the appearance of small and medium-sized lymphocytes.

Stem cell processing

After collection the stem cell harvest is processed with removal of red cells and concentration of the mononuclear cells. Autologous collections may be 'purged' by chemotherapy or antibodies in an attempt to remove residual malignant cells. Allogeneic collections may be treated with antibodies to remove T cells to reduce graft-versus-host disease (GVHD). $CD34^+$ stem cells may be selected from both types of harvest (Fig. 21.3).

Conditioning

Prior to infusion of haemopoietic stem cells patients receive chemotherapy, sometimes in combination with total body irradiation (TBI; Fig. 21.1) in a procedure called ***conditioning***. This is designed to eradicate the patient's haemopoietic and immune system and, if present, malignancy. In addition, in the setting of allogeneic SCT it helps to suppress the host immune system and thereby prevent rejection of the 'foreign' stem cells. An important development that has occurred in SCT is a major shift from ***myeloablative*** conditioning regimes to ***non-myeloablative*** conditioning. Non-myeloabalative conditioning does not completely ablate the patient's bone marrow and is discussed more fully later (p. 262).

TBI is usually used in patients with malignant disease and is administered as a single dose or in smaller doses over several days (fractionated). The most commonly used drug is cyclophosphamide but busulfan, melphalan, cytosine arabinoside, etoposide or nitrosoureas are given in some protocols. At least 36 h are allowed for the elimination of the drugs from the circulation following the last dose of chemotherapy before donor stem cells are infused. Conditioning therapy is often complicated by mucositis and patients sometimes need parenteral nutrition. Trials are taking place in which monoclonal antibodies directed against specific antigens such as CD45 are attached to toxins or radioactive isotopes in an attempt to selectively target white cells as an aid to conditioning.

Post-transplant engraftment and immunity

After a period of typically 1–3 weeks of severe pancytopenia, the first signs of successful engraftment are monocytes and neutrophils in the blood with a subsequent increase in platelet count (Fig. 21.4). A reticulocytosis also begins and natural killer (NK) cells are among the earliest donor-derived lymphocytes to appear. G-CSF may be used to reduce the period of neutropenia. Engraftment is usually quicker following PBSC transplantation compared with BMT.

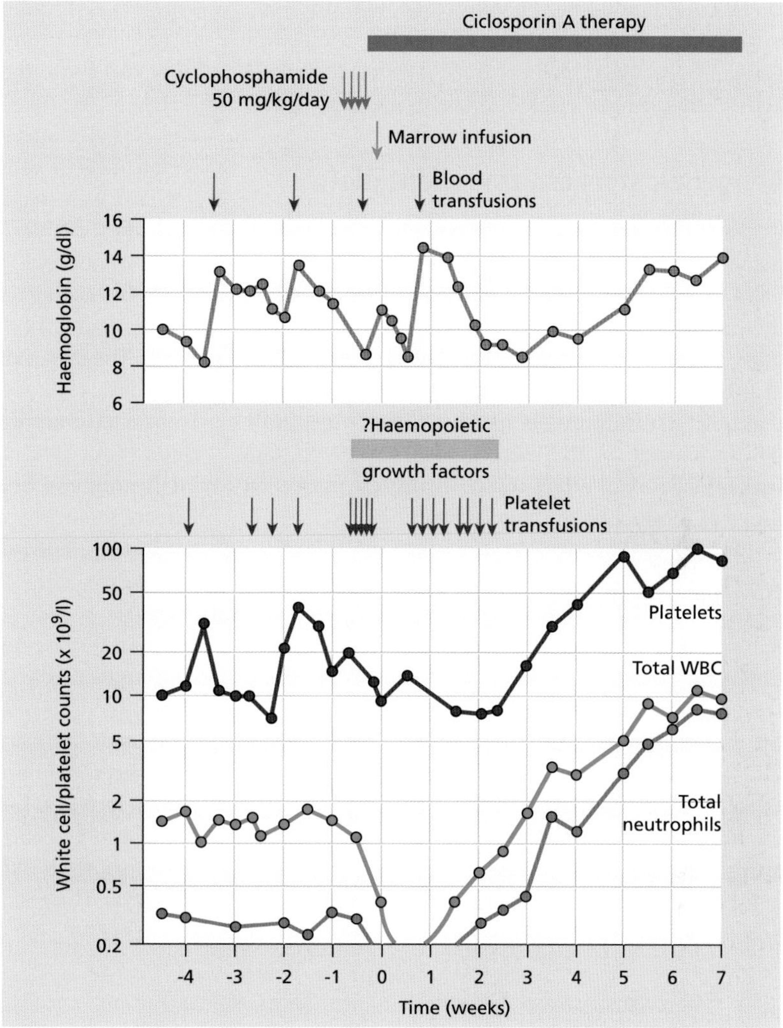

Fig. 21.4 Typical haematological chart of a patient undergoing allogeneic marrow transplantation for aplastic anaemia. WBC, white blood cells.

The marrow cellularity gradually returns to normal but the marrow reserve remains impaired for 1–2 years. There is profound immunodeficiency for 3–12 months with a low level of CD4 helper cells and a raised CD8 : CD4 ratio for 6 months or more. Immune recovery is quicker after autologous and syngeneic SCT than following allogeneic SCT. The patient's blood group changes to that of the donor and antigen-specific immunity becomes that of the donor after approximately 60 days.

Autologous stem cell transplantation

This allows the delivery of a high dose of chemotherapy, with or without radiotherapy, which otherwise would result in prolonged bone marrow aplasia. Stem cells are harvested and stored before the treatment is given and are then reinfused to 'rescue' the patient from the myeloablative effects of the treatment (Fig. 21.1). A limitation of the procedure is that tumour cells contaminating the stem cell harvest may be reintroduced into the patient. Nevertheless, autografting has a major role in the treatment of haematological diseases such as lymphoma and myeloma and is under investigation in other diseases such as acute leukaemia and severe autoimmune diseases. The major problem associated with autografting is recurrence of the original disease.

GVHD is not an issue. Procedure-related mortality is generally well below 5%. Trials of autologous bone marrow cell transfer to treat myocardial infarct and other non-haemopoietic diseases are in progress.

Allogeneic stem cell transplantation

In this procedure, stem cells harvested from another person are infused into the patient. The procedure has a significant morbidity and mortality and one of the major reasons is the immunological incompatibility between donor and patient despite matching of the human leucocyte antigens (HLA). This may manifest as immunodeficiency, GVHD or graft failure. Paradoxically, there is also a graft-versus-leukaemia (GVL) effect which probably underlies much of the success of the procedure.

The human leucocyte antigen system

Allografting would be impossible without the ability to perform HLA typing. The short arm of chromosome 6 contains a cluster of genes known as the major histocompatibility complex (MHC) or the HLA region (Fig. 21.5a). Genes in this region encode the HLA antigens and several other molecules including complement components, tumour necrosis factor (TNF) and proteins associated with antigen processing. HLA proteins are divided into two types: class I and II (Table 21.3). Their role is to bind intracellular peptides and 'present' these to T lymphocytes for antigen recognition. Class I molecules (HLA-A, -B and -C) present antigen to $CD8^+$ T cells and class II molecules (HLA-DR, -DQ and -DP) present to $CD4^+$ T cells (Fig. 21.5b).

Class I antigens are present on most nucleated cells and on the cell surface they are associated with β_2-microglobulin. Class II antigens have a more restricted tissue distribution and comprise α and β chains, both encoded by genes in the MHC locus. The inheritance of the four loci (HLA-A, -B, -C and -DR) is closely linked, one set of loci is inherited from each parent so that there is approximately a one in four chance of two siblings having identical HLA antigens (Fig. 21.6a). Crossing-over of genes during meiosis accounts for occasional unexpected disparities. The inheritance is independent of sex or blood group.

Human leucocyte antigen and transplantation

The natural role of HLA molecules is in directing T-lymphocyte responses and the greater the HLA mismatch the more severe is the immune response between transplanted cells. HLA typing is critical in donor selection for allogeneic SCT.

Minor histocompatibility antigens are peptides that are presented by HLA molecules and are able to act as antigens in SCT either because they are

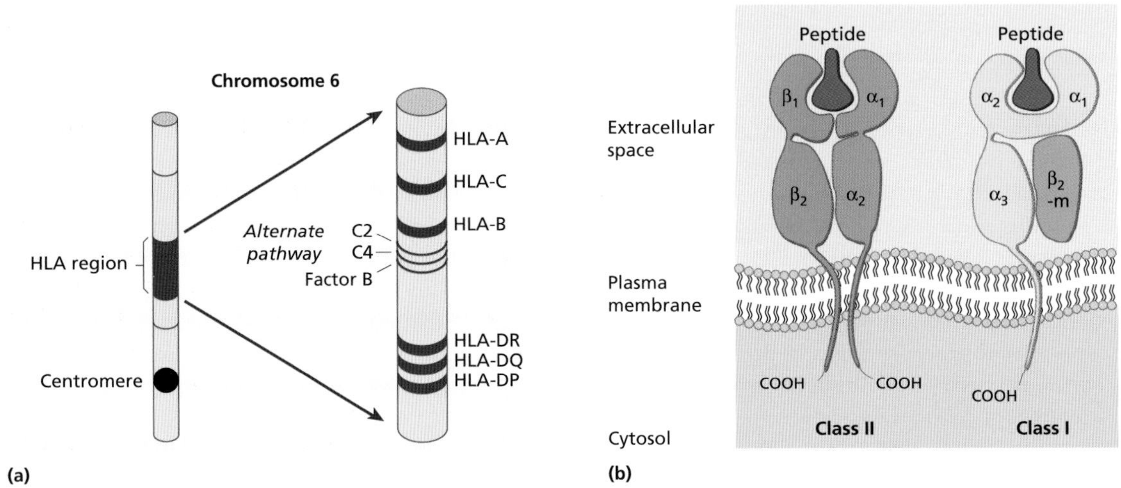

Fig. 21.5 **(a)** The human leucocyte antigen (HLA) complex. **(b)** HLA class I and II molecules showing protein domains and bound peptide.

Table 21.3 The human leucocyte antigens.

	Class I	Class II
Antigens	HLA-A, -B, -C	HLA-DR, -DP, -DQ
Distribution	All nucleated cells, platelets	B lymphocytes Monocytes Macrophages Activated T cells
Structure	Large polypeptide chain (MHC coded) and a β_2-microglobulin	Two polypeptide chains (α and β) both MHC coded
Interacts with	CD8 lymphocytes	CD4 lymphocytes

HLA, human leucocyte antigen; MHC, major histocompatibility complex.

polymorphic in the population or because they are encoded on the Y chromosome and therefore represent novel antigens when a female immune system engrafts in a male. They are likely to be important antigens in GVHD and the GVL reaction (see below).

HLA typing may be carried out by serological or molecular techniques. Serological testing involves the use of antibodies that are specific for individual HLA alleles or small families of alleles. Positivity may be detected by direct binding of a labelled antibody or by the use of complement to kill target cells that bind antibody (the two-stage lymphocytotoxicity test).

Molecular testing is performed on DNA. The most widely used methods use PCR sequence-specific primers or PCR sequence-specific oligonucleotide probes. Both methods use DNA primers or probes that react with polymorphic sequence motifs present within the nucleotide sequence of the *HLA* allele.

The nomenclature for *HLA* alleles is now standardized. A single antigenic specificity defined by serological typing (e.g. *HLA-A*) can be divided into different alleles by DNA sequencing. Each allele is given in numerical designation. The gene name is followed by an asterisk. The first two subsequent digits indicate the allele group. The third and fourth digits list subtypes. Subsequent digits indicate minor differences in non-coding regions. As an example, alleles at the *HLA-A* loci are written as *HLA-A*0101* to *HLA-A*8001*, where the first two digits after the asterisk indicate the type of the allele and the last two digits indicate the subtype. The type often corresponds to the serological antigen carried by the alleles (e.g. HLA-A2 for the *HLA-A*0201* to *HLA-A*0230* alleles). The nomenclature for the class II genes is similar but complicated by the fact that there may be more than one *HLA-DRB* gene on each chromosome (Fig. 21.6b).

Further cellular tests of histocompatibility that are sometimes employed, particularly in unrelated donor SCT, are limiting dilution analyses of cytotoxic T-lymphocyte or helper T-lymphocyte precursors (CTLp and HTLp). A higher value indicates greater mismatch and appears to correlate with increased GVHD.

When searching for an unrelated donor the aim is to match HLA-A, -B and -DR between recipient and donor and this is then called a 6/6 match. Occasionally a single mismatch (5/6) can be tolerated but it is rare to accept a donor with a greater mismatch than this. An exception is when a donor with only a single HLA haplotype match, usually a parent or sibling, is used in a ***haploidentical SCT***. Such transplants usually require a stem cell graft that is heavily depleted of T cells in order to limit the development of GVHD. There are over 4 million volunteer donors on international registries and the chance of identifying a matched unrelated donor for a patient lacking an HLA identical sibling (depending on the ethnic group) is usually greater than 50%.

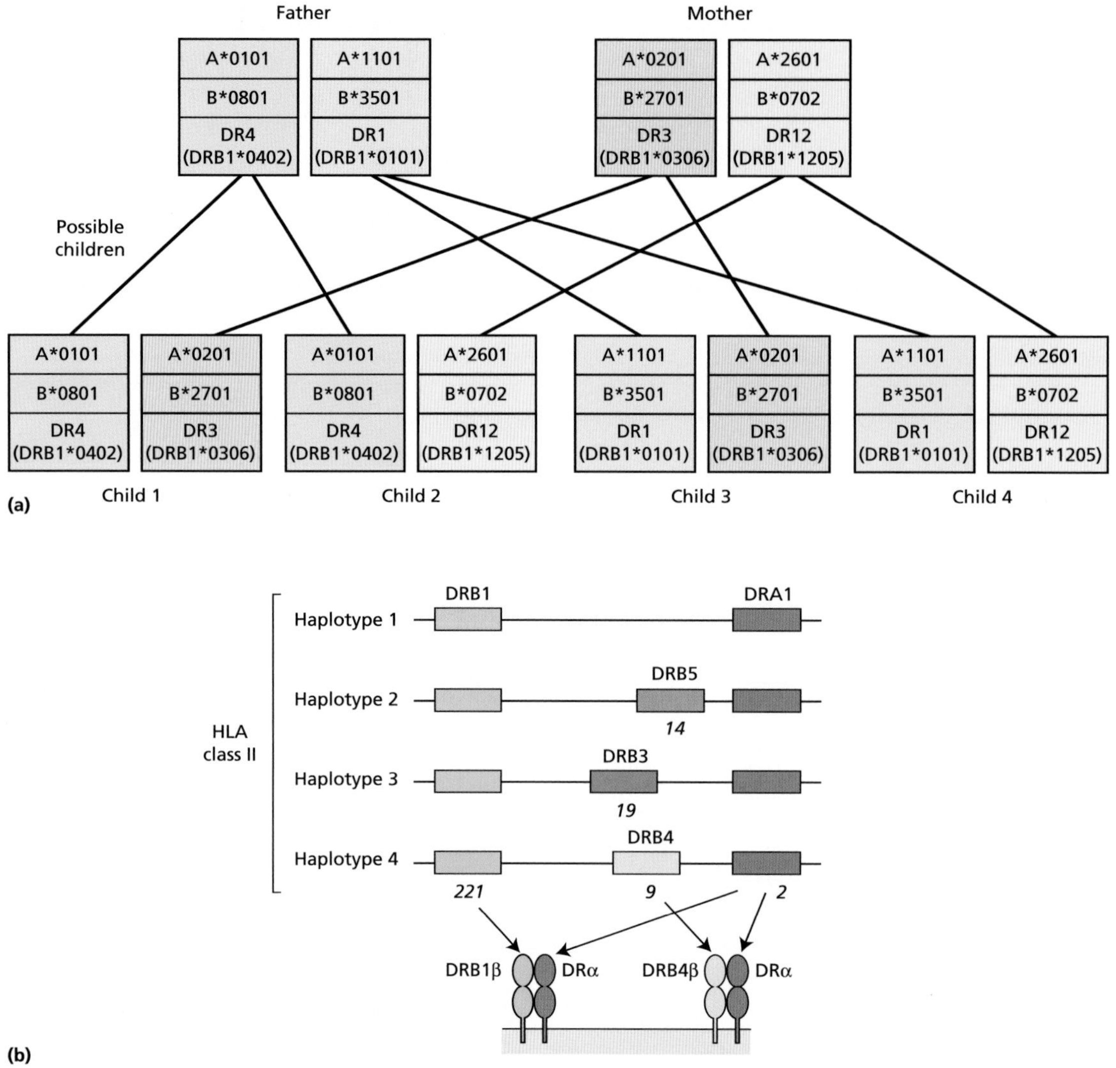

Fig. 21.6 **(a)** An example of the possible pattern of inheritance of the A, B and DR (*DRB1*) series alleles of the human leucocyte antigen (HLA) complex. **(b)** Molecular genetics of the HLA class II gene complex. There are four major haplotypes of MHC class II genes in the population and each individual may have up to two (one on each chromosome). The *DRA1* gene codes for the DRα protein and the *DRB1*, *DRB3*, *DRB4* and *DRB5* genes encode DRβ chains. Expression from the *DRB1* gene is higher than from the other genes. The number of alleles at each gene is shown underneath the gene in italics. Alleles at each locus have a standard nomenclature (e.g. the alleles at the *DRB1* gene are termed *DRB1*0101* to *DRB1*1608*). It is now known that the DR51, DR52 and DR53 antigens, which are defined by serological testing, are encoded from the *DRB5*, *DRB4* and *DRB3* genes, respectively.

Complications (Table 21.4)

Graft-versus-host disease

This is caused by donor-derived immune cells, particularly T lymphocytes, reacting against recipient tissues. Its incidence is increased with increasing age of donor and recipient and if there is any degree of HLA mismatch between them. GVHD prophylaxis is usually given as ciclosporin (intravenously or orally for 6–12 months) and methotrexate (three

Table 21.4 Complications of stem cell transplantation.

Early (usually <100 days)	Late (usually >100 days)
Infections, especially bacterial, fungal, herpes simplex virus, CMV	Infections, especially varicella-zoster, capsulate bacteria
Haemorrhage	Chronic GVHD (arthritis, malabsorption, hepatitis, scleroderma, sicca syndrome, lichen planus, pulmonary disease, serous effusions)
Acute GVHD (skin, liver, gut)	Chronic pulmonary disease
Graft failure	Autoimmune disorders
Haemorrhagic cystitis	Cataract
Interstitial pneumonitis	Infertility
Others: veno-occlusive disease, cardiac failure	Second malignancies

CMV, cytomegalovirus; GVHD, graft-versus-host disease.

Table 21.5 Acute graft-versus-host disease: clinical staging (Seattle system).

Stage	Skin	Liver (bilirubin, μmol/L)	Gut (diarrhoea, L/day)
I	Rash <25%	20–35	0.5–1.0
II	Rash 25–50%	35–80	1.0–1.5
III	Erythroderma	80–150	1.5–2.5
IV	Bullae, desquamation	>150	>2.5; severe pain, ileus

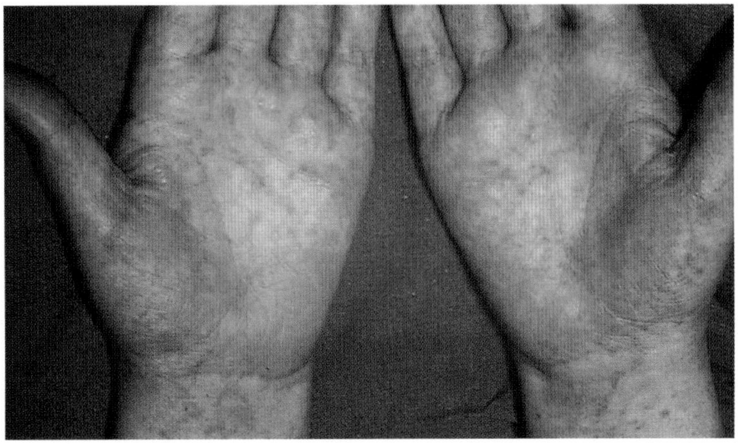

Fig. 21.7 Widespread erythematous skin rash in acute graft-versus-host disease following bone marrow transplantation.

or four injections). An alternative is to remove T cells from the donor stem cell infusion. In addition, anti-T-cell antibodies may be given to the patient.

In ***acute GVHD***, occurring in the first 100 days, the skin, gastrointestinal tract or liver are affected (Table 21.5). The skin rash typically affects the face, palms, soles and ears but may in severe cases affect the whole body (Fig. 21.7). The diagnosis is usually confirmed by skin biopsy which shows initially single cell necrosis in the basal layer of the epidermis; lymphocyte infiltration may be scanty. Diarrhoea may lead to fluid and electrolyte depletion. Typically, bilirubin and alkaline phosphatase are raised but the other hepatic enzymes are relatively normal. Acute GVHD is usually treated by high doses of corticosteroids which are effective in the majority of cases.

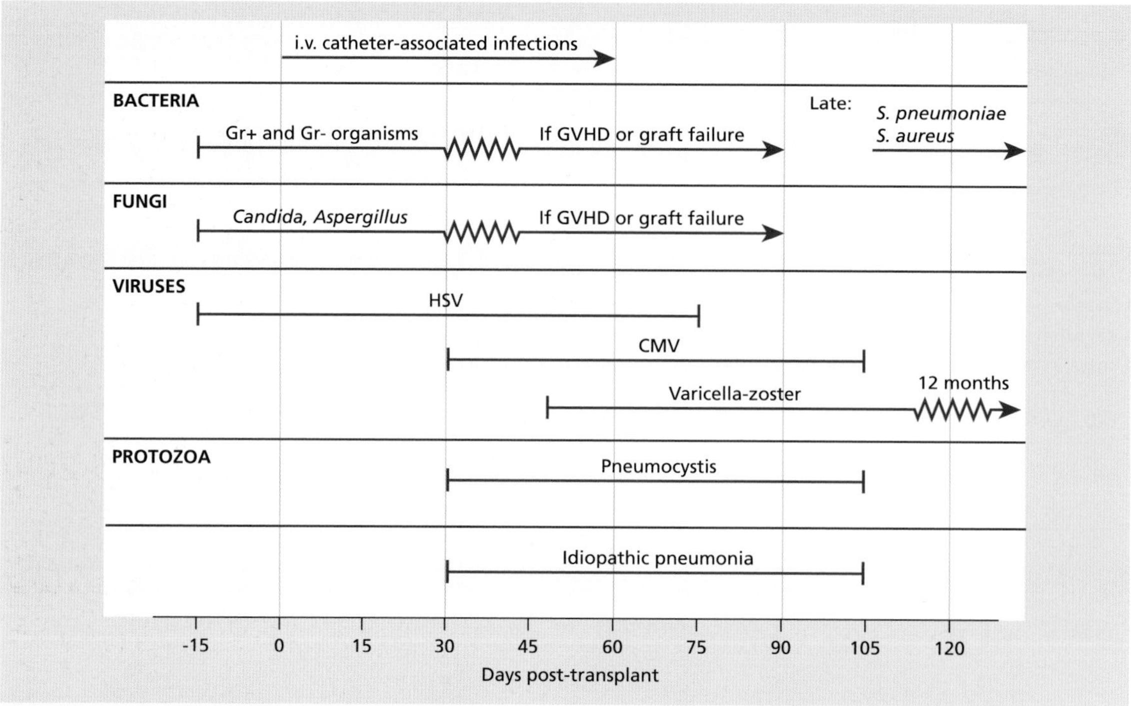

Fig. 21.8 Time sequence for development of different types of infection following allogeneic bone marrow transplantation. CMV, cytomegalovirus; Gr+, Gr–, Gram-positive or -negative; GVHD, graft-versus-host disease; HSV, herpes simplex virus.

In ***chronic GVHD***, occurring after 100 days and usually evolving from acute GVHD, these tissues are involved but also the joints and other serosal surfaces, the oral mucosa and lacrimal glands. Features of scleroderma, Sjögren's syndrome and lichen planus may develop. The immune system is impaired (including hyposplenism) with risk of infection. Malabsorption and pulmonary abnormalities are frequent. Drugs such as ciclosporin, azathioprine, mycophenolate mofetil, thalidomide or corticosteroids are used although response may be poor.

Infections

In the early post-transplant period, bacterial or fungal infections are frequent (Fig. 21.8). These may be reduced by reverse barrier nursing with laminar or positive pressure air flow and the use of skin and mouth antiseptics. Prophylactic therapy with aciclovir, antifungal agents and oral antibiotics is often added. If a fever or other evidence of an infection occurs, broad-spectrum intravenous antibiotics are commenced immediately after blood cultures and other appropriate microbiological specimens have been taken. Failure of response to antibacterial agents is usually an indication to commence systemic antifungal therapy with amphotericin B, caspofungin or voriconazole (p. 151). Fungal infections, especially *Candida* and *Aspergillus* species (Fig. 21.9) are a particular problem because of the prolonged neutropenia. Fluconazole is effective in reducing the risk of *Candida* infection and itraconazole may provide some prophylaxis against both organisms. The standard formulation of amphotericin is nephrotoxic and the newer preparations such as liposomal amphotericin are better tolerated.

Viral infections, particularly with the herpes group of viruses, are frequent with herpes simplex, cytomegalovirus (CMV) and varicella zoster virus (VZV) occurring at different peak intervals (Fig. 21.8).

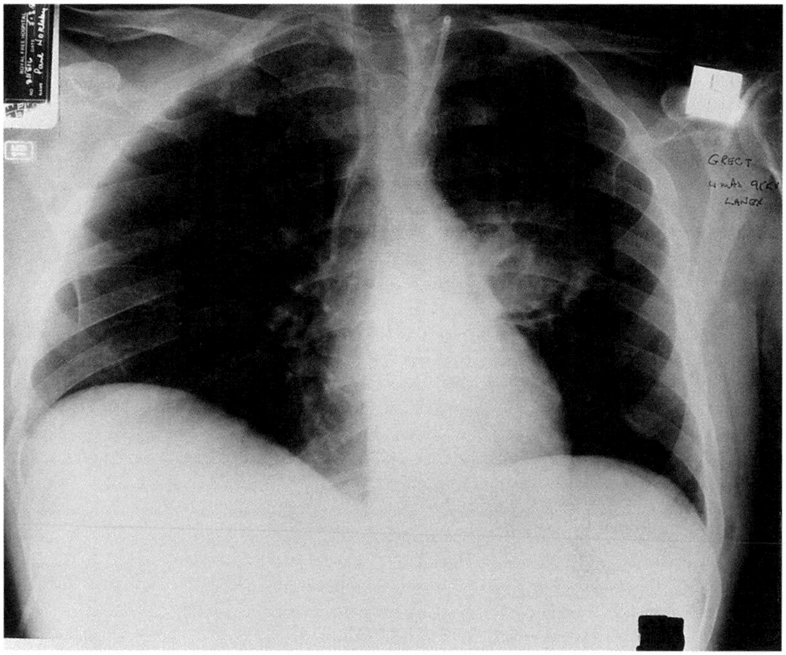

(a)

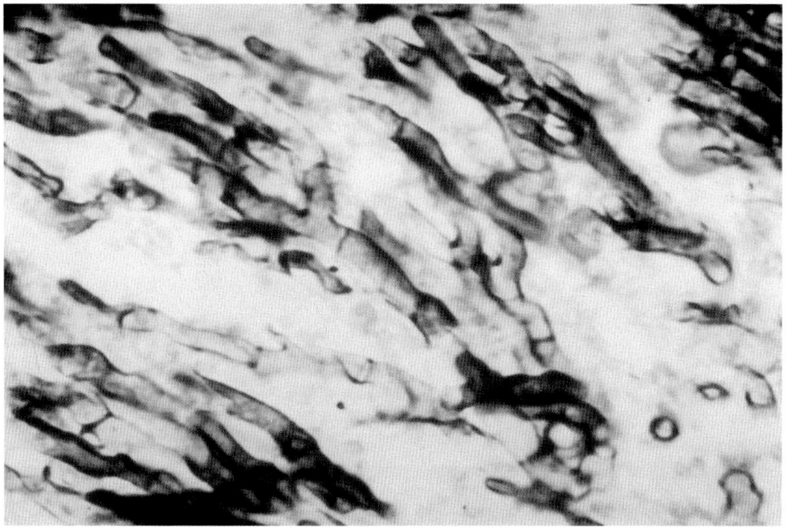

(b)

Fig. 21.9 **(a)** Chest radiograph showing an aspergilloma in a patient following stem cell transplantation. **(b)** Cytology of sputum illustrates the branching septate hyphae of *Aspergillus* (methenamine silver stain).

CMV presents a particular threat and is associated with a potentially fatal interstitial pneumonitis as well as with hepatitis and falling blood counts. The infection may be caused by reactivation of CMV in the recipient or a new infection transmitted by the donor. In CMV-seronegative patients with CMV-seronegative donors, CMV-negative blood products or filtered blood must be given. Aciclovir may be useful in prophylaxis. Most centres screen patients regularly for evidence of CMV reactivation following allogeneic transplantation using polymerase chain reaction (PCR) or antibody-based tests. If these tests become positive, ganciclovir may suppress the virus before disease occurs. Ganciclovir, foscarnet and CMV immunoglobulin may be tried for established CMV infection.

Pneumocystis carinii is another cause of pneumonitis that may be prevented by prophylactic co-trimoxazole. VZV infection is also frequent post-SCT but occurs later with a median onset at 4–5 months. Rarely, disseminated VZV infection occurs. Intravenous aciclovir is indicated. Epstein–Barr virus (EBV) infections and EBV-associated lymphoproliferative disease are less frequent after SCT than after solid organ transplants.

Interstitial pneumonitis

This is one of the most frequent causes of death post-SCT (Fig. 21.10). CMV is a frequent agent but other herpes viruses and *P. carinii* account for other cases; in many, no cause other than the previous radiation and chemotherapy can be implicated. Bronchoalveolar lavage or open lung biopsy may be needed to establish the diagnosis.

Blood product support

Platelet concentrates are given to maintain a count of 10×10^9/L or more. Platelets and blood transfusions given in the post-transplant period must be irradiated prior to administration in order to kill any lymphocytes that might cause GVHD.

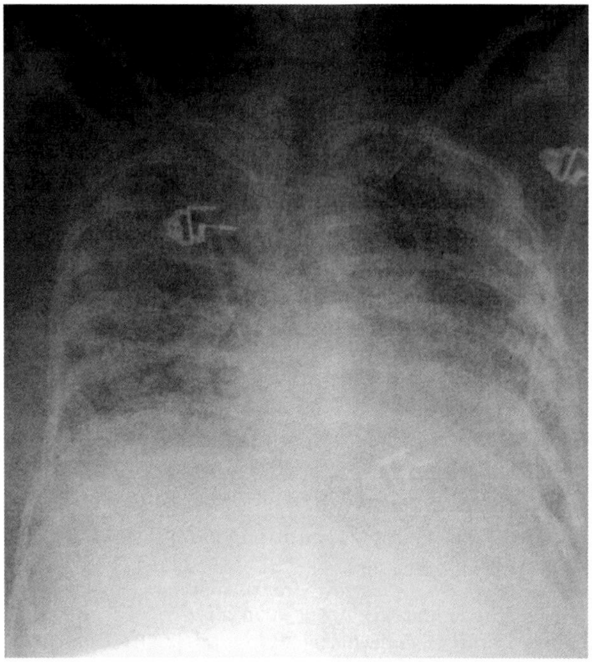

(a)

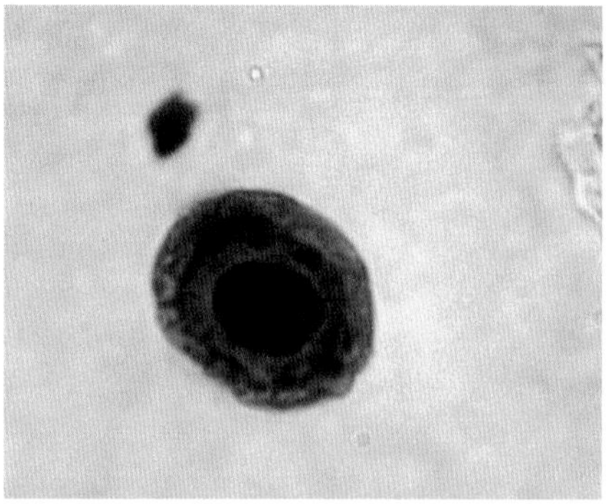

(b)

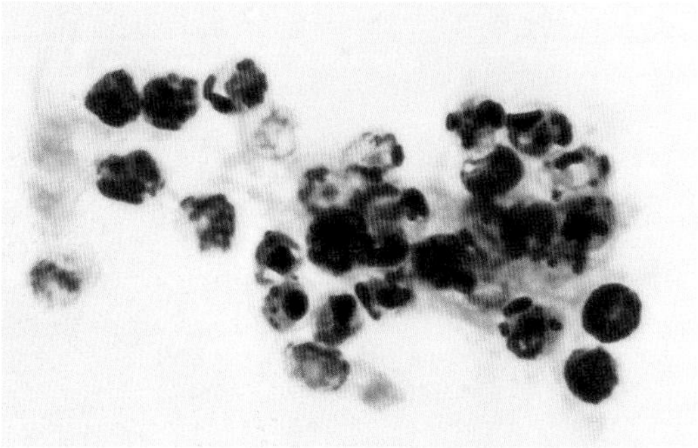

(c)

Fig. 21.10 **(a)** Chest radiograph showing interstitial pneumonitis following bone marrow transplantation. Widespread diffuse mottling can be seen. The patient had received total body irradiation and had grade III graft-versus-host disease. No infective cause of the pneumonitis was identified. Possible causes include pneumocystis, cytomegalovirus, herpes zoster, fungal infection or a combination of these. **(b)** Sputum cytology: intranuclear CMV inclusion body in a pulmonary cell. Papanicolaou stain. **(c)** *Pneumocystis carinii* in bronchial washings, Gram–Weigert stain.

Other complications of allogeneic transplantation

Graft failure

The risk of graft failure is increased if the patient has aplastic anaemia or if T-cell depletion of donor marrow is used as GVHD prophylaxis. This suggests that donor T cells are needed to overcome host resistance to engraftment of stem cells.

Haemorrhagic cystitis

This is usually caused by the cyclophosphamide metabolite acrolein. Mesna is given in an attempt to prevent this. Certain viruses (e.g. adenovirus or polyomavirus) may also cause this complication.

Other complications

These include veno-occlusive disease of the liver (manifest as jaundice, hepatomegaly and ascites or weight gain) and cardiac failure as a result of the conditioning regime (especially high doses of cyclophosphamide) and previous chemotherapy on the heart. Haemolysis because of ABO incompatibility between donor and recipient may cause problems in the first weeks. Microangiopathic haemolytic anaemia may also occur.

Late complications

Relapse of the original disease (e.g. acute or chronic leukaemia) may occur. Bacterial infections are frequent, especially with Gram-negative or encapsulated organisms affecting the respiratory tract. Oral penicillin is given prophylactically to reduce this risk. VZV and fungal infections are also frequent. The use of prophylactic co-trimoxazole and oral aciclovir for 3–6 months reduces the risk of *Pneumocystis* and herpes infections, respectively.

Delayed pulmonary complications include restrictive pneumonitis and bronchiolitis obliterans. Endocrine complications include hypothyroidism, growth failure with low growth hormone levels in children, impaired sexual development and infertility. These endocrine problems are more marked if TBI has been used. Clinically apparent autoimmune disorders are infrequent and include myasthenia, rheumatoid arthritis, anaemia, thrombocytopenia or neutropenia. Autoantibodies are frequently detected in the absence of symptoms. Second malignancies (especially non-Hodgkin's lymphoma) occur with a six- or sevenfold incidence compared with controls. CNS complications include neuropathies and eye problems caused by chronic GVHD (sicca syndrome) or cataracts.

Umbilical cord transplants

Fetal blood contains a large number of haemopoietic stem cells and umbilical cord blood has been used successfully as a source of stem cells. The main problem is the small amount of blood and therefore limited number of stem cells that can be collected from each sample and this limits the application of umbilical blood transplants to children or small adults. *Ex vivo* expansion of progenitor cells or administration of two or more cord units may be of value in the future. The immunological properties of cord blood cells are under investigation.

Graft-versus-leukaemia effect and donor leucocyte infusions

After allogeneic transplantation the donor immune system helps to eradicate the patient's leukaemia, a phenomenon known as the ***graft-versus-leukaemia*** (GVL) effect. Evidence includes the decreased relapse rate in patients with severe GVHD, the increased relapse rate in identical twins and, most convincingly, the ability of ***donor leucocyte infusions*** (DLI) to cure relapsed leukaemia in some patients. Graft-versus-lymphoma and -myeloma effects also exist. The principle of DLI is that peripheral blood mononuclear cells are collected from the original allograft donor and directly infused into the patient at the time of leukaemia relapse (Fig. 13.6).

There is a large difference in the outcome of different diseases treated by DLI. Chronic myeloid leukaemia (CML) is most sensitive whereas acute lymphoblastic leukaemia rarely responds. In CML the response to DLI is better in cases of early relapse. PCR is used to monitor serial blood samples for evidence of recurrence of the *BCR-ABL* transcript before karyotypic or clinical relapse occurs (Fig. 13.6). DLI can then be used in cases of molecular relapse. The response to DLI may take several weeks but usually results in a permanent cure. The mechanism is unclear but a T-cell-mediated

Table 21.6 Vectors used in gene therapy.

Vector	Properties
Viral vectors	
Retroviral	Integrate into DNA; infect variety of cell types. Only infect dividing cells
Adenovirus	Do not integrate, therefore transient expression. Infect dividing and non-dividing cells. Often provoke immune response
Adeno-associated virus	Limited integration sites
Herpes virus	Can carry large genes; no integration. Can infect resting cells
Non-viral vectors	
Liposomal	Relatively simple and cheap to make
Naked DNA	Low efficiency of entry into cells
Ballistic (gene gun)	

alloreactive immune response is likely to be a major component.

Non-myeloablative transplants

In order to reduce the morbidity and mortality of allogeneic transplantation, a number of low-intensity ***non-myeloablative conditioning regimens*** have been introduced which do not completely destroy the host bone marrow. These can include agents such as fludarabine, low-dose irradiation, antilymphocyte globulin and low doses of busulfan or cyclophosphamide. The aim in these 'mini-transplants' is to use enough immunosuppression to allow donor stem cells to engraft without completely eradicating host marrow stem cells. DLIs are commonly used at a late stage in order to encourage complete donor engraftment. Such regimes rely heavily on the ability of the GVL effect to cure the underlying malignant disease (Fig. 21.11) and extend the age range and increase the treatment indications for allogeneic transplantation.

Gene therapy and SCT

The ability to introduce novel genes into cells using appropriate vectors offers the opportunity to manipulate stem cells before reinfusion. Gene therapy vectors may be viral or non-viral and their relative properties are shown in Table 21.6. Many different genes are being investigated for possible expression in cells such as haemopoietic stem cells and specific differentiated populations such as T lymphocytes. These include genes to correct specific inborn errors of metabolism, genes such as neomycin to 'mark' specific populations for subsequent analysis, 'suicide' genes such as thymidine kinase that render cells susceptible to ganciclovir and resistance genes to protect normal stem cells from high-dose chemotherapy. Unfortunately, haemopoietic stem cells are difficult to transfect because they are relatively rare and few are in cell cycle at any particular time. Therefore the sustained correction of metabolic disorders following the introduction of transduced autologous haemopoietic progenitors remains a difficult problem.

Bibliography

Appelbaum F.R. (2003) The current status of hematopoietic cell transplantation. *Annu Rev Med* **54**,491–512.

Appelbaum F.R., Blume K.G., Forman S.J., Donnall T.E. (2003) *Thomas' Hematopoietic Cell Transplantation*. Blackwell Science, Oxford.

Copelan E.A. (2006) Hematopoietic stem-cell transplantation. *N Engl J Med* **354**,1813–26.

Diaconescu R., Flowers C.R., Storer B. *et al.* (2004) Morbidity and mortality with nonmyeloablative compared with myeloablative conditioning before hematopoietic cell transplantation from HLA-matched related disorders. *Blood* **104**,1550–8.

Hebart H. and Einsele H. (2004) Clinical aspects of CMV infection after stem cell transplantation. *Hum Immunol* **65**,432–6.

Jacobsohn D.A., Duerst R., Tse W., Kletzel M. (2004) Reduced intensity haemopoetic stem-cell transplantation for treatment of non-malignant diseases in children. *Lancet* **364**,156–62.

Little A-M., Marsh S.G.E., Madrigal J.A. (2005) Histocompatibility. In: Hoffbrand A.V., Tuddenham E.G.D., Catovsky D. (eds) *Postgraduate Haematology*, 5th edn. Blackwell Publishing, Oxford: pp. 395–418.

Mathur A. and Martin J.F. (2004) Stem cells and repair of the heart. *Lancet* **364**,183–92.

Peggs K.S. and Mackinnon S. (2004) Immune reconstitution following haematopoietic stem cell transplantation. *Br J Haematol* **124**,407–20.

Peggs K.S., Mackinnon S., Linch D.C. (2005) The role of allogeneic transplantation in non-Hodgkin's lymphoma. *Br J Haematol* **128**,153–68.

Wollert K.C., Meyer G.P., Lote J. *et al.* (2004) Intracoronary autologous bone-marrow cell transfer after myocardial infarction: the BOOST randomised controlled clinical trial. *Lancet* **364**,141–8.

CHAPTER 22

22 Platelets, blood coagulation and haemostasis

The normal haemostatic response to vascular damage depends on closely linked interaction between the blood vessel wall, circulating platelets and blood coagulation factors (Fig. 22.1).

An efficient and rapid mechanism for stopping bleeding from sites of blood vessel injury is clearly essential for survival. Nevertheless, such a response needs to be tightly controlled to prevent extensive clots developing and to break down such clots once damage is repaired. The haemostatic system thus represents a delicate balance between procoagulant and anticoagulant mechanisms allied to a process for

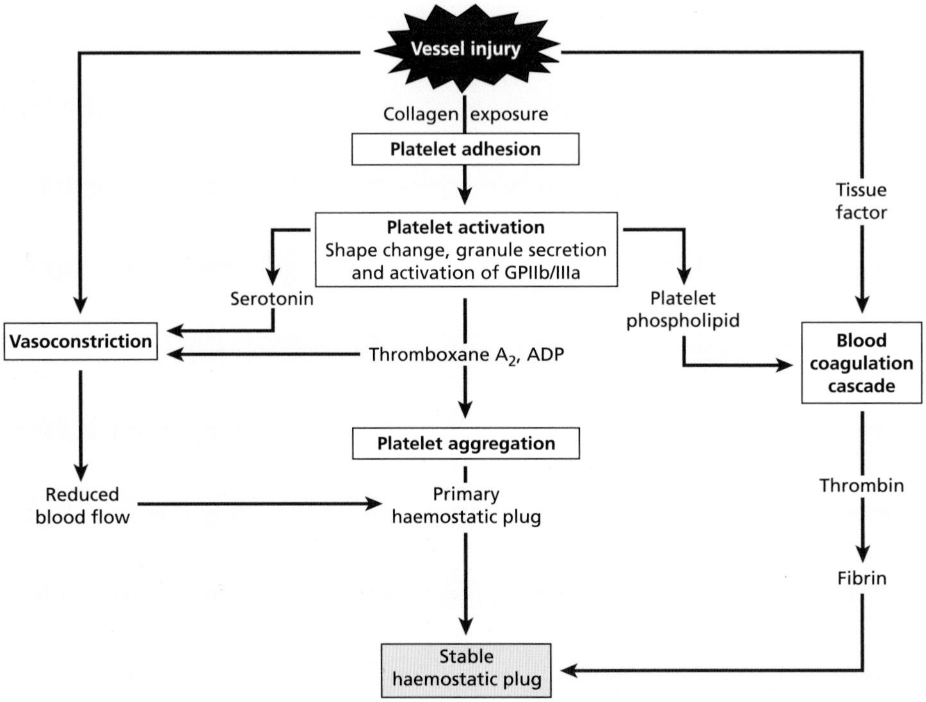

Fig. 22.1 The involvement of blood vessels, platelets and blood coagulation in haemostasis. ADP, adenosine diphosphate.

fibrinolysis. The five major components involved are platelets, coagulation factors, coagulation inhibitors, fibrinolysis and blood vessels. These are described later in the haemostatic response section on p. 275.

Components of haemostatic response

Platelets

Platelet production

Platelets are produced in the bone marrow by fragmentation of the cytoplasm of megakaryocytes, one of the largest cells in the body. The precursor of the megakaryocyte—the megakaryoblast—arises by a process of differentiation from the haemopoietic stem cell (Fig. 22.2). The megakaryocyte matures by endomitotic synchronous replication (i.e. DNA replication in the absence of nuclear or cytoplasmic division) enlarging the cytoplasmic volume as the number of nuclear lobes increase in multiples of two. A picture of mature polyploid megakaryocytes is shown in Fig. 22.3. Very early on invaginations of plasma membrane are seen, called the demarcation membrane, which evolves through the development of the megakaryocyte into a highly branched network. At a variable stage in development, most commonly at the eight nucleus stage, the cytoplasm becomes granular. Mature megakaryocytes are extremely large, with an eccentric placed single lobulated nucleus and a low nuclear to cytoplasmic ratio. Platelets form by fragmentation of megakaryocyte cytoplasm, approximately each megakaryocyte giving rise to 1000–5000 platelets. The time interval from differentiation of the human stem cell to the production of platelets averages approximately 10 days.

Thrombopoietin is the major regulator of platelet production and is constitutively produced by the liver and kidneys. Thrombopoietin increases the number and rate of maturation of megakaryocytes via c-Mpl receptor. Platelet levels start to rise 6 days after the start of therapy and remain high for 7–10 days. Unfortunately, thrombopoietin is not available for routine clinical practice. Platelets also have c-Mpl receptors for thrombopoietin and remove it from the circulation. Therefore, levels are high in thrombocytopenia as a result of marrow aplasia and vice versa.

The normal platelet count is approximately 250×10^9/L (range $150–400 \times 10^9$/L) and the normal platelet lifespan is 7–10 days. Up to one-third of the marrow output of platelets may be trapped at any one time in the normal spleen but this rises to 90% in cases of massive splenomegaly (p. 286).

Platelet structure

Platelets are extremely small and discoid, 3.0 × 0.5 μm in diameter, with a mean volume 7–11 fL. The ultrastructure of platelets is represented in

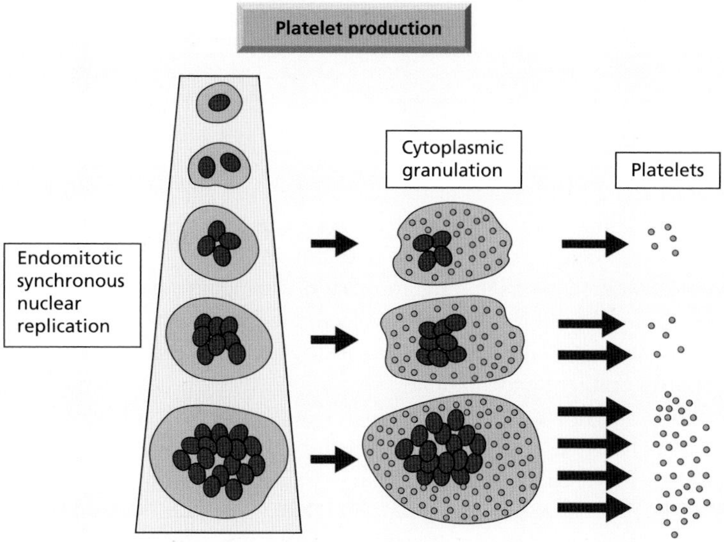

Fig. 22.2 Simplified diagram to illustrate platelet production from megakaryocytes.

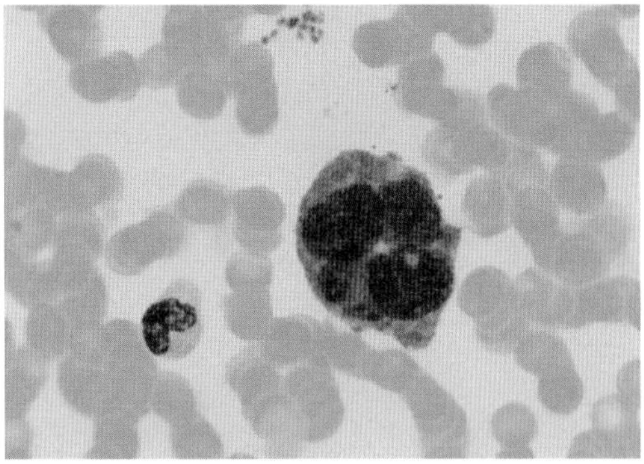

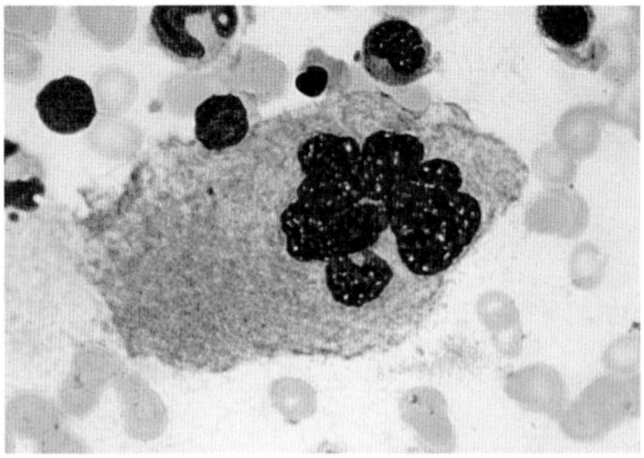

Fig. 22.3 Megakaryocytes: (a) immature form with basophilic cytoplasm; (b) mature form with many nuclear lobes and pronounced granulation of the cytoplasm.

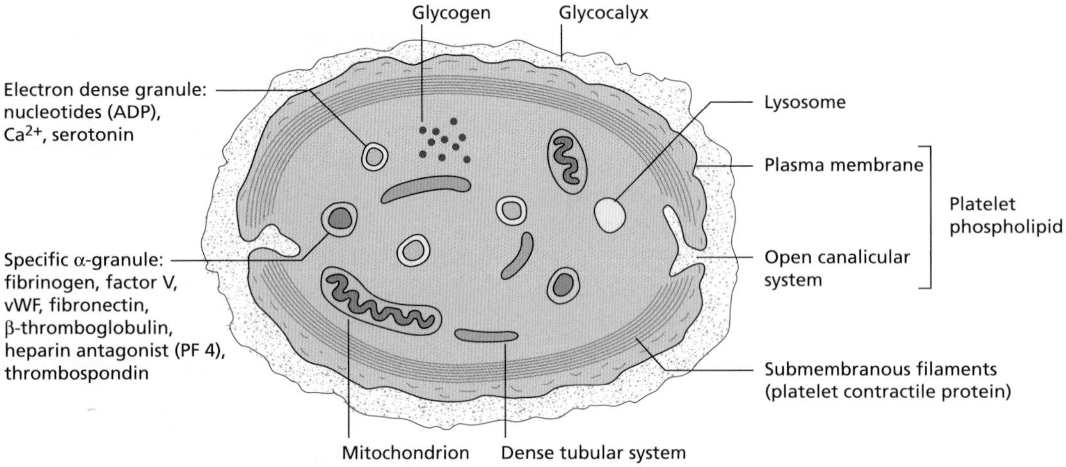

Fig. 22.4 The ultrastructure of platelets. ADP, adenosine diphosphate; PF, platelet factor; VWF, von Willebrand factor.

Fig. 22.4. The glycoproteins of the surface coat are particularly important in the platelet reactions of adhesion and aggregation which are the initial events leading to platelet plug formation during haemostasis. Adhesion to collagen is facilitated by glycoprotein Ia (GPIa). Glycoproteins Ib (defective in Bernard–Soulier syndrome) and IIb/IIIa (defective in thrombasthenia) are important in the attachment of platelets to von Willebrand factor (VWF) and hence to vascular subendothelium (Fig. 22.5) where metabolic interactions occur (Fig. 22.6). The binding site for IIb/IIIa is also the receptor for fibrinogen which is important in platelet–platelet aggregation.

The plasma membrane invaginates into the platelet interior to form an open membrane (canalicular) system which provides a large reactive surface to which the plasma coagulation proteins may be selectively absorbed. The membrane phospholipids (previously known as platelet factor 3) are of particular importance in the conversion of coagulation factor X to Xa and prothrombin (factor II) to thrombin (factor IIa) (Fig. 22.7).

The platelet contains three types of storage

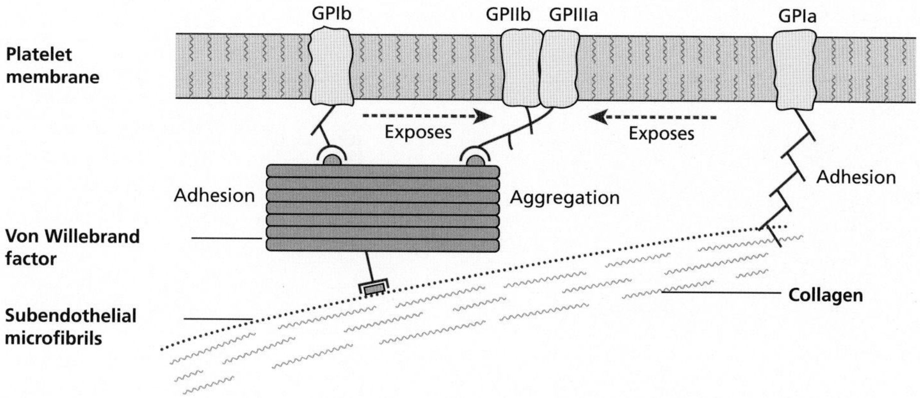

Fig. 22.5 Platelet adhesion. The binding of glycoprotein (GP) Ib (which consists of four proteins: GPIbα, GPIbβ, GPIX, GPV) to von Willebrand factor leads to adhesion to the subendothelium and also exposes the GPIIb/IIIa ($\alpha_{IIb}\beta_3$ integrin) binding sites to fibrinogen and von Willebrand factor leading to platelet aggregation. The GPIa site permits direct adhesion to collagen.

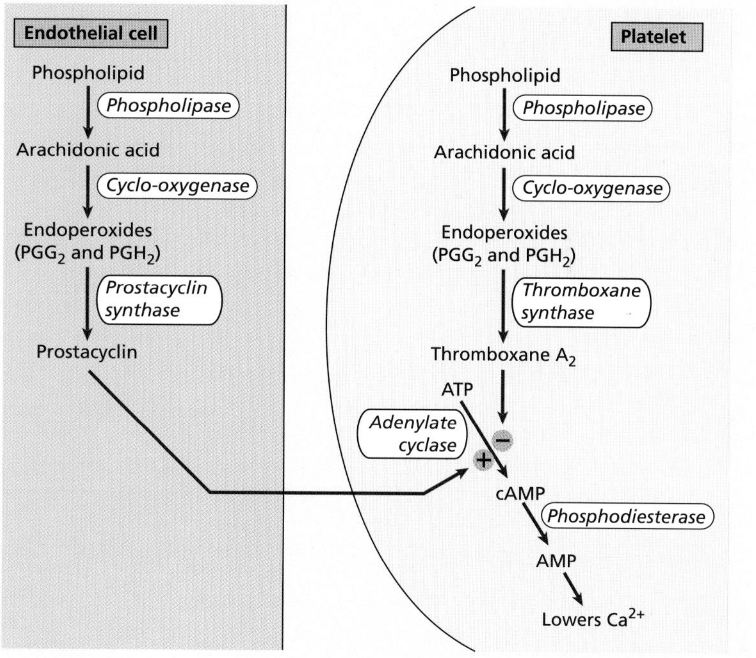

Fig. 22.6 The synthesis of prostacyclin and thromboxane. The opposing effects of these agents are mediated by changes in the concentration of cyclic adenosine monophosphate (cAMP) in platelets via stimulation or inhibition of the enzyme adenylate cyclase. cAMP controls the concentration of free calcium ions in the platelet which are important in the processes which cause adhesion and aggregation. High levels of cAMP lead to low free calcium ion concentrations and prevent aggregation and adhesion. ATP, adenosine triphosphate; Ca, calcium; PG, prostaglandin (G_2 and H_2).

granules: dense, α and lysosomes. The more frequent specific α granules contain a heparin antagonist (PF4), platelet-derived growth factor (PDGF), β-thromboglobulin, fibrinogen, VWF and other clotting factors. Dense granules are less common and contain adenosine diphosphate (ADP), adenosine triphosphate (ATP), 5-hydroxytryptamine (5-HT) and calcium. Lysosomes contain hydrolytic enzymes and peroxisomes contain catalase. During the release reaction described below, the contents of

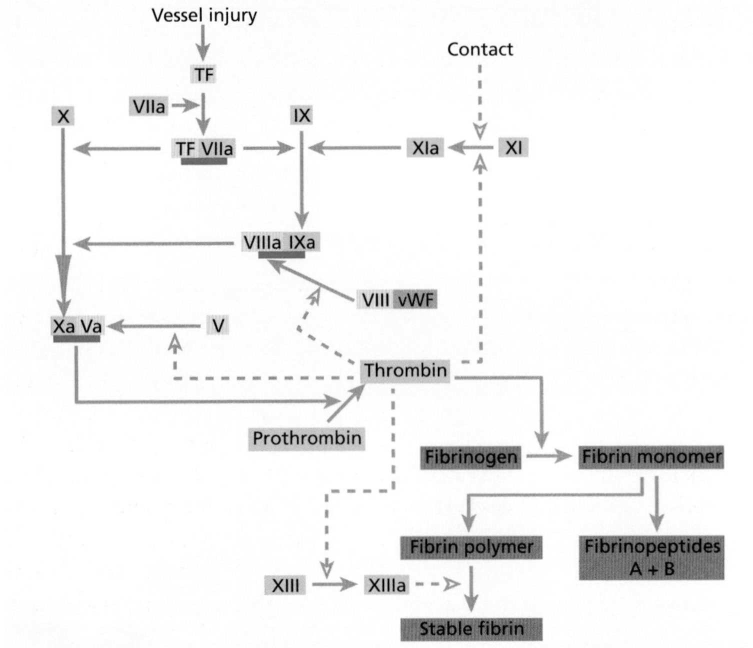

Fig. 22.7 The pathway of blood coagulation initiated by tissue factor (TF) on the cell surface. When plasma comes into contact with TF, factor VII binds to TF. The complex of TF and activated VII (VIIa) activates X and IX. TF pathway inhibitor (TFPI) is an important inhibitor of TF/VIIa. VIIIa–IXa complex greatly amplifies Xa production from X. The generation of thrombin from prothrombin by the action of Xa–Va complex leads to fibrin formation. Thrombin also activates XI (dashed line), V and XIII. Thrombin cleaves VIII from its carrier von Willebrand factor (VWF), greatly increasing the formation of VIIIa–IXa and hence of Xa–Va. Pale green, serine proteases; yellow, cofactors.

the granules are discharged into the open canalicular system.

Platelets are also rich in signalling and cytoskeletal proteins which support the rapid switch from quiescent to activation that follows vessel damage.

Platelet antigens

Several platelet surface proteins have been found to be important antigens in platelet-specific autoimmunity and they have been termed human platelet antigens (HPA). In most cases, two different alleles exist, termed a or b alleles (e.g. HPA-1a). Platelets also express ABO and human leucocyte antigen (HLA) class I but not class II antigens.

Platelet function

The main function of platelets is the formation of mechanical plugs during the normal haemostatic response to vascular injury. In the absence of platelets, spontaneous leakage of blood through small vessels may occur. The immobilization of platelets at the sites of vascular injury requires specific platelet–vessel wall (adhesion) and platelet—platelet (aggregation) interactions. The blood flow conditions determine the specific receptor ligand interactions.

Platelet adhesion and activation

Following blood vessel injury, platelets adhere to the exposed subendothelial matrix proteins via specific adhesive glycoproteins (GP). Under condition of high shear, e.g. arterioles, the exposed subendothelial matrix is initially coated with VWF multimers. The platelets than make contact with VWF via the GPIb-XI-V complex on platelets. This initiates platelet rolling in the direction of blood flow over the exposed VWF with activation of GPIIb/IIIa receptors. Firm adhesion is established by the slower but stronger interaction of other glycoproteins including activated GPIIb/IIIa with VWF and GPVI and integrin $\alpha1/\beta2$ with collagen and other components of the subendothelial matrix. Under static or low shear conditions, platelets adhere predominantly to collagen of the subendothelium. Collagen binds initially to GPIa/IIa, cross-links many of these integrin molecules, and in this way activates platelets.

This ligand receptor binding results in a complex cascade of signals which result in platelet activation. The events that follow are shape change and spreading, activation of GPIIb/IIIa and granule secretion. Platelets become more spherical and extrude long pseudopodia which enhance platelet vessel wall and platelet–platelet interaction. The end result of spreading is a flattened spread out platelet with granules and organelles in the centre, resulting in a characteristic fried egg appearance. These changes are brought about by the actin cytoskeleton. The granules are secreted from the centre of the cell.

Von Willebrand factor VWF is involved in platelet adhesion to the vessel wall and to other platelets (aggregation) (Fig. 22.5). It also carries factor VIII (see below) and used to be referred to as factor VIII-related antigen (VIII-Rag). It is a large cysteine-rich glycoprotein, with multimers made up on average of 2–50 subunits, with a molecular weight (MW) of $0.8–20 \times 10^6$. VWF is encoded by a gene on chromosome 12 and is synthesized both in endothelial cells and megakaryocytes, and stored in Weiberl–Palade bodies and platelet α granules respectively. Plasma VWF is almost entirely derived from endothelial cells, with two distinct pathways of secretion. The majority is continuously secreted and a minority is stored in Weibel–Palade bodies. The stored VWF can rise the plasma levels and it can be released under the influence of several secretagogues, like stress, exercise, adrenaline and infusion of desmopressin (1-deamieno-8-D-arginine vasopressin, DDAVP). The VWF released from Weibel–Palade bodies is in the form of large and ultra large multimers, the most adhesive and reactive form of VWF. They are in turn cleaved in plasma to monomeric VWF and smaller multimers by the specific plasma metalloprotease, ADAMTS-13.

Platelet aggregation

It is characterized by cross-linking of platelets through active GPIIb/IIIa receptors with fibrinogen bridges. A resting platelet has about 50–80 000 GPIIb/IIIa receptors, which do not bind fibrinogen, VWF or other ligands. Stimulation of a platelet leads to an increase in GPIIb/IIIa molecules, due to binding of α-granule membrane (rich in receptors) with the plasma membrane, activation of surface-exposed GPIIb/IIIa, enabling platelet cross-linking with fibrinogen bridges. Binding brings about molecular conformational changes resulting in a firm connection and further activation of the platelet.

Platelet release reaction and amplification

Primary activation by various agonists induces intracellular signalling, leading to the release of α and δ- granules. α-Granule contents play an important role in platelet aggregate formation and stabilization and, in addition, the ADP released from dense granules plays a major positive feedback role in promoting platelet activation. TXA2 is the second of the two major platelet positive feedback loops important in secondary amplification of platelet activation to firm a stable platelet aggregate. It is formed *de novo* upon activation of cytosolic phospholipase A_2 (PL_{A2}) which is the rate limiting step. This liberates arachidonic acid from the membrane phospholipids, and is metabolized by cycloxogenase to TXA2. It is a labile substance and lowers platelet cyclic adenosine monophosphate (cAMP) levels and initiates the release reaction (Fig. 22.6). Thromboxane A_2 not only potentiates platelet aggregation, but also has powerful vasoconstrictive activity. The release reaction is inhibited by substances that increase the level of platelet cAMP. One such substance is the prostaglandin prostacyclin (PGI_2) which is synthesized by vascular endothelial cells. It is a potent inhibitor of platelet aggregation and prevents their deposition on normal vascular endothelium.

Clot formation and retraction

The highly localized enhancement of ongoing platelet activation by ADP and TXA2 results in a platelet plug large enough to plug the area of endothelial injury. In this platelet plug the platelets are completely degranulated and adherent to each other. This is followed by clot retraction which is mediated by GPIIb/IIIa receptors which link the cytoplasmic actin filaments to the surface bound fibrin polymers.

Platelet procoagulant activity

After platelet aggregation and release, the exposed membrane phospholipid (platelet factor 3) is available for two reactions in the coagulation cascade. Both phospholipid-mediated reactions are calcium-ion dependent. The first (tenase) involves factors IXa, VIIIa and X in the formation of factor Xa (Fig. 22.7). The second (prothrombinase) results in the formation of thrombin from the interaction of factors Xa, Va and prothrombin (II). The phospholipid surface forms an ideal template for the crucial concentration and orientation of these proteins.

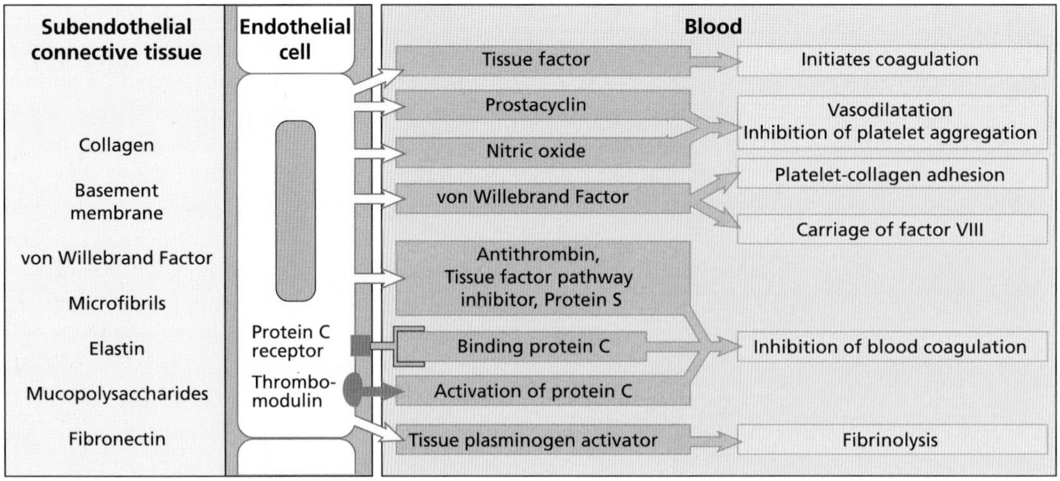

Fig. 22.8 The endothelial cell forms a barrier between platelets and plasma clotting factors and the subendothelial connected tissues. Endothelial cells produce substances that can initiate coagulation, cause vasodilatation, inhibit platelet aggregation or haemostasis, or activate fibrinolysis.

Growth factor

PDGF found in the specific granules of platelets stimulates vascular smooth muscle cells to multiply and this may hasten vascular healing following injury.

Natural inhibitors of platelet function

Nitric oxide (NO) is constitutively released from endothelial cells and also from macrophages and platelets. It has a short half-life of 3–5 s. It inhibits platelet activation and promotes vasodilatation. Prostacyclin synthesized by endothelial cells also inhibits platelet function (Fig. 22.8) and causes vasodilatation by raising cyclic guanosine monophosphate (GMP) levels. The transmembrane protein PECAM-1 is expressed also on endothelial cells. It is its own ligand and inhibits platelet activation by collagen.

Blood coagulation

The coagulation cascade

Blood coagulation involves a biological amplification system in which relatively few initiation substances sequentially activate by proteolysis a cascade of circulating precursor proteins (the coagulation factor enzymes) which culminates in the generation of thrombin; this, in turn, converts soluble plasma fibrinogen into fibrin (Fig. 22.7). Fibrin enmeshes the platelet aggregates at the sites of vascular injury and converts the unstable primary platelet plugs to firm, definitive and stable haemostatic plugs. A list of the coagulation factors appears in Table 22.1. They are assembled from a small number of molecules or domains (Fig. 22.9). The operation of this enzyme cascade requires local concentration of circulating coagulation factors at the site of injury.

Surface-mediated reactions occur on exposed collagen, platelet phospholipid and tissue factor. With the exception of fibrinogen, which is the fibrin clot subunit, the coagulation factors are either enzyme precursors or cofactors (Table 22.1). All the enzymes, except factor XIII, are serine proteases (i.e. their ability to hydrolyse peptide bonds depends upon the amino acid serine at their active centre; Fig. 22.10). The scale of amplification achieved in this system is dramatic, (e.g. 1 mol of activated factor XI through sequential activation of factors IX, X and prothrombin may generate up to 2×10^8 mol of fibrin).

Coagulation *in vivo*

The generation of thrombin *in vivo* is a complex network of amplification and negative feedback loops

Table 22.1 The coagulation factors.

Factor number	Descriptive name	Active form
I	Fibrinogen	Fibrin subunit
II	Prothrombin	Serine protease
III	Tissue factor	Receptor/cofactor*
V	Labile factor	Cofactor
VII	Proconvertin	Serine protease
VIII	Antihaemophilic factor	Cofactor
IX	Christmas factor	Serine protease
X	Stuart–Prower factor	Serine protease
XI	Plasma thromboplastin antecedent	Serine protease
XII	Hageman (contact) factor	Serine protease
XIII	Fibrin-stabilizing factor	Transglutaminase
	Prekallikrein (Fletcher factor)	Serine protease
	HMWK (Fitzgerald factor)	Cofactor*

HMWK, high molecular weight kininogen.
* Active without proteolytic modification.

to ensure a localized and limited production. The generation of thombin is dependant on three enzyme complexes, each consisting of protease, cofactor, phospholipids (PL) and calcium. They are extrinsic Xase (VIIa, TF, PL, Ca^{2+}) and intrinsic Xase (IXa, VIIIa, PL, Ca^{2+}) generating FXa, prothrombinase complex (Xa, Va, PL, Ca^{2+}) generating thrombin. The generation of thrombin following vascular injury occurs in two waves of very different magnitude with different functions. During the initiation phase small amounts are generated (picomolar concentrations) which prepares the coagulation cascade for the second larger thrombin burst in the amplification when micromolar concentrations are produced, i.e. a million-fold higher concentration than produced during the initiation phase.

Initiation

Coagulation is initiated by the interaction of the membrane bound TF exposed by vascular injury, with plasma factor VIIa. One to two per cent of the total factor VII circulates in the activated form, but does not express proteolytic activity unless bound to TF. The factor VIIa-tissue factor (extrinsic factor Xase) complex activates both factor IX and factor X. The factor Xa, in the absence of its cofactor, forms small amounts of thrombin from prothrombin. This is insufficient to initiate significant fibrin polymerization, it activates the coenzymes, factor V and factor VIII, platelets and factor XI.

Amplification

The initiation pathway or extrinsic Xase is rapidly inactivated by TFPI which forms a quaternary complex of VIIa, TF, Xa and TFPI. The thrombin generation is now dependant on the traditional intrinsic pathway which has been primed by the small amounts of thrombin generated during initiation. In the amplification phase the intrinsic Xase formed by IXa and VIIIa on phospholipid surface in the presence of Ca^{2+} activates sufficient Xa which then in combination with Va, PL and Ca^{2+} forms the prothrombinase complex and results in the explosive generation of thrombin which acts on fibrinogen to form the fibrin clot.

In the 'classic' pathway formulated to explain *in vitro* coagulation testing, initiation of the pathway required contact reactions between factor XII, kallikrein and high molecular weight kininogen (HMWK) leading to the activation of factor XI. However, the lack of abnormal bleeding in individuals with hereditary deficiencies of these contact factors suggests that these reactions are not required for physiological coagulation *in vivo*.

Factor XI does not seem to have a role in the physiological initiation of coagulation. It has a

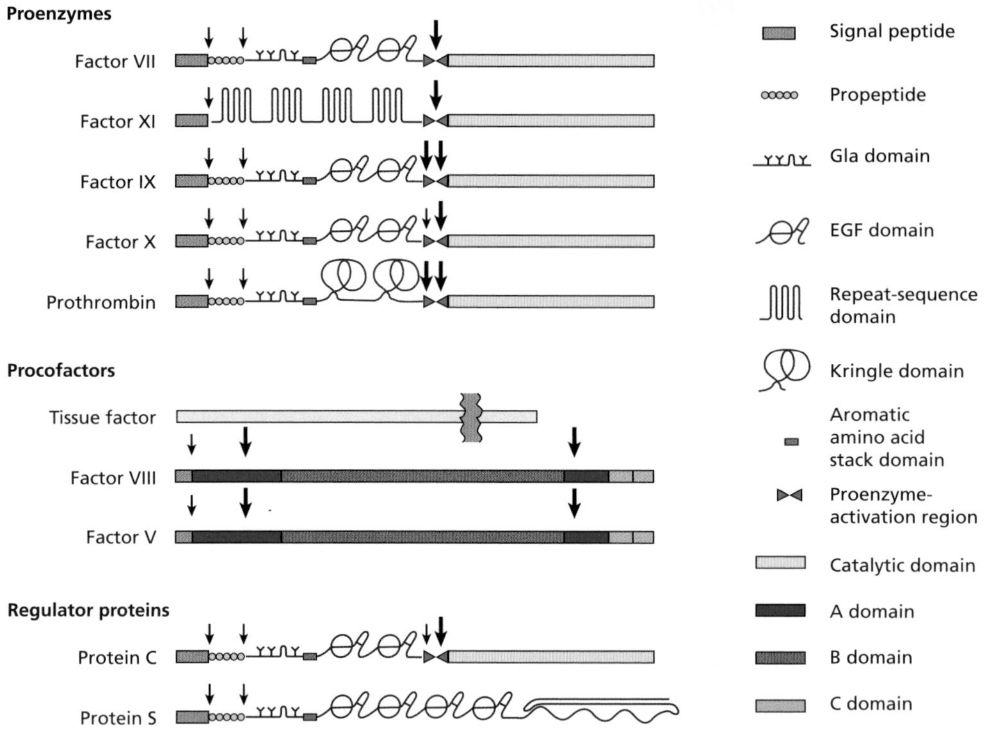

Fig. 22.9 Domains of the enzymes, receptors and cofactors involved in blood coagulation and regulation. The components of blood coagulation are proenzymes, procofactors and regulator proteins. The proenzymes, including protein C, contain a catalytic domain, an activation region and a signal peptide. The vitamin K-dependent proteins include a propeptide and a γ-carboxyglutamic acid (Gla) domain. Other important domains include the epidermal growth factor-like (EGF) domain, the kringle domain and the repeat-sequence domain. Tissue factor is an integral membrane protein unrelated to other known proteins. Factors V and VIII have marked similarities in structure. Sites of intracellular peptide bonds cleaved during synthesis are indicated by thin arrows, and sites of peptide bonds cleaved during protein activation are indicated by thick arrows. The transmembrane domain of tissue factor is shown within the phospholipid bilayer. (From B. Furie and B.C. Furie 1992, courtesy of the *New England Journal of Medicine* with permission.)

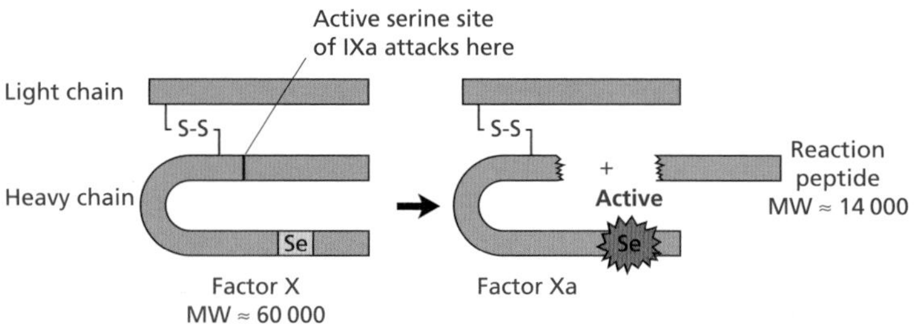

Fig. 22.10 Serine (Se) protease activity. This example shows the activation of factor X by factor IX.

supplementary role in the activation of factor IX (see above) and may be important at major sites of trauma or at operations and potentially causes excess bleeding in factor XI deficient individuals.

Thrombin hydrolyses fibrinogen, releasing fibrinopeptides A and B to form fibrin monomers (Fig. 22.11). Fibrin monomers link spontaneously by hydrogen bonds to form a loose insoluble fibrin

Table 22.2 The coagulation factors.

Factor	Plasma half-life (h)	Plasma concentration (mg/L)	Comments
II	65	100	Prothrombin group: vitamin K needed for synthesis; require Ca^{2+} for activation
VII	5	0.5	
IX	25	5	
X	40	10	
I	90	3000	Thrombin interacts with them; increase in inflammation, pregnancy, oral contraceptives
V	15	10	
VIII	10	0.1	
XI	45	5	
XII	50	30	

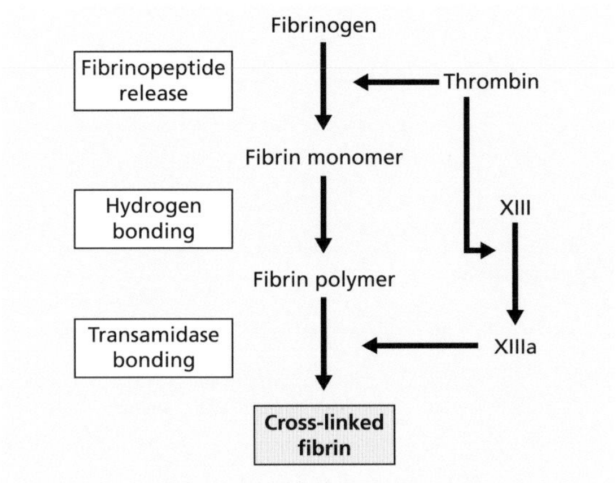

Fig. 22.11 The formation and stabilization of fibrin.

polymer. Factor XIII is also activated by thrombin together with calcium. Activated factor XIII stabilizes the fibrin polymers with the formation of covalent bond cross-links.

Fibrinogen has a MW 340 000 and consists of two identical subunits, each containing three dissimilar polypeptide chains (Aα, Bβ and γ) which are linked by disulphide bonds. After cleavage by thrombin of fibrinopeptides A and B, fibrin monomer consists of three paired α, β and γ chains.

Some of the properties of the coagulation factors are listed in Table 22.2. The activity of factors II, VII, IX and X is dependent upon vitamin K which is responsible for carboxylation of a number of terminal glutamic acid residues on each of these molecules (see Fig. 24.7).

The serine protease coagulation factors along with those of the fibrinolytic system (see below) have a high degree of homology and contain characteristic structural domains (Fig. 22.9), such as the kringles which are concerned with substrate binding and the carboxylated glutamic acid (Gla) residues which bind to phospholipid. There are also regions of homology with fibronectin (finger regions) and with epidermal growth factor. Although factor VIII and V cofactors are not protease enzymes, they circulate in a precursor form that requires limited cleavage by thrombin for expression of full cofactor activity.

Physiological limitation of blood coagulation

Unchecked blood coagulation would lead to dangerous occlusion of blood vessels (thrombosis) if the protective mechanisms of coagulation factor inhibitors, blood flow and fibrinolysis were not in operation.

Coagulation factor inhibitors

It is important that the effect of thrombin is limited to the site of injury. The first inhibitor to act is tissue factor pathway inhibitor (TFPI) which is synthesized in endothelial cells and is present in plasma and platelets and accumulates at the site of injury caused by local platelet activation. This inhibits Xa and VIIa and tissue factor to limit the main *in vivo* pathway by forming the quaternary complex. There is direct inactivation of thrombin and other serine protease factors by other circulating inhibitors of which antithrombin is the most potent. It inactivates serine proteases by combining with them by peptide bonding to form high molecular weight stable complexes

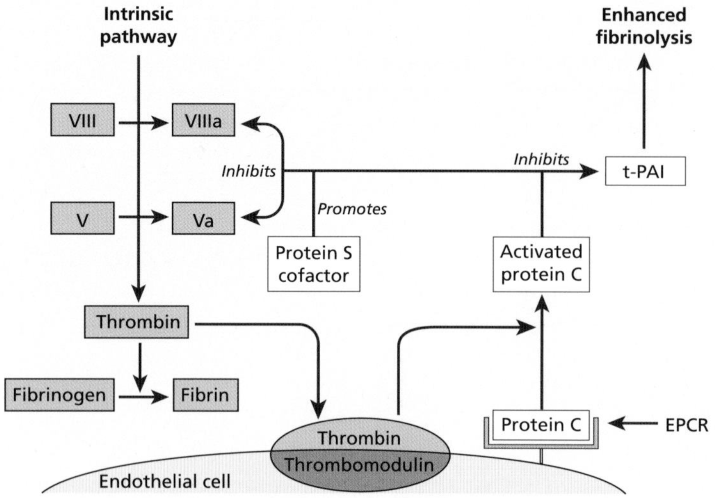

Fig. 22.12 Activation and action of protein C by thrombin which has bound to thrombomodulin on the endothelial cell surface. Protein S is a cofactor that facilitates binding of activated protein C to the platelet surface. The inactivation of factors Va and VIIIa results in the inhibition of blood coagulation. The inactivation of tissue plasminogen activator inhibitor (tPAI) enhances fibrinolysis. EPCR, endothelial protein C receptor.

(Fig. 25.6). Heparin potentiates its action markedly. Another protein, heparin cofactor II, also inhibits thrombin. α_2-Macroglobulins, α_2-antiplasmin, C_1 esterase inhibitor and α_1-antitrypsin also exert inhibitory effects on circulating serine proteases.

Protein C and protein S

These are inhibitors of coagulation cofactors V and VIII. Thrombin binds to an endothelial cell surface receptor, thrombomodulin. The resulting complex activates the vitamin K-dependent serine protease protein C which is able to destroy activated factors V and VIII, thus preventing further thrombin generation. The action of protein C is enhanced by another vitamin K-dependent protein, S, which binds protein C to the platelet surface (Fig. 22.12). An endothelial protein C receptor localizes protein C to the endothelial surface, promoting protein C activation by the thrombin–thrombomodulin complex (Fig. 22.12). In addition, activated protein C enhances fibrinolysis (Fig. 22.12).

As with other serine proteases, activated protein C is subject to inactivation by serum protease inactivators (serpins), e.g. antithrombin.

Blood flow

At the periphery of a damaged area of tissue, blood flow rapidly achieves a dilution and dispersal of activated factors before fibrin formation has occurred. Activated factors are destroyed by liver parenchymal cells and particulate matter is removed by liver Kupffer cells and other reticuloendothelial cells.

Fibrinolysis

Fibrinolysis (like coagulation) is a normal haemostatic response to vascular injury. Plasminogen, a β-globulin proenzyme in blood and tissue fluid, is converted to the serine protease plasmin by activators either from the vessel wall (intrinsic activation) or from the tissues (extrinsic activation) (Fig. 22.13). The most important route follows the release of tissue plasminogen activator (tPA) from endothelial cells. tPA is a serine protease that binds to fibrin. This enhances its capacity to convert thrombus-bound plasminogen into plasmin. This fibrin dependence of tPA action strongly localizes plasmin generation by tPA to the fibrin clot. Release of tPA

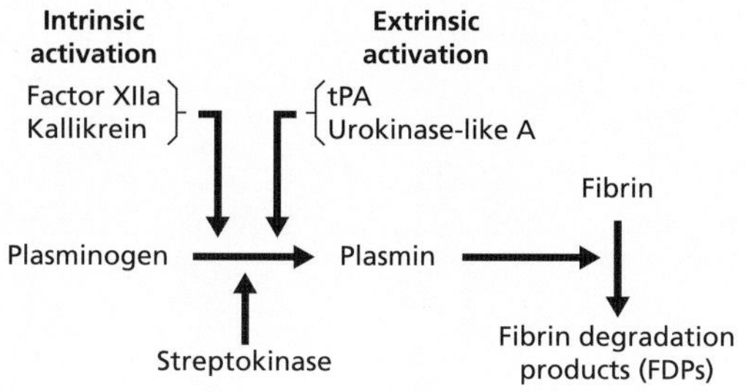

Fig. 22.13 The fibrinolytic system. tPA, tissue plasminogen activator.

occurs after such stimuli as trauma, exercise or emotional stress. Activated protein C stimulates fibrinolysis by destroying plasma inhibitors of tPA (Fig. 22.12). On the other hand, thrombin inhibits fibrinolysis by activating thrombin-activated fibrinolysis inhibitor (TAFI).

Plasmin generation at the site of injury limits the extent of the evolving thrombus. The split products of fibrinolysis are also competitive inhibitors of thrombin and fibrin polymerization. Normally, α_2-antiplasmin inhibits any local free plasmin.

Fibrinolytic agents are widely used in clinical practice (p. 317). Therapeutic recombinant tPA has been synthesized using recombinant DNA technology. The bacterial agent streptokinase is a peptide produced by haemolytic streptococci and forms a complex with plasminogen, which converts other plasminogen molecules to plasmin. Urokinase is a tPA initially isolated from human urine.

Plasmin is capable of digesting fibrinogen, fibrin, factors V and VIII and many other proteins. Cleavage of peptide bonds in fibrin and fibrinogen produces a variety of split (degradation) products (Fig. 22.13). Large amounts of the smallest fragments D and E can be detected in the plasma of patients with disseminated intravascular coagulation (p. 298).

Inactivation of plasmin

Tissue plasminogen activator is inactivated by plasminogen activator inhibitor (PAI). Circulating plasmin is inactivated by potent inhibitors α_2-antiplasmin and α_2-macroglobulin.

Endothelial cells

The endothelial cell has an active role in the maintenance of vascular integrity. This cell provides the basement membrane that normally separates collagen, elastin and fibronectin of the subendothelial connective tissue from the circulating blood (Fig. 22.8). Loss or damage to the endothelium results in both haemorrhage and activation of the haemostatic mechanism. The endothelial cell also has a potent inhibitory influence on the haemostatic response, largely through the synthesis of PGI_2 and NO, which have vasodilatatory properties and inhibit platelet aggregation. In contrast, endothelins are a family of vasoactive peptides that can activate fibrinolysis via the release of tPA. Synthesis of tissue factor which initiates haemostasis only occurs in endothelial cells following activation and its natural inhibitor, tFPI, is also synthesized. Synthesis of prostacyclin, VWF, plasminogen activator, antithrombin and thrombomodulin, the surface protein responsible for activation of protein C, provides agents that are vital to both platelet reactions and blood coagulation (Fig. 22.8).

Haemostatic response

Vasoconstriction

An immediate vasoconstriction of the injured vessel and reflex constriction of adjacent small arteries and arterioles is responsible for an initial slowing of blood flow to the area of injury. When there is widespread damage this vascular reaction prevents exsanguination. The reduced blood flow allows contact activation of platelets and coagulation factors. The vasoactive amines and thromboxane A_2 liberated from platelets, and the fibrinopeptides liberated during fibrin formation, also have vasoconstrictive activity (Fig. 22.1).

Platelet reactions and primary haemostatic plug formation

Following a break in the endothelial lining, there is an initial adherence of platelets to exposed connective tissue, potentiated by VWF. Collagen exposure and thrombin produced at the site of injury cause the adherent platelets to release their granule contents and also activate platelet prostaglandin synthesis leading to the formation of thromboxane A_2. Released ADP causes platelets to swell and aggregate. Additional platelets from the circulating blood are drawn to the area of injury. This continuing platelet aggregation promotes the growth of the haemostatic plug which soon covers the exposed connective tissue. The unstable primary haemostatic plug produced by these platelet reactions in the first minute or so following injury is usually sufficient to provide temporary control of bleeding. It seems likely that prostacyclin, produced by endothelial and smooth muscle cells in the vessel wall adjacent to the area of damage, is important in limiting the extent of the initial platelet plug.

Stabilization of the platelet plug by fibrin

Definitive haemostasis is achieved when fibrin formed by blood coagulation is added to the platelet mass and by platelet-induced clot retraction/compaction.

Following vascular injury, the formation of extrinsic Xase (VIIa, TF, PL and Ca^{2+}) initiates the coagulation cascade. Platelet aggregation and release reactions accelerate the coagulation process by providing abundant membrane phospholipid. Thrombin generated at the injury site converts soluble plasma fibrinogen into fibrin, potentiates platelet aggregation and secretion and also activates factor XI and XIII and cofactors V and VIII. The fibrin component of the haemostatic plug increases as the fused platelets autolyse and after a few hours the entire haemostatic plug is transformed into a solid mass of cross-linked fibrin. Nevertheless, because of incorporation of plasminogen and tPA (p. 273), this plug begins to autodigest during the same time frame.

Tests of haemostatic function

Defective haemostasis with abnormal bleeding may result from:

1 A vascular disorder;

2 Thrombocytopenia or a disorder of platelet function; or

3 Defective blood coagulation.

A number of simple tests are employed to assess the platelet, vessel wall and coagulation components of haemostasis.

Blood count and blood film examination

As thrombocytopenia is a common cause of abnormal bleeding, patients with suspected bleeding disorders should initially have a blood count including platelet count and blood film examination. In addition to establishing the presence of thrombocytopenia, the cause may be obvious (e.g. acute leukaemia).

Screening tests of blood coagulation

Screening tests provide an assessment of the 'extrinsic' and 'intrinsic' systems of blood coagulation and also the central conversion of fibrinogen to fibrin (Table 22.3).

The prothrombin time (PT) measures factors VII, X, V, prothrombin and fibrinogen. Tissue thromboplastin (a brain extract) and calcium are added to citrated plasma. The normal time for clotting is 10–14 s. It may be expressed as the international normalized ratio (INR) (p. 314).

The activated partial thromboplastin time (APTT) measures factors VIII, IX, XI and XII in addition to factors X, V, prothrombin and fibrinogen. Three substances—phospholipid, a surface activator (e.g. kaolin) and calcium—are added to citrated plasma. The normal time for clotting is approximately 30–40 s.

Prolonged clotting times in the PT and APTT because of factor deficiency are corrected by the addition of normal plasma to the test plasma (50 : 50 mix). If there is no correction or incomplete

Table 22.3 Screening tests used in the diagnosis of coagulation disorders.

Screening tests	Abnormalities indicated by prolongation	Most common cause of disorder
Thrombin time (TT)	Deficiency or abnormality of fibrinogen or inhibition of thrombin by heparin or FDPs	Disseminated intravascular coagulation Heparin therapy
Prothrombin time (PT)	Deficiency or inhibition of one or more of the following coagulation factors: VII, X, V, II, fibrinogen	Liver disease Warfarin therapy DIC
Activated partial thromboplastin time (APTT or PTTK)	Deficiency or inhibition of one or more of the following coagulation factors: XII, XI, IX (Christmas disease), VIII (haemophilia), X, V, II, fibrinogen	Haemophilia, Christmas disease (+ conditions above)
Fibrinogen quantitation	Fibrinogen deficiency	Disseminated intravascular coagulation, liver disease

FDPs, fibrin degradation products.

NB. Platelet count and the tests of platelet function are also used in screening patients with a bleeding disorder.

correction with normal plasma, the presence of an inhibitor of coagulation is suspected.

The thrombin (clotting) time (TT) is sensitive to a deficiency of fibrinogen or inhibition of thrombin. Diluted bovine thrombin is added to citrated plasma at a concentration giving a clotting time of 14–16 s with normal subjects.

Specific assays of coagulation factors

Most factor assays are based on an APTT or PT in which all factors except the one to be measured are present in the substrate plasma. This usually requires a supply of plasma from patients with hereditary deficiency of the factor in question or artificially produced factor-deficient plasma. The corrective effect of the unknown plasma on the prolonged clotting time of the deficient substrate plasma is then compared with the corrective effect of normal plasma. Results are expressed as a percentage of normal activity.

A number of chemical, chromogenic and immunological methods are available for quantification of other proteins such as fibrinogen, VWF and factor VIII. Factor XIII activity can be assessed by testing for clot solubility in urea.

Bleeding time

The bleeding time is a useful test for abnormal platelet function including the diagnosis of VWF deficiency. It has largely been replaced by the platelet function analysis-100 (PFA-100) test (see below). It will be prolonged in thrombocytopenia but is normal in vascular causes of abnormal bleeding. The test involves the application of pressure to the upper arm with a blood pressure cuff, after which small incisions are made in the flexor surface forearm skin. Bleeding stops normally in 3–8 min.

Tests of platelet function

The most valuable investigation is platelet aggregometry which measures the fall in light absorbance in platelet-rich plasma as platelets aggregate. Initial (primary) aggregation is caused by an external agent, the secondary response to aggregating agents released from the platelets themselves. The five external aggregating agents most commonly used are ADP, collagen, ristocetin, arachidonic acid and adrenaline. The pattern of response to each agent helps to make the diagnosis (see Fig. 23.1). Flow cytometry is now increasingly used in routine practice to identify platelet glyoprotein defects.

In the PFA-100 test, citrated blood is aspirated through a capillary tube onto a membrane coated with collagen/ADP or collagen/adrenaline. Blood flow is maintained. Platelets begin to adhere and aggregate, primarily via VWF interactions with GPIb and GPIIb/IIIa, resulting in occlusion of the aperture.

The PFA-100 analysis may give false negative results with relatively common platelet defects. Full platelet function tests and VWF screening may be required to exclude abnormal platelet function, even if the PFA-100 test is normal.

Test of fibrinolysis

Increased levels of circulating plasminogen activator may be detected by demonstrating shortened euglobulin clot lysis times. A number of immunological methods are available to detect fibrinogen or fibrin degradation products (including D-dimers) in serum. In patients with enhanced fibrinolysis, low levels of circulating plasminogen may be detected.

Bibliography

Aird W.C. (2003) Endothelial cell heterogeneity. *Crit Care Med* **31**,S221–30.

Dahlback B. and Villoutreic B.O. (2003) Molecular recognition in the protein C anticoagulant pathway. *J Thromb Haemost* **1**,1525–34.

Harrison P. (2005) The role of PFA-100 testing in the investigation and management of haemostatic defects in children and adults. *Br J Haematol* **130**,3–10.

Italiano J.E. Jr. and Shivdasani R.A. (2003) Megakaryocytes and beyond: the birth of platelets. *J Thromb Haemost* **1**,1174–82.

Kemball-Cook, G., Tuddenham E.G.D., McVey J.H. (2005) Normal haemostasis. In: Hoffbrand A.V., Catovsky D., Tuddenham E. (eds) *Postgraduate Haematology*, 5th edn. Blackwell Publishing, Oxford: pp. 783–801.

Michelson A.D. (ed.) (2002) *Platelets*. Academic Press, San Diego, CA.

Watson, S.P. and Harrison P. (2005) The vascular function of platelets. In: Hoffbrand A.V., Catovsky D., Tuddenham E. (eds) *Postgraduate Haematology*, 5th edn. Blackwell Publishing, Oxford: pp. 808–824.

CHAPTER 23

23 Bleeding disorders caused by vascular and platelet abnormalities

Abnormal bleeding may result from:
1 Vascular disorders;
2 Thrombocytopenia;
3 Defective platelet function; or
4 Defective coagulation.
The pattern of bleeding is relatively predictable depending on the aetiology. Vascular and platelet disorders tend to be associated with bleeding from mucous membranes and into the skin whereas in coagulation disorders the bleeding is often into joints or soft tissue (Table 23.1).

The first three categories are discussed in this chapter and the disorders of blood coagulation follow in Chapter 24.

Table 23.1 Clinical differences between diseases of platelets/vessel walls or coagulation factors.

Finding	Platelet/vessel walls	Coagulation
Mucosal bleeding	Common	Rare
Petechiae	Common	Rare
Deep haematomas	Rare	Characteristic
Bleeding from skin cuts	Persistent	Minimal
Sex of patient	Equal	>80% male

Vascular bleeding disorders

The vascular disorders are a heterogeneous group of conditions characterized by easy bruising and spontaneous bleeding from the small vessels. The underlying abnormality is either in the vessels themselves or in the perivascular connective tissues. Most cases of bleeding caused by vascular defects alone are not severe. Frequently, the bleeding is mainly in the skin causing petechiae, ecchymoses or both (Fig. 23.1). In some disorders there is also bleeding from mucous membranes. In these conditions the standard screening tests are normal. The bleeding time is normal and the other tests of haemostasis are also normal. Vascular defects may be inherited or acquired.

Inherited vascular disorders

Hereditary haemorrhagic telangiectasia

In this uncommon disorder, which is transmitted as an autosomal dominant trait. There are dilated microvascular swellings which appear during childhood and become more numerous in adult life. These telangiectasia develop in the skin, mucous membranes (Fig. 23.1a) and internal organs. Pulmonary and cerebral arteriovenous malformations are seen in a minority of cases. Recurrent epistaxes are frequent and recurrent gastrointestinal tract haemorrhage

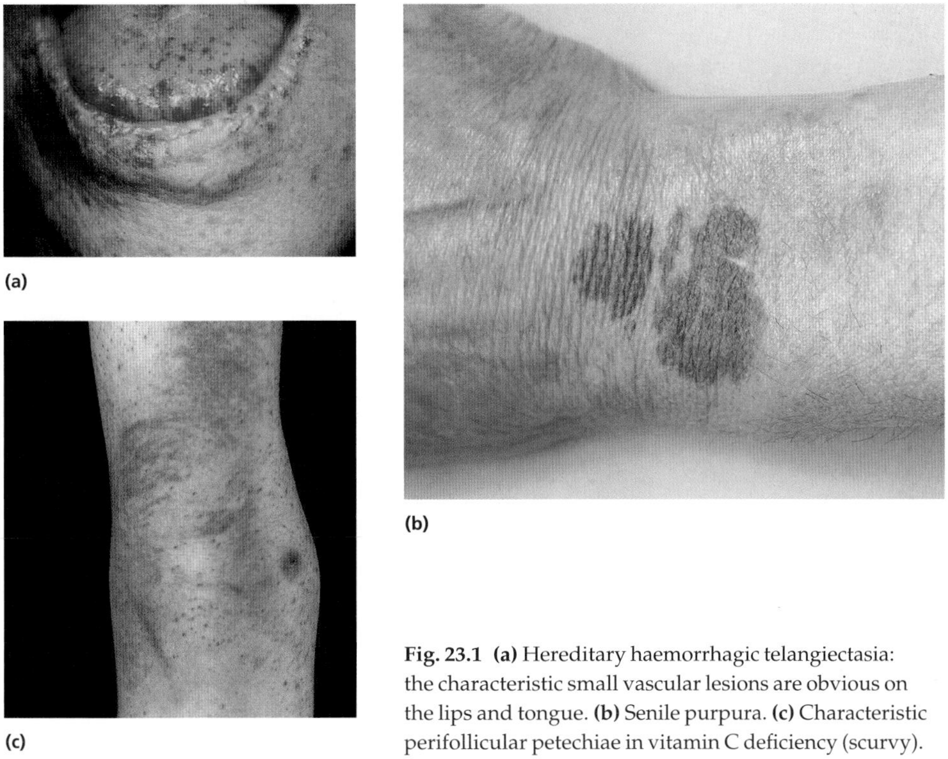

Fig. 23.1 **(a)** Hereditary haemorrhagic telangiectasia: the characteristic small vascular lesions are obvious on the lips and tongue. **(b)** Senile purpura. **(c)** Characteristic perifollicular petechiae in vitamin C deficiency (scurvy).

may cause chronic iron deficiency anaemia. Treatment is with embolization, laser treatment, oestrogens, tranexamic acid and iron supplementation.

Connective tissue disorders

In the Ehlers–Danlos syndrome there are hereditary collagen abnormalities with purpura resulting from defective platelet aggregation, hyperextensibility of joints and hyperelastic friable skin. Pseudoxanthoma elasticum is associated with arterial haemorrhage and thrombosis. Mild cases may present with superficial bruising and purpura following minor trauma.

Giant cavernous haemangioma

These congenital malformations occasionally cause chronic activation of coagulation leading to laboratory features of disseminated intravascular coagulation (DIC) and in some cases thrombocytopenia.

Acquired vascular defects

1 Simple easy bruising is a common benign disorder which occurs in otherwise healthy women, especially those of child-bearing age.

2 Senile purpura caused by atrophy of the supporting tissues of cutaneous blood vessels is seen mainly on dorsal aspects of the forearms and hands (Fig. 23.1b).

3 Purpura associated with infections. Many bacterial, viral or rickettsial infections may cause purpura from vascular damage by the organism or as a result of immune complex formation (e.g. measles, dengue fever or meningococcal septicaemia).

4 The Henoch–Schönlein syndrome is usually seen in children and often follows an acute upper respiratory tract infection. It is an immunoglobulin A (IgA)-mediated vasculitis. The characteristic purpuric rash accompanied by localized oedema and itching is usually most prominent on the buttocks and extensor surfaces of the lower legs and elbows (Fig. 23.2). Painful joint swelling, haematuria and abdominal pain may also occur. It is usually a self-limiting condition but occasional patients develop renal failure.

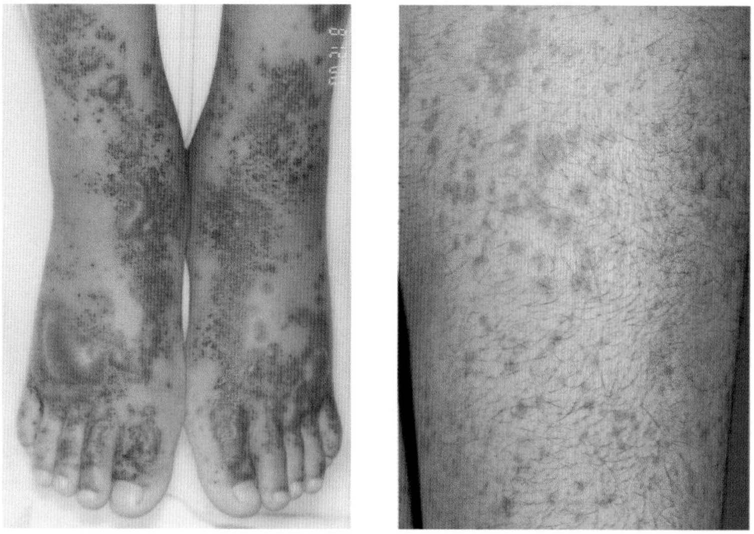

(a) (b)

Fig. 23.2 Henoch–Schönlein purpura: **(a)** unusually severe purpura on legs with bullous formation in a 6-year-old child; and **(b)** early urticarial lesions.

5 Scurvy. In vitamin C deficiency, defective collagen may cause perifollicular petechiae, bruising and mucosal haemorrhage (Fig. 23.1c).

6 Steroid purpura. The purpura, which is associated with long-term steroid therapy or Cushing's syndrome, is caused by defective vascular supportive tissue.

Tranexamic acid and aminocaproic acid are useful antifibrinolytic drugs that may reduce bleeding resulting from vascular disorders or thrombocytopenia but are contraindicated in the presence of haematuria because they might lead to clots obstructing the renal tract.

Thrombocytopenia

Abnormal bleeding associated with thrombocytopenia or abnormal platelet function is characterized by spontaneous skin purpura (Fig. 23.3) and mucosal haemorrhage and prolonged bleeding after

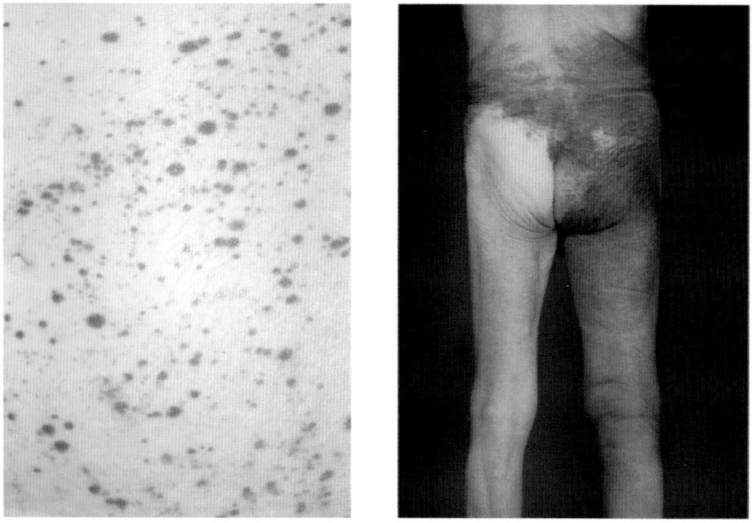

(a) (b)

Fig. 23.3 **(a)** Typical purpura; and **(b)** massive subcutaneous haemorrhage in a patient with drug-induced thrombocytopenia.

Table 23.2 Causes of thrombocytopenia.

Failure of platelet production
Selective megakaryocyte depression
rare congenital defects
drugs, chemicals, viral infections
Part of general bone marrow failure
cytotoxic drugs
radiotherapy
aplastic anaemia
leukaemia
myelodysplastic syndromes
myelofibrosis
marrow infiltration (e.g. carcinoma, lymphoma)
multiple myeloma
megaloblastic anaemia
HIV infection
Increased consumption of platelets
Immune
autoimmune
idiopathic
associated with systemic lupus erythematosus, chronic lymphocytic leukaemia or lymphoma
infections: HIV, other viruses, malaria
drug-induced
heparin
post-transfusional purpura
feto-maternal alloimmune thrombocytopenia
Disseminated intravascular coagulation
Thrombotic thrombocytopenic purpura
Abnormal distribution of platelets
Splenomegaly
Dilutional loss
Massive transfusion of stored blood to bleeding patients

HIV, human immunodeficiency virus.

Table 23.3 Thrombocytopenia as a result of drugs or toxins.

Bone marrow suppression
Predictable (dose-related)
ionizing radiation, cytotoxic drugs, ethanol
Occasional
chloramphenicol, co-trimoxazole, idoxuridine, penicillamine, organic arsenicals, benzene, etc.
Immune mechanisms (proven or probable)
Analgesics, anti-inflammatory drugs, gold salts
Antimicrobials
penicillins, rifamycin, sulphonamides, trimethoprim, para-aminosalicylate
Sedatives, anticonvulsants
diazepam, sodium valproate, carbamazepine
Diuretics
acetazolamide, chlorathiazides, frusemide
Antidiabetics
chlorpropamide, tolbutamide
Others
digitoxin, heparin, methyldopa, oxyprenolol, quinine, quinidine
Platelet aggregation
Ristocetin, heparin (p. 313)

trauma (Table 23.1). The main causes of thrombocytopenia are listed in Tables 23.2 and 23.3.

Failure of platelet production

This is the most common cause of thrombocytopenia and is usually part of a generalized bone marrow failure (Table 23.2). Selective megakaryocyte depression may result from drug toxicity or viral infection. Rarely, it is congenital as a result of mutation of the c-MPL thrombopoietin receptor, in association with absent radii, or in May–Hegglin anomaly, with large inclusions in granulocytes, or Wiskott–Aldrich syndrome (WAS) with eczema and immune deficiency. Diagnosis of these causes of thrombocytopenia is made from the clinical history, peripheral blood count, the blood film and bone marrow examination.

Increased destruction of platelets

Autoimmune (idiopathic) thrombocytopenic purpura

Autoimmune (idiopathic) thrombocytopenic purpura (ITP) may be divided into chronic and acute forms.

Chronic idiopathic thrombocytopenic purpura

This is a relatively common disorder. The highest incidence has been considered to be in women aged 15–50 years although some reports suggest an increasing incidence with age. It is the most common cause of thrombocytopenia without anaemia or neutropenia. It is usually idiopathic but may

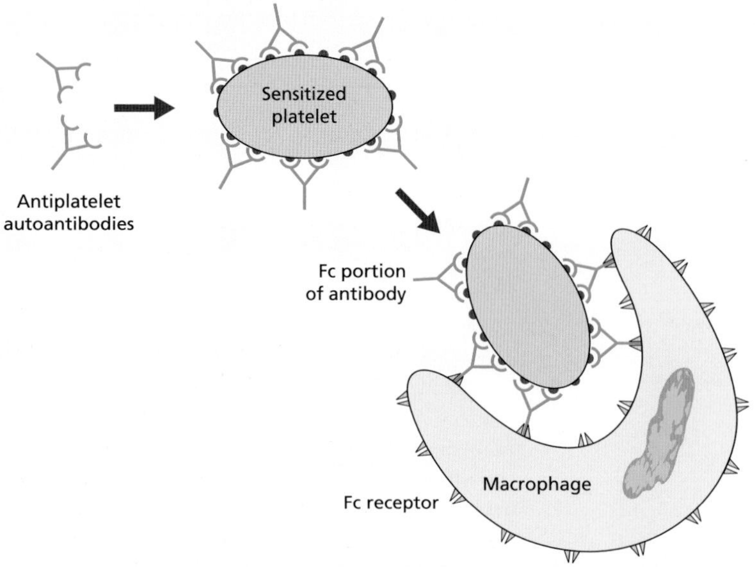

Fig. 23.4 The pathogenesis of thrombocytopenia in autoimmune thrombocytopenic purpura.

be seen in association with other diseases such as systemic lupus erythematosus (SLE), human immunodeficiency virus (HIV) infection, chronic lymphocytic leukaemia (CLL), Hodgkin's disease or autoimmune haemolytic anaemia (Table 23.2).

Pathogenesis

Platelet autoantibodies (usually IgG) result in the premature removal specific to platelets from the circulation by macrophages of the reticuloendothelial system, especially the spleen (Fig. 23.4). In many cases, the antibody is directed against antigen sites on the glycoprotein (GP) IIb–IIIa or Ib complex. The normal lifespan of a platelet is 7–10 days but in ITP this is reduced to a few hours. Total megakaryocyte mass and platelet turnover are increased in parallel to approximately five times normal.

Clinical features

The onset is often insidious with petechial haemorrhage, easy bruising and, in women, menorrhagia. Mucosal bleeding (e.g. epistaxes or gum bleeding) occurs in severe cases but fortunately intracranial haemorrhage is rare. The severity of bleeding in ITP is usually less than that seen in patients with comparable degrees of thrombocytopenia from bone marrow failure; this is attributed to the circulation of predominantly young, functionally superior platelets in ITP. Chronic ITP tends to relapse and remit spontaneously so the course may be difficult to predict. Many asymtomatic cases are discovered by a routine blood count.

The spleen is not palpable unless there is an associated disease causing splenomegaly.

Diagnosis

1 The platelet count is usually $10–50 \times 10^9/L$. The haemoglobin concentration and white cell count are typically normal unless there is iron deficiency anaemia because of blood loss.

2 The blood film shows reduced numbers of platelets, those present often being large.

3 The bone marrow shows normal or increased numbers of megakaryocytes.

4 Sensitive tests are able to demonstrate specific antiglycoprotein GPIIb/IIIa or GPIb antibodies on the platelet surface or in the serum in most patients. Platelet-associated IgG assays are less specific.

Treatment

As this is a chronic disease the aim of treatment should be to maintain a platelet count above the level at which spontaneous bruising or bleeding

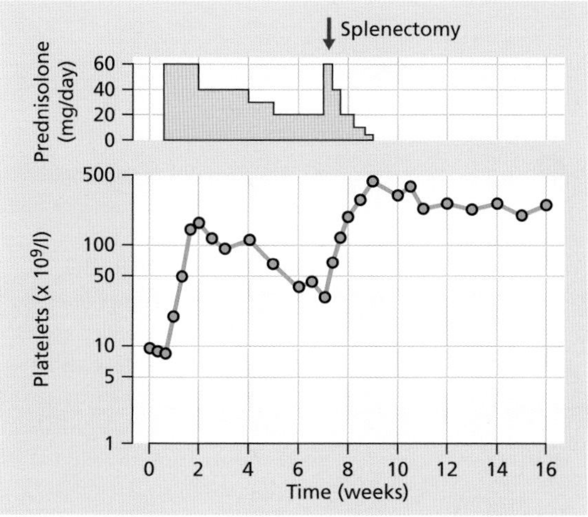

Fig. 23.5 Response to prednisolone in chronic immune thrombocytopenic purpura with subsequent relapse and response to splenectomy.

occurs with the minimum of intervention. In general, a platelet count above 50×10^9/L does not require treatment.

1 *Corticosteroids* Eighty per cent of patients remit on high-dose corticosteroid therapy. Prednisolone 1 mg/kg/day is the usual initial therapy in adults and the dosage is gradually reduced after 10–14 days. In poor responders the dosage is reduced more slowly but splenectomy or alternative immunosuppression is considered.

2 *Splenectomy* (Fig. 23.5) This operation is recommended in patients who have symptoms and still have platelets $<30 \times 10^9$/L after 3 months of steroid therapy or who require unacceptably high doses of steroids to maintain a platelet count above 30×10^9/L. Good results occur in most of the patients, but in patients with ITP refractory to steroids or immunoglobulin there may be little benefit. Splenunculi must be removed otherwise subsequent relapse of ITP can occur.

3 *High-dose intravenous immunoglobulin therapy* is able to produce a rapid rise in platelet count in the majority of patients. A regimen of 400 mg/kg/day for 5 days or 1 g/kg/day for 2 days is recommended. It is particularly useful in patients with life-threatening haemorrhage, in steroid-refractory ITP, during pregnancy or prior to surgery. The mechanism of action may be blockage of Fc receptors on macrophages or modification of autoantibody production.

4 *Immunosuppressive drugs* (e.g. vincristine, cyclophosphamide, azathioprine, mycophenolate mofetil or ciclosporin alone or in combination) are usually reserved for those patients who do not respond sufficiently to steroids and splenectomy.

5 *Monoclonal antibody* Rituximab (anti-CD20) produces responses in approximately 50%, which are often durable.

6 *Other treatments* that may elicit a remission include danazol (an androgen which may virilize in women) and intravenous anti-D immunoglobulin. It is often necessary to combine two drugs (e.g. danazol and an immunosuppressive agent).

7 *Platelet transfusions* Platelet concentrates are beneficial in patients with acute life-threatening bleeding. Their benefit will only last a few hours.

8 *Stem cell transplatation* has cured some severe cases.

Acute idiopathic thrombocytopenic purpura

This is most common in children. In approximately 75% of patients the episode follows vaccination or an infection such as chickenpox or infectious mononucleosis. Most cases are caused by non-specific immune complex attachments. Spontaneous remissions are usual but in 5–10% of cases the disease becomes chronic (lasting >6 months). Fortunately, morbidity and mortality in acute ITP is very low.

The diagnosis is one of exclusion and there is debate as to the need for bone marrow aspiration. If the platelet count is over 30×10^9/L no treatment is necessary unless the bleeding is severe. Those with counts below 20×10^9/L may be treated with steroids and/or intravenous immunoglobulin, especially if there is significant bleeding.

Infections

It seems likely that the thrombocytopenia associated with many viral and protozoal infections is immune-mediated. In HIV infection, reduced platelet production is also involved (p. 328).

Post-transfusion purpura

Thrombocytopenia occurring approximately 10 days after a blood transfusion has been attributed to antibodies in the recipient developing against the human

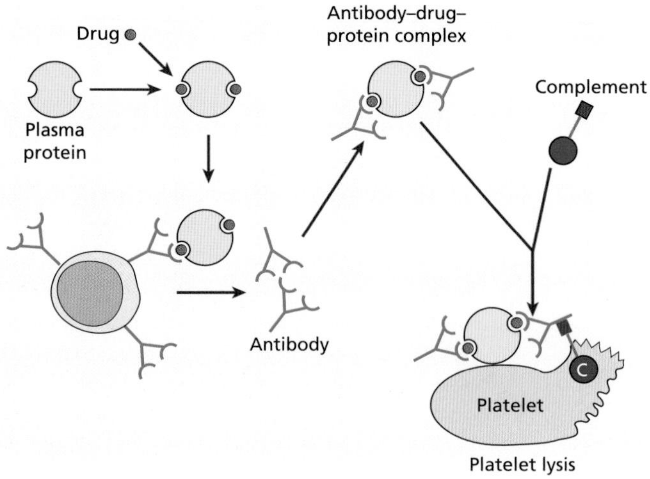

Fig. 23.6 Usual type of platelet damage caused by drugs in which an antibody–drug–protein complex is deposited on the platelet surface. If complement is attached and the sequence goes to completion, the platelet may be lysed directly. Otherwise it is removed by reticuloendothelial cells because of opsonization with immunoglobulin and/or the C3 component of complement.

platelet antigen-1a (HPA-1a) (absent from the patient's own platelets) on transfused platelets. The reason why the patient's own platelets are then destroyed is unknown. Treatment is with intravenous immunoglobulin, plasma exchange or corticosteroids.

Drug-induced immune thrombocytopenia

An immunological mechanism has been demonstrated as the cause of many drug-induced thrombocytopenias (Fig. 23.6). Quinine (including that in tonic water), quinidine and heparin are particularly common causes (Table 23.3).

The platelet count is often less than $10 \times 10^9/L$, and the bone marrow shows normal or increased numbers of megakaryocytes. Drug-dependent antibodies against platelets may be demonstrated in the sera of some patients. The immediate treatment is to stop all suspected drugs but platelet concentrates should be given to patients with dangerous bleeding.

Thrombotic thrombocytopenic purpura and haemolytic uraemic syndrome

Thrombotic thrombocytopenic purpura (TTP) occurs in familial or acquired forms. There is deficiency of a ADAMTS13 metalloprotease which breaks down ultra large von Willebrand factor multimers (ULVWF) (Fig. 23.7). In the familial forms more than 50 ADAMTS13 mutations have been reported whereas in acquired forms it follows the development of an inhibitory IgG autoantibody, the presence of which may be stimulated by infection, autoimmune/connective tissue disease, certain drugs, stem cell transplantation or cardiac surgery. ULVWF multimeric strings secreted from Weibel–Palade bodies are anchored to the endothelial cells, and passing platelets adhere via their GPIbα receptors. Increasing platelet aggregation onto the ULVWF multimeric strings has the potential to form large, occlusive, platelet thrombi. These strings are capable of emobolising to microvessels downstream contributing to organ ischemia (Fig. 23.8). In the closely related haemolytic uraemic syndrome (HUS) ADAMTS13 levels are normal.

TTP has traditionally been described as pentad of thrombocytopenia, microangiopathic hamolytic anaemia, neurologic abnormalities, renal failure and fever. The microvascular thrombosis causes variable degrees of tissue ischaemia and infarction and is responsible for the microangiopathic haemolytic anaemia and thrombocytopenia. In current clinical practice, thombocytopenia, schistocytosis, and an impressively elevated serum lactate dehydrogenase (LDH) value are sufficient to suggest the diagnosis. The serum LDH is derived both from ischaemic or necrotic tissue cells and lysed red cells. Coagulation tests are normal in contrast to the findings in DIC (Fig. 24.8). The serum LDH is raised. ADAMTS13 is absent or severly reduced in plasma. Treatment is with plasma exchange, using fresh frozen plasma (FFP) or cryosupernatant. This removes the large molecular weight VWF multimers and the antibody and provides ADAMTS13.

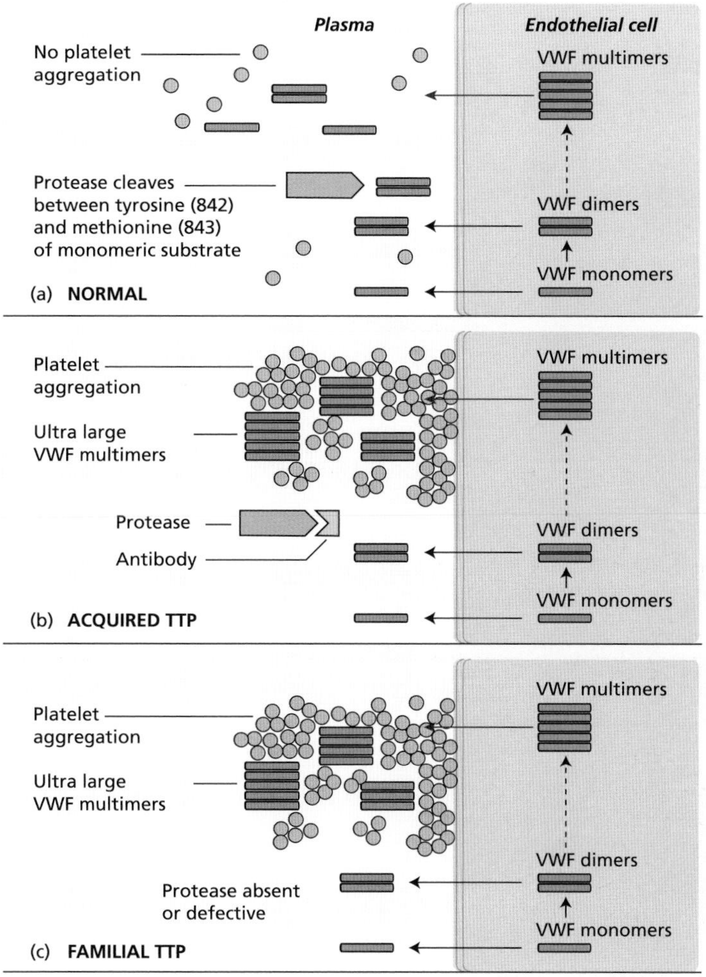

Fig. 23.7 Proposed pathogenesis of thrombotic thrombocytopenic purpura (TTP). Von Willebrand factor (VWF) consists of a series of VWF multimers each of molecular weight (MW) 250 kDa which are covalently linked. **(a)** Under physiological circumstances a metalloprotease ADAMTS13 cleaves high molecular weight multimers at a Tyr-842–Met-843 bond and the resulting VWF has an MW of 500–20 000 kDa. **(b)** In non-familial TTP, an antibody develops to the metalloprotease and so blocks cleavage of VWF multimers. **(c)** In congenital forms of TTP, the protease appears to be absent. In both cases, the resultant ultra large VWF multimers can bind platelets under high shear stress conditions and lead to platelet aggregation.

The platelet count and serum LDH are useful for monitoring the response to treatment. More recently, rituximab (anti-CD20) has been found effective in therapy, used in conjunction with plasma infusions or with plasma exhange. In refractory cases and chronic relapsing cases, high-dose corticosteroids, vincristine, intravenous immunoglobulin, rituximab and immunosuppressive therapy with azathioprine or cyclophosphamide have been used. In untreated cases mortality may approach 90%. Relapses are frequent.

HUS in children has many common features but organ damage is limited to the kidneys. There is also usually diarrhoea. Fits are frequent. Many cases are associated with *Escherichia coli* infection with verotoxin 0157 or with other organisms, especially *Shigella*. Supportive renal dialysis and control of hypertension and fits are the mainstays of treatment. Platelet transfusions are contraindicated in HUS and TTP.

Disseminated intravascular coagulation

Thrombocytopenia may result from an increased rate of platelet destruction through consumption of platelets because of their participation in DIC (p. 298).

Increased splenic pooling

The major factor responsible for thrombocytopenia in splenomegaly is platelet 'pooling' by the spleen. In splenomegaly, up to 90% of platelets may be

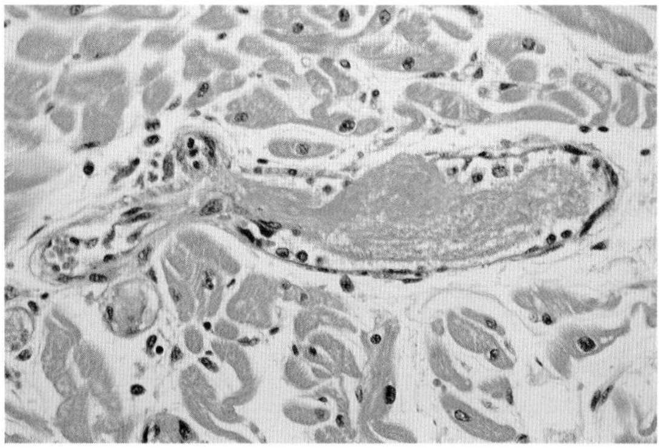

(a)

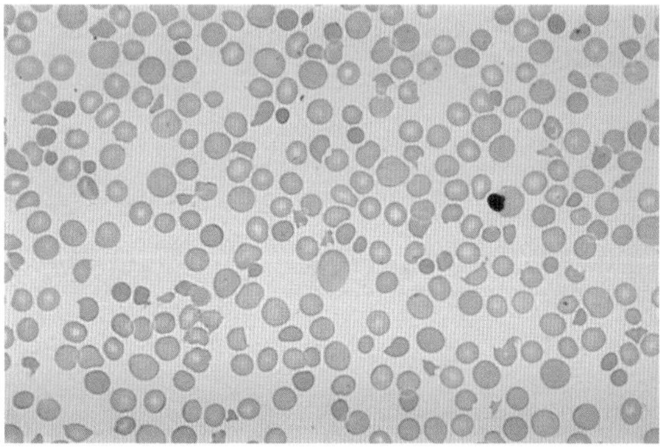

(b)

Fig. 23.8 Thrombotic thrombocytopenic purpura. **(a)** Platelet thrombus in a small cardiac vessel with minor endothelial and inflammatory reaction. (Courtesy of Dr J.E. McLaughlin) **(b)** Peripheral blood film showing red cell fragmentation.

sequestered in the spleen whereas normally this accounts for approximately one-third of the total platelet mass (Fig. 23.9). Platelet lifespan is normal and in the absence of additional haemostatic defects, the thrombocytopenia of splenomegaly is not usually associated with bleeding.

Massive transfusion syndrome

Platelets are unstable in blood stored at 4°C and the platelet count rapidly falls in blood stored for more than 24 h. Patients transfused with massive amounts of stored blood (more than 10 units over a 24-h period) frequently show abnormal clotting and thrombocytopenia. These should be corrected by the use of platelet transfusions and FFP.

Disorders of platelet function

Disorders of platelet function are suspected in patients who show skin and mucosal haemorrhage and in whom the bleeding time is prolonged despite a normal platelet count. These disorders may be hereditary or acquired.

Hereditary disorders

Rare inherited disorders may produce defects at each of the different phases of the platelet reactions leading to the formation of the haemostatic platelet plug.

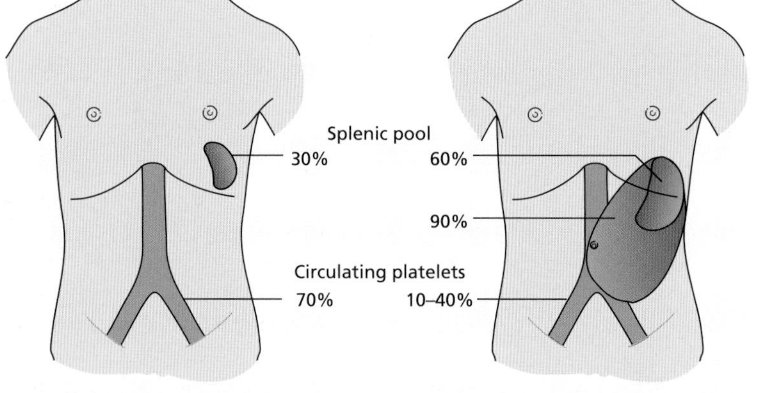

Fig. 23.9 The platelet distribution between the circulation and spleen in normal individuals (left), and in patients with moderate or massive splenomegaly (right).

Thrombasthenia (Glanzmann's disease)
This autosomal recessive disorder leads to failure of primary platelet aggregation because of a deficiency of membrane GPIIb (gene on chromosome 17). It usually presents in the neonatal period and, characteristically, platelets fail to aggregate *in vitro* to any agonist except ristocetin.

Bernard–Soulier syndrome
In this disease the platelets are larger than normal and there is a deficiency of GPIb (chromosome 23). There is defective binding to VWF, defective adherence to exposed subendothelial connective tissues and platelets do not aggregate with ristocetin. There is a variable degree of thrombocytopenia.

Storage pool diseases
In the rare grey platelet syndrome, the platelets are larger than normal and there is a virtual absence of α granules with deficiency of their proteins. In the more common β-storage pool disease there is a deficiency of dense granules.

Platelet function is abnormal in von Willebrand disease because of an inherited defect in VWF (p. 295).

Acquired disorders

Antiplatelet drugs
Aspirin therapy is the most common cause of defective platelet function. It produces an abnormal bleeding time and, although purpura may not be obvious, the defect may contribute to the associated gastrointestinal haemorrhage. The cause of the aspirin defect is inhibition of cyclo-oxygenase with impaired thromboxane A_2 synthesis (see Fig. 25.8). There is consequent impairment of the release reaction and aggregation with adrenaline and adenosine diphosphate (ADP). After a single dose the defect lasts 7–10 days, i.e. the life of the platelet. Aspirin is contraindicated in patients with gastrointestinal or genitourinary bleeding, retinal bleeding, peptic ulcer, haemophilia or severe hypertension. Dipyridamole inhibits platelet aggregation by blocking reuptake of adenosine and is usually used as an adjunct to oral anticoagulants. Clopidogrel inhibits binding of ADP to its platelet receptor and is mainly used for prevention of thrombotic events (e.g. after coronary stenting or angioplasty) in patients with a history of symptomatic atherosclerotic disease. Intravenous agents abciximab, eptifibatide and tirofiban are inhibitors of GPIIb/IIIa receptor sites and may be used in patients undergoing percutaneous coronary intervention with unstable angina and acute coronary syndromes. There is a risk of transient thrombocytopenia with these agents, especially with abciximab, and platelet transfusions may be needed.

Hyperglobulinaemia
Hyperglobulinaemia associated with multiple myeloma or Waldenström's disease may cause interference with platelet adherence, release and aggregation.

Myeloproliferative and myelodysplastic disorders
Intrinsic abnormalities of platelet function occur in many patients with essential thrombocythaemia and other myeloproliferative and myelodysplastic diseases and in paroxysmal nocturnal haemoglobinuria.

Uraemia
This is associated with various abnormalities of platelet function. Heparin, dextrans, alcohol and radiographic contrast agents may also cause defective function.

Diagnosis of platelet disorders

Patients with suspected platelet or blood vessel abnormalities should initially have a blood count and blood film examination (Fig. 23.10). Bone marrow examination is often needed in thrombocytopenic patients to determine whether or not there is a failure of platelet production. The marrow may also reveal one of the conditions associated with defective production (Table 23.2). In children and young adults with isolated thrombocytopenia, the marrow test is often not performed. In the elderly, the test is needed particularly to exclude myelodysplasia. In patients with thrombocytopenia, a negative drug history, normal or excessive numbers of marrow megakaryocytes and no other marrow abnormality or splenomegaly, ITP is the usual

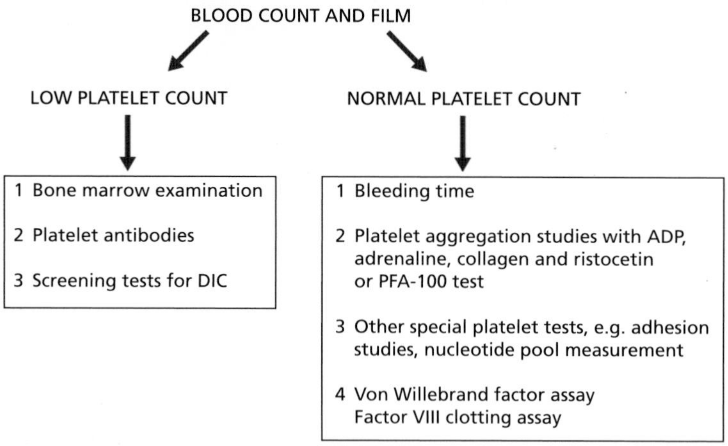

Fig. 23.10 Laboratory tests for platelet disorders. NB. Some intrinsic platelet functional disorders are associated with thrombocytopenia (e.g. Bernard–Soulier syndrome). ADP, adenosine diphosphate; DIC, disseminated intravascular coagulation.

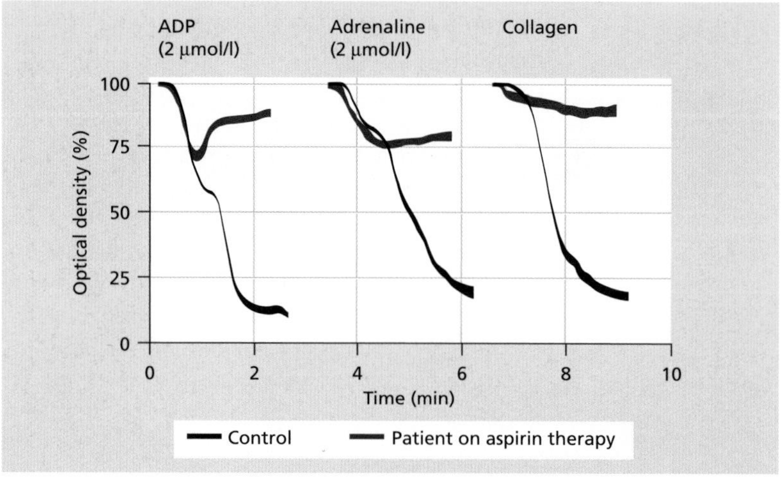

Fig. 23.11 Defective platelet aggregation in a patient on aspirin therapy. There is no secondary phase aggregation with adenosine diphosphate (ADP) and reduced responses to both adrenaline and collagen. Similar results are obtained in α-storage granule deficiency and cyclo-oxygenase deficiency.

diagnosis. Testing for platelet antibodies in serum or on the surface of platelets has not proved reliable in distinguishing ITP from other causes of thrombocytopenia. Screening tests for DIC are also useful, as are tests for an underlying disease (e.g. SLE or HIV infection).

When the blood count, including platelet count and blood film examination, are normal, a PFA-100 (platelet function analysis) or, much less frequently, a bleeding time is used to detect abnormal platelet function. In most patients with abnormal platelet function demonstrated by prolonged bleeding time, or the PFA-100 test, the defect is acquired and associated either with systemic disease (e.g. uraemia) or with aspirin therapy. The very rare hereditary defects of platelet function require more elaborate *in vitro* tests to define the specific abnormality. These include platelet aggregation studies (Fig. 23.11) and nucleotide pool measurements. If von Willebrand disease is suspected, assay of VWF and coagulation factor VIII are required.

Platelet transfusions

Transfusion of platelet concentrates are indicated in the following circumstances:

1 Thrombocytopenia or abnormal platelet function when bleeding or before invasive procedures and there is no alternative therapy available (e.g. steroids or high-dose immunoglobulin). The platelet count should be above $50 \times 10^9/L$ before, for example, liver biopsy or lumbar puncture.

2 Prophylactically in patients with platelet counts of less than $5–10 \times 10^9/L$. If there is infection, potential bleeding sites or coagulopathy, the count should be kept above $20 \times 10^9/L$).

The indications for transfusion of platelet concentrates are discussed further on p. 349.

Bibliography

Balduini C.L., Cattaneo M., Fabris F. *et al.* (2003) Inherited thrombocytopenias: a proposed diagnostic algorithm from the Italian Gruppo di Studio delle Piastrine. *Haematologica* **88**,582–92.

British Committee for Standards in Haematology, Blood Transfusion Task Force (2003) Guidelines for the use of platelet transfusions. *Br J Haematol* **122**,10–23.

British Committee for Standards in Haematology, General Haematology Task Force (2003) Guidelines for the investigation and management of idiopathic thrombocytopenic purpura in adults, children and in pregnancy. *Br J Haematol* **120**,574–96.

Fakhouri F., Vernant J.P., Veyradier A. *et al.* (2005) Efficiency of curative and prophylactic treatment with rituximab in ADAMTS13-deficient thrombotic thrombocytopenic purpura: a study of 11 cases. *Blood* **106**,1932–7.

George J.N. (2006) Clinical practice. Thrombotic thrombocytopenic purpura. *N Engl J Med* **354**,1927–35.

Keeling D., Davidson S., Watson H. (2006) The management of heparin-induced thrombocytopenia. *Br J Haematol* **133**,258–69.

Levy G.G., Motto D.G., Ginsburg D. (2005) ADAMTS13 turns 3. *Blood* **106**,11–7.

Mannucci P.M., Canciani M.T., Forza I. *et al.* (2001) Changes in health and disease of the metalloprotease that cleaves von Willebrand factor. *Blood* **98**,2730–5.

Moake J.L. (2002) Thrombotic microangiopathies. *N Engl J Med* **347**,589–600.

Provan D. and Newland A. (2002) Fifty years of idiopathic thrombocytopenic purpura (ITP): management of refractory ITP in adults. *Br J Haematol* **118**,933–44.

Vesely S.K., George J.N., Lammle B. *et al.* (2003) ADAMTS13 activity in thrombotic thrombocytopenic purpura-hemolytic uremic syndrome: relation to presenting features and clinical outcomes in a prospective cohort of 142 patients. *Blood* **102**,60–8.

CHAPTER 24

24 Coagulation disorders

Hereditary coagulation disorders

Hereditary deficiencies of each of the coagulation factors have been described. Haemophilia A (factor VIII deficiency), haemophilia B (Christmas disease, factor IX deficiency) and von Willebrand disease (VWD) are the most common; the others are rare.

Haemophilia A

Haemophilia A is the most common of the hereditary clotting factor deficiencies. The prevalence is of the order of 30–100 per million population. The inheritance is sex-linked (Fig. 24.1) but up to 33% of patients have no family history and result from spontaneous mutation.

Molecular genetics

The factor VIII gene is situated near the tip of the long arm of the X chromosome (Xq2.6 region). It is extremely large and consists of 26 exons. The factor VIII protein includes a triplicated region $A_1A_2A_3$ with 30% homology with each other, a duplicated homology region C_1C_2 and a heavy glycosylated B domain which is removed when factor VIII is activated by thrombin. The protein is synthesized in the liver and spleen.

The defect is an absence or low level of plasma factor VIII. Approximately half of the patients have missense or frameshift mutations or deletions in the factor VIII gene. In others a characteristic 'flip-tip' inversion is seen in which the factor VIII gene is broken by an inversion at the end of the X chromosome (Fig. 24.2). This mutation leads to a severe clinical form of haemophilia A.

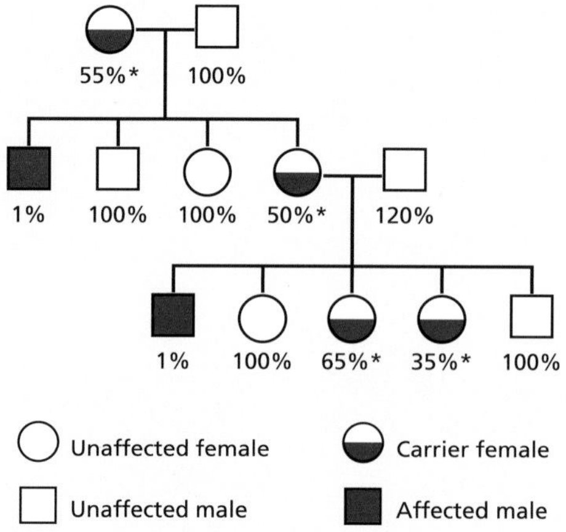

Fig. 24.1 A typical family tree in a family with haemophilia. Note the variable levels of factor VIII activity in carriers (*) because of random inactivation of X chromosome (Lyonization). The percentages show the degree of factor VIII activity as a percentage of normal.

Clinical features

Infants may suffer from profuse post-circumcision haemorrhage or develop joint and soft tissue bleeds

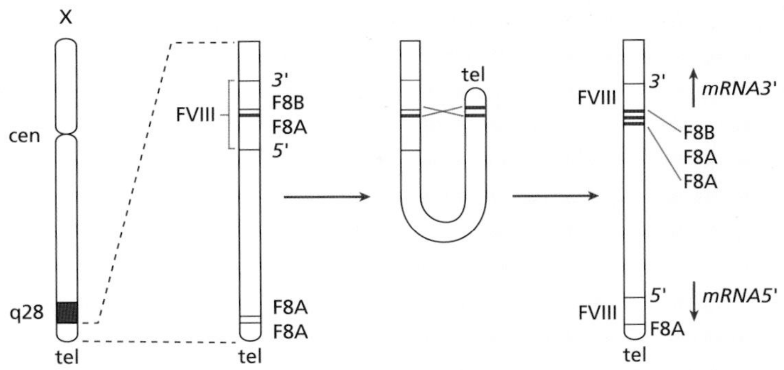

Fig. 24.2 The mechanism of the flip-tip inversion leading to disruption of the factor VIII gene. (Left) The orientation of the factor VIII gene is shown with the three copies of gene A in this region in (one within in intron 22 and two near the telomere). (Middle) During spermatogenesis at meiosis, the single X pairs with the Y chromosome in the homologous regions. The X chromosome is longer than the Y and there is nothing to pair with most of the long arm of X. The chromosome undergoes homologous recombination between the A genes. (Right) The final result is that the factor VIII gene is disrupted. cen, centromeric end; tel, telomere; the arrows indicate the direction of transcription from the A gene.

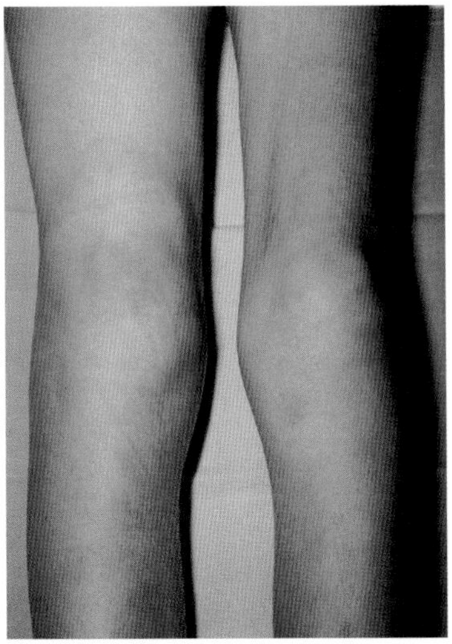

Fig. 24.3 Haemophilia A: acute haemarthrosis of the left knee joint with swelling of the suprapatellar region. There is wasting of the quadriceps muscles, particularly on the right.

and excessive bruising when they start to be active. Recurrent painful haemarthroses and muscle haematomas dominate the clinical course of severely affected patients and if poorly treated may lead to progressive joint deformity and disability (Figs 24.3–24.6). Local pressure can cause entrapment neuropathy or ischaemic necrosis. Prolonged bleeding occurs after dental extractions. Spontaneous haematuria and gastrointestinal haemorrhage, sometimes with obstruction resulting from intramucosal bleeding, can also occur. The clinical severity of the disease correlates with the extent of the factor VIII deficiency (Table 24.1). Operative and post-traumatic haemorrhage are life-threatening both in severely and mildly affected patients. Although not common, spontaneous intracerebral haemorrhage occurs more frequently than in the general population and is an important cause of death in patients with severe disease.

Haemophilic pseudotumours are large encapsulated haematomas with progressive cystic swelling from repeated haemorrhage. They may occur in fascial and muscle planes, large muscle groups and in the long bones, pelvis and cranium. These result from repeated subperiosteal haemorrhages with bone destruction and new bone formation.

As a result of human immunodeficiency virus (HIV) present in concentrates made from human plasma during the early 1980s, over 50% of haemophiliacs treated in the USA or Western Europe became infected with HIV. Acquired immune deficiency syndrome (AIDS) has been a common cause of death in severe haemophilia. Thrombocytopenia from HIV infection may exacerbate bleeding episodes.

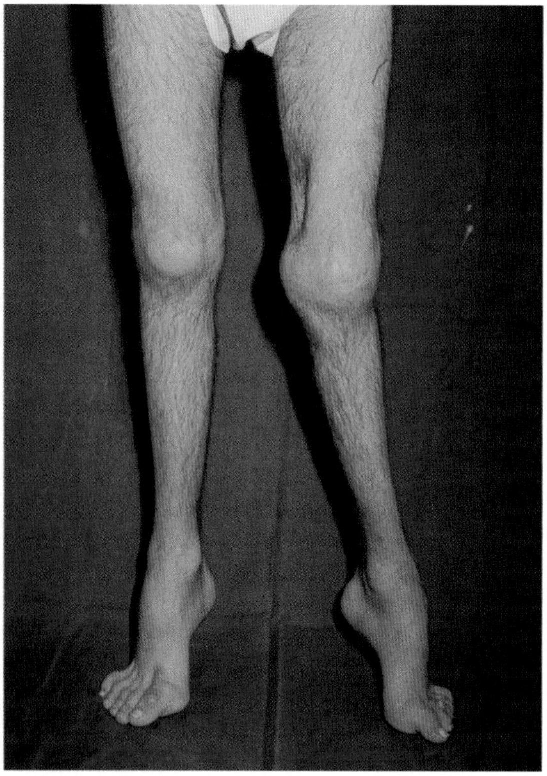

Fig. 24.4 Haemophilia A showing severe disability. The left knee is swollen with posterior subluxation of the tibia on the femur. The ankles and feet show residual deformities of talipes equinus, with some cavus and associated toe clawing. There is generalized muscle wasting. The scar on the medial side of the left lower thigh is the site of a previously excised pseudotumour.

Many patients were infected with hepatitis C virus before testing of donors and blood products became possible. This is causing an increasing amount of morbidity including chronic hepatitis, cirrhosis and hepatoma. Hepatitis B transmission may also be a risk.

Laboratory findings (Table 24.2)

The following tests are abnormal:

1 Activated partial thromboplastin time (APTT).

2 Factor VIII clotting assay.

The bleeding time and prothrombin time (PT) tests are normal.

Carrier detection and antenatal diagnosis

Until recently, carrier detection and antenatal diagnosis were limited to measuring plasma levels of factor VIII and von Willebrand factor (VWF). Carriers are now better detected with DNA probes. A known specific mutation can be identified or restriction fragment length polymorphisms within or close to the factor VIII gene allows the mutant allele to be tracked. Chorionic biopsies at 8–10 weeks' gestation provide sufficient fetal DNA for analysis. Antenatal diagnosis is also possible following the demonstration of low levels of factor VIII in fetal blood obtained at 16–20 weeks' gestation from the umbilical vein by ultrasound-guided needle aspiration.

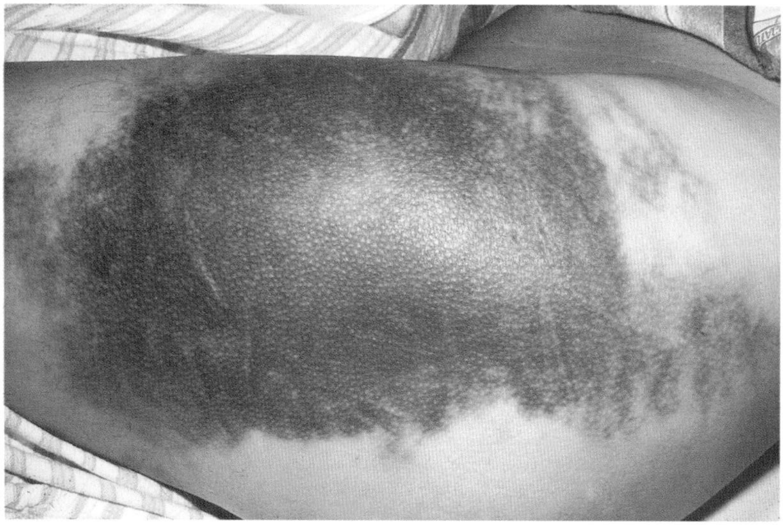

Fig. 24.5 Haemophilia A: massive haemorrhage in the area of the right buttock.

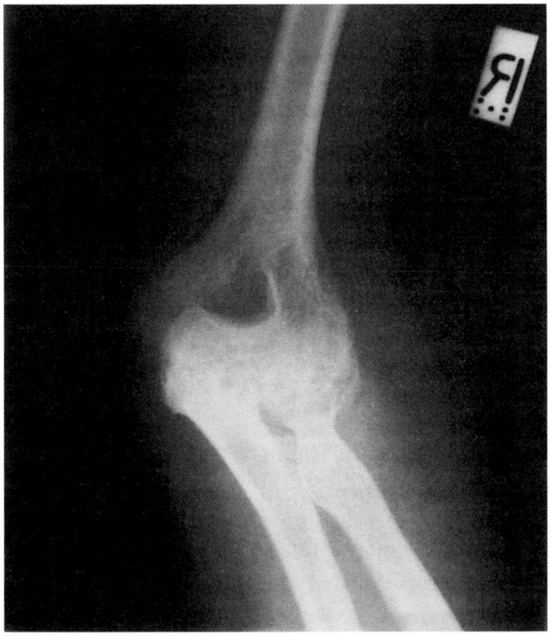

Fig. 24.6 Haemophilia A: radiographic appearances of the right elbow joint in a 25-year-old male. The joint space has been destroyed and there is bony ankylosis. Subchondral cystic areas are prominent.

Treatment

Most patients attend specialized haemophilia centres where there is a multidisciplinary team dedicated to their care. Bleeding episodes are treated with factor VIII replacement therapy and spontaneous bleeding is usually controlled if the patient's factor VIII level is raised to 30–50% of normal. Guidelines exist for the plasma level to be achieved for different types of haemorrhage. For major surgery, serious post-traumatic bleeding or when haemorrhage is occurring at a dangerous site, the factor VIII level should be elevated to 100% and then maintained above 50% when acute bleeding has stopped, until healing has occurred. On average, factor VIII infusion produces a plasma increment of 2 U/dL per unit infused per kilogram body weight. Roughly, the dose to be infused (units) = (weight (kg) × increment needed (U/dL))/2.

Recombinant factor VIII (five different commercial preparations) and immunoaffinity-purified factor VIII preparations, which are heat or solvent-detergent treated, are now available for clinical use and virtually eliminate the risk of viral transmission.

DDAVP (desmopressin) provides an alternative means of increasing the plasma factor VIII level in milder haemophiliacs. Following the intravenous administration of this drug, there is a 2–4-fold rise maximum at 30–60 min in the patient's own factor VIII by release from endothelial cells and this rise is proportional to the resting level. DDAVP may also be taken subcutaneously or nasally—this has been used as immediate treatment for mild haemophilia after accidental trauma or haemorrhage. DDAVP has an antidiuretic action and should be avoidedin the elderly; fluid restitution is advised after its use.

Local supportive measures used in treating haemarthroses and haematomas include resting the affected part and the prevention of further trauma.

Table 24.1 Correlation of coagulation factor activity and disease severity in haemophilia A or B.

Coagulation factor activity (percentage of normal)	Clinical manifestations
<2	Severe disease Frequent spontaneous bleeding into joints, muscles, internal organs from early life Joint deformity and crippling if not adequately treated
2–10	Moderate disease Bleeding after minor trauma Occasional spontaneous episodes
>10–30	Mild disease Minor bleeding after significant trauma, surgery

Table 24.2 Main clinical and laboratory findings in haemophilia A, factor IX deficiency (haemophilia B, Christmas disease) and von Willebrand disease.

	Haemophilia A	Factor IX deficiency	von Willebrand disease
Inheritance	Sex-linked	Sex-linked	Dominant (incomplete)
Main sites of haemorrhage	Muscle, joints, post-trauma or postoperative	Muscle, joints, post-trauma or postoperative	Mucous membranes, skin cuts, post-trauma or postoperative
Platelet count	Normal	Normal	Normal
Bleeding time	Normal	Normal	Prolonged
Prothrombin time	Normal	Normal	Normal
Partial thromboplastin time	Prolonged	Prolonged	Prolonged or normal
Factor VIII	Low	Normal	May be moderately reduced
Factor IX	Normal	Low	Normal
VWF	Normal	Normal	Low or abnormal function (Table 24.3)
Ristocetin-induced platelet aggregation	Normal	Normal	Impaired

VWF, von Willebrand factor.

Prophylactic treatment

The increased availability of factor VIII concentrates that may be stored in domestic refrigerators has dramatically altered haemophilia treatment. At the earliest suggestion of bleeding, the haemophilic child may be treated at home. This advance has reduced the occurrence of crippling haemarthroses and the need for inpatient care. Severely affected patients are now reaching adult life with little or no arthritis. After the first spontaneous joint bleed, most boys with severe haemophilia are started on prophylactic factor VIII three times a week, aiming to keep their factor VIII levels above 1%. This may require the placement of a vascular access device such as Port-a-Cath if venous access is difficult.

Haemophiliacs are advised to have regular conservative dental care. Haemophilic children and their parents often require extensive help with social and psychological matters. With modern treatment the lifestyle of a haemophilic child can be almost normal but certain activities such as body contact sports are to be avoided.

Gene therapy

Because it is only necessary to maintain factor levels >1% to prevent most of the mortality and morbidity of factor VIII or IX deficiency, there is great interest in gene-based therapy. Various viral vectors (retroviral, adeno-associated) as well as non-viral vectors are being explored. Phase 1 trials have been carried out for both haemophilia A and B.

Inhibitors

One of the most serious complications of haemophilia is the development of antibodies (inhibitors) to infused factor VIII which occurs in 5–10% of (mainly severe) patients, especially children. This renders the patient refractory to further replacement therapy so that tremendous doses have to be given to achieve a significant rise in plasma factor VIII activity. Immunosuppression and immune tolerance regimes have been used in an attempt to eradicate the antibody. Recombinant activated factor VII (VIIa) and activated prothrombin complex concentrates (FEIBA—factor VIII inhibitor bypassing activity) can be useful in the treatment of bleeding episodes.

Factor VIIa complexes with tissue factor exposed at the site of injury and produces local haemostasis. The process is independent of factor VIII or IX and is not affected by their inhibitors. Factor VIIa has a short half-life and therefore frequent doses may be needed. In the longer term, immunosuppression with cyclophosphamide, intravenous immunoglobulin and high-dose factor VIII has also been successful.

Factor IX deficiency

The inheritance and clinical features of factor IX deficiency (Christmas disease, haemophilia B) are identical to those of haemophilia A. Indeed, the two disorders can only be distinguished by specific coagulation factor assays. The incidence is one-fifth that of haemophilia A. Factor IX is coded by a gene close to the gene for factor VIII near the tip of the long arm of the X chromosome. Its synthesis, like that of prothrombin, factor VII, factor X and protein C, is vitamin K-dependent. Carrier detection and antenatal diagnosis is performed as for haemophilia A. The principles of replacement therapy are similar to those of haemophilia A. Bleeding episodes are treated with high-purity factor IX concentrates. Because of its longer biological half-life, infusions do not have to be given as frequently as factor VIII concentrates in haemophilia A. Recombinant factor IX is available. Higher doses are needed compared with plasma-derived factor IX.

Laboratory findings (Table 24.2)

The following tests are abnormal:

1 APTT

2 Factor IX clotting assay

As in haemophilia A, the bleeding time and PT tests are normal.

Von Willebrand disease

In this disorder there is either a reduced level or abnormal function of VWF resulting from a point mutation or major deletion. VWF is produced in endothelial cells and megakaryocytes. It has two roles (Chapter 22). It promotes platelet adhesion to damaged endothelium and it is the carrier molecule for factor VIII, protecting it from premature destruction. The latter property explains the occasional reduced factor VIII levels found in VWD.

Chronic elevation of VWF is part of the acute phase response to injury, inflammation, neoplasia or pregnancy. VWF is synthesized as a large 300-kDa protein which then forms multimers up to 10^6 Da in weight. Three types of VWD have been described (Table 24.3). Type 2 is divided into four subtypes depending on the type of functional defect. Type 1 accounts for 75% of cases.

VWD is the most common inherited bleeding disorder. Usually, the inheritance is autosomal dominant with varying expression. The severity of the bleeding is variable. Typically, there is mucous membrane bleeding (e.g. epistaxes, menorrhagia), excessive blood loss from superficial cuts and abrasions, and operative and post-traumatic haemorrhage. The severity is variable in the different types. Haemarthroses and muscle haematomas are rare, except in type 3 disease.

Laboratory findings (Table 24.2)

1 The bleeding time can be prolonged. This test is usually replaced by the PFA-100 test (see p. 277).

2 Factor VIII levels are often low. If low, a factor VIII VWF binding assay is performed.

Table 24.3 Classification of von Willebrand disease.

Type 1	Quantitative partial deficiency
Type 2	Functional abnormality
Type 3	Complete deficiency

Secondary classification of type 2 VWD

Subtype	Platelet-associated function	Factor VIII binding capacity	High MW VWF multimers
2A	Decreased	Normal	Absent
2B	Increased affinity for GPIb	Normal	Usually reduced/absent
2M	Decreased	Normal	Normal or ultra large
2N	Normal	Reduced	Normal

GPIb, glycoprotein Ib; MW, molecular weight; VWD, von Willebrand disease; VWF, von Willebrand factor.

3 The APTT may be prolonged.
4 VWF levels are usually low.
5 There is defective platelet aggregation by patient plasma in the presence of ristocetin (VWF: Rco). Aggregation to other agents (adenosine diphosphate (ADP), thrombin or adrenaline) is usually normal.
6 Collagen-binding function (VWF: CB) is usually reduced.
7 Multimer analysis is useful for diagnosing different subtypes (Table 24.3).
8 The platelet count is normal except for type 2B disease (where it is low).

Treatment

Options are as follows:
1 Local measures and antifibrinolytic agent (e.g. tranexamic acid for mild bleeding).
2 DDAVP infusion for those with type 1 VWD. This releases VWF from endothelial stage sites 30 min after intravenous infusion.
3 High-purity factor VWF concentrates for patients with very low VWF levels. Factor VIII concentrate may also be given for more rapid correction.

Hereditary disorders of other coagulation factors

All these disorders (deficiency of fibrinogen, prothrombin, factors V, VII, combined V and VIII, factors X, XI, XIII) are rare. In most the inheritance is autosomal recessive. Factor XI deficiency is seen mainly in Ashkenazi Jews and occurs in either sex. The bleeding risk is not related to severity of the deficiency, and is absent from muscles and joints. The severity is poorly related to the factor XI level in plasma. It usually causes excess bleeding only after trauma such as surgery, and is treated by factor XI concentrate or fresh frozen plasma. Factor XIII deficiency produces a severe bleeding tendency, characteristically with umbilical stump bleeding. Specific concentrates or recombinant preparation of factors VII, XI and XIII are now available.

Acquired coagulation disorders

The acquired coagulation disorders (Table 24.4) are more common than the inherited disorders. Unlike the inherited disorders, multiple clotting factor deficiencies are usual.

Table 24.4 The acquired coagulation disorders.

Deficiency of vitamin K-dependent factors
Haemorrhagic disease of the newborn
Biliary obstruction
Malabsorption of vitamin K (e.g. tropical sprue, gluten-induced enteropathy)
Vitamin K-antagonist therapy (e.g. coumarins, indandiones)
Liver disease
Disseminated intravascular coagulation
Inhibition of coagulation
Specific inhibitors (e.g. antibodies against factor VIII)
Non-specific inhibitors (e.g. antibodies found in systemic lupus erythematosus, rheumatoid arthritis)
Miscellaneous
Diseases with M-protein production
L-Asparaginase
Therapy with heparin, defibrinating agents or thrombolytics
Massive transfusion syndrome

Vitamin K deficiency

Fat-soluble vitamin K is obtained from green vegetables and bacterial synthesis in the gut. Deficiency may present in the newborn (haemorrhagic disease of the newborn) or in later life.

Deficiency of vitamin K is caused by an inadequate diet, malabsorption or inhibition of vitamin K by drugs such as warfarin which act as vitamin K antagonists. Warfarin is associated with a decrease in the functional activity of factors II, VII, IX and X and proteins C and S, but immunological methods show normal levels of these factors. The non-functional proteins are called PIVKA (proteins formed in vitamin K absence). Conversion of PIVKA factors to their biologically active forms is a post-translational event involving carboxylation of glutamic acid residues in the N-terminal region where these factors show strong sequence homology (Fig. 24.7). Gamma-carboxylated glutamic acid binds calcium ions through which it forms

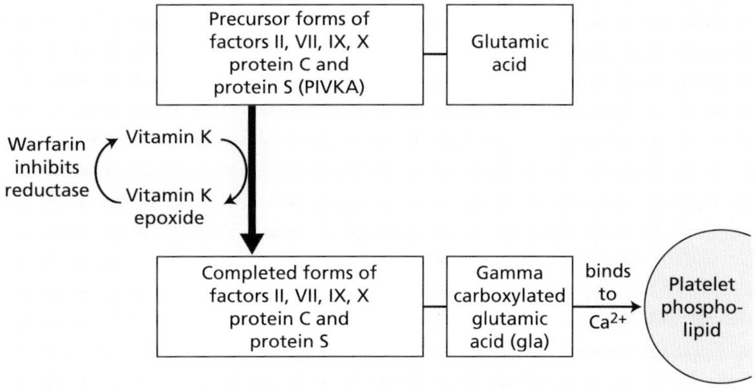

Fig. 24.7 The action of vitamin K in γ-carboxylation of glutamic acid in coagulation factors which are then able to bind Ca^{2+} and attach to the platelet phospholipid.

a complex with phospholipid. In the process of carboxylation, vitamin K is converted to vitamin K epoxide which is cycled back to the reduced form by reductases. Warfarin interferes with the reduction of vitamin K epoxide leading to a functional vitamin K deficiency.

Haemorrhagic disease of the newborn

Vitamin K-dependent factors are low at birth and fall further in breast-fed infants in the first few days of life. Liver cell immaturity, lack of gut bacterial synthesis of the vitamin and low quantities in breast milk may all contribute to a deficiency which may cause haemorrhage, usually on the second to fourth day of life, but occasionally during the first 2 months.

Diagnosis

The PT and APTT are both abnormal. The platelet count and fibrinogen are normal with absent fibrin degradation products.

Treatment

1 Prophylaxis. For many years vitamin K has been given to all newborn babies as a single intramuscular injection of 1 mg. This remains the most appropriate and safest treatment. Following epidemiological evidence suggesting a possible link between intramuscular vitamin K and an increased risk of childhood tumours (which has not been substantiated), some centres recommended an oral regimen but this is less effective in prevention and repeat doses are needed up to day 28.

2 In bleeding infants: vitamin K 1 mg intramuscularly is given every 6 h with, initially, fresh frozen plasma if haemorrhage is severe.

Vitamin K deficiency in children or adults

Deficiency resulting from obstructive jaundice, pancreatic or small bowel disease occasionally causes a bleeding diathesis in children or adults.

Diagnosis

Both PT and APTT are prolonged. There are low plasma levels of factors II, VII, IX and X.

Treatment

1 Prophylaxis: vitamin K 5 mg/day orally.

2 Active bleeding or prior to liver biopsy: vitamin K 10 mg slowly intravenously. Some correction of PT is usual within 6 h. The dose should be repeated on the next 2 days after which optimal correction is usual.

Liver disease

Multiple haemostatic abnormalities contribute to a bleeding tendency and may exacerbate haemorrhage from oesophageal varices.

1 Biliary obstruction results in impaired absorption of vitamin K and therefore decreased synthesis of factors II, VII, IX and X by liver parenchymal cells.

2 With severe hepatocellular disease, in addition to a deficiency of these factors, there are often reduced levels of factor V and fibrinogen and increased amounts of plasminogen activator.

3 Functional abnormality of fibrinogen (dysfibrinogenaemia) is found in many patients.

4 Decreased thrombopoietin production from the liver contributes to thrombocytopenia.

5 Hypersplenism associated with portal hypertension frequently results in thrombocytopenia.

6 Disseminated intravascular coagulation (DIC; see below) may be related to release of thromboplastins from damaged liver cells and reduced concentrations of antithrombin, protein C and α_2-antiplasmin. In addition, there is impaired removal of activated clotting factors and increased fibrinolytic activity.

Disseminated intravascular coagulation

Widespread inappropriate intravascular deposition of fibrin with consumption of coagulation factors and platelets occurs as a consequence of many disorders which release procoagulant material into the circulation or cause widespread endothelial damage or platelet aggregation (Table 24.5). It may be associated with a fulminant haemorrhagic or thrombotic syndrome with organ dysfunction or run a less severe and more chronic course. The main clinical presentation is with bleeding but 5–10% of patients manifest microthrombotic lesions (e.g. with gangrene of limbs).

Pathogenesis (Fig. 24.8)

The key event underlying DIC is increased activity of tissue factor. This can come from its release into the circulation from damaged tissues present on tumour cells or from up-regulation of tissue factor on circulating monocytes or endothelial cells

Table 24.5 Causes of disseminated intravascular coagulation.

Infections
Gram-negative and meningococcal septicaemia
Clostridium welchii septicaemia
Severe Falciparum malaria
Viral infection—varicella, HIV, hepatitis, cytomegalovirus
Malignancy
Widespread mucin-secreting adenocarcinoma
Acute promyelocytic leukaemia
Obstetric complications
Amniotic fluid embolism
Premature separation of placenta
Eclampsia; retained placenta
Septic abortion
Hypersensitivity reactions
Anaphylaxis
Incompatible blood transfusion
Widespread tissue damage
Following surgery or trauma
After severe burns
Vascular abnormalities
Kasabach–Merritt syndrome
Leaking prosthetic valves
Cardiac bypass surgery
Vascular aneurysms
Miscellaneous
Liver failure
Pancreatitis
Snake and invertebrate venoms
Hypothermia
Heat stroke
Acute hypoxia
Massive blood loss

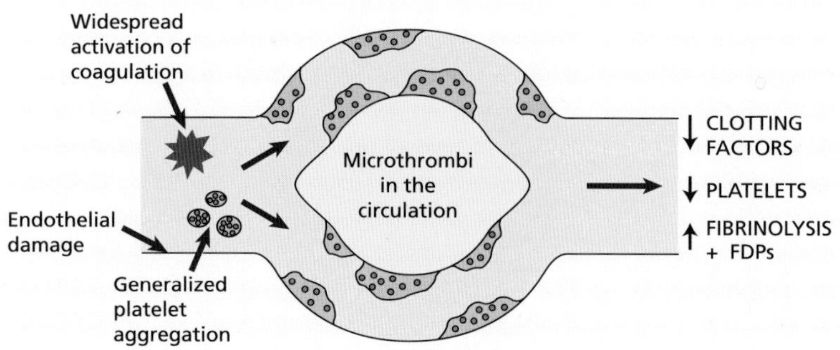

Fig. 24.8 The pathogenesis of disseminated intravascular coagulation and the changes in clotting factors, platelets and fibrin degradation products (FDPs) that occur in this syndrome.

in response to pro-inflammatory cytokines (e.g. interleukin-1, tumour necrosis factor, endotoxin).

1 DIC may be triggered by the entry of procoagulant material into the circulation in the following situations: severe trauma, amniotic fluid embolism, premature separation of the placenta, widespread mucin-secreting adenocarcinomas, acute promyelocytic leukaemia (AML type M_3), liver disease, severe falciparum malaria, haemolytic transfusion reaction and some snake bites.

2 DIC may also be initiated by widespread endothelial damage and collagen exposure (e.g. endotoxaemia, Gram-negative and meningococcal septicaemia, septic abortion), certain virus infections and severe burns or hypothermia.

In addition to its role in the deposition of fibrin in the microcirculation, intravascular thrombin formation produces large amounts of circulating fibrin monomers which form complexes with fibrinogen. Intense fibrinolysis is stimulated by thrombi on vascular walls and the release of split products interferes with fibrin polymerization, thus contributing to the coagulation defect. The combined action of thrombin and plasmin normally causes depletion of fibrinogen and all coagulation factors. Intravascular thrombin also causes widespread platelet aggregation and deposition in the vessels. The bleeding problems which may be a feature of DIC are compounded by thrombocytopenia caused by consumption of platelets.

Clinical features

These are dominated by bleeding, particularly from venepuncture sites or recent wounds (Fig. 24.9a). There may be generalized bleeding in the gastrointestinal tract, the oropharynx, into the lungs, urogenital tract and in obstetric cases vaginal bleeding may be particularly severe. Less frequently, microthrombi may cause skin lesions, renal failure, gangrene of the fingers or toes (Fig. 24.9b) or cerebral ischaemia.

Some patients may develop subacute or chronic DIC, especially with mucin-secreting adenocarcinoma. Compensation by the liver may render some of the coagulation tests normal.

Laboratory findings (Table 24.6)

In many acute syndromes the blood may fail to clot because of gross fibrinogen deficiency.

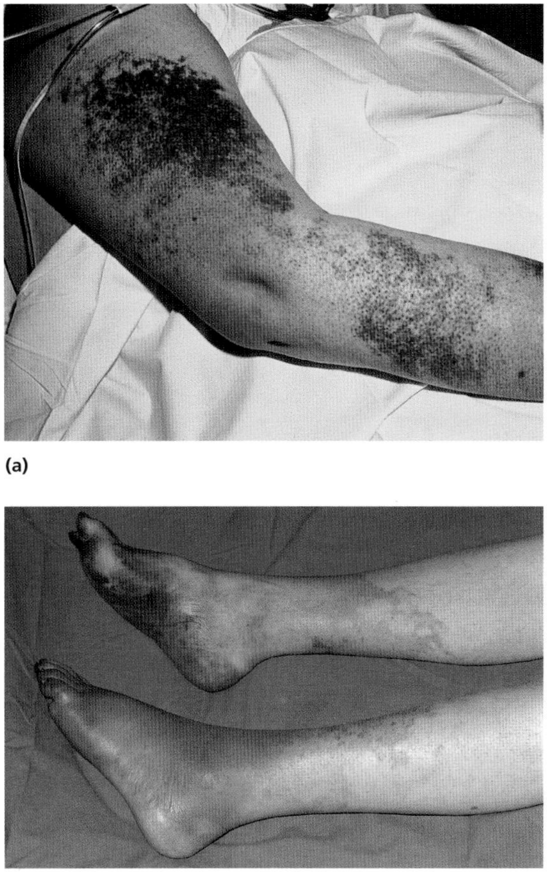

(a)

(b)

Fig. 24.9 Clinical features of disseminated intravascular coagulation: **(a)** indurated and confluent purpura of the arm; **(b)** peripheral gangrene with swelling and discoloration of the skin of the feet in fulminant disease.

Tests of haemostasis

1 The platelet count is low.

2 Fibrinogen concentration low.

3 The thrombin time is prolonged.

4 High levels of fibrin degradation products such as D-dimers are found in serum and urine.

5 The PT and APTT are prolonged in the acute syndromes.

Blood film examination

In many patients there is a haemolytic anaemia ('microangiopathic') and the red cells show prominent fragmentation because of damage caused when passing through fibrin strands in small vessels (p. 69).

Table 24.6 Haemostasis tests: typical results in acquired bleeding disorders.

	Platelet count	Prothrombin time	Activated partial thromboplastin time	Thrombin time
Liver disease	Low	Prolonged	Prolonged	Normal (rarely prolonged)
DIC	Low	Prolonged	Prolonged	Grossly prolonged
Massive transfusion	Low	Prolonged	Prolonged	Normal
Oral anticoagulants	Normal	Grossly prolonged	Prolonged	Normal
Heparin	Normal (rarely low)	Mildly prolonged	Prolonged	Prolonged
Circulating anticoagulant	Normal	Normal or prolonged	Prolonged	Normal

DIC, Disseminated intravascular coagulation.

Table 24.7 Indications for the use of fresh frozen plasma (National Institutes of Health Consensus Guidelines).

Coagulation factor deficiency (where specific or combined factor concentrate is not available)
Reversal of warfarin effect
Multiple coagulation defects (e.g. in patients with liver disease, DIC)
Massive blood transfusion with coagulopathy and clinical bleeding
Thrombotic thrombocytopenic purpura
Deficiencies of antithrombin*, protein C* or protein S
Some patients with immunodeficiency syndromes

DIC, disseminated intravascular coagulation.
* Antithrombin and protein C concentrates now available.

Treatment

Treatment of the underlying cause is most important. The management of patients who are bleeding differs from that of patients with thrombotic problems.

Bleeding

Supportive therapy with fresh frozen plasma (Table 24.7) and platelet concentrates is indicated in patients with dangerous or extensive bleeding. Cryoprecipitate provides a more concentrated source of fibrinogen and red cell transfusions may be required.

Thrombosis

The use of heparin or antiplatelet drugs to inhibit the coagulation process is considered in those with thrombotic problems such as dermal ischaemia. Fibrinolytic inhibitors should not be considered because failure to lyse thrombi in organs such as the kidney may have adverse effects. Antithrombin concentrates or recombinant human protein C may be used to inhibit DIC in severe cases with sepsis (e.g. meningococcal septicaemia). There is reduced activated protein C (APC) in severe sepsis and recombinant human APC has been found to reduce mortality in this setting.

Coagulation deficiency caused by antibodies

Circulating antibodies to coagulation factors are occasionally seen with an incidence of approximately 1 per millon per year. Alloantibodies to factor VIII occur in 5–10% of haemophiliacs. Factor VIII autoantibodies may also result in a bleeding syndrome. These immunoglobulin G (IgG) antibodies occur rarely post-partum, in certain immunological disorders (e.g. rheumatoid arthritis), in cancer and in old age. Treatment usually consists of a combination of immunosuppression and treatment with factor replacement, usually as human factor VIII, recombinant VIIa or activated prothrombin complex concentrate (FEIBA).

Another protein known as the lupus anticoagulant interferes with lipoprotein-dependent stages of coagulation and is usually detected by prolongation of the APTT test (Table 24.6). This inhibitor is detected in 10% of patients with systemic lupus erythematosus (SLE) and in patients with other autoimmune diseases who frequently have antibodies to other lipid-containing antigens (e.g. cardiolipin). The antibody is not associated with a bleeding tendency but there is an increased risk of arterial or venous thrombosis and, as with other causes of thrombophilia, an association with recurrent miscarriage (Chapter 25).

Massive transfusion syndrome

Many factors may contribute to a bleeding disorder following massive transfusion. Blood loss results in reduced levels of platelets, coagulation factors and inhibitors. Further dilution of these factors occurs during replacement with red cells.

Management

Platelet concentrates are given to maintain a platelet count $>50 \times 10^9/L$ or $80–100 \times 10^9/L$ in cerebral injury or polytrauma. The PT and APTT should be kept to less than 1.5 times normal with fresh frozen plasma given initially at 15 mL/kg. Cryoprecipitate is given to keep fibrinogen at least 1 g/L. Recombinant VIIa is increasingly used in patients with massive blood loss after trauma or surgery to reduce haemorrhage.

The results of haemostasis screening tests in acquired bleeding disorders are shown in Table 24.6 and a summary of the indications for use of fresh frozen plasma in Table 24.7.

Thromboelastography: near-patient testing

Thromboelastography (TEG) is a technique for a global assessment of haemostatic function of a single blood sample in which the reaction of platelets with the protein coagulation cascade is observed from the time of the initial platelet fibrin interaction

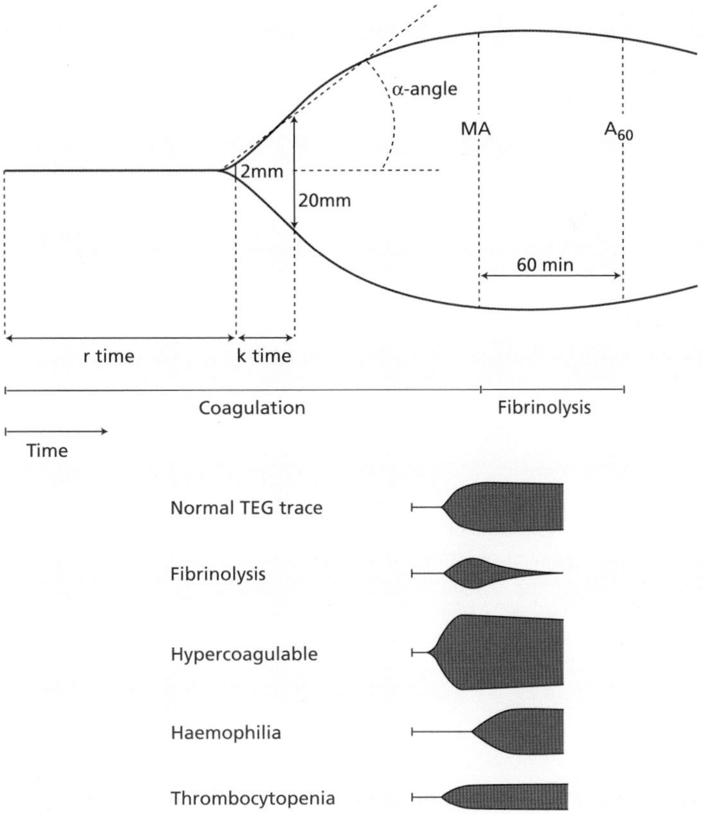

Fig. 24.10 Thromboelastography (TEG): normal trace and appearances in different pathological states. α-angle, speed of solid clot formation; A_{60}, measure of clot lysis or retraction at 60 min; k, clot formation time; MA, absolute strength of fibrin clot; r, rate of initial fibrin formation. (From S.V. Mallett and D.J.A. Cox (1992). Thromboelastography. *Br J Anaesth* **69**,307–13 with permission)

through platelet aggregation, clot strengthening and fibrin cross-linkage to eventual clot lysis. It is suited as a monitor of haemostasis in surgery (e.g. of the liver or heart) associated with haemostatic defects. Freshly drawn blood is placed in a cuvette which is oscillated, the motion being transferred to a pin which writes on heat-sensitive paper. As fibrin strands form, the fibrin clot affects movement of the pin. The normal trace shows the rate of initial fibrin formation, the time to formation of a clot (coagulation time), strength of the fibrin clot, clot lysis index or retraction. Typical patterns showing results in fibrinolysis, hypercoagulability, haemophilia and thrombocytopenia are shown in Fig. 24.10.

The platelet function analyser (PFA-100) may also be useful in testing platelet function before and during surgery (p. 277).

Bibliography

Bernard G.R., Vincent J.L., Laterre P.F. *et al.* (2001) Efficacy and safety of recombinant human activated protein C for severe sepsis. *N Engl J Med* **344**,699–709.

Blumberg N., Francis C., Heal J. (eds) (2006) Clinical uses of plasma and plasma fractions. *Best Pract Res Clin Haematol* **19**,1–258.

Deldado J., Jimenez-Yuste V., Hernandez-Navarro F. *et al.* (2003) Acquired haemophilia: review and meta-analysis focused on therapy and prognostic factors. *Br J Haematol* **121**,21–35.

Erber W.N. and Perry D.J. (2006) Plasma and plasma products in the treatment of massive haemorrhage. *Best Pract Res Clin Haematol* **19**,97–112.

Favaloro E.J. (2001) Utility of the PFA-100® for assessing bleeding disorders and monitoring therapy: a review of analytical variables, benefits and limitations. *Haemophilia* **7**,170–9.

Haemophilia A database: http://europium.csc.mrc.ac.uk

Haemophilia database: http://www.unds.ac.uk/mdgen

Hay C.R.M., Brown S., Collins P.W. *et al.* (2006) The diagnosis and management of factor VIII and IX inhibitors: a guideline from the United Kingdom Haemophilia Centre Doctors Organisation. *Br J Haematol* **133**,591–605.

Josephson C.D. and Abshire T.C. (2006) Clinical uses of plasma and plasma fractions: plasma-derived products for hemophilias A and B, and for von Willebrand disease. *Best Pract Res Clin Haematol* **19**,35–49.

Laffan M., Brown S.A. Collins P.W. *et al.* (2004) The diagnosis of von Willebrand disease: a guideline from the UK Haemophilia Centre Doctors' Organization. *Haemophilia* **10**,199–217.

Lee C.A., Berntorp E.E., Hoots W.K. (eds) (2005) *Textbook of Haemophilia*. Blackwell Publishing, Oxford.

Levi M. (2004) Current understanding of disseminated intravascular coagulation. *Br J Haematol* **124**,567–76.

Mannucci P.M. (2003) Hemophilia: treatment options in the twenty-first century. *J Thromb Haemost* **1**,1349–55.

Mannucci P.M. (2004) Treatment of von Willebrand's Disease. *N Engl J Med* **351**,683–94.

Mittal S. and Watson H.G. (2006) A critical appraisal of the use of recombinant factor VIIa in acquired bleeding conditions. *Br J Haematol* **133**,355–63.

O'Shaughnessy D.F., Atterbury C., Bolton Maggs P. *et al.* for the British Committee for Standards in Haematology, Blood Transfusion Task Force. (2004) Guidelines for the use of fresh-frozen plasma, cryoprecipitate and cryosupernatant. *Br J Haematol* **126**,11–28.

Pasi K.J., Collins P.W., Keeling D.M. *et al.* (2004) Management of von Willebrand disease: a guideline from the UK Haemophilia Centre Doctors' Organization. *Haemophilia* **10**,218–31.

Peyvandi F. and Mannucci P.M. (2005) Congenital bleeding: autosomal recessive disorders. In: Hoffbrand A.V., Tuddenham E., Catovsky D. (eds) *Postgraduate Haematology*, 5th edn. Blackwell Publishing, Oxford: pp. 842–58.

Plug I., Mausev-Bunshoten P., Bröcker-Vriends A.H.J.T. *et al.* (2006) Bleeding in causes of haemophilia. *Blood* **108**,52–6.

Roberts H.R., Monroe D.M., White G.C. (2004) The use of recombinant factor VIIa in the treatment of bleeding disorders. *Blood* **104**,3858–64.

Salooja N. and Perry D.J. (2002) Thromboelastography. *Blood Coagul Fibrinolysis* **12**,327–37.

United Kingdom Haemophilia Centre Doctors' Organization. (2003) Guidelines on the selection and use of therapeutic products to treat haemophilia and other hereditary bleeding disorders. *Haemophilia* **9**,1–23.

CHAPTER 25

25 Thrombosis and antithrombotic therapy

Thrombi are solid masses or plugs formed in the circulation from blood constituents. Platelets and fibrin form the basic structure. Their clinical significance results from ischaemia from local vascular obstruction or distant embolization. Thrombi are involved in the pathogenesis of myocardial infarction, cerebrovascular disease, peripheral arterial disease and deep vein occlusion.

Thrombosis, both arterial and venous, is more common as age increases and is frequently associated with risk factors (e.g. surgery or pregnancy). The term thrombophilia is used to describe the inherited or acquired disorders of the haemostatic mechanism that predispose to thrombosis.

Arterial thrombosis

Pathogenesis

Atherosclerosis of the arterial wall, plaque rupture and endothelial injury expose blood to subendothelial collagen and tissue factor. This initiates the formation of a platelet nidus on which platelets adhere and aggregate.

Platelet deposition and thrombus formation are important in the pathogenesis of atherosclerosis. Platelet-derived growth factor (PDGF) stimulates the migration and proliferation of smooth muscle cells and fibroblasts in the arterial intima. Regrowth of endothelium and repair at the site of arterial damage and incorporated thrombus result in thickening of the vessel wall.

As well as blocking arteries locally, emboli of platelets and fibrin may break away from the primary thrombus to occlude distal arteries. Examples are carotid artery thrombi leading to cerebral thrombosis and transient ischaemic attacks (TIAs) and heart valve and chamber thrombi leading to systemic emboli and infarcts (Fig. 25.1).

Clinical risk factors

The risk factors for arterial thrombosis are related to the development of atherosclerosis and are listed in Table 25.1. The identification of patients at risk is largely based on clinical assessment. A number of epidemiological studies have resulted in the construction of coronary artery thrombosis risk profiles based on sex, age, elevated blood pressure, high levels of serum cholesterol, glucose intolerance, cigarette smoking and electrocardiogram (ECG) abnormalities. These profiles have allowed pre-symptomatic assessment of young and apparently fit subjects and are valuable in counselling a change in lifestyle or for recommending medical therapy in individuals at risk. The Northwick Park Heart Study showed

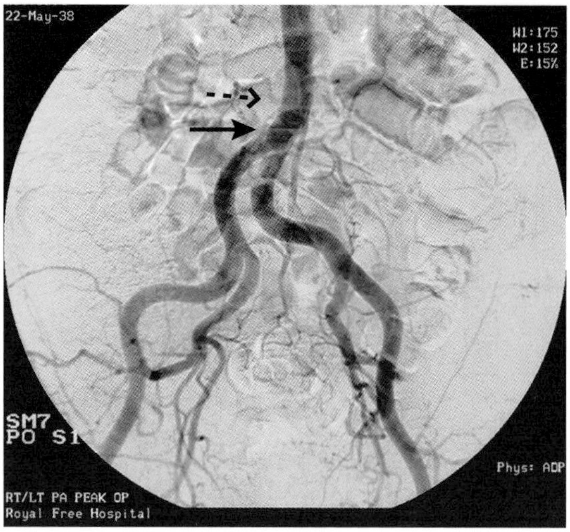

Fig. 25.1 Arteriogram showing saddle embolus at the aortic bifurcation (dotted arrow) and embolus in the left common iliac artery (solid arrow).

Table 25.1 Risk factors in arterial thrombosis (atherosclerosis).

Positive family history
Male sex
Hyperlipidaemia
Hypertension
Diabetes mellitus
Gout
Polycythaemia
Hyperhomocysteinaemia
Cigarette smoking
ECG abnormalities
Elevated factor VII
Elevated fibrinogen
Lupus anticoagulant
Collagen vascular diseases
Behçet's disease

ECG, electrocardiogram.

that elevated plasma levels of factor VII and fibrinogen are the strongest independent predictors of coronary events. Hyperhomocysteinaemia has been recognized more recently as a risk factor for peripheral and coronary arterial disease and stroke.

Venous thrombosis

Pathogenesis and risk factors

Virchow's triad suggests that there are three components that are important in thrombus formation:

Table 25.2 Risk factors for venous thrombosis.

Related to coagulation abnormality
Hereditary haemostatic disorders
Factor V Leiden
Prothrombin G20210A variant
Protein C deficiency
Antithrombin deficiency
Protein S deficiency
Abnormal fibrinogen
Abnormal plasminogen
Hereditary or acquired haemostatic disorders
Raised plasma levels of factor VII, VIII, IX or XI
Raised plasma levels of fibrinogen
Raised plasma levels of homocysteine
Glucosylceramide deficiency
Coagulation factor IX concentrates
Lupus anticoagulant
Oestrogen therapy (oral contraceptive and HRT)
Heparin-induced thrombocytopenia
Pregnancy and puerperium
Surgery, especially abdominal and hip
Major trauma
Malignancy
Myocardial infarct
Thrombocythaemia
Related to stasis
Cardiac failure
Stroke
Prolonged immobility
Pelvic obstruction
Nephrotic syndrome
Dehydration
Hyperviscosity, polycythaemia
Varicose veins
Related to unknown factors
Age
Obesity
Sepsis
Paroxysmal nocturnal haemoglobinuria
Behçet's disease

HRT, hormone replacement therapy.

1 Slowing down of blood flow;
2 Hypercoagulability of the blood; and
3 Vessel wall damage.

For venous thrombosis, increased systemic coagulability and stasis are most important, vessel wall damage being less important than in arterial thrombosis, although it may be important in patients with sepsis and indwelling catheters. Stasis allows the completion of blood coagulation at the site of initiation of the thrombus (e.g. behind the valve pockets of the leg veins in immobile patients).

Table 25.2 lists a number of recognized risk factors.

Hereditary disorders of haemostasis

The prevalence of inherited disorders associated with increased risk of thrombosis is at least as high as that of hereditary bleeding disorders. A hereditary 'thrombophilia' should be particularly suspected in young patients who suffer from spontaneous thrombosis, recurrent deep vein thromboses (Fig. 25.2) or

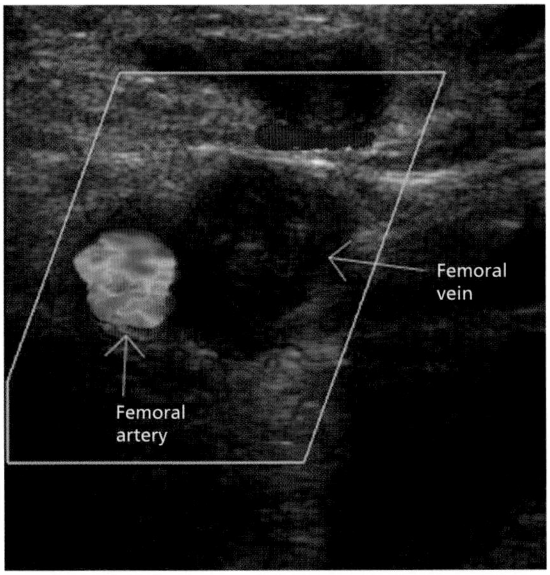

(a)

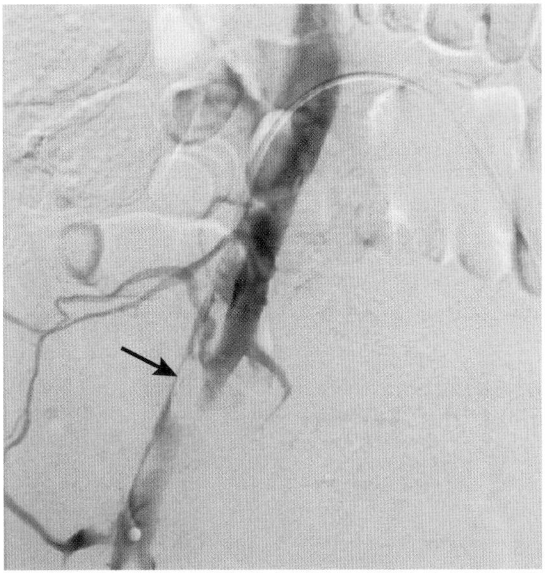

(b)

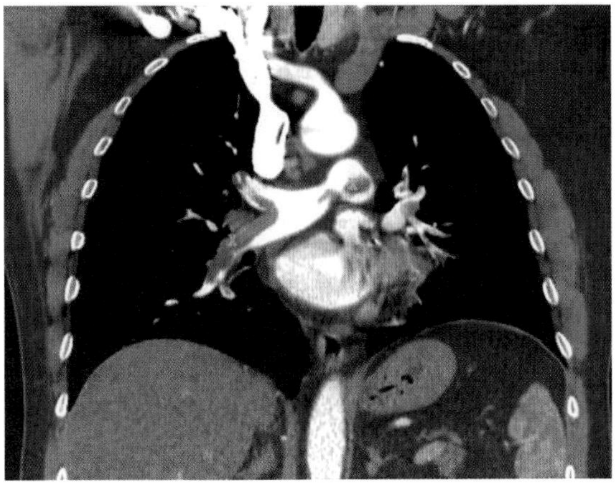

(c)

Fig. 25.2 Diagnostic imaging of deep vein thrombosis (DVT) and pulmonary embolus (PE). **(a)** Colour power Doppler ultrasound of the right femoral vessels with compression shows normal flow in the femoral artery but absent flow in the vein because of thrombus. A normal vein would collapse with compression of the probe. (Courtesy of Dr Tony Young) **(b)** Femoral venogram demonstrating extensive thrombus within the right external iliac vein. (Courtesy of Drs I.S. Francis and A.F. Watkinson) **(c)** Computed tomography (CT) pulmonary angiography: a coronal image shows bilateral filling defects (green crosses) in the central central pulmonary arteries indicating pulmonary emboli. (Courtesy of Dr Tony Young) an unusual site of thrombosis (e.g. axillary, splanchnic veins, sagittal sinus). Several abnormalities are now well characterized (Table 25.2).

Factor V Leiden gene mutation (activated protein C resistance)

This is the most common inherited cause of an increased risk of venous thrombosis. It occurs in approximately 4% of Caucasian factor V alleles. It was first recognized because of a failure to see prolongation in the activated partial thromboplastin time (APTT) test when activated protein C was added to the plasma of certain patients. Protein C breaks down activated factor V so activated protein C should slow the clotting reaction and prolong the APTT. In 1994, the underlying reason for this phenomenon was recognized to be a genetic polymorphism in the factor V gene (replacement of arginine at position 506 with glutamine—Arg506Gln) which makes factor V less susceptible to cleavage by activated protein C (Fig. 25.3). This is called the factor V Leiden mutation. The frequency of factor V Leiden in the general population in Western countries means that it cannot be regarded as a rare mutation but as a genetic polymorphism that is maintained in the population (Fig. 25.4). Presumably, individuals with this allele have been 'selected', probably because of reduced bleeding tendency. It does not increase the risk of arterial thrombosis.

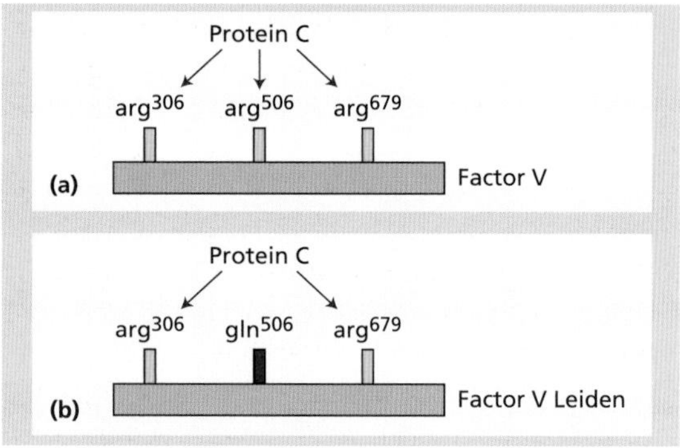

Fig. 25.3 The genetic basis of factor V Leiden. **(a)** Activated protein C inactivates factor Va by proteolytic cleavage at three sites in the Va heavy chain. **(b)** In the factor V Leiden mutation the Arg506Gln polymorphism leads to glutamine at position 506 with less efficient inactivation of factor V and increased risk of thrombosis.

Patients who are heterozygous for factor V Leiden are at an approximately 5–8-fold increased risk of thrombosis compared to the general population. Individuals who are homozygous have a 30–140-fold risk. Following venous thrombosis they have a higher risk of re-thrombosis compared to individuals with deep vein thrombosis (DVT) but normal factor V.

The incidence of factor V Leiden in patients with venous thrombosis is approximately 20–40%. Polymerase chain reaction (PCR) screening for the mutation is relatively simple and the test is widely performed. The absolute risk of thrombosis will depend on many other factors and it is difficult to advise individual patients of their risk. At present it is not recommended to start anticoagulation therapy in individuals with the Leiden mutation, even if homozygous, with no history of thrombosis. A small minority of patients with activated protein C resistance do not have factor V Leiden and have other mutations of factor V.

Antithrombin deficiency

Inheritance is autosomal dominant. There are recurrent venous thromboses usually starting in early adult life. Arterial thrombi occur occasionally. Antithrombin concentrates are available and are used to prevent thrombosis during surgery or childbirth. Many molecular variants of antithrombin have been categorized and are associated with varying degrees of risk of thrombosis.

Protein C deficiency

Inheritance is autosomal dominant with variable penetrance. Protein C levels in heterozygotes are approximately 50% of normal. Characteristically, many patients develop skin necrosis as a result of dermal vessel occlusion when treated with warfarin, thought to be caused by reduction of protein C levels even further in the first day or two of warfarin therapy before reduction in the levels of the vitamin K-dependent clotting factors, especially factor VII. Rarely, infants may be born with homozygous deficiency and characteristically present with severe disseminated intravascular coagulation (DIC) or purpura fulminans in infancy. Protein C concentrates are available.

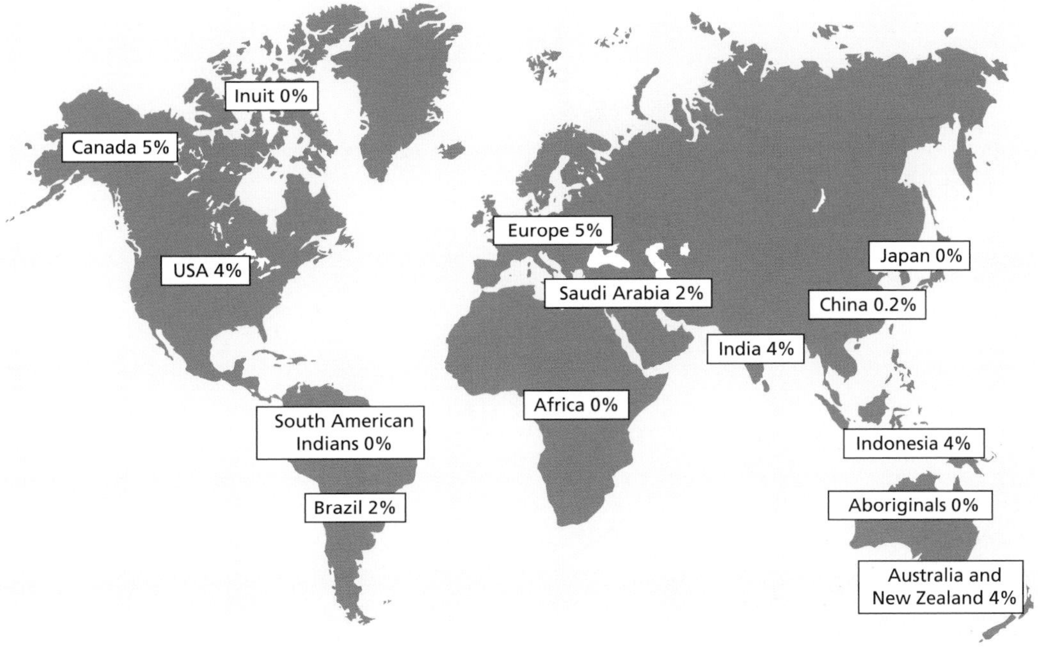

Fig. 25.4 The incidence of carriers of factor V Leiden in different countries.

Protein S deficiency

Protein S deficiency has been found in a number of families with a thrombotic tendency. It is a cofactor for protein C and the clinical features are similar to protein C deficiency, including a tendency to skin necrosis with warfarin therapy. The inheritance is autosomal dominant.

Prothrombin allele G20210A

Prothrombin allele G20210A is a variant (prevalence 2–3% in the population) that leads to increased plasma prothrombin levels and increases thrombotic risk by at least twofold. It is probable that the cause of venous thrombosis with this mutation and with high levels of factors VIII, IX and XI is that sustained generation of thrombin results in prolonged down-regulation of fibrinolysis through activation of thrombin-activated fibrinolysis inhibitor (p. 274).

Hyperhomocyst(e)inaemia

Higher levels of plasma homocysteine may be genetic or acquired and are associated with increased risk for both venous and arterial thrombosis. However, recent large trials show no evidence that lowering the levels reduces these risks.

Homocysteine is derived from dietary methionine and is removed by either remethylation to methionine or conversion to cysteine via a *trans*-sulphuration pathway (Fig. 25.5). Classic homocystinuria is a rare autosomal recessive disorder caused by deficiency of cystathione β-synthase, the enzyme responsible for *trans*-sulphuration. Vascular disease and thrombosis are major features of the disease. Heterozygous cystathione β-synthase deficiency is present in approximately 0.5% of the population and leads to a moderate increase in homocysteine. Methylene tetrahydrofolate reductase (MTHR) is involved in the remethylation pathway and a common thermolabile variant of the enzyme may be responsible for mild homocysteinaemia (above 15 μmol/L) although this may only be seen in the presence of folate deficiency (p. 46). Acquired risk factors for hyperhomocysteinaemia include deficiencies of folate, vitamin B_{12} or vitamin B_6, drugs (e.g. ciclosporin), renal damage

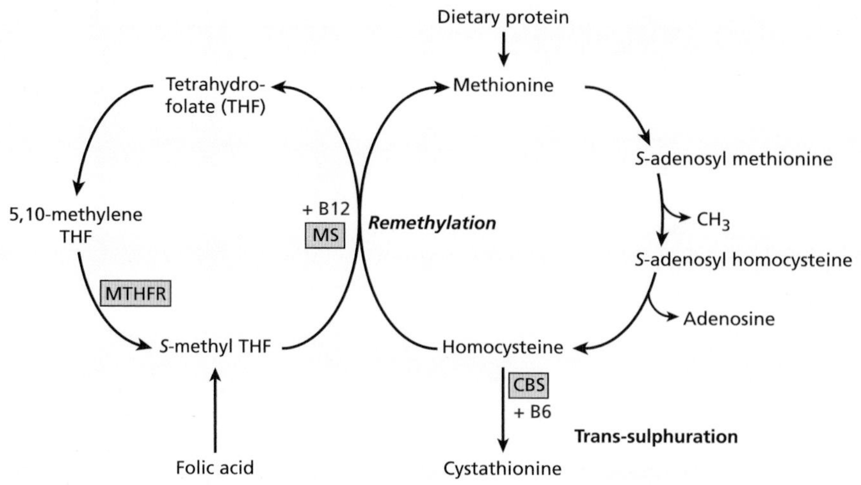

Fig. 25.5 The metabolism of homocysteine. Homocysteine is derived from dietary methionine and is metabolized either by the *trans*-sulphuration or remethylation pathways. *Trans*-sulphuration proceeds using the cystathionine β-synthase (CBS) enzyme with vitamin B_6 as a cofactor. Remethylation involves the action of methionine synthase (MS) on 5-methyl-THF with vitamin B_{12} as a cofactor. In addition, methylene-tetrahydrofolate reductase (MTHFR) is involved in this cycle.

and smoking. The levels also increase with age and are higher in men and post-menopausal females.

Defects of fibrinogen

Defects of fibrinogen are usually clinically silent or cause excess bleeding. Thrombosis is a rare association.

Hereditary or acquired disorders of haemostasis

High factor VIII or fibrinogen levels are also associated arterial thrombosis.

The combination of multiple risk factors is associated with increased risk of thrombosis. If these are persistent they may represent a reason for extended anticoagulation.

Acquired risk factors

These may cause thrombosis in patients without another identifiable abnormality but are most likely to do so if an inherited predisposing abnormality (e.g. factor V Leiden) is also present.

Postoperative venous thrombosis

This is more likely to occur in the elderly, obese, those with a previous or family history of venous thrombosis, and in those in whom major abdominal or hip operations are performed.

Venous stasis and immobility

These factors are probably responsible for the high incidence of postoperative venous thrombosis and for venous thrombosis associated with congestive cardiac failure, myocardial infarction and varicose veins. In atrial fibrillation, thrombin generation from accumulation of activated clotting factors leads to a high risk of systemic embolization. The use of muscle relaxants during anaesthesia may also contribute to venous stasis. Venous thrombosis also has a higher frequency after prolonged aeroplane journeys.

Malignancy

Patients with carcinoma of the ovary, brain and pancreas have a particularly increased risk of venous thrombosis but there is an increased risk with all cancers. The tumours produce tissue factor and a pro-coagulant that directly activates factor X. Mucin-secreting adenocarcinomas may be associated with DIC.

Inflammation

This up-regulates procoagulant factors, down-regulates anticoagulant pathways, particularly protein C. Thrombosis is particularly likely in inflammatory bowel disease, Behçet's disease, systemic tuberculosis, systemic lupus erythematosus (SLE) and diabetes.

Blood disorders

Increased viscosity, thrombocytosis, altered platelet membrane receptors and responses are possible factors for the high incidence of thrombosis in patients with polycythaemia vera and essential thrombocythaemia. There is a high incidence of venous thrombosis, including thrombi in large veins (e.g. the hepatic vein) in patients with paroxysmal nocturnal haemoglobinuria. An increased tendency to venous thrombosis has been observed in patients with sickle cell disease and patients with post splenectomy thrombocytosis.

Oestrogen therapy

Oestrogen therapy, particularly high-dose therapy, is associated with increased plasma levels of factors II, VII, VIII, IX and X and depressed levels of antithrombin and tissue plasminogen activator in the vessel wall. There is a high incidence of postoperative venous thrombosis in women on high-dose oestrogen therapy and full-dose oestrogen-containing oral contraceptives. The risk is much less with low-dose oestrogen contraceptive preparations. Hormone replacement therapy also increases the risk of thrombosis, largely obviated by the use of low oestrogen preparations.

The antiphospholipid syndrome

This may be defined as the occurrence of thrombosis or recurrent miscarriage in association with laboratory evidence of persistent antiphospholipid antibody. One antiphospholipid antibody is the 'lupus anticoagulant' (LA) which was initially detected in patients with SLE, and is identified by a prolonged plasma APTT which does not correct with a 50 : 50 mixture of normal plasma. A second test dependent on limiting quantities of phospholipid (e.g. the dilute Russell's viper venom test) is also used in diagnosis. The antibody represents part of the spectrum of antiphospholipid antibody syndrome (APS) and whereas lupus anticoagulants are reactive in the fluid phase, the other antiphospholipid antibodies (APAs), such as anticardiolipin antibodies (ACA) and antibodies to β_2-glycoprotein (β_2-GPI), are identified by solid phase immunoassay. Both solid phase assays and coagulation tests for LA should be used in the diagnosis of APS.

Table 25.3 Clinical associations of lupus anticoagulant and anticardiolipin antibodies.

Venous thrombosis deep venous thrombosis/pulmonary embolism renal, hepatic, retinal veins
Arterial thrombosis
Recurrent fetal loss
Thrombocytopenia
Livedo reticularis

NB. Recurrent fetal loss may also occur in other types of thrombophilia.

As well as patients with SLE, APS is also found in other autoimmune disorders particularly of connective tissues, lymphoproliferative diseases, post-viral infections, with certain drugs including phenothiazines and as an 'idiopathic' phenomenon in otherwise healthy subjects. Paradoxically, in view of its name, it is associated with venous and arterial thrombosis. The arterial thrombosis may cause peripheral limb ischaemia, stroke or myocardial infarct. As with other causes of thrombophilia, recurrent abortion caused by placental infarction is also associated (Table 25.3). Thrombocytopenia may be present and livedo reticularis is a frequent dermal manifestation. Treatment is with anticoagulation where indicated. It is usual to maintain an international normalized ratio (INR) of between 2.0 and 3.0 with warfarin but higher levels may be needed if previous arterial or major DVT has occurred or recurrence of thrombosis occurs on warfarin therapy. Low-dose heparin and aspirin are useful in the management of recurrent miscarriage.

Collagen vascular diseases and Behçet's syndrome are also associated with arterial and venous thrombosis, whether or not the lupus anticoagulant is present (p. 300).

Factor IX concentrates

Venous thrombosis may complicate the use of factor IX concentrates which contain trace amounts of activated coagulation factors. Patients with liver disease who are unable to clear these activated factors are especially at risk.

Glucosylceramide deficiency

Reduced plasma levels of the glycolipid glucosylceramide are a potential risk factor for venous thrombosis, particularly in young male patients. The glycolipid modulates the protein C pathway.

Investigation of thrombophilia

Many of the conditions associated with an increased thrombotic risk are obvious following clinical examination. A full assessment is indicated, particularly in patients who have recurrent or spontaneous DVT or pulmonary emboli, in patients who have thrombosis at a young age and in those patients with a familial tendency to thrombosis or thrombosis at an unusual site. It is also needed in women with recurrent fetal loss. With the increasing recognition of systemic causes of thrombophilia, the indications for thrombophilia screening are widening. The following laboratory tests are used in diagnosis.

Screening tests

1 Blood count and erythrocyte sedimentation rate (ESR)—to detect elevation in haematocrit, white cell count, platelet count, fibrinogen and globulins.

2 Blood film examination—may provide evidence of myeloproliferative disorder; leucoerythroblastic features may indicate malignant disease.

3 Prothrombin time (PT) and APTT—a shortened APPT is often seen in thrombotic states and may indicate the presence of activated clotting factors. A prolonged APTT test, not corrected by the addition of normal plasma, suggests a 'lupus anticoagulant' or an acquired inhibitor to a coagulation factor.

4 Anticardiolipin and anti-β_2-GPI antibodies.

5 Thrombin time and reptilase time—prolongation suggests an abnormal fibrinogen.

6 Fibrinogen assay.

7 Activated protein C (APC) resistance test and DNA analysis for factor V Leiden.

8 Antithrombin—immunological and functional assays.

9 Protein C and protein S—immunological and functional assays.

10 Prothrombin gene analysis for the G20210A variant.

11 Plasma homocysteine estimation.

In many patients even full investigation yields no abnormalities and treatment with oral anticoagulants may remain empirical.

12 Test for CD59 and CD55 expression (paroxysmal nocturnal haemoglobinuria) in red cells if paroxysmal nocturnal haemoglobinuria is suspected.

Diagnosis of venous thrombosis

Deep vein thrombosis

Clinical suspicion DVT is suspected in those with previous DVT, cancer or confined to bed. In the leg, unilateral thigh or calf swelling or tenderness, pitting oedema and the presence of collateral superficial non-varicose veins are important signs.

Serial compression ultrasound This is the most reliable and practical method for patients with first suspicion of DVT in the legs and other sites (Fig. 25.2a). It can be combined with spectral, colour (Fig. 25.2) or power Doppler (duplex) scanning which improves accuracy by focusing on individual veins. It does not distinguish between acute and chronic thrombi. Persisting venous obstruction detected by ultrasonography at the completion of warfarin therapy is associated with an increased risk of recurrent thrombosis.

Contrast venography This most sensitive procedure is reserved for patients with highly suggestive clinical findings but negative ultrasonography. Iodinated contrast medium is injected into a vein peripheral to the suspected DVT. This permits direct demonstration by X-ray of the site, size and extent of the thrombus (Fig. 25.2b). However, it is a painful invasive technique, with a risk of contrast reaction and procedure-induced DVT.

Plasma D-dimer concentration The concentration of these fibrin breakdown products is raised when there is a fresh venous thrombosis. It is a useful assay when recurrent thrombosis is suspected and also may be combined with the tests above for diagnosis of a first event. A negative result is useful in emergency departments for excluding DVT in patients with equivocal clinical features. D-dimer elevation in cancer, inflammation after surgery or trauma limits its usefulness.

Magnetic resonance imaging (MRI) This may also be used but is expensive. Impedance plethysmography is less sensitive and accurate and is falling out of use.

Pulmonary embolus

Clinical suspicion This is particularly suspected in patients with chest symptoms, especially if there are signs of or previous history of DVT, immobilization for more than 2 days or recent (<4 weeks) surgery, haemoptysis or cancer.

Chest X-ray This is often normal but may show evidence of pulmonary infarction or pleural effusion.

Ventilation perfusion (VQ) scintigraphy This detects areas of the lung being ventilated but not perfused.

Computed tomography (CT) pulmonary angiography Fine slices of the lung are scanned by spiral CT so that filling defects in the pulmonary arteries are visualized (Fig. 25.2c).

Magnetic resonance pulmonary angiography Gadolinium-enhanced MRI is a relatively new, expensive but accurate technique.

Pulmonary angiography This is the traditional reference method but is invasive with complications, albeit uncommon, such as arrhythmia or contrast reaction.

Electrocardiogram This is performed to determine whether there is right heart 'strain' which occurs only in relatively severe cases.

Anticoagulant drugs

Anticoagulant drugs are used widely in the treatment of venous thromboembolic disease. Their value in the treatment of arterial thrombosis is less well established.

Heparin

This acidic, unfractionated mucopolysaccharide of average molecular weight (MW) 15 000–18 000 is an inhibitor of blood coagulation because of its action in potentiating the activity of antithrombin (see below). As it is not absorbed from the gastrointestinal tract it must be given by injection. It is inactivated by the liver and excreted in the urine. The effective biological half-life is approximately 1 h (Table 25.4).

Table 25.4 Comparison of unfractionated heparin with low molecular weight heparin.

	Unfractionated heparin	Low molecular weight heparin
Mean molecular weight in kilodaltons (range)	15 (4–30)	4.5 (2–10)
Anti-Xa : anti-IIa	1 : 1	2 : 1 to 4 : 1
Inhibits platelet function	Yes	No
Bioavailability	50%	100%
Half-life		
intravenous	1 h	2 h
subcutaneous	2 h	4 h
Elimination	Renal and hepatic	Renal
Monitoring	APTT	Xa assay (usually not needed)
Frequency of heparin-induced thrombocytopenia	High	Low
Osteoporosis	Yes	Less frequent

APTT, activated partial thromboplastin time.

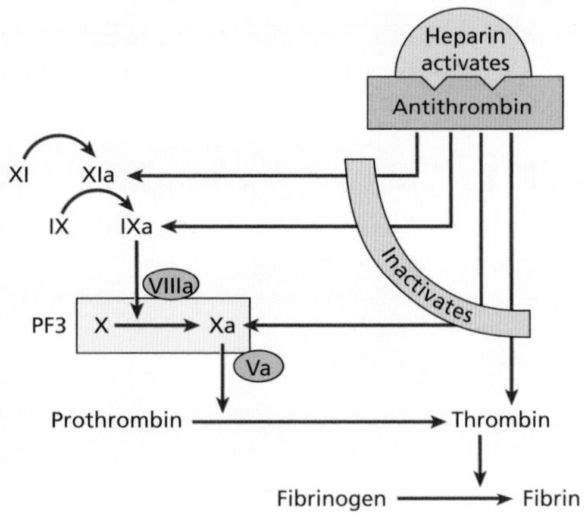

Fig. 25.6 The action of heparin. This activates antithrombin which then forms complexes with activated serine protease coagulation factors (thrombin, Xa, IXa and XIa) and so inactivates them.

Mode of action

Heparin dramatically potentiates the formation of complexes between antithrombin and activated serine protease coagulation factors, thrombin (IIa) and factors IXa, Xa and XIa (Fig. 25.6). This complex formation inactivates these factors irreversibly. In addition, heparin impairs platelet function.

Low molecular weight heparin (LMWH) preparations (MW 2000–10 000) are produced by enzymatic or chemical depolymerization of unfractionated heparin. They have a greater ability to inhibit factor Xa than to inhibit thrombin and interact less with platelets compared with standard heparin, and so may have a lesser tendency to cause bleeding. They also have greater bioavailability and a more prolonged half-life in plasma, making once-daily administration in prophylaxis or treatment feasible (Table 25.4).

Indications

Heparin is routinely used in DVT, pulmonary embolism and unstable angina pectoris. It is also widely used in the prophylaxis of venous thrombosis and is the drug of choice for women requiring anticoagulation in pregnancy because it does not cross the placenta. It is also used during cardiopulmonary bypass surgery, for maintaining the patency of indwelling venous lines and in some case of DIC if the manifestations are predominantly vaso-occlusive. There is some evidence that LMWH (or warfarin) may improve the survival in cancer patients over and above the protection from venous thrombosis but the exact mechanisms, types of cancer improved and optimum treatment regimes remain to be elucidated.

Administration and laboratory control

Standard heparin

Continuous intravenous infusion This provides the smoothest control of heparin therapy and is the treatment of choice where rapid reversal of anticoagulation by protamine sulphate may be required (e.g. in surgical patients or late pregnancy). It is still preferred by many for treatment of acute pulmonary embolus. In an adult, dosage of 30 000–40 000 units over 24 h (1000–2000 units/h with a loading dose of 5000 units) is usually satisfactory. Therapy is monitored by maintaining the APTT at 2–3 times the upper limit of the normal value. It is usual to start warfarin therapy within 2 days of starting heparin therapy and to discontinue heparin when the INR has been above 2.0 on two successive days. For acute coronary syndromes, both unfractionated heparin and LMWH are of benefit when used with aspirin in the prevention of mural thrombosis, systemic embolization and venous thrombosis.

Subcutaneous heparin Intermittent subcutaneous injections are preferred when heparin is given as prophylaxis against venous thrombosis (e.g. for surgical procedures). The usual dosage is 5000 units 12-hourly preoperatively followed by this dosage 8–12-hourly for 7 days or until the patient is mobile. LMWH (see below) is usually perferred as it can be given once daily.

Low molecular weight heparin

LMWH is given by subcutaneous injection and, as it has a longer half-life than standard heparin, it can be given once a day in prophylaxis, or once or twice a day in treatment (Table 25.4). Compared with unfractionated heparin, LMWH has a more predictable dose–response which avoids the need for routine monitoring. There is less risk of thrombocytopenia or osteoporosis. It is the treatment of choice for preventing or treating DVT. It is used increasingly for treatment of pulmonary embolus and unstable angina. Although routine monitoring is not required, measurement of anti-Xa peak levels 4 h after injection allows dose adjustment in selected patients (e.g. in pregnancy, renal failure, gross obesity and in children). Typical treatment regimens are 200 anti-Xa units/kg once daily or 100 anti-Xa units/kg twice daily). LMWH is preferred to unfractionated heparin for therapy of DVT including pulmonary embolism. Many patients with uncomplicated DVTs may now be managed at home with regular LMWH injections once or twice daily according to the preparation. LMWH is the preferred treatment for the prevention of DVT in both medical and surgical patients. It is also the preferred anticoagulant in pregnancy because it does not cross the placenta. Typical once daily subcutaneous dosage in prophylaxis is 2000–2500 units (moderate risk patients) or 4000–5000 units (high-risk patients).

Complications

Unfractionated heparin is associated with a number of side-effects. The risk of these complications appears to be reduced by approximately 50% by the use of LMWH.

Bleeding during heparin therapy

Bleeding may be because of excessive prolonged anticoagulation or to an antiplatelet functional effect of heparin. Intravenous heparin has a half-life of less than 1 h and it is usually only necessary to stop the infusion. Protamine is able to inactivate heparin immediately and for severe bleeding a dose of 1 mg/100 units heparin provides effective neutralization. However, protamine itself may act as an anticoagulant when in excess.

Heparin-induced thombocytopenia

A mild lowering of the platelet count may occur in the first 24 h as a result of platelet clumping. This is of no clinical consequence (heparin-induced thombocytopenia, HIT, type 1). The important HIT, type 2, may occur in up to 5% of patients who are treated with unfractionated heparin and paradoxically presents with thrombosis. It results from the binding of heparin to platelets followed by the generation of an immunoglobulin G (IgG) antibody to the heparin–platelet factor 4 (PF4) complex, which leads to platelet activation (Fig. 25.7). Typically, it presents as a fall of >50% in the platelet count 5 or more days after starting heparin treatment or earlier if heparin has been given previously. Diagnosis is difficult but assays have recently been developed to allow the detection of antibodies to immobilized heparin–PF4 complex. Heparin therapy must be discontinued. Thrombin inhibitors such as hirudin or lepirudin or argatroban appear promising as alternatives and the heparinoid danaparoid may also be used. LMWH is less likely than unfractionated heparin to cause HIT but there is cross-reactivity of the antibody. Warfarin therapy in some cases causes skin necrosis and should be delayed until alternative anticoagulation has been achieved.

Osteoporosis

This occurs with long-term (>2 months) heparin therapy, especially in pregnancy. The drug complexes minerals from the bones but the exact pathogenesis is unknown.

Oral anticoagulants

These are derivatives of coumarin or indandione. Warfarin, a coumarin, is most widely used. The drugs are vitamin K antagonists (p. 297) and so treatment results in decreased biological activity of the vitamin K-dependent factors II, VII, IX and X. Oral anticoagulants block the post-ribosomal γ-carboxylation of glutamic acid residues of these proteins (Fig. 24.7). After warfarin is given, factor VII levels fall considerably within 24 h but prothrombin has a longer plasma half-life and only falls to 50% of normal at 3 days; the patient is fully anticoagulated only after this period.

Principles of oral anticoagulation

A typical starting regimen for warfarin would be 10 mg on day 1, 5 mg on day 2 and then 5 mg on the third day. After this the dosage should be adjusted according to the PT. The usual maintenance dosage

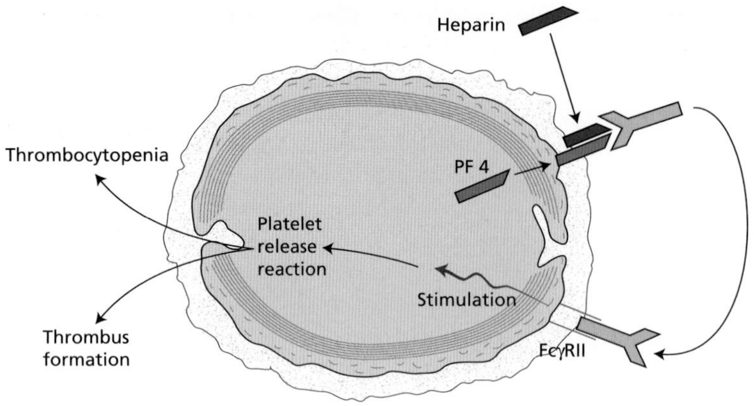

Fig. 25.7 Mechanism of heparin-induced thrombocytopenia (HIT). Platelet factor 4 (PF4) is released from α granules and forms a complex on the platelet surface with heparin. Immunoglobulin G antibodies (usually IgG_2) develop against this complex and once bound can activate the platelet through the platelet immunoglobulin receptor Fc-γRII. This leads to platelet stimulation, further release of PF4 and the platelet release reaction with consequent thrombocytopenia and thrombus development.

Table 25.5 Oral anticoagulant control tests. Target levels recommended by the British Society for Haematology (2000).

Target INR	Clinical state
2.5 (2.0–3.0)	Treatment of DVT, pulmonary embolism, atrial fibrillation, recurrent DVT off warfarin; symptomatic inherited thrombophilia, cardiomyopathy, mural thrombus, cardioversion
3.5 (3.0–4.0)	Recurrent DVT while on warfarin, mechanical prosthetic heart valves, antiphospholipid syndrome (some cases)

DVT, deep vein thrombosis; INR, international normalized ratio.

of warfarin is 3–9 mg/day but individual responses vary greatly. Lower loading dosage is recommended for the elderly or those with liver disease.

The indications and recommended ranges for INR with warfarin treatment are summarized in Table 25.5. The effect of oral anticoagulants is monitored by the PT. The INR is used and is based on the ratio of the patient's PT to a mean normal PT with correction for the 'sensitivity' of the thromboplastin used. This is calibrated against a primary World Health Organization (WHO) standard thromboplastin.

Warfarin crosses the placenta and is teratogenic. Heparin is preferred for pregnant patients because it does not cross the placenta and its action is short-lived.

It is usual to continue warfarin for 3–6 months for established DVT, pulmonary embolism and following xenograft heart valves. Long-term therapy is given for recurrent venous thrombosis, for embolic complications of rheumatic heart disease or atrial fibrillation, and with prosthetic valves and arterial grafts. It is also given long term in patients with a severe cause of thrombophilia (e.g. the lupus anticoagulant and a history of thrombosis).

Drug interactions

Approximately 97% of warfarin in the circulation is bound to albumin and only a small fraction of warfarin is free and can enter the liver parenchymal cells; it is this free fraction that is active. In the liver cells, warfarin is degraded in microsomes to an inactive water-soluble metabolite which is conjugated and excreted in the bile and partially reabsorbed to be also excreted in urine. Drugs that affect the albumin binding or excretion of warfarin (or of other oral anticoagulants) or those that decrease the absorption of vitamin K will interfere with the control of therapy (Table 25.6).

Table 25.6 Drugs and other factors that interfere with the control of anticoagulant therapy.

Potentiation of oral anticoagulants	Inhibition of oral anticoagulants
Drugs that increase the effect of coumarins	**Drugs that depress the action of coumarins**
Reduced coumarin binding to serum albumin	*Acceleration of hepatic microsomal degradation of coumarin*
Sulfonamides	Barbiturates
Inhibition of hepatic microsomal degradation of coumarin	Rifampicin
Cimetidine	*Enhanced synthesis of clotting factors*
Allopurinol	Oral contraceptives
Tricyclic antidepressants	**Hereditary resistance to oral anticoagulants**
Metronidazole	
Sulfonamides	**Pregnancy**
Alteration of hepatic receptor site for drug	
Thyroxine	
Quinidine	
Decreased synthesis of vitamin K factors	
High doses of salicylates	
Some cephalosporins	
Liver disease	
Decreased synthesis of vitamin K factors	
Decreased absorption of vitamin K	
e.g. malabsorption, antibiotic therapy, laxatives	

NB. Patients are also more likely to bleed if taking antiplatelet agents (e.g. NSAIDs, dipyridamole or aspirin); alcohol in large amounts enhances warfarin action.

Management of warfarin overdose

If the INR is in excess of 4.5 without bleeding, warfarin should be stopped for 1 or 2 days and the dose adjusted according to the INR. The long half-life of warfarin (40 h) delays the full impact of dose changes for 4–5 days. If the INR is very high (e.g. >8) without bleeding, an oral dose of 0.5–2.5 mg vitamin K may be given. Mild bleeding usually only needs an INR assessment, drug withdrawal and subsequent dosage adjustment (Table 25.7). More serious bleeding may need cessation of therapy, vitamin K therapy or the infusion of fresh frozen plasma or prothrombin concentrates. Vitamin K is the specific antidote; an oral or intravenous dose of 2.5 mg is usually effective. Higher doses result in resistance to further warfarin therapy for 2–3 weeks.

Management of surgery

For minor surgery (e.g. dental extraction) anticoagulation can be maintained and mouth rinses with tranexamine acid given. For major surgery, warfarin is stopped to get an INR <1.5 and LMWH given when the INR falls to <2.0 (except on the day or surgery) and continued until the INR is >2.0 after restarting warfarin.

New anticoagulants

Traditional anticoagulant therapy has disadvantages. LMWH has to be given subcutaneously and warfarin requires frequent monitoring and dose adjustment and there is interaction with drugs and food.

Factor Xa inhibitors: Fondaparinux, a synthetic analogue of the antithrombin-binding pentasaccharide of heparin, is an indirect irreversible factor Xa inhibitor. It is given subcutaneously, has a plasma half-life of 17 h and does not require laboratory monitoring. Extensive trials have demonstrated that

Table 25.7 Recommendations on the management of bleeding and excessive anticoagulation by the British Committee for Standards in Haematology (third edition 1998; 2005 update).

INR 3.0–6.0 (target INR 2.5)	Reduce warfarin dose or stop
INR 4.0–6.0 (target INR 3.5)	Restart warfarin when INR <5.0
INR 6.0–8.0 No bleeding or minor bleeding	Stop warfarin* Restart when INR <5.0
INR >8.0 No bleeding or minor bleeding	Stop warfarin Restart warfarin when INR <5.0 If other risk factors for bleeding give 0.5–2.5 mg vitamin K orally
Major bleeding	Stop warfarin Give prothrombin complex concentrate 50 units/kg, in preference FFP 15 mL/kg (when available) Give 5 mg vitamin K (i.v. or oral)

FFP, fresh frozen plasma; INR, international normalized ratio; i.v., intravenous.
* 1 mg vitamin K may be given orally to rapidly reduce the INR to the therapeutic range within 24 h in all patients with an INR above the therapeutic range and no bleeding.

it is an effective antithrombotic agent in selected patients for prevention and treatment of both venous and arterial thromboembolic disorders. It also reduces major bleeding and may improve long-term mortality and morbity e.g. in acute coronary syndromes. *Idraparinux*, a chemically modified analogue of fondaparinux has a longer half-life and, as a once weekly injection, it may be more convenient than LMWH in treatment and prophylaxis, and has the potential to replace warfarin in selected patients.

Direct thrombin inhibitors These include recombinant hirudins, bivalirudin, argatroban, melagratan and ximelagratan.

Bivalirudin has been used as an alternative to heparin in patients undergoing percutaneous coronary interventions and is associated with less bleeding and a reduced need for adjunctive treatment with glycoprotein IIb/IIIa antagonists in patients undergoing stenting.

Ximelagratan, a lipophilic pro-drug may be given orally and following absorption is rapidly converted to melagratan. *Melagratan* may be given subcutaneously. Routine anticoagulation monitoring is unnecessary. Approximately 6–10% of patients develop reversible increases in liver enzymes. Ximelagratan has been compared with either LMWH or warfarin in large numbers of clinical trials. It is as effective as conventional therapy in preventing venous thrombous in orthopoedic and general surgery without an increased risk of major haemorrhage. It has had similar success in the treatment of acute venous thrombosis, myocardial infarction and severe recurrent myocardial ischaemia and in the prevention of stroke and systemic arterial embolism in patients with atrial fibrillation.

Before they are licensed, more data on their effectiveness and safety in a more diverse spectrum of patients are necessary. No specific antidote is available for either the pentasaccharides or ximelagatran.

Graduated compression stockings

These are used postoperatively and during long aeroplane flights to reduce the risk of DVT. After a DVT, they reduce the risk of post-thrombotic syndrome.

Inferior vena cava filter

This can provide short-term protection against pulmonary embolism when a DVT in the legs is diagnosed but anticoagulation is contraindicated (e.g. ongoing or very recent intracranial or gastrointestinal bleeding or where there is recurrent pulmonary embolism despite adequate anticoagulation).

Table 25.8 Fibrinolytic agents—plasminogen activators.

Streptokinase (SK)
Tissue plasminogen activator (tPA)
Single-chain urokinase-type plasminogen activator (SCU-PA)
Acylated plasminogen–streptokinase activator complex (APSAC)

Fibrinolytic agents

A number of fibrinolytic agents are able to lyse fresh thrombi (Table 25.8). They may be used systemically for patients with acute myocardial infarction, major pulmonary embolism or iliofemoral thrombosis, and locally in patients with acute peripheral arterial occlusion.

Administration of thrombolytic agents has been simplified with standardized dosage regimens. The therapy is most effective in the first 6 h after symptoms begin but is still of benefit up to 24 h. Streptokinase is given in a loading dose of 250 000 units followed by a maintenance dose 100 000 units/h for 12–48 h. In acute myocardial infarction, streptokinase is given as a single dose of 1500 000 units over 60 min. Aspirin therapy is also given and the value of additional heparin therapy is under study.

The use of laboratory tests for monitoring and control of short-term thrombolytic therapy is now considered unnecessary. However, certain clinical complications exclude the use of thrombolytic agents (Table 25.9).

Recombinant tissue plasminogen activator (tPA) has a particularly high affinity for fibrin and this allows lysis of thrombi with less systemic activation of fibrinolysis. Acylated plasminogen streptokinase activator complex (APSAC) and single-chain urokinase-type plasminogen activator (SCU-PA) are two other fibrinolytic agents.

Antiplatelet drugs

Antiplatelet agents are gaining an increasing role in clinical medicine. It is now clear that aspirin is valuable in the secondary prevention of vascular disease. Several other agents are being used for different indications (Table 25.10). The sites of action of the antiplatelet drugs are illustrated in Fig. 25.8.

Aspirin Aspirin inhibits platelet cyclo-oxygenase irreversibly, thus reducing the production of platelet thromboxane A_2. It has been suggested that vascular endothelial cyclo-oxygenase is less sensitive to aspirin than platelet cyclo-oxygenase. Low-dose therapy (e.g. 75 mg/day) is more effective than standard doses at enhancing the prostacyclin : thromboxane A_2 ratio and may have a greater antithrombotic effect. It is used in patients who have a history of coronary artery or cerebrovascular disease. It may also be useful in preventing thrombosis in patients with thrombocytosis.

Dipyridamole (Persantin) This drug is a phosphodiesterase inhibitor thought to elevate cyclic adenosine

Table 25.9 Contraindications to thrombolytic therapy.

Absolute contraindications	Relative contraindications
Active gastrointestinal bleeding	Traumatic cardiopulmonary resuscitation
Aortic dissection	Major surgery in the past 10 days
Head injury or cerebrovascular accident in the past 2 months	Past history of gastrointestinal bleeding
Neurosurgery in the past 2 months	Recent obstetric delivery
Intracranial aneurysm or neoplasm	Prior arterial puncture
Proliferative diabetic retinopathy	Prior organ biopsy
	Serious trauma
	Severe arterial hypertension (systolic pressure >200 mmHg, diastolic pressure >110 mmHg)
	Bleeding diathesis

Table 25.10 Antiplatelet therapy in patients with an acute coronary syndrome and in those undergoing percutaneous coronary intervention (PCI). (After Lange R.A. and Hillis L.D. (2004) Antiplatelet therapy for ischemic heart disease. *N Engl J Med* **350**,277–80)

Drug	Target/patient group	Duration
Acute coronary syndrome		
Aspirin	All	Life long
Clopidogrel	All	9–12 months
Glycoprotein IIb/IIIa inhibitors		
Abciximab	None	–
Eptifibatide	High risk	48–72 h
Tirofiban	High risk	48–72 h
Patients undergoing PCI		
Aspirin	All	Life long
Clopidogrel	All	9–12 months
Abciximab	High risk	12 h after PCI
Eptifibatide	High risk	18–24 h after PCI
Tirofiban	None	–

monophosphate (cAMP) levels in circulating platelets which decreases their sensitivity to activating stimuli. Dipyridamole has been shown to reduce thromboembolic complications in patients with prosthetic heart valves and to improve the results in coronary bypass operations.

Sulfinpyrazone This drug is a competitive inhibitor of cyclo-oxygenase. It has been effective in reducing the frequency of blockage in arteriovenous shunts in chronic dialysis patients.

Ticlopidine This is an antiplatelet drug that was used following coronary angioplasty. Side-effects include neutropenia or thrombocytopenia. It has been replaced by clopidogrel except in patients intolerant of clopidogrel.

Clopidogrel This adenosine diphospate (ADP) receptor antagonist is an antiplatelet agent in use for reduction of ischaemic events in patients with

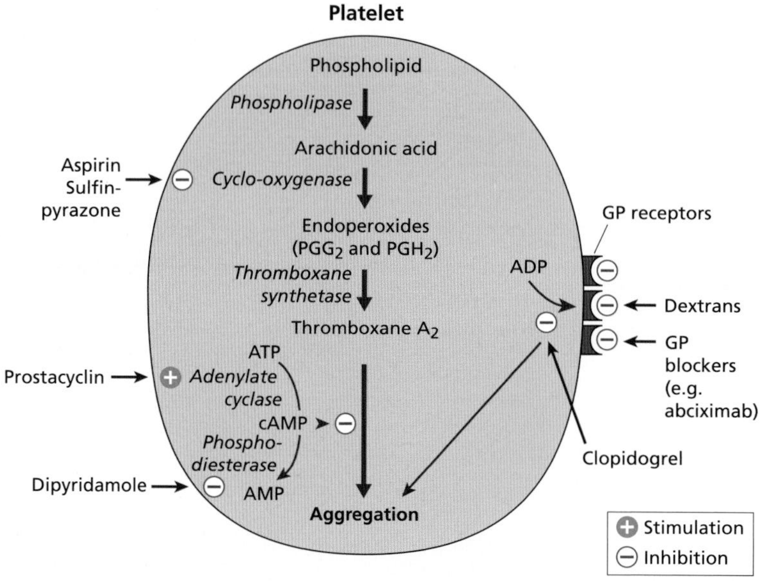

Fig. 25.8 Sites of action of antiplatelet drugs. Aspirin acetylates the enzyme cyclo-oxygenase irreversibly. Sulfinpyrazone inhibits cyclo-oxygenase reversibly. Dipyridamole inhibits phosphodiesterase, increases cyclic adenosine monophosphate (cAMP) levels and inhibits aggregation. Inhibition of adenosine uptake by red cells allows adenosine accumulation in plasma which stimulates platelet adenylate cyclase. Prostacyclin (epoprostenol) stimulates adenylate cyclase. The lipid-soluble β-blockers inhibit phospholipase. Calcium-channel antagonists block the influx of free calcium ions across the platelet membrane. Dextrans coat the surface interfering with adhesion and aggregation. GP, glycoprotein.

ischaemic stroke, myocardial infarction or peripheral vascular disease. It is used after coronary artery stenting or angioplasty and in patients requiring long-term antiplatelet therapy who are intolerant or allergic to aspirin.

Glycoprotein IIb/IIIa inhibitors: abciximab, eptifibatide, tirofiban These drugs are monoclonal antibodies that inhibit the platelet GPIIb/IIIa receptor. They are used in conjunction with heparin and aspirin for the prevention of ischaemic complications in high-risk patients undergoing percutaneous transluminal coronary angioplasty. They can be used once only.

Specific antithrombotic agents Intravenous prostacyclin has been used in clinical trials in patients with peripheral vascular disease and thrombotic thrombocytopenic purpura. It has also reduced arteriovenous shunt blockage in haemodialysis patients.

Bibliography

Baglin T.P., Keeling D.M., Watson H.G. (2006) Guidelines on oral anticoagulation (warfarin): third edition – 2005 update. *Br J Haematol* **132**,277–85.

Baglin T., Barrowcliffe T.W., Cohen A., Greave M. (2006) Guidelines on the use and monitoring of heparin. *Br J Haematol* **133**,19–34.

Bates S.M. and Weitz J.I. (2006) The status of new anticoagulants. *Br J Haematol* **134**,3–19.

Bønaa K.H., Njølstad I., Ueland P.M. *et al.* (2006) Homocysteine lowering and myocardial infarction. *N Engl J Med* **354**,1573–88.

Bounameaux H. and de Moerloose P. (2004) Is laboratory monitoring of low-molecular-weight heparin therapy necessary? No. *J Thromb Haemost* **2**,551–4.

Fedullo P.F. and Tapson V.F. (2003) The evaluation of suspected pulmonary embolism. *N Engl J Med* **349**,1247–56.

The Fifth Organization to assess strategies in acute ischemic syndromes investigators (2006) Comparison of fondaparinux and enoxaparin in acute coronary syndromes. *N Engl J Med* **354**,1464–76.

Geerts W.H., Pineo G.F., Heit J.A. *et al.* (2004) Prevention of venous thromboembolism: the Seventh ACCP Conference on antithrombotic and thrombolytic therapy. *Chest* **126**,338S–400S.

Greaves M., Cohen H., MacHin S.J., Mackie I. (2000) Guidelines on the investigation and management of the antiphospholipid syndrome *Br J Haematol* **109**,704–15.

Hasan H.I. and Matson M.B. (2006) Inferior vena cava filters: current concepts. *Thrombus* **10**,9–11.

Hirsh J., Guyatt, G., Albers G.W., Schünemann H.J. (eds) (2004) The Seventh ACCP Conference on antithrombotic and thrombolytic therapy: evidence-based guidelines. *Chest* **126**(Suppl.),172S–3S.

Hirsh J., O'Donnell M., Weitz J.I. (2005) New anticoagulants. *Blood* **105**,453–63.

The HOPE-2 Investigators (2006) Homocysteine lowering and cardiovascular events after acute myocardial infarction. *N Engl J Med* **354**,1567–77.

Keeling D.M., Mackie I.J., Moody A., Watson H.G. (2004) The diagnosis of deep vein thrombosis in symptomatic outpatients and the potential for clinical assessment and D-dimer assays to reduce the need for diagnostic imaging. *Br J Haematol* **124**,15–25.

Kujovich J.L. (2004) Hormones and pregnancy: thromboembolic risks for women. *Br J Haematol* **126**,443–54.

Kyrle P.A. and Eichinger S. (2005) Deep vein thrombosis. *Lancet* **365**,1163–74.

Lane D.A. and Grant P.J. (2000) Role of hemostatic gene polymorphisms in venous and arterial thrombotic disease. *Blood* **95**,1517–32.

Lange R.A. and Hillis L.D. (2004) Antiplatelet therapy for ischemic heart disease. *N Engl J Med* **350**,277–80. Erratum in (2004) *N Engl J Med* **351**,200.

Lecumberri R., Paramo J.A., Rocha E. (2005) Anticoagulant treatment and survival in cancer patients: the evidence from clinical studies. *Haematologica* **90**,1258–66.

Lissalde-Lavigne G., Cochery-Nouvellon E., Mercier E. *et al.* (2005) The association between hereditary thrombophilias and pregnancy loss. *Haematologica* **90**,1223–30.

Lockshin M.D. and Erkan D. (2003) Treatment of the antiphospholipid syndrome. *N Engl J Med* **349**,1177–9.

Love C.D.O. (2006) Can haematological tests predict cardiovascular risk? The 2005 Kettle Lecture. *Br J Haematol* **133**,232–50.

Schulman S. (2003) Clinical practice. Care of patients receiving long-term anticoagulant therapy. *N Engl J Med* **349**,675–83.

Stein P.D., Fowler S.E., Goodman L.R. *et al.* (2006) Multidetector computed tomography for acute pulmonary embolism. *N Engl J Med* **354**,2317–27.

Stein P.D., Hull R.D., Patel K.C. *et al.* (2004) D-dimer for the exclusion of acute venous thrombosis and pulmonary embolism: a systematic review. *Ann Intern Med* **140**,589–602.

Wells P.S., Anderson D.R., Rodger M. *et al.* (2003) Evaluation of D-dimer in the diagnosis of suspected deep-vein thrombosis. *N Engl J Med* **349**,1227–35.

Wood K. (ed) For the British Committee for Standards in Haematology. (2000) *Standard Haematology Practice 2: Guidelines in Oral Anticoagulation*. Blackwell Science, Oxford: pp. 104–29.

CHAPTER 26

26 Haematological changes in systemic disease

Anaemia of chronic disorders

Many of the anaemias seen in clinical practice occur in patients with systemic disorders and are the result of a number of contributing factors. The anaemia of chronic disorders (also discussed on p. 39) is of central importance and occurs in patients with a variety of chronic inflammatory and malignant diseases (Table 26.1). Usually, both the erythrocyte sedimentation rate (ESR) and C-reactive protein (CRP) are raised. It may be complicated by additional features which may be because of disease affecting particularly one or other system. The characteristic features are described in Chapter 3.

The pathogenesis of this anaemia appears to be related to the decreased release of iron from macrophages to plasma and so to erythroblasts caused by hepcidin, reduced red cell lifespan and an inadequate erythropoietin response to anaemia. The plasma levels of various cytokines, especially interleukin-1 (IL-1), IL-6 and tumour necrosis factor (TNF) are raised and reduce erythropoietin secretion. The anaemia is corrected by the successful treatment of the underlying disease. It does not respond to iron therapy despite the low serum iron. Responses to recombinant erythropoietin therapy may be obtained (e.g. in rheumatoid arthritis or cancer). In many conditions the anaemia is complicated by anaemia from other causes (e.g. iron or folate deficiency, renal failure, bone marrow infiltration, hypersplenism or endocrine abnormality).

Table 26.1 Causes of anaemia of chronic disorders.

Chronic inflammatory diseases
Infectious (e.g. pulmonary abscess, tuberculosis, osteomyelitis, pneumonia, bacterial endocarditis)
Non-infectious (e.g. rheumatoid arthritis, systemic lupus erythematosus and other connective tissue diseases, sarcoid, Crohn's disease, cirrhosis)

Malignant disease
(e.g. carcinoma, lymphoma, sarcoma, myeloma)

Malignant diseases (other than primary bone marrow diseases)

Anaemia

Contributing factors include anaemia of chronic disorders, blood loss and iron deficiency, marrow infiltration (Fig. 26.1) often associated with a leucoerythroblastic blood film (nucleated red cells and granuloctye precursors in the blood film), folate deficiency, haemolysis and marrow suppression from radiotherapy or chemotherapy (Table 26.2). Other causes of a leucoerythroblastic anaemia include

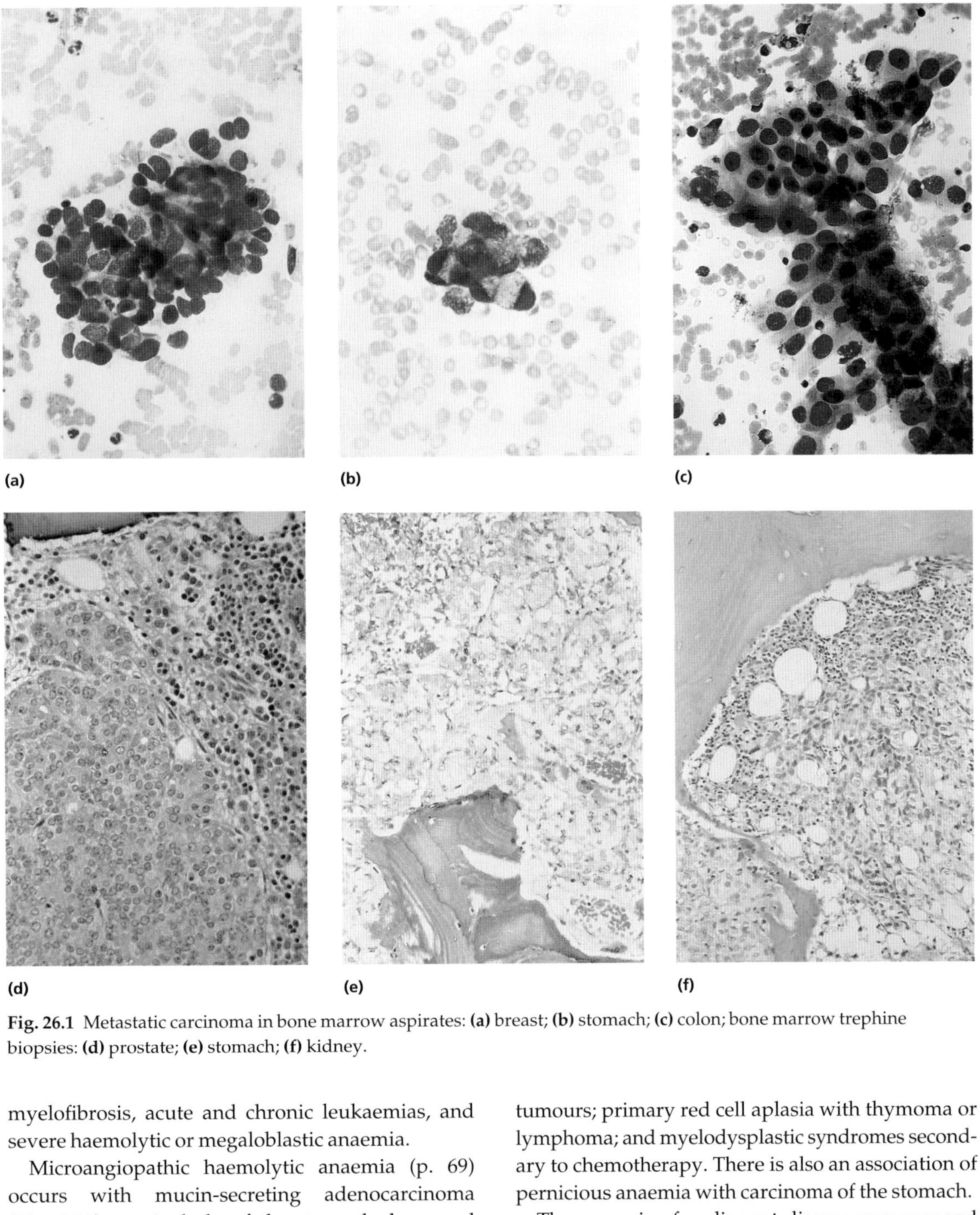

Fig. 26.1 Metastatic carcinoma in bone marrow aspirates: **(a)** breast; **(b)** stomach; **(c)** colon; bone marrow trephine biopsies: **(d)** prostate; **(e)** stomach; **(f)** kidney.

myelofibrosis, acute and chronic leukaemias, and severe haemolytic or megaloblastic anaemia.

Microangiopathic haemolytic anaemia (p. 69) occurs with mucin-secreting adenocarcinoma (Fig. 26.2), particularly of the stomach, lung and breast. Less common forms of anaemia with malignant disease include autoimmune haemolytic anaemia with malignant lymphoma and rarely with other tumours; primary red cell aplasia with thymoma or lymphoma; and myelodysplastic syndromes secondary to chemotherapy. There is also an association of pernicious anaemia with carcinoma of the stomach.

The anaemia of malignant disease may respond partly to erythropoietin. Folic acid should only be given if there is definite megaloblastic anaemia caused by the deficiency; it might 'feed' the tumour.

Table 26.2 Haematological abnormalities in malignant disease.

Haematological abnormality	Tumour or treatment associated
Pancytopenia	
Marrow hypoplasia	Chemotherapy, radiotherapy
Myelodysplasia	Chemotherapy, radiotherapy
Leucoerythroblastic	Metastases in marrow
Megaloblastic	Folate deficiency
	B_{12} deficiency (carcinoma of stomach)
Red cells	
Anaemia of chronic disorders	Most forms
Iron deficiency anaemia	Especially gastrointestinal, uterine
Pure red cell aplasia	Thymoma
Immune haemolytic anaemia	Lymphoma, ovary, other tumours
Microangiopathic haemolytic anaemia	Mucin-secreting carcinoma
Polycythaemia	Kidney, liver, cerebellum, uterus
White cells	
Neutrophil leucocytosis	Most forms
Leukaemoid reaction	Disseminated tumours, those with necrosis
Eosinophilia	Hodgkin's disease, others
Monocytosis	Various tumours
Platelets and coagulation	
Thrombocytosis	Gastrointestinal tumours with bleeding, others
Disseminated intravascular coagulation	Mucin-secreting carcinoma, prostate
Activation of fibrinolysis	Prostate
Acquired inhibitors of coagulation	Most forms
Paraprotein interfering with platelet function	Lymphomas, myeloma
Tumour cell procoagulants—tissue factor and cancer procoagulant (density activates factor X)	Especially ovarian, pancreas, brain, colon

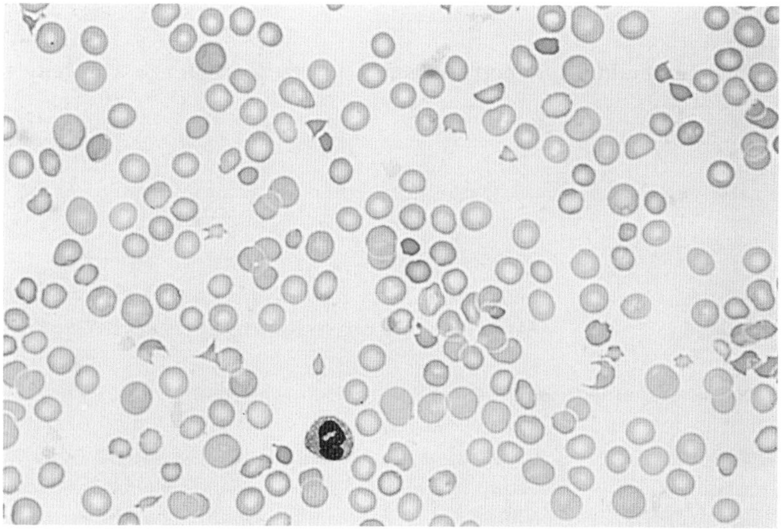

Fig. 26.2 Peripheral blood film in metastatic mucin-secreting adenocarcinoma of the stomach showing red cell polychromasia and fragmentation and thrombocytopenia. The patient had disseminated intravascular coagulation.

Polycythaemia

Secondary polycythaemia is occasionally associated with renal, hepatic, cerebellar and uterine tumours (p. 236).

White cell changes

Leukaemoid reactions (p. 102) may occur with tumours showing widespread necrosis and inflammation. Hodgkin's disease is associated with a variety of white cell abnormalities including eosinophilia, monocytosis and leucopenia. In non-Hodgkin's lymphoma, malignant cells may circulate in the blood (p. 194).

Platelet and blood coagulation abnormalities

Patients with malignant disease may show either thrombocytosis or thrombocytopenia. Disseminated tumours, particularly mucin-secreting adenocarcinomas, are associated with disseminated intravascular coagulation (DIC; p. 298) and generalized haemostatic failure. Activation of fibrinolysis occurs in some patients with carcinoma of the prostate. Occasional patients with malignant disease have spontaneous bruising or bleeding caused by an acquired inhibitor of one or other coagulation factor, most frequently factor VIII, or to a paraprotein interfering with platelet function.

Cancer patients have a high incidence (estimated at 15%) of venous thromboembolism. This is increased by surgery and some drugs, most recently thalidomide. It is most common in ovarian, brain, pancreatic and colon cancers. It may be difficult to manage with oral anticoagulation because of bleeding, interruptions with chemotherapy and thrombocytopenia, anorexia or vomiting. Liver disease and drug interactions can cause further complications so daily low molecular weight heparin injections may be preferable to warfarin.

Rheumatoid arthritis (and other connective tissue disorders)

In patients with rheumatoid arthritis, the anaemia of chronic disorders is proportional to the severity of the disease. It is complicated in some patients by iron deficiency caused by gastrointestinal bleeding related to therapy with salicylates, non-steroidal anti-inflammatory agents or corticosteroids. Bleeding into inflamed joints may also be a factor. Marrow hypoplasia may follow therapy with gold. In Felty's syndrome, splenomegaly is associated with neutropenia (Fig. 26.3). Anaemia and thrombocytopenia may also be present. In systemic lupus erythematosus (SLE) there may be anaemia of chronic disorders and 50% of patients are leucopenic with reduced neutrophil and lymphocyte counts often associated with circulating immune complexes. Renal impairment and drug-induced gastrointestinal blood loss also contribute to the anaemia. Autoimmune haemolytic anaemia (typically with immunoglobulin G (IgG) and the C3 component of complement on the surface of the red cells) occurs in 5% of patients and may be the presenting feature of the syndrome. There may be autoimmune

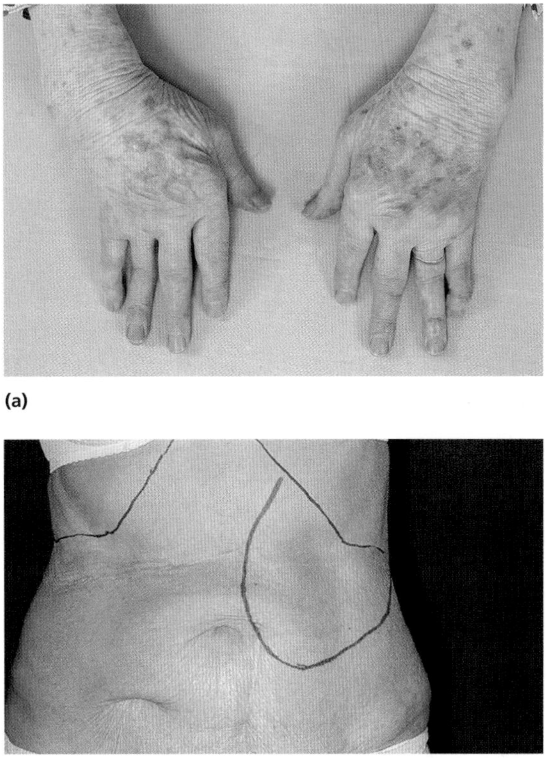

(a)

(b)

Fig. 26.3 Felty's syndrome: **(a)** the typical deformities of rheumatoid arthritis of the hand and **(b)** splenomegaly.

thrombocytopenia in 5% of patients. The lupus anticoagulant is described on p. 300. This circulating anticardiolipin interferes with blood coagulation by altering the binding of coagulation factors to platelet phospholipid and predisposes to both arterial and venous thrombosis and recurrent abortions. The antibody may be responsible for a false positive Wassermann reaction. Tests for antinuclear factor (ANF) and anti-DNA antibodies are usually positive.

Patients with temporal arteritis and polymyalgia rheumatica have a markedly elevated ESR, pronounced red cell rouleaux in the blood film and a polyclonal immunoglobulin response. These and other collagen vascular disorders are associated with anaemia of chronic disorders.

Renal failure

Anaemia

A normochromic anaemia is present in most patients with chronic renal failure. Generally, there is a 2 g/dL fall in haemoglobin level for every 10 mmol/L rise in blood urea. There is impaired red cell production as a result of defective erythropoietin secretion (see Fig. 2.5). Uraemic serum has also been shown to contain factors that inhibit proliferation of erythroid progenitors but, in view of the excellent response to erythropoietin in most patients, the clinical relevance of these is doubtful. Variable shortening of red cell lifespan occurs and in severe uraemia the red cells show abnormalities including spicules (spurs) and 'burr' cells (Fig. 26.4). Increased red cell 2,3-diphosphoglycerate (2,3-DPG) levels in response to the anaemia and hyperphosphataemia result in decreased oxygen affinity and a shift of the haemoglobin oxygen dissociation curve to the right (p. 18), which is augmented by uraemic acidosis. The patient's symptoms are therefore relatively mild for the degree of anaemia.

Other factors may complicate the anaemia of chronic renal failure (Table 26.3): the anaemia of chronic disorders, iron deficiency from blood loss during dialysis or caused by bleeding because of defective platelet function, and folate deficiency in some chronic dialysis patients. Aluminium excess in patients on chronic dialysis also inhibits erythropoiesis. Patients with polycystic kidneys usually have retained erythropoietin production and may have less severe anaemia for the degree of renal failure.

Treatment

Erythropoietin therapy has been found to correct the anaemia in patients on dialysis or in chronic renal failure, providing that iron and folate deficiency, aluminium excess and infections have been corrected. The dosage of erythropoietin usually required is 50–150 units/kg three times a week intravenously or by subcutaneous infusion. The response is faster after intravenous administration, but greater with the subcutaneous route.

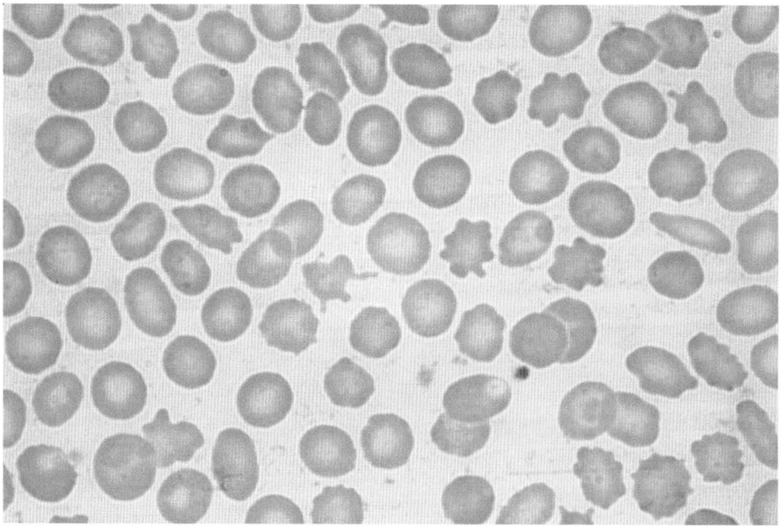

Fig. 26.4 Peripheral blood film in chronic renal failure showing red cell acanthocytosis and numerous 'burr' cells.

Table 26.3 Haematological abnormalities in renal failure.

Anaemia
Reduced erythropoietin production
Aluminium excess in dialysis patients
Anaemia of chronic disorders
Iron deficiency
blood loss (e.g. dialysis, venesection, defective platelet function)
Folate deficiency
chronic haemodialysis without replacement therapy
Abnormal platelet function
Thrombocytopenia
Immune complex-mediated (e.g. systemic lupus erythematosus, polyarteritis nodosa)
Some cases of acute nephritis and following allograft
Haemolytic uraemic syndrome and thrombotic thrombocytopenic purpura
Thrombosis
Some cases of the nephrotic syndrome
Polycythaemia
In renal allograft recipients
Rarely in renal cell carcinoma, cysts, arterial disease

Maintenance by 75 units/kg/week subcutaneously is typical. Complications of therapy have been initial transient flu-like symptoms, hypertension, clotting of the dialysis lines and, rarely, fits. A poor response to erythropoietin suggests iron or folate deficiency, infection, aluminium toxicity or hyperparathyroidism.

Platelet and coagulation abnormalities

A bleeding tendency with purpura, gastrointestinal or uterine bleeding occurs in 30–50% of patients with chronic renal failure and is marked in patients with acute renal failure. The bleeding is out of proportion to the degree of thrombocytopenia and has been associated with abnormal platelet or vascular function, which can be reversed by dialysis. Correction of the anaemia with erythropoietin also improves the bleeding tendency. Immune complex-mediated thrombocytopenia occurs in some patients with acute nephritis, SLE and polyarteritis nodosa and also following renal allografts. Renal allografts may also lead to polycythaemia in 10–15% of patients.

The haemolytic uraemic syndrome and thrombotic thrombocytopenic purpura are discussed on p. 284. Patients with the nephrotic syndrome have an increased risk of venous thrombosis.

Liver disease

The haematological abnormalities in liver disease are listed in Table 26.4. Chronic liver disease is associated with anaemia that is mildly macrocytic and often accompanied by target cells, mainly as a result of increased cholesterol in the membrane (Fig. 26.5a). Contributing factors to the anaemia may include blood loss (e.g. bleeding varices) with iron deficiency, dietary folate deficiency and direct suppression of haemopoiesis by alcohol. Alcohol may have an inhibiting effect on folate metabolism and is occasionally associated with (ring) sideroblastic changes which disappear when alcohol is withdrawn.

Haemolytic anaemia may occur in patients with alcohol intoxication (Zieve's syndrome) (Fig. 26.5b) and in Wilson's disease (caused by copper oxidation of red cell membranes) and autoimmune haemolytic anaemia is found in some patients with

Table 26.4 Haematological abnormalities in liver disease.

Liver failure ± obstructive jaundice ± portal hypertension
Refractory anaemia—usually mildly macrocytic, often with target cells; may be associated with:
Blood loss and iron deficiency
Alcohol (± ring sideroblastic change)
Folate deficiency
Haemolysis (e.g. Zieve's syndrome, Wilson's disease, immune hypersplenism from portal hypertension)
Bleeding tendency
Deficiency of vitamin K-dependent factors; also of factor V and fibrinogen
Thrombocytopenia hypersplenism, immune platelet function defects
Functional abnormalities of fibrinogen
Increased fibrinolysis
Portal hypertension—haemorrhage from varices
Viral hepatitis
Aplastic anaemia
Tumours
Polycythaemia
Neutrophil leucocytosis and leukaemoid reactions

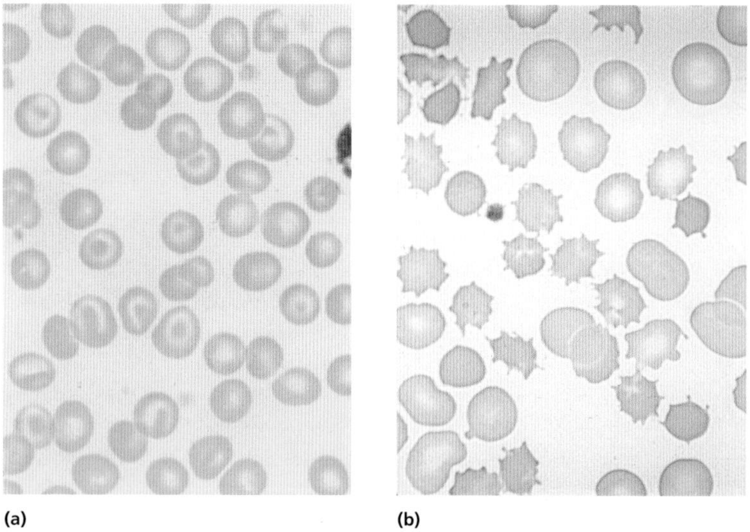

Fig. 26.5 Liver disease: peripheral blood film showing: **(a)** macrocytosis and target cells; and **(b)** marked acanthocytosis and echinocytosis in Zieve's syndrome.

chronic immune hepatitis. Haemolysis may also occur in end-stage liver disease because of abnormal red cell membranes resulting from lipid changes. Viral hepatitis (usually non-A, non-B, non-C) is associated with aplastic anaemia.

The acquired coagulation abnormalities associated with liver disease are described on p. 297. There are deficiencies of vitamin K-dependent factors (II, VII, IX and X) and, in severe disease, of factor V and fibrinogen. Thrombocytopenia may occur from hypersplenism or from immune complex-mediated platelet destruction. Abnormalities of platelet function may also be present. Dysfibrinogenaemia with abnormal fibrin polymerization may occur as a result of excess sialic acid in the fibrinogen molecules. A consumptive coagulopathy may be superimposed. These haemostatic defects may contribute to major blood loss from bleeding varices caused by portal hypertension.

Hypothyroidism

A moderate anaemia is usual and may be caused by lack of thyroxine. T_3 and T_4 potentiate the action of erythropoietin. There is also a reduced oxygen need and thus reduced erythropoietin secretion. The anaemia is often macrocytic and the mean corpuscular volume (MCV) falls with thyroxine therapy. Autoimmune thyroid disease, especially myxoedema or Hashimoto's disease, is associated with pernicious anaemia. Iron deficiency may also be present, particularly in women with menorrhagia.

Infections

Haematological abnormality is usually present in patients with infections of all types (Table 26.5). The effect of inflammation as a prothrombotic stimulus is also discussed on p. 308.

Bacterial infections

Acute bacterial infections are the most common cause of neutrophil leucocytosis. Toxic granulation, Döhle bodies and metamyelocytes may be present in the blood. Leukaemoid reactions with a white cell count $>50 \times 10^9/L$ and granulocyte precursors in the blood may occur in severe infections, particularly in infants and young children. The neutrophil alkaline phosphatase (NAP) score is raised in contrast to the low NAP score in chronic myeloid leukaemia. Mild anaemia is common if the infection is prolonged. Severe haemolytic anaemia occurs in bacterial septicaemias, particularly those caused by Gram-negative organisms, where there is usually associated DIC (p. 298). DIC dominates the clinical picture with certain infections (e.g. bacterial meningitis). The acute phase response to infections is accompanied by a rise in coagulation factors

Table 26.5 Blood abnormalities associated with infections.

Haematological abnormality	Infection associated
Anaemia	
Anaemia of chronic disorders	Chronic infections especially tuberculosis
Aplastic anaemia	Viral hepatitis
Transient red cell aplasia	Human parvovirus
Marrow fibrosis	Tuberculosis
Immune haemolytic anaemia	Infectious mononucleosis, *Mycoplasma pneumoniae*
Direct red cell damage or microangiopathic	Bacterial septicaemia (associated DIC), *Clostridium perfringens*, malaria, bartonellosis
	Viruses—haemolytic uraemic syndrome and TTP
Hypersplenism	Chronic malaria, tropical splenomegaly syndrome, leishmaniasis, schistosomiasis
White cell changes	
Neutrophil leucocytosis	Acute bacterial infections
Leukaemoid reactions	Severe bacterial infections particularly in infants
	Tuberculosis
Eosinophilia	Parasitic diseases (e.g. hookworm, filariasis, schistosomiasis, trichinosis)
	Recovery from acute infections
Monocytosis	Chronic bacterial infections: tuberculosis, brucellosis, bacterial endocarditis, typhoid
Neutropenia	Viral infections—HIV, hepatitis, influenza
	Fulminant bacterial infections (e.g. typhoid, miliary tuberculosis)
Lymphocytosis	Infectious mononucleosis, toxoplasmosis, cytomegalovirus, rubella, viral hepatitis, pertussis, tuberculosis, brucellosis
Lymphopenia	HIV infection
	Legionella pneumonophilia
Thrombocytopenia	
Megakaryocytic depression, immune complex-mediated and direct interaction with platelets	Acute viral infections particularly in children (e.g. measles, varicella, rubella, malaria, severe bacterial infection)
Prothrombotic state	All with prolonged inflammation

DIC, disseminated intravascular coagulation; HIV, human immunodeficiency virus; TTP, thrombotic thrombocytopenic purpura.

and a fall in natural anticoagulants. Recombinant human activated protein C reduces the death rate of severe DIC.

Clostridium perfringens organisms produce an α toxin, a lecithinase acting directly on the circulating red cells (Fig. 26.6). Haemolysis in bartonellosis (Oroya fever) is caused by direct red cell infection. With severe acute bacterial infections there may be thrombocytopenia. *Mycoplasma pneumoniae* infections are associated with autoimmune haemolytic anaemia of the 'cold' type (p. 67).

Chronic bacterial infections are associated with the anaemia of chronic disorders. In tuberculosis, additional factors in the pathogenesis of anaemia include marrow replacement and fibrosis associated with miliary disease and reactions to anti-tuberculous therapy (e.g. isoniazid is a pyridoxine antagonist and may cause sideroblastic anaemia). Disseminated tuberculosis is associated with leukaemoid reactions and patients with involvement of bone marrow may show leucoerythroblastic changes in the peripheral blood film.

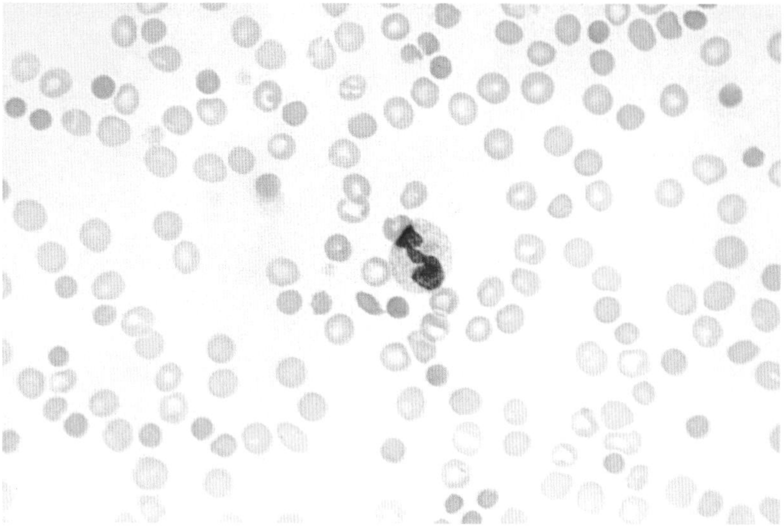

Fig. 26.6 Peripheral blood film in a patient with haemolytic anaemia in clostridial septicaemia showing red cell contraction and spherocytosis.

Viral infections

Acute viral diseases are often associated with a mild anaemia. An immune haemolytic anaemia with an anti-i autoantibody is associated with infectious mononucleosis (p. 68). Viral infections, as well as syphilis, have been associated with paroxysmal cold haemoglobinuria (p. 70). Viruses have also been linked to the pathogenesis of the haemolytic uraemic syndrome, thrombotic thrombocytopenic purpura (pp. 284 and 285) and the haemophagocytic syndrome (p. 106). Aplastic anaemia may occur with viral A or more usually non-A, non-B, non-C hepatitis. Transient red cell aplasia is associated with human parvovirus infection and this may result in severe anaemia in patients with a haemolytic anaemia because of the shortened red cell survival (e.g. in hereditary spherocytosis or sickle cell disease; p. 247).

Acute thrombocytopenia is not uncommon in rubella, morbilli and varicella infections. Rubella and cytomegalovirus (CMV) infections may cause a reactive lymphocytosis similar to that found in infectious mononucleosis. CMV may be responsible for a post-transfusion mononucleosis-like syndrome, CMV being transmitted by leucocytes. CMV infections in infants are associated with massive hepatosplenomegaly. In bone marrow transplant recipients or other immunosuppressed patients, CMV infections may cause pancytopenia as well as other severe disorders (e.g. pneumonitis or hepatitis; p. 258).

HIV infection

This is associated with a wide range of haematological changes. These are caused by marrow defects and immune cytopenias directly resulting from HIV infection, the effects of opportunistic infections or lymphoma and the side-effects of drugs used to treat HIV itself or drugs for the complicating infection or lymphoma.

Thrombocytopenia and neutropenia may be immune or secondary to marrow dysfunction. The marrow may be hypercellular with prominent plasma cells and lymphocytes, normocellular, hypocellular or fibrotic. Dysplastic features are common, with ineffective thrombopoiesis or granulocyte formation accounting at least in part for the cytopenia. The myelodysplasia does not show the chromosome abnormalities found in classic myelodysplasia and does not appear to be pre-leukaemic. Thrombocytopenia is treated if necessary by corticosteroids, high-dose gammaglobulin infusions or by other therapies for immune thrombocytopenia (p. 281), or by antiretroviral therapy.

Anaemia is also common, like the other cytopenias, and more severe as the disease progresses. It is usually multifactorial in origin—the anaemia of chronic disorders, marrow dysplasia and drug therapy, especially zidovudine. Serum vitamin B_{12} is often low, most likely because of intestinal malabsorption, but the anaemia does not respond to vitamin B_{12} therapy. Blood transfusions or recombinant erythropoietin injections are needed.

Increased plasma cells in the marrow and polyclonal increase in immunoglobulins are frequent. A paraprotein is present in 5–10% but appears benign. Non-Hodgkin's lymphoma, in over 90% high grade, both systemically and in the central nervous system, occurs in HIV infected individuals with over 100 times the frequency expected in the general population. Diffuse large B-cell lymphomas are most common, with 20% confined to the central nervous system. Approximately one-third are Burkitt's lymphoma. Hodgkin's disease, usually of poor prognosis type, is also increased in frequency. EBV infection appears to underlie this as well as Burkitt's lymphoma. Treatment of lymphomas in the setting of HIV is with standard regimens. Continuation of antiretroviral therapy exaggerates the tendency to cytopenia induced by chemotherapy so prophylaxis against opportunistic infections is important. The bone marrow may indeed reveal the presence of opportunistic infection (Fig. 26.7a,b).

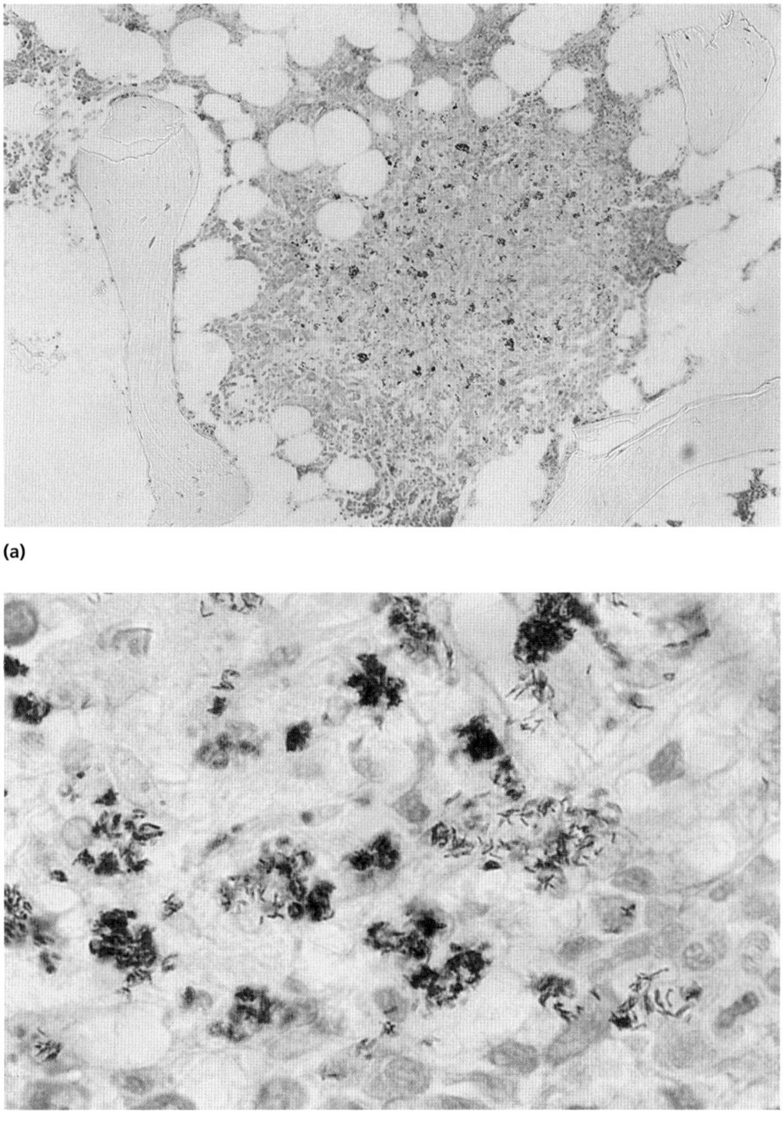

(a)

(b)

Fig. 26.7 Human immunodeficiency virus (HIV) infection: bone marrow trephine biopsy. **(a)** Granuloma showing positivity with Ziehl-Nielsen stain. **(b)** Higher power shows large numbers of acid-fast bacilli

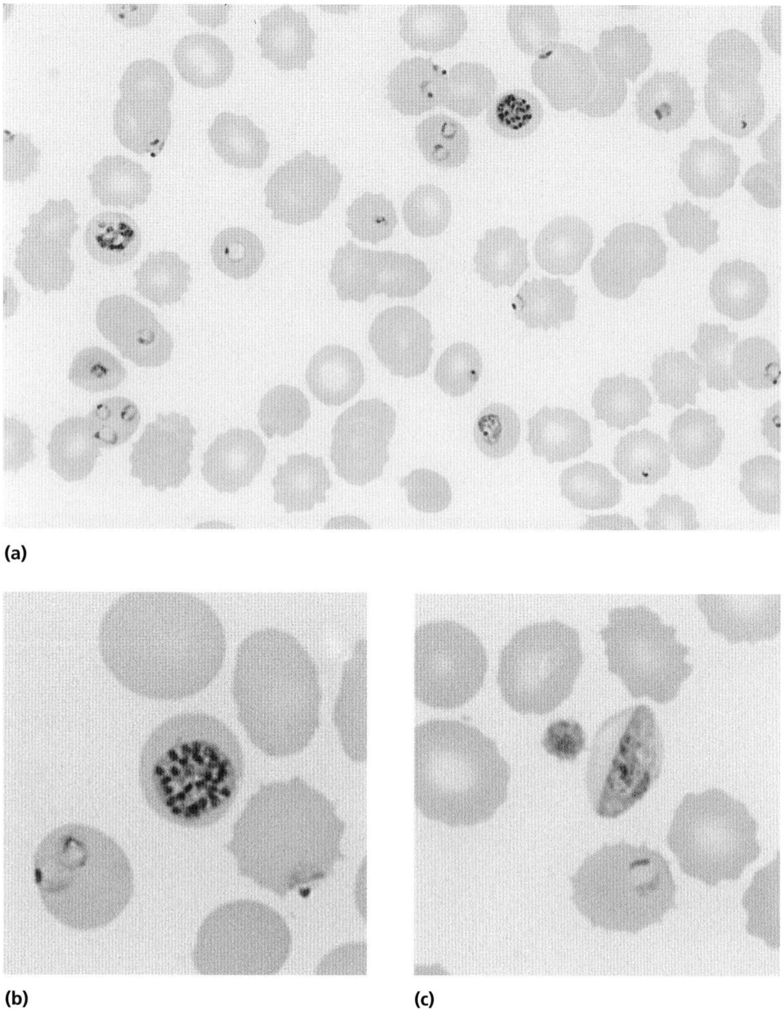

Fig. 26.8 Malaria: peripheral blood in severe *Plasmodium falciparum* infection showing: **(a)** many ring forms and a meront; and at higher magnification: **(b)** a meront; and **(c)** a gametocyte.

Malaria

Some degree of haemolysis is seen in all types of malarial infection. The most severe abnormalities are found in *Plasmodium falciparum* infections (Fig. 26.8). In the worst cases, DIC occurs and intravascular haemolysis is marked with haemoglobinuria. This may be associated with quinine therapy ('blackwater fever'). Thrombocytopenia is commonly found in acute malaria. Patients with chronic malaria have an anaemia of chronic disorders; hypersplenism may contribute to the anaemia and result in moderate thrombocytopenia and neutropenia. Tropical splenomegaly (p. 125) is probably a chronic immune reaction to malaria. Dyserythropoiesis in the marrow, folate deficiency and protein-calorie malnutrition may contribute to the anaemia.

Toxoplasmosis

Toxoplasmosis in children and adults is associated with lymphadenopathy and large numbers of atypical lymphocytes in the blood. Congenital disease may be confused with hydrops fetalis in a severely anaemic hydropic infant with gross hepatosplenomegaly, thrombocytopenia or a leucoerythroblastic blood film.

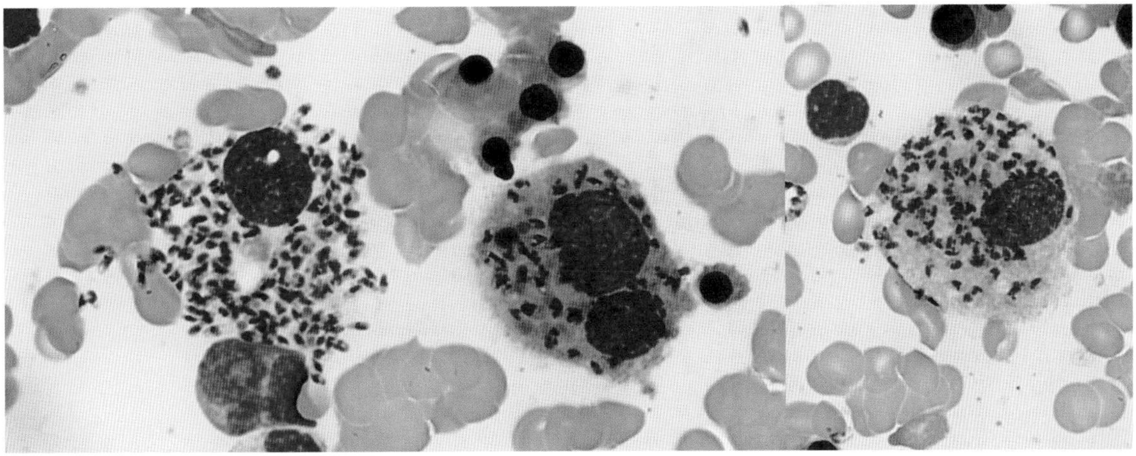

Fig. 26.9 Kala-azar: bone marrow aspirates showing macrophages containing Leishman–Donovan bodies.

Kala-azar (visceral leishmaniasis)

The visceral form of leishmaniasis is associated with pancytopenia, hepatosplenomegaly and lymphadenopathy. Bone marrow or splenic aspirates may show large numbers of parasitized macrophages (Fig. 26.9).

Other parasitic diseases

In the acute phase of both African and South American trypanosomiasis, organisms are found in the peripheral blood (Fig. 26.10). Microfilariae of bancroftian filariasis and loiasis are also detected during blood film examination (Fig. 26.11). In chronic schistosomiasis, hypersplenism follows the splenic enlargement associated with portal hypertension. In many parasitic diseases there is eosinophilia (Table 26.5).

Inborn errors of metabolism

Gaucher's, Tay–Sachs and Niemann–Pick diseases all result from hereditary deficiency of the enzymes required for glycolipid breakdown.

Gaucher's disease

Gaucher's disease is an uncommon autosomal recessive disorder characterized by an accumulation of glucosylceramide in the lysosomes of

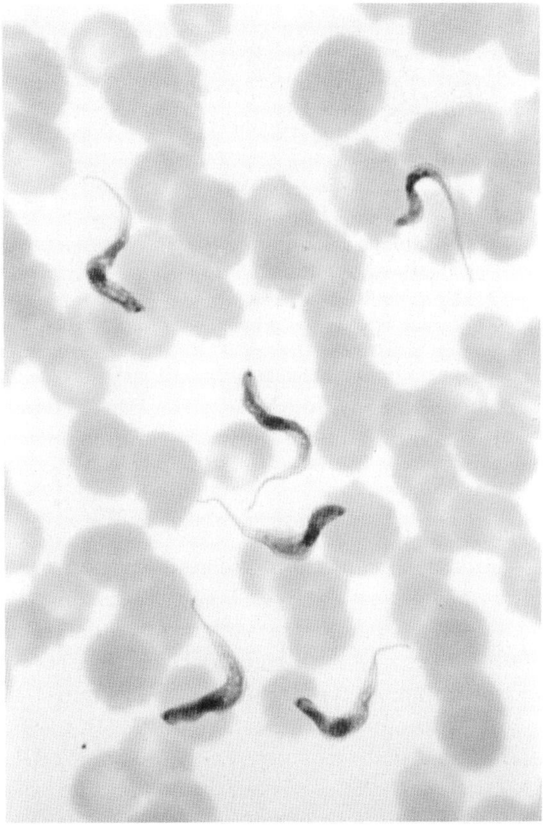

Fig. 26.10 African trypanosomiasis: blood film showing *Trypanosoma brucei*.

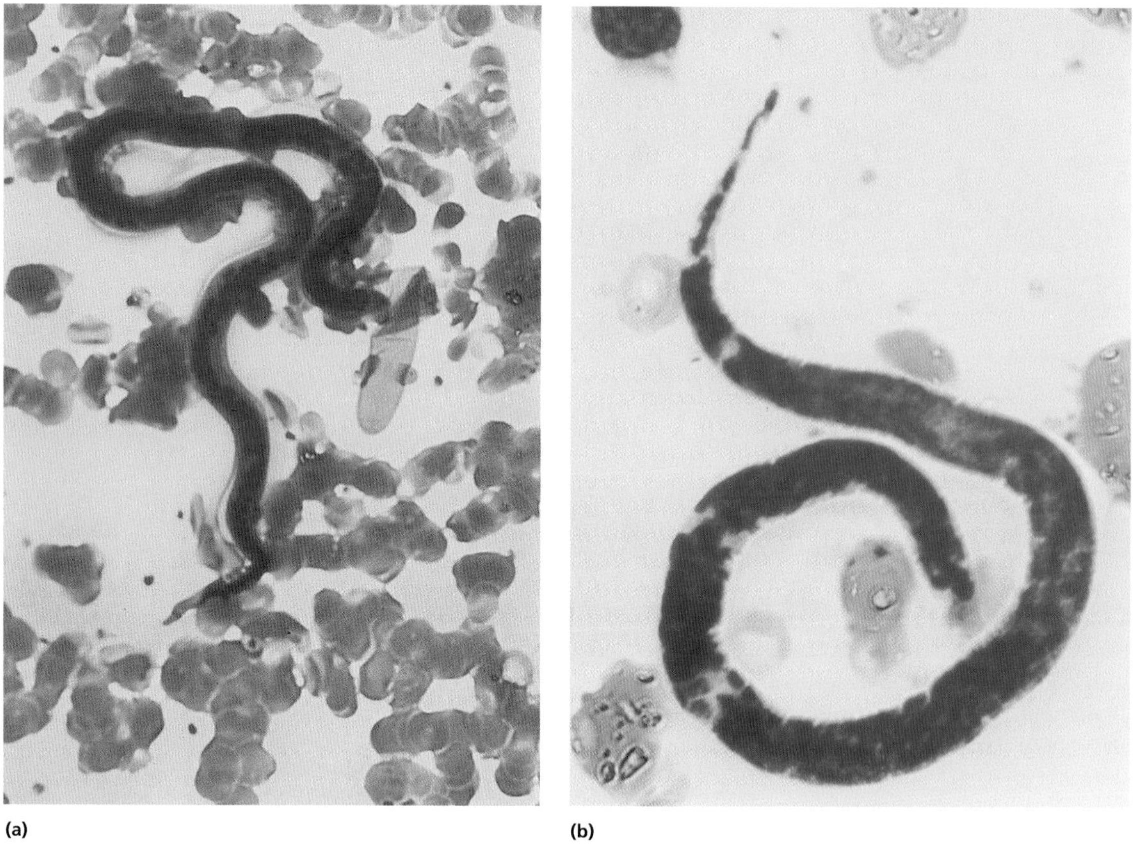

Fig. 26.11 Peripheral blood films showing microfilariae of: **(a)** *Wuchereria bancrofti*; and **(b)** *Loa loa*.

reticuloendothelial cells as a result of deficiency of glucocerebrosidase (Fig. 26.12). Three types occur: a chronic adult type (type I); an acute infantile neuronopathic type (type II); and a subacute neuronopathic type with onset in childhood or adolescence (type III). Type I is caused by a variety of mutations in the glucocerebrosidase gene, one type of which (a single base pair substitution in codon 444) is particularly common in Ashkenazi Jews and explains the high incidence of the disease in this group. In type I the outstanding physical sign is splenomegaly. Moderate liver enlargement and pingueculae (conjunctival deposits) are other characteristic findings. In many cases, bone deposits cause bone pain and pathological fractures. Expansion of the lower end of the femur may produce the 'Erlenmeyer flask deformity' (Fig. 26.13c).

The clinical manifestations are caused by the accumulation of glucocerebroside-laden macrophages in the spleen, liver and bone marrow (Fig. 26.13a,b,e). Gaucher's disease at all ages is commonly associated with marked anaemia, leucopenia and thrombocytopenia occurring singly or in combination. Polyclonal hypergammaglobulinemia or monoclonal gammopathy are frequent. Diagnosis is made by assay of white cell glucocerebrosidase and DNA analysis. Lysosomal enyzmes, chitotriosidase and acid phosphatase are raised and useful in monitoring therapy. Pulmonary activation-regulated cytokine (PARC), angiotensin-converting enzyme (ACE) and ferritin are also elevated.

Enzyme replacement therapy with glucocerebrosidase made by recombinant technology and given intravenously is very effective in treating the

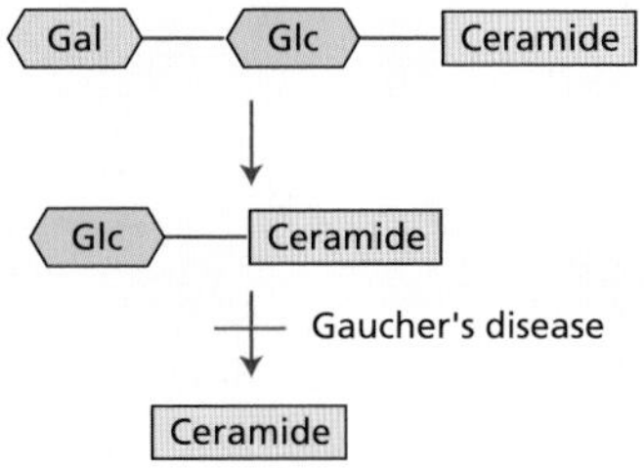

Fig. 26.12 Gaucher's disease results from a deficiency of glucocerebrosidase. Gal, Galactose; Glc, glucose.

disease with shrinkage of spleen, rise in blood count and improved bone structure (Fig. 26.13d,f). An oral drug, miglustat, is useful in mild forms. It reduces the amount of substrate being produced in lysosomes and may be used in combination with the intravenous enzyme. Splenectomy can result in haematological improvement but following this operation there is often increased deposition of cerebroside in extrasplenic tissue, particularly bones. Stem cell transplantation has been carried out successfully in severely affected patients, usually with type II or III disease.

Niemann–Pick disease

Niemann–Pick disease shows certain clinical and pathological similarities to Gaucher's disease. It is caused by a sphingomyelinase deficiency. The majority of patients are infants who die in the first few years of life although occasional patients survive to adult life. Massive hepatosplenomegaly occurs and there is usually lung and nervous system involvement with retarded physical and mental development. A 'cherry-red' spot is commonly seen in the retina of affected infants. Pancytopenia is a regular feature and in marrow aspirates 'foam cells' of similar size to Gaucher cells are seen. Chemical analysis of the tissues reveals that the disorder is caused by an accumulation of sphingomyelin and cholesterol.

Non-specific monitoring of systemic disease

The inflammatory response to tissue injury includes changes in plasma concentrations of proteins known as acute phase proteins. These proteins include fibrinogen and other clotting factors, complement components and CRP (p. 334), haptoglobin, serum amyloid A (SAA) protein, ferritin and others. The rise in these liver-derived proteins is part of a wider response which includes fever, leucocytosis and increased immune reactivity. The acute phase response is mediated by cytokines (e.g. IL-1; see Fig. 7.4) and TNF, released from macrophages and possibly other cells. Patients with chronic disease may show periodic or continuous evidence of the acute phase response depending upon the extent of inflammation. Quantitative measurements of acute phase proteins are valuable indicators of the presence and extent of inflammation and of its response to treatment. When short-term (less than 24 h) changes in the inflammatory response are expected CRP is the test of choice (Table 26.6). Long-term changes in the acute phase proteins are monitored by either the ESR or plasma viscosity. These tests are influenced by plasma proteins which are either slowly responding acute phase reactants (e.g. fibrinogen) or are not acute phase proteins (e.g. immunoglobulins).

Erythrocyte sedimentation rate

This commonly used but non-specific test measures the speed of sedimentation of red cells in plasma over a period of 1 h. The speed is mainly dependent on the plasma concentration of large proteins (e.g. fibrinogen and immunoglobulins). The normal range in men is 1–5 mm/h and in women 5–15 mm/h but there is a progressive increase in old age. The ESR is raised in a wide variety of systemic inflammatory and neoplastic diseases and in pregnancy.

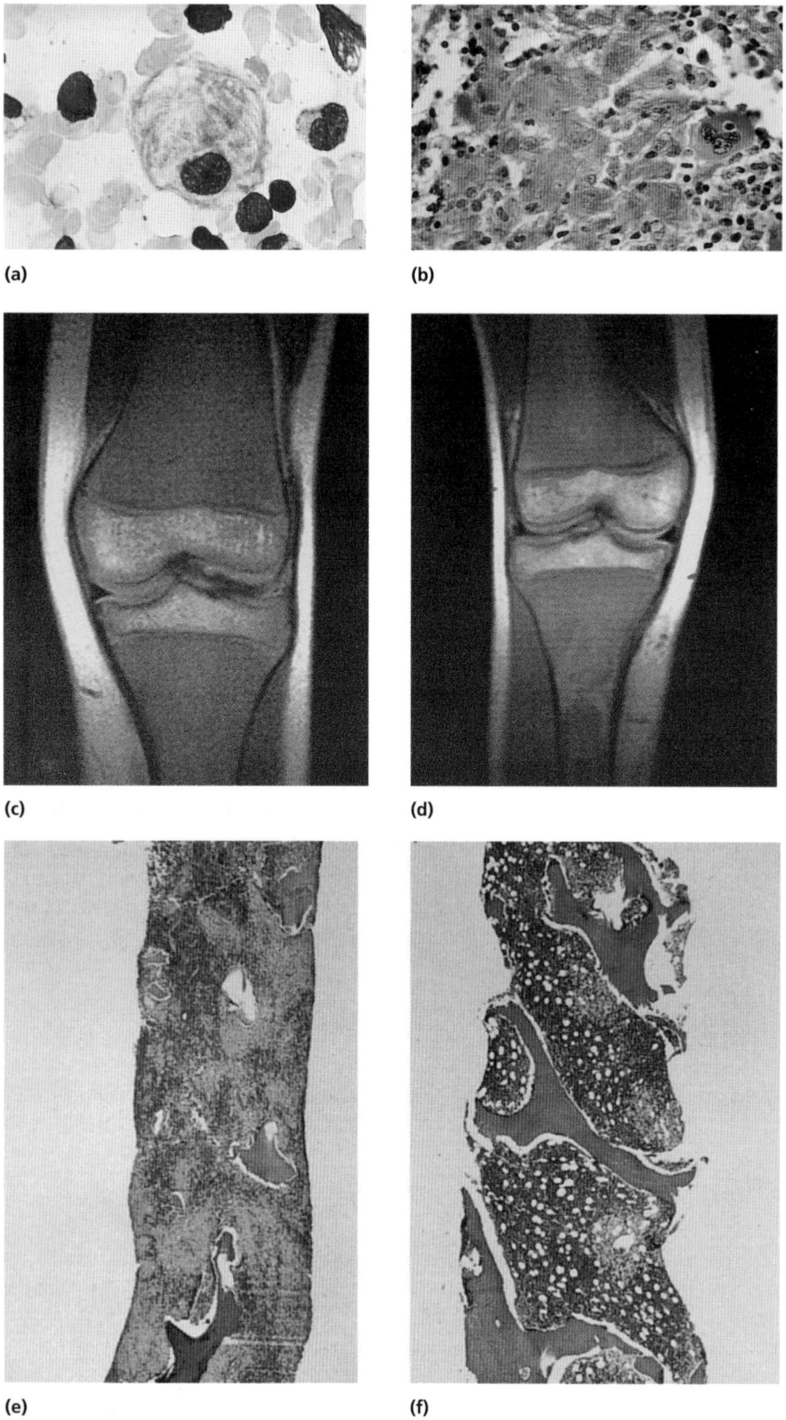

Fig. 26.13 Gaucher's disease: **(a)** bone marrow aspirate—a Gaucher cell with 'fibrillar' cytoplasmic pattern; **(b)** spleen histology—pale clusters of Gaucher cells in the reticuloendothelial cord; **(c)** magnetic resonance imaging (MRI) scan of the left knee of a patient before treatment showing Erlenmeyer flask deformity with expansion of the marrow and thinning of the cortical bone; **(d)** following a year of glucocerebrosidase therapy with subsequent remodelling of bone; and bone marrow trephine biopsy before **(e)** and after **(f)** 2 years of glucocerebrosidase therapy.

Table 26.6 Advantages and disadvantages of the tests used to monitor the acute phase response.

Advantages	Disadvantages
*CRP**	
Specific test of acute phase protein	More than one protein required to measure acute (CRP) and chronic inflammation
Fast response (6 h) to change in disease activity	Costly when assayed in small numbers
High sensitivity—owing to large incremental change	Sophisticated equipment and antisera required
Can be measured on stored serum	
Small sample volumes	
Automated analysis	
ESR and plasma viscosity	
Useful in chronic disease	Not sensitive to acute changes (<24 h)
ESR inexpensive, easy, no electrical power required	Not specific for acute phase response
Plasma viscosity—result obtained quickly (15 min)	Slow to change with alteration in disease activity and insensitive to small changes in activity
Plasma viscosity not affected by anaemia	Fresh samples (<2 h) required for ESR

ESR, erythrocyte sedimentation rate.
* C-reactive protein (CRP) is normally present in low concentrations (<5 mg/L). Levels are not influenced by anaemia, pregnancy or heart failure. During severe acute infection the plasma concentration may rise 100-fold.

It is useful for diagnosing and monitoring temporal arteritis and polymyalgia rheumatica and for monitoring patients with Hodgkin's disease. High values (>100 mm/h) have a 90% predictive value for serious disease including infections, collagen vascular disease or malignancy (particularly myeloma). A raised ESR is associated with marked rouleaux formation of red cells in the peripheral blood film (see Fig. 18.4). Changes in the ESR can be used to monitor the response to therapy.

Lower than expected readings occur in polycythaemia vera because of the high red cell concentration. Higher than expected values may occur in severe anaemia because of the low red cell concentration.

Plasma viscosity

In many laboratories measurement of ESR has been replaced by plasma viscosity measurement. Plasma viscosity is affected by the concentration of plasma proteins of large molecular size, especially those with pronounced axial asymmetry—fibrinogen and some immunoglobulins. Normal values at room temperature are usually in the range of 1.50–1.70 mPa/s. Lower levels are found in neonates because of lower levels of proteins, particularly fibrinogen. Viscosity increases only slightly in the elderly as fibrinogen increases. There is no difference in values between men and women. Other advantages over the ESR test include independence from the effects of anaemia and results that are available within 15 min.

C-reactive protein

Phylogenetically CRP is a crude 'early' immunoglobulin which initiates the inflammatory reaction. CRP–antigen complexes can substitute for antibody in the fixation of Clq and trigger the complement cascade initiating the inflammatory response to antigens or tissue damage, Subsequent binding of C3b on the surface of microorganisms opsonizes them for phagocytosis.

After tissue injury, an increase in CRP, SAA protein and other acute phase reactants may be detected within 6–10 h. Increase in fibrinogen may not occur until 24–48 h following injury. Immunoassays of CRP are now widely used for early detection of acute inflammation or tissue injury and for the monitoring of remission (e.g. response of infection to an antibiotic).

Table 26.6 lists the advantages and disadvantages of the tests used to assess the acute phase response.

Bibliography

Desnick R.J. and Schuchman E.H. (2003) Enzyme replacement and enhancement therapies: lessons from lysosomal disorders. *Nat Rev Genet* **3**,954–66. Erratum in: (2003) *Nat Rev Genet* **4**,157.

Ganz T. (2003) Hepcidin, a key regulator of iron metabolism and mediator of anemia of inflammation. *Blood* **102**,783–8.

Ludwig H., Rai K., Blade J. *et al.* (2002) Management of disease-related anemia in patients with multiple myeloma or chronic lymphocytic leukemia: epoetin treatment recommendations. *Hematol J* **3**,121–30.

Spivak J.L. (2000) The blood in systemic disorders. *Lancet* **355**,1707–12.

Vellodi A. (2005) Lysosomal storage disorders. *Br J Haematol* **128**,413–31.

Weiss G. and Goodnough L.T. (2005) Anemia of chronic disease. *N Engl J Med* **352**,1011–23.

Wraith J.E. (2001) Advances in the treatment of lysosomal storage disease. *Dev Med Child Neurol* **43**,639–46.

CHAPTER 27

27 Blood transfusion

Blood transfusion consists of the 'safe' transfer of blood components (Fig. 27.1) from a donor to a recipient.

Blood donor

This should be voluntary. The measures to protect donors are listed in Table 27.1.

Red cell antigens and blood group antibodies

Approximately 400 red blood cell group antigens have been described. The clinical significance of blood groups in blood transfusion is that individuals who lack a particular blood group antigen may produce antibodies reacting with that antigen which may

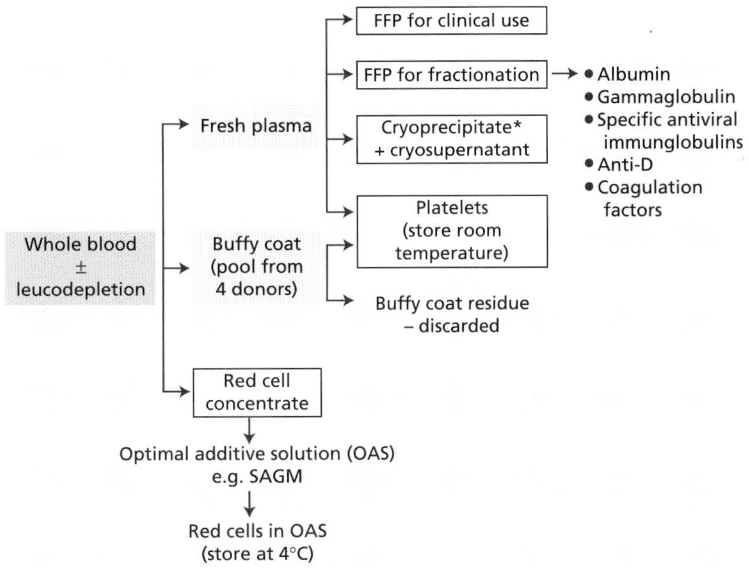

Fig. 27.1 The preparation of blood components from whole blood. FFP, fresh frozen plasma; SAGM, saline-adenine-glucose-mannitol. * Cryoprecipitate is mainly a source of fibrinogen. Cryosupernatant is used for plasma exchange in thrombotic thrombocytopenic purpura.

Table 27.1 Measures to protect the donor.

Age 17–70 years (maximum 60 at first donation)
Weight above 50 kg (7 st 12 lb)
Haemoglobin >13 g/dL for men, >12 g/dL for women
Minimum donation interval of 12 weeks (16 weeks advised) and three donations per year maximum
Pregnant and lactating women excluded because of high iron requirements
Exclusion of those with:
known cardiovascular disease, including hypertension
significant respiratory disorders
epilepsy and other CNS disorders
gastrointestinal disorders with impaired absorption
Insulin-dependent diabetes
Chronic renal disease
Ongoing medical investigation or clinical trials
Exclusion of any donor returning to occupations such as driving bus, plane or train, heavy machine or crane operator, mining, scaffolding, etc. because delayed faint would be dangerous

CNS, central nervous system.

lead to a transfusion reaction. The different blood group antigens vary greatly in their clinical significance with the ABO and Rh (formerly Rhesus) groups being the most important. Some other systems are listed in Table 27.2.

Blood group antibodies

Naturally occurring antibodies occur in the plasma of subjects who lack the corresponding antigen and who have not been transfused or been pregnant. The most important are anti-A and anti-B. They are usually immunoglobulin M (IgM), and react optimally at cold temperatures (4°C) so, although reactive at 37°C, are called cold antibodies.

Immune antibodies develop in response to the introduction—by transfusion or by transplacental passage during pregnancy—of red cells possessing antigens that the subject lacks. These antibodies are commonly IgG, although some IgM antibodies may also develop—usually in the early phase of an immune response. Immune antibodies react optimally at 37°C (warm antibodies). Only IgG antibodies are capable of transplacental passage from mother to fetus. The most important immune antibody is the Rh antibody, anti-D.

ABO system

This consists of three allelic genes: A, B and O. The A and B genes control the synthesis of specific enzymes responsible for the addition of single carbohydrate residues (*N*-acetyl galactosamine for group A and D-galactose for group B) to a basic antigenic glycoprotein or glycolipid with a terminal sugar L-fucose on the red cell, known as the H substance (Fig. 27.2). The O gene is an amorph and does not transform the H substance. Although there are six possible genotypes, the absence of a specific anti-O prevents the serological recognition of more than four phenotypes (Table 27.3). The two major subgroups of A (A_1 and A_2) complicate the issue but are of minor clinical significance. A_2 cells react more

Table 27.2 Clinically important blood group systems.

Systems	Frequency of antibodies	Cause of haemolytic transfusion reaction	Cause of haemolytic disease of newborn
ABO	Almost universal	Yes (common)	Yes (usually mild)
Rh	Common	Yes (common)	Yes
Kell	Occasional	Yes (occasional)	Anaemia not haemolysis
Duffy	Occasional	Yes (occasional)	Yes (occasional)
Kidd	Occasional	Yes (occasional)	Yes (occasional)
Lutheran	Rare	Yes (rare)	No
Lewis	Occasional	Yes (rare)	No
P	Occasional	Yes (rare)	Yes (rare)
MN	Rare	Yes (rare)	Yes (rare)
Li	Rare	Unlikely	No

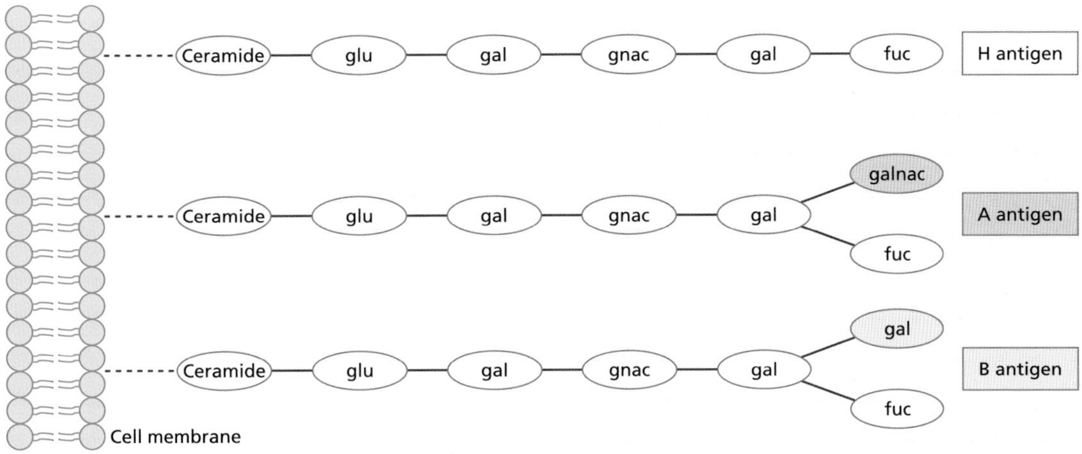

Fig. 27.2 Structure of ABO blood group antigens. Each consists of a chain of sugars attached to lipids or proteins which are an integral part of the cell membrane. The H antigen of the O blood group has a terminal fucose (fuc). The A antigen has an additional *N*-acetyl galactosamine (galnac), and the B antigen has an additional galactose (gal). glu, glucose.

Table 27.3 The ABO blood group system.

Phenotype	Genotype	Antigens	Naturally occurring antibodies	Frequency (UK) (%)
O	OO	O	Anti-A, anti-B	46
A	AA or AO	A	Anti-B	42
B	BB or BO	B	Anti-A	9
AB	AB	AB	None	3

weakly than A_1 cells with anti-A and patients who are A_2B can be wrongly grouped as B.

The A, B and H antigens are present on most body cells including white cells and platelets. In the 80% of the population who possess secretor genes, these antigens are also found in soluble form in secretions and body fluids (e.g. plasma, saliva, semen and sweat).

Naturally occurring antibodies to A and/or B antigens are found in the plasma of subjects whose red cells lack the corresponding antigen (Table 27.3; Fig. 27.3).

Rhesus system

The Rh blood group locus is composed of two related structural genes, *RhD* and *RhCE*, which encode the membrane proteins that carry the D, Cc and Ee antigens. The *RhD* gene may be either present or absent, giving the Rh D+ or Rh D– phenotype, respectively. Alternative RNA splicing from the *RhCE* gene generates two proteins, which encode the C, c, E or e antigens (Fig. 27.4). A shortened nomenclature for Rh phenotype is commonly used (Table 27.4).

Rh antibodies rarely occur naturally; most are immune (i.e. they result from previous transfusion or pregnancy). Anti-D is responsible for most of the clinical problems associated with the system and a simple subdivision of subjects into Rh D+ and Rh D– using anti-D is sufficient for routine clinical purposes. Anti-C, anti-c, anti-E and anti-e are occasionally seen and may cause both transfusion reactions and haemolytic disease of the newborn. Anti-d does not exist. Rh haemolytic disease of the newborn is described in Chapter 28.

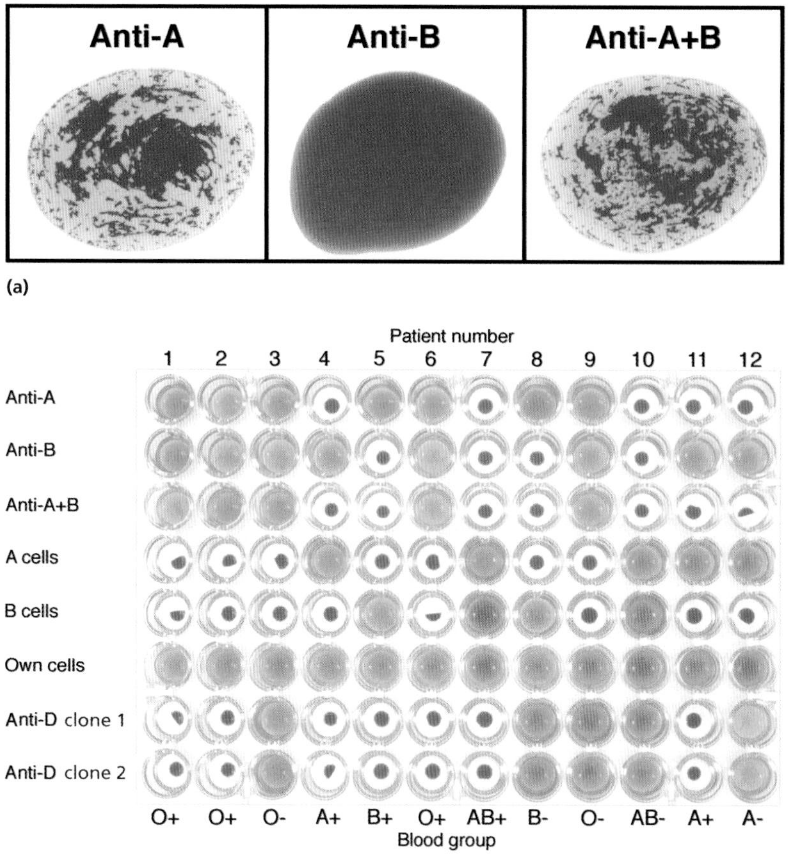

Fig. 27.3 **(a)** The ABO grouping in a group A patient. The red cells suspended in saline agglutinate in the presence of anti-A or anti-A + B (serum from a group O patient). **(b)** Routine grouping in a 96-well microplate. Positive reactions show as sharp agglutinates; in negative reactions the cells are dispersed. Rows 1–3, patient cells against antisera; rows 4–6, patient sera against known cells; rows 7–8, anti-D against patient cells.

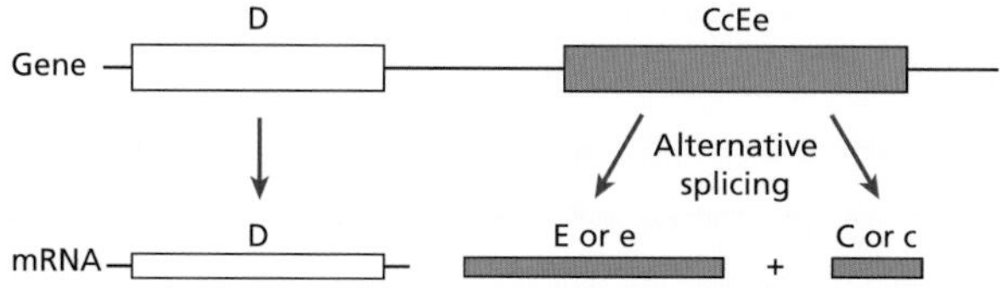

Fig. 27.4 Molecular genetics of the rhesus blood group. The locus consists of two closely linked genes, *RhD* and *RhCcEe*. The *RhD* gene codes for a single protein which contains the RhD antigen whereas *RhCcEe* mRNA undergoes alternative splicing to three transcripts. One of these encodes the E or e antigen whereas the other two (only one is shown) contain the C or c epitope. A polymorphism at position 226 of the *RhCcEe* gene determines the Ee antigen status whereas the C or c antigens are determined by a four amino acid allelic difference. Some individuals do not have an *RhD* gene and are therefore RhD–.

Other blood group systems

Other blood group systems are less frequently of clinical importance. Although naturally occurring antibodies of the P, Lewis and MN system are not uncommon, they usually only react at low temperatures and hence are of no clinical consequence. Immune antibodies against antigens of these systems are detected infrequently. Many of the antigens are of low antigenicity and others (e.g. Kell),

Table 27.4 The most common Rh genotypes in the UK population.

CDE nomenclature	Short symbol	Caucasian frequency (%)	Rh D status
cde/cde	rr	15	Negative
CDe/cde	R_1r	31	Positive
CDe/CDe	R_1R_1	16	Positive
cDE/cde	R_2r	13	Positive
CDe/cDE	R_1R_2	13	Positive
cDE/cDE	R_2R_2	3	Positive
Other genotypes		9	Positive (almost all)

although comparatively immunogenic, are of relatively low frequency and therefore provide few opportunities for isoimmunization except in multiply transfused patients.

Hazards of allogeneic blood transfusion

A large number of measures are taken to protect the recipient (Table 27.5).

Infection

Donor selection and testing of all donations are designed to prevent transmission of diseases (Table 27.6). The main risk is from viruses that have long incubation periods and especially those that are carried for many years by asymptomatic individuals. Some viruses that are transfusion transmissible show cell-associated latency and, if in white cells, can cause infection in the recipient after allogeneic transfusion. Live viruses causing acute infection can be transmitted in the pre-symptomatic viraemic phase if blood is collected during that short period.

Table 27.5 Measures to protect recipient.

Donor selection
Donor deferral/exclusion
Stringent arm cleaning
Microbiological testing of donations (Table 27.6)
Immunohaematological testing of donations
Diversion of first 20–30 mL of blood collected
Leucodepletion of cellular products
Post-collection viral inactivation
Monitoring and testing for bacterial contamination
Pathogen inactivation
Safest possible sources of donor for plasma products

Table 27.6 Microbiological testing in England and Wales.

1 Human immunodeficiency virus (HIV) 1 and 2
2 Hepatitis B virus (HBV)
3 Hepatitis C virus (HCV)
4 Human T-cell leukaemia viruses (HTLV)
5 Cytomegalovirus (CMV)—for immunosuppressed recipients
6 Malaria—antibody screening of potentially exposed donors
7 Chagas' disease—antibody screening of potentially exposed donors
8 Bacteria—all donations tested for antibody to syphilis17p

Individual infections (Table 27.7)

Hepatitis

Donors with a history of hepatitis are deferred for 12 months. If there is a history of jaundice, they can be accepted if markers for HBV and HCV are negative.

Human immunodeficiency virus (HIV)

This can be transmitted by cells or plasma. Male homosexuals, bisexuals, intravenous drug users and prostitutes are excluded, as are their sexual partners and partners of haemophiliacs. Inhabitants of large areas of sub-Saharan Africa and South-East Asia where HIV infection is particularly common are also excluded. Rare transmission occurs when the donor is incubating the infection but is not yet positive for the antigen-antibody test used (window period transmission).

Table 27.7 Infections agents reported to have been transmitted by blood transfusion.

Viruses	
Hepatitis viruses	Hepatitis A virus (HAV)
	Hepatitis B virus (HBV)
	Hepatitis C virus (HCV)
	Hepatitis D virus (HDV) (requires coinfection with HBV)
Retroviruses	Human immunodeficiency virus (HIV) 1 + 2 (+ other subtypes)
	Human T-cell leukaemia virus (HTLV) I + II
Herpes viruses	Human cytomegalovirus (CMV)
	Epstein–Barr virus (EBV)
	Human herpesvirus 8 (HHV-8)
Parvoviruses	Parvovirus B19
Miscellaneous viruses	GBV-C—previously referred to as hepatitis G virus (HGV)
	Transfusion transmitted virus (TTV)
	West Nile virus
Bacteria	
Endogenous	*Treponema pallidum* (syphilis)
	Borrelia burgdorferi (Lyme disease)
	Brucella melitensis (brucellosis)
	Yersinia enterocolitical/Salmonella spp.
Exogenous	Environmental species—staphyloccocal spp./pseudomonas/*Serratia* spp.
Rickettsiae	*Rickettsia rickettsii* (Rocky Mountain spotted fever)
	Coxiella burnettii (Q fever)
Protozoa	
	Plasmodium spp. (malaria)
	Trypanosoma cruzi (Chagas' disease)
	Toxoplasma gondii (toxoplasmosis)
	Babesia microti/divergens (babesiosis)
	Leishmania spp. (leishmaniasis)
Prions	
	New variant Creuzfeldt–Jacob disease (nvCJD)

Human T-cell leukaemias viruses

Human T-cell leukaemias virus type I (HTLVI) is associated with adult T-cell leukaemia or tropical spastic paraperesis. Human T-cell leukaemia virus type II (HLTVII) has no known association with any clinical condition. Screening for both is mandatory in the UK despite the low prevalence, approximately 1 in 50 000 untested donors.

Cytomegalovirus

Post-infusion cytomegalovirus (CMV) infection is usually subclinical but may give an infectious mononucleosis syndrome. Immunosuppressed individuals are at risk of pneumonitis and a potentially fatal disease. These are premature babies (<1500 g), bone marrow and other organ transplant recipients, and pregnant women (the fetus is at risk). For such recipients, CMV negative blood or blood components must be given.

Other infections

Syphilis is more likely to be transmitted by platelets (stored at room temperature) than blood (stored at 4°C). However, all donations are tested. Malarial parasites are viable in blood stored at 4°C, so in endemic areas all recipients are given antimalarial drugs. In non-endemic areas, donors are carefully vetted for travel to tropical areas and in some centres tests for malarial antibodies are performed. Chagas' disease is a significant problem with blood transfusion in Latin America. **Bacterial infections** resulting from skin commensals are most frequently transmitted by platelets stored for more than 3 days.

Prions The risk of new variant Creuzfeldt–Jacob disease (nvCJD) is considered a threat to blood safety only in the UK. Plasma for fractionation and fresh frozen plasma for infants or children is obtained from the USA. It is unknown how many people could be infected with nvCJD. There are three reports of possible transmission by blood transfusion, so recipients of blood or blood components are now excluded as blood donors in the UK. No screening tests for prions are yet available.

Techniques in blood group serology

The most important technique is based on the agglutination of red blood cells. Saline agglutination is important in detecting IgM antibodies, usually at room temperature and 4°C (e.g. anti-A, anti-B; Fig. 27.3). Addition of colloid to the incubation or proteolytic enzyme treatment of red cells increases the sensitivity of the indirect antiglobulin test, as does low ionic strength saline (LISS). These latter methods can detect a range of IgG antibodies.

The antiglobulin (Coombs') test is a fundamental and widely used test in both blood group serology and general immunology. Antihuman globulin (AHG) is produced in animals following the injection of human globulin, purified complement or specific immunoglobulin (e.g. IgG, IgA or IgM). Monoclonal preparations are also now available. When AHG is added to human red cells coated with immunoglobulin or complement components, agglutination of the red cells indicates a positive test (Fig. 27.5).

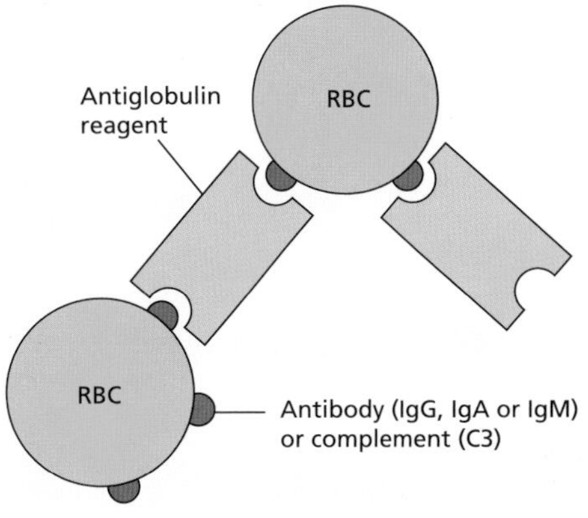

Fig. 27.5 The antiglobulin test for antibody or complement on the surface of red blood cells (RBC). The antihuman globulin (Coombs') reagent may be broad spectrum or specific for immunoglobulin G (IgG), IgM, IgA or complement (C3).

The antiglobulin test may be either direct or indirect. The direct antiglobulin test (DAT) is used for detecting antibody or complement on the red cell surface where sensitization has occurred *in vivo*. The AHG reagent is added to washed red cells and agglutination indicates a positive test. A positive test occurs in haemolytic disease of the newborn, autoimmune or drug-induced immune haemolytic anaemia and haemolytic transfusion reactions.

The indirect antiglobulin test (IAT) is used to detect antibodies that have coated the red cells *in vitro*. It is a two-stage procedure: the first step involves the incubation of test red cells with serum; in the second step, the red cells are washed and the AHG reagent is added. Agglutination implies that the original serum contained antibody which has coated the red cells *in vitro*. This test is used as part of the routine antibody screening of the recipient's serum prior to transfusion and for detecting blood group antibodies in a pregnant woman.

Most of the above methods were originally developed for tube techniques. These were replaced by 96-well microplates but most laboratories now use gel-based technology (Fig. 27.6).

Cross-matching and pre-transfusion tests

A number of steps are taken to ensure that patients receive compatible blood at the time of transfusion.

From the patient

1 The ABO and Rh blood group is determined.

2 Serum is screened for important antibodies by an indirect antiglobulin test on a large panel of antigenically-typed group O red cells.

If a red cell alloantibody is discovered, donor blood is selected lacking the relative antigen. The most likely are Rh D, C, c, E, e and K.

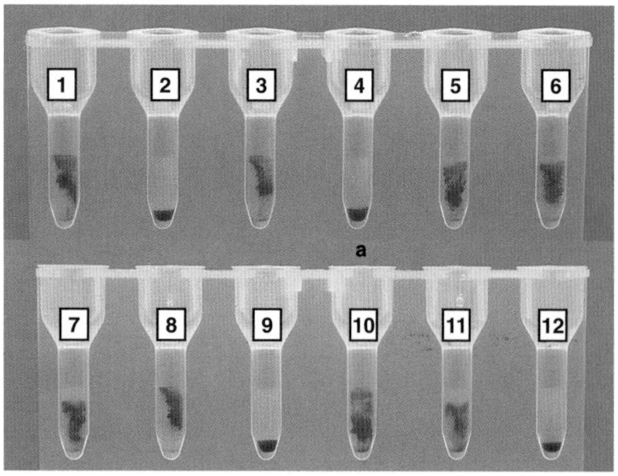

Fig. 27.6 Patient antibody screening using the microcolumn (gel) system: 10 tests with two controls (tube 11 is the positive control and tube 12 the negative control) are shown. The patient's serum is tested against screening cells with known red cell phenotype. Tubes 1, 3, 5–8 and 10 show positive results. The patient's serum contained anti-Fy[a]. (Courtesy of Mr G. Hazlehurst)

Table 27.8 Techniques used in compatibility testing. Donor cells tested against recipient serum and agglutination detected visually or microscopically after mixing and incubation at the appropriate temperature.

For detecting clinically significant IgM antibodies
Saline 37°C
For detecting immune antibodies (mainly IgG)
Indirect antiglobulin test at 37°C
Low ionic strength saline at 37°C
Enzyme-treated red cells at 37°C

Ig, immunoglobulin.

From the donor

An appropriate ABO and Rh unit is selected. Donor (blood) testing is described on p. 341.

The cross-match

The techniques that may be used are described in Table 27.8.

Electronic cross-match

In this, a patient has group and antibody screen performed as two separate occasions. If both are negative and no blood has been transfused between the test, ABO and Rh compatible blood is issued directly without wet testing.

Complications of blood transfusion

(Table 27.9)

Haemolytic transfusion reactions

Haemolytic transfusion reactions may be immediate or delayed. Immediate life-threatening reactions associated with massive intravascular haemolysis are the result of complement-activating antibodies of IgM or IgG classes, usually with ABO specificity. Reactions associated with extravascular haemolysis (e.g. immune antibodies of the Rh system which are unable to activate complement) are generally less severe but may still be life-threatening. The cells become coated with IgG and are removed in the reticuloendothelial system. In mild cases, the only signs of a transfusion reaction may be a progressive unexplained anaemia with or without jaundice. In some cases where the pre-transfusion level of an antibody was too low to be detected in a cross-match, a patient may be reimmunized by transfusion of incompatible red cells and this will lead to a delayed transfusion reaction with accelerated clearance of the red cells. There may be rapid appearance of anaemia with mild jaundice.

Clinical features of a major haemolytic transfusion reaction

Haemolytic shock phase This may occur after only a few millilitres of blood have been transfused or up to 1–2 h after the end of the transfusion. Clinical features include urticaria, pain in the lumbar region, flushing, headache, precordial pain, shortness of breath, vomiting, rigours, pyrexia and a fall in blood pressure. If the patient is anaesthetized this shock phase is masked. There is increasing evidence of red cell destruction and haemoglobinuria, jaundice and disseminated intravascular coagulation (DIC) may occur. Moderate leucocytosis (e.g. 15–20 × 10^9/L is usual.

The oliguric phase In some patients with a haemolytic reaction there is renal tubular necrosis with acute renal failure.

Table 27.9 Complications of blood transfusion

Early	Late
Haemolytic reactions: immediate or delayed	Transmission of infection (Table 27.7)
Reactions caused by infected blood	Transfusional iron overload
Allergic reactions to white cells, platelets or proteins	Immune sensitization e.g. to red cells, platelets or Rh D antigen
Pyrogenic reactions (to plasma proteins or caused by HLA antibodies)	Transfusion-associated graft-versus-host disease
Circulatory overload	
Bacterial contamination	
Air embolism	
Thrombophlebitis	
Citrate toxicity	
Hyperkalaemia	
Clotting abnormalities (after massive transfusion)	
TRALI	
Post-transfusion purpura	

CMV, cytomegalovirus; HIV, human immunodeficiency virus; HLA, human leucocyte antigen; TRALI, transfusion-related acute lung injury.

Diuretic phase Fluid and electrolyte imbalance may occur during the recovery from acute renal failure.

Investigation of an immediate transfusion reaction

If a patient develops features suggesting a severe transfusion reaction the transfusion should be stopped and investigations for blood group incompatibility and bacterial contamination of the blood must be initiated.

1 Most severe reactions occur because of clerical errors in the handling of donor or recipient blood specimens. Therefore it must be established that the identity of the recipient (from the patient's wristband) is the same as that on the compatibility label and that this corresponds with the actual unit being transfused.

2 The unit of donor blood and post-transfusion samples of the patient's blood should be sent to the laboratory who will:

(a) repeat the group on pre- and post-transfusion samples and on the donor blood, and repeat the cross-match;

(b) perform a direct antiglobulin test on the post-transfusion sample;

(c) check the plasma for haemoglobinaemia;

(d) perform tests for DIC; and

(e) examine the donor sample directly for evidence of gross bacterial contamination and set up blood cultures from it at 20 and 37°C. If the clinical picture is suggestive of bacterial infection blood cultures must be taken from the patient and broad spectrum intravenous antibodies started.

3 A post-transfusion sample of urine must be examined for haemoglobinuria.

4 Further samples of blood are taken 6 h and/or 24 h after transfusion for a blood count and bilirubin, free haemoglobin and methaemalbumin estimations.

5 In the absence of positive findings, the patient's serum is examined 5–10 days later for red cell or white cell antibodies.

Management of patients with major haemolysis

The principal object of initial therapy is to maintain the blood pressure and renal perfusion. Intravenous dextran, plasma or saline and frusemide are sometimes needed. Hydrocortisone 100 mg intravenously and an antihistamine may help to alleviate shock. In the event of severe shock, support with intravenous adrenaline 1 : 10 000 in small incremental doses may be required. Further compatible transfusions may be required in severely affected patients. If acute renal failure occurs this is managed in the usual way, if necessary with dialysis until recovery occurs.

Other transfusion reactions

Febrile reactions because of white cell antibodies Human leucocyte antigen (HLA) antibodies (see below and Chapter 21) are usually the result of sensitization by pregnancy or a previous transfusion. They produce rigors, pyrexia and, in severe cases, pulmonary infiltrates. They are minimized by giving leucocyte-depleted (i.e. filtered) packed cells (see below).

Febrile or non-febrile non-haemolytic allergic reactions These are usually caused by hypersensitivity to donor plasma proteins and if severe can result in anaphylactic shock. The clinical features are urticaria, pyrexia and, in severe cases, dyspnoea, facial oedema and rigors. Immediate treatment is with antihistamines and hydrocortisone. Adrenaline is also useful. Washed red cells or frozen red cells may be needed for further transfusions if the majority of plasma-removed blood (e.g. saline, adenine, glucose, mannitol (SAGM) blood) causes reactions.

Post-transfusion circulatory overload The management is that of cardiac failure. These reactions are prevented by a slow transfusion of packed red cells or of the blood component required, accompanied by diuretic therapy.

Transfusion of bacterially contaminated blood This is very rare but may be serious. It can present with circulatory collapse.

Graft-versus-host disease This may occur when live lymphocytes are transfused to an immunocompromised patient. It is prevented by irradiation of the blood product. It is uniformly fatal.

Transfusion related acute lung injury (TRALI) This presents as pulmonary infiltrates with chest symptoms depending on severity. It is caused by positive transfer of leucoagglutins in donor plasma causing endothelial and epithelial injury. Most of the donors are multiparous women. Management is supportive.

Post-transfusion purpura This is a rare problem of severe thrombocytopenia 7–10 days after transfusion of a platelet-containing product, usually red cells. It is caused by an antibody in the recipient (previously transfused or pregnant) anti HPA-1a against a platelet-specific antigen HPA-Ia (PI^{AI}). Both transfused and recipient platelets are destroyed by the immune complexes. It is usually self-limiting but immunoglobulin or plasma exchange may be needed.

Viral transmission Post-transfusion hepatitis may be caused by one of the hepatitis viruses, although CMV and Epstein–Barr virus (EBV) have also been implicated. Post-transfusion hepatitis and HIV infection is seen rarely now because of routine screening of all blood donations.

Other infections Toxoplasmosis, malaria and syphilis may be transmitted by blood transfusion. Transfusion-transmitted nvCJD has probably occurred in three cases in the UK.

Post-transfusional iron overload Repeated red cell transfusions over many years, in the absence of blood loss, cause deposition of iron initially in reticuloendothelial tissue at the rate of 200–250 mg/unit of red cells. After 50 units in adults, and lesser amounts in children, the liver, myocardium and endocrine glands are damaged with clinical consequences. This is a major problem in thalassaemia major and other severe chronic refractory anaemias (Chapter 6).

Reduction of blood product use

In light of transfusion risks, and limited resources, appropriate use of blood component is of ever increasing importance.

Preoperative correction of anaemia (particularly iron deficiency) and cessation of anti-platelet therapies (e.g. aspirin) where possible, together with lower trigger levels for red cell transfusions (7–8 g/dL in most surgical patients) can all help to reduce blood use.

In surgery the use of alternative fluid replacement, intraoperative or post-operative cell salvage, biological alternatives (e.g. erythopoetin, recombinant clotting factors, recombinant activated clotting factor VII (VIIa) or fibrin glue) all may help.

Blood components

A blood donation is taken by an aseptic technique into plastic bags containing an appropriate amount of anticoagulant—usually citrate, phosphate, dextrose (CPD). The citrate anticoagulates the blood by combining with the blood calcium. Three components are made by initial centrifugation of whole blood: red cells, buffy coat and plasma (Fig. 27.1).

Red cells are stored at 4–6°C for up to to 35 days, depending on the preservative. After the first 48 h there is a slow progressive K^+ loss from the red cells into the plasma. In cases where infusion of K^+ could be dangerous, fresh blood should be used (e.g. for exchange transfusion in haemolytic disease of the newborn). During red cell storage there is a fall in 2,3-diphosphoglycerate (2,3-DPG) but after transfusion 2,3-DPG levels return to normal within 24 h. Optimum additive solutions have been developed to increase the shelf life of plasma-depleted red cells by maintaining both adenosine triphosphate (ATP) and 2,3-DPG levels.

Platelets and plasma may also be collected by apharesis.

Leucodepletion

In many countries, including Britain, blood products are now routinely filtered to remove the majority of white cells, a process known as leucodepletion. This is usually performed soon after collection and prior to processing and is more effective than filtration of blood at the bedside. A blood component is defined as leucocyte depleted if there are less than 5×10^6/L white cells present.

Leucodepletion reduces the incidence of febrile transfusion reactions and HLA alloimmunization. It is effective at preventing transmission of CMV infection and in addition should reduce the theoretical possibility of transmission of nvCJD in countries where this has been reported.

Red cells

Packed (plasma-depleted) red cells are the treatment of choice for most transfusions (Fig. 27.7a). In older subjects, a diuretic is often given simultaneously and the infusion should be sufficiently slow to avoid circulatory overload. Iron chelation therapy should be considered with patients on a regular transfusion programme to avoid iron overload.

Recombinant erythropoietin is widely used to reduce transfusion requirements (e.g. in patients on dialysis, cancer patients and myelodysplasia). Factor VIIa can reduce transfusion need in patients with major haemorrhage (e.g. at surgery or after trauma).

Red cell substitutes are under development but have not yet proven clinically valuable. These synthetic oxygen-carrying substitutes are often fluorinated hydrocarbons and stromal-free pyridoxylated and polymerized haemoglobin solutions.

Autologous donation and transfusion

Anxiety over acquired immune deficiency syndrome (AIDS) and other infections has increased the demand for autotransfusion. There are three ways of administering an autologous transfusion:

1 ***Predeposit*** Blood is taken from the potential recipient in the weeks immediately prior to elective surgery.

2 ***Haemodilution*** Blood is removed immediately prior to surgery once the patient has been anaesthetized and then reinfused at the end of the operation.

3 ***Salvage*** Blood lost during the operation is collected during heavy blood loss and then reinfused.

Autotransfusion is the safest form of transfusion with regard to transmission of viral disease though it has a higher risk of bacterial contamination and of clerical errors. The individual involved must be fit enough to donate blood and the predicted operative replacement transfusion should be 2–4 units. Larger replacement transfusions would require blood to be collected over a longer period and red cells stored in the frozen state, which is both labour intensive and expensive. The high cost and initial restriction of its use to patients undergoing elective surgery means that it will benefit only a minor proportion of the total number of blood recipients.

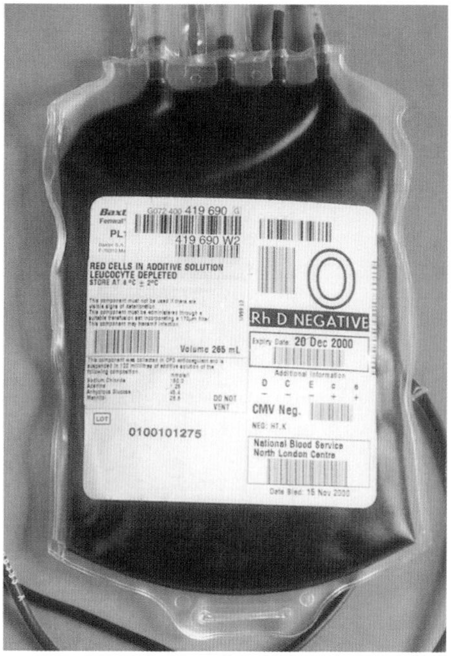

(a)

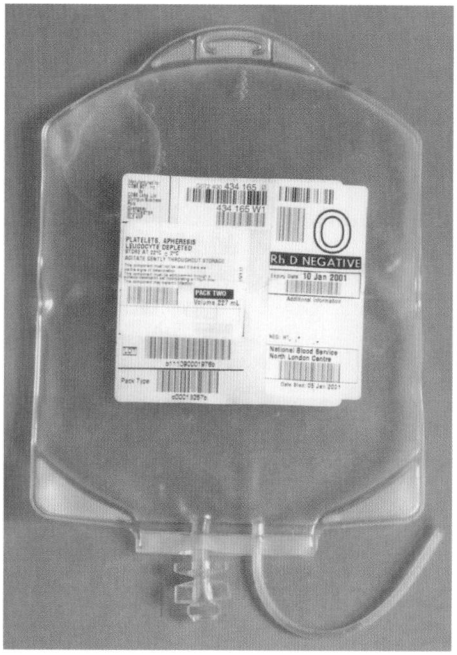

(b)

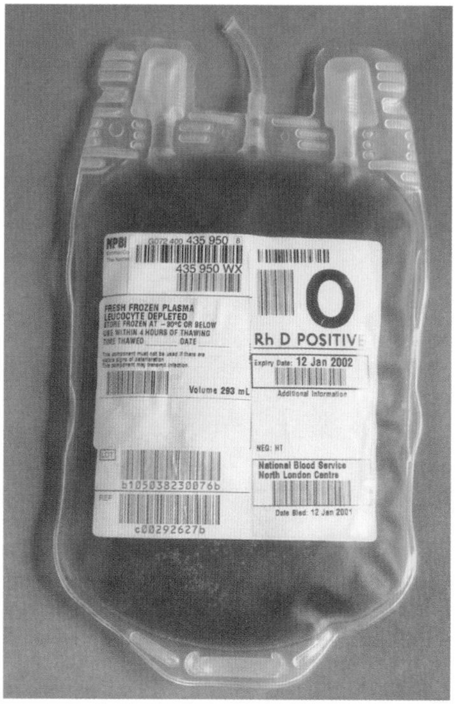

(c)

Fig. 27.7 Blood components: **(a)** plasma-depleted red cells; **(b)** platelets; and **(c)** fresh frozen plasma.

Preoperative autotransfusion is largely reserved for those patients with multiple antibodies.

Granulocyte concentrates

These are prepared as buffy coats or on blood cell separators from normal healthy donors or from patients with chronic myeloid leukaemia. They have been used in patients with severe neutropenia ($<0.5 \times 10^9/L$) who are not responding to antibiotic therapy but it is not usually possible to give sufficient amounts. They may transmit CMV infection and must be irradiated to eliminate the risk of causing GVHD.

Platelet concentrates

These are harvested by cell separators or from individual donor units of blood (Fig. 27.7b). They are stored at room temperature. Platelet transfusion is used in patients who are thrombocytopenic or have disordered platelet function and who are actively bleeding (therapeutic use) or are at serious risk of bleeding (prophylactic use).

For prophylaxis, the platelet count should be kept above $5–10 \times 10^9/L$ unless there are additional risk factors such as sepsis, drug use or coagulation disorders for which the threshold should be higher. For invasive procedures (e.g. liver biopsy or lumbar puncture) the platelet count should be raised to above $50 \times 10^9/L$. For brain or eye surgery the count should be $>100 \times 10^9/L$.

Therapeutic use is indicated in bleeding associated with platelet disorders. In massive haemorrhage the count should be kept above $50 \times 10^9/L$.

Platelet transfusions should be avoided in autoimmune thrombocytopenic purpura unless there is serious haemorrhage. They are contraindicated in heparin-induced thrombocytopenia, thrombotic thrombocytopenic purpura and haemolytic uraemic syndrome (p. 284).

Refractoriness to platelet transfusions is defined by a poor platelet increment post-transfusion ($<7.5 \times 10^9/L$ at 1 h or $<4.5 \times 10^9/L$ at 24 h). The causes are either immunological (mostly HLA alloimmunization) or non-immunological (sepsis, hypersplenism, DIC, drugs). Platelets express HLA class I (but not class II) antigens and HLA-matched or cross-match-compatible platelets are needed for patients with HLA antibodies.

Preparations from human plasma

Fresh frozen plasma (FFP)

Rapidly frozen plasma separated from fresh blood is stored at less than –30°C. Frozen plasma is usually prepared from single donor units though pooled products are also available. Its main use is for the replacement of coagulation factors (e.g. when specific concentrates are unavailable) or after massive transfusions, in liver disease and DIC, after cardiopulmonary bypass surgery, to reverse a warfarin effect, and in thrombotic thrombocytopenic purpura (see p. 284). Virally inactivated forms of FFP are now available.

Human albumin solution (4.5%)

It is a useful plasma volume expander when a sustained osmotic effect is required prior to the administration of blood, but it should not be given in excess. It is also used for fluid replacement in patients undergoing plasmapheresis and sometimes for fluid replacement in selected patients with hypoalbuminaemia.

Human albumin solution (20%) (salt-poor albumin)

It may be used in severe hypoalbuminaemia when it is necessary to use a product with minimal electrolyte content. Principal indications for its use are patients with nephrotic syndrome or liver failure.

Cryoprecipitate

This is obtained by thawing FFP at 4°C and contains concentrated factor VIII and fibrinogen. It is stored at less than –30°C or, if lyophylized, at 4–6°C, and was used widely as replacement therapy in haemophilia A and von Willebrand disease before more purified preparations of factor VIII became available. Its main use is in fibrinogen replacement in disseminated intravascular coagulation (DIC) or massive transfusion or hepatic failure.

Freeze-dried factor VIII concentrates

These are also used for treating haemophilia A or von Willebrand disease. The small volume makes them ideal for children, surgical cases, patients at risk from circulatory overload and for those on home treatment. Their use is declining as recombinant forms of factor VIII become widely available.

Freeze-dried factor IX–prothrombin complex concentrates

A number of preparations are available that contain variable amounts of factors II, VII, IX and X. They are mainly used for treating factor IX deficiency (Christmas disease) but are also used in patients with liver disease or in haemorrhage following overdose with oral anti-coagulants or in patients with factor VIII inhibitors. There is a risk of thrombosis.

Protein C concentrate

This is used in severe sepsis with disseminated intravascular coagulation (e.g. meningococcal septicaemia) to reduce thrombosis resulting from depletion of protein C.

Immunoglobulin

Pooled immunoglobulin is a valuable source of antibodies against common viruses. It is used in hypogammaglobulinaemia for protection against viral and bacterial disease. It may also be used in immune thrombocytopenia and other acquired immune disorders (e.g. post-transfusion purpura or alloimmune neonatal thrombocytopenia).

Specific immunoglobulin

This may be obtained from donors with high titres of antibody (e.g. anti-RhD, antihepatitis B, antiherpes zoster or antirubella).

Acute blood loss

After a single episode of blood loss, there is initial vasoconstriction with a reduction in total blood volume. The plasma volume rapidly expands and the haemoglobin and packed cell volume fall and there is a rise in neutrophils and platelets. The reticulocyte response begins on the second or third day and lasts 8–10 days. The haemoglobin begins to rise by about the seventh day but, if iron stores have become depleted, the haemoglobin may not rise subsequently to normal. Clinical assessment is needed to gauge whether blood transfusion is needed. This is usually unnecessary in adults at losses less than 500 mL unless haemorrhage is continuing and may not be needed with losses of up to 1.5 L. Blood transfusion is not without risks and should not be undertaken lightly. The problems of massive blood loss and massive transfusion are considered on p. 301.

Bibliography

American Association of Blood Banks (2002) *American Association of Blood Banks Technical Manual*, 14th edn. AABB, Bethesda, MD.

Ashford P., Gozzard D., Jones J. *et al.* for the British Committee for Standards in Haematology, Blood Transfusion Task Force. (2000) Guidelines for blood bank computing. *Transfus Med* **10**,307–14.

Barbara J.A.J. (2002) Transfusion transmitted infections. Transfusion alternatives. *Transfus Med* **4**,42–7.

Blumberg N., Francis C., Heal J. (eds) (2006) Clinical, use of plasma and plasma fractions. *Clin Haematol* **19**,1–258.

British Committee for Standards in Haematology, Blood Transfusion Task Force (1996) Guidelines for pretransfusion compatibility procedures in blood transfusion laboratories. *Transfus Med* **6**,273–83.

British Committee for Standards in Haematology, Blood Transfusion Task Force (1998) Guidelines on the clinical use of leucocyte-depleted blood components. *Transfus Med* **8**,59–72.

British Committee for Standards in Haematology, Blood Transfusion Task Force (2003) Guidelines for the use of platelet transfusions. *Br J Haematol* **122**,10–23.

British Committee for Standards in Haematology, Blood Transfusion Task Force (2004) Guidelines for the use of fresh-frozen plasma, cryoprecipitate and cryosupernatant. *Br J Haematol* **126**,11–28.

British Committee for Standards in Haematology Guidelines (1999) The administration of blood and blood components and the management of transfused patients. *Transfus Med* **9**,227–38.

Chang T.M.S. (2000) Red blood cell substitutes. *Clin Haematol* **13**,651–68.

Daniels G. (2002) *Human Blood Groups*, 2nd edn. Blackwell Science, Oxford.

Daniels G., Poole J., de Silva M. *et al.* (2002) The clinical significance of blood group antibodies. *Transfus Med* **12**,287–95.

Gibson B.E., Todd A., Roberts I. *et al.* for the British Committee for Standards in Haematology Transfusion Task Force: Writing Group (2004) Transfusion guidelines for neonates and older children. *Br J Haematol* **124**,433–53.

Llewelyn CA., Hewitt P.E., Knight R.S. *et al.* (2004) Possible transmission of variant Creutzfeldt–Jakob disease by blood transfusion. *Lancet* **363**,417–21.

Klein H. and Anstee D. (2005) *Mollison's Blood Transfusion in Clinical Medicine*, 11th edn. Blackwell Publishing, Oxford.

Murphy M.F. and Pamphilon D.H. (eds) (2005) *Practical Transfusion Medicine*, 2nd edn. Blackwell Publishing, Oxford.

Murphy M.F., Wallington T.B., Kelsey P. *et al.* for the British Committee for Standards in Haematology, Blood Transfusion Task Force (2001) Guidelines for the clinical use of red cell transfusions. *Br J Haematol* **113**,24–31.

National Institute for Clinical Excellence (2003) Full guidance on the use of antenatal anti-D prophylaxis for RhD–negative women (http://www.nice.org.uk).

Roberts HR., Monroe D.M., White G.C. (2004) The use of recombinant factor VIIa in the treatment of bleeding disorders. *Blood* **104**,3858–64.

Stainsky D., Cohen H., Jones H. *et al.* (2004) *Serious Hazards of Blood Transfuions Annual Report 2003* (http://www.shotuk.org/SHOT%20Report%202003.pdf).

UK Blood Transfusion Services (2002) *Guidelines for the Blood Transfusion Services in the United Kingdom*, 6th edn. The Stationery Office of London (or http://www.transfusionguidelines.org.uk).

Webert K.E. and Blajchman M.A. (2003) Transfusion-related acute lung injury. *Transfus Med Rev* **17**,252–62.

CHAPTER 28

28 Pregnancy and neonatal haematology

Haematology of pregnancy

Pregnancy places extreme stresses on the haematological system and an understanding of the physiological changes that result is obligatory in order to interpret any need for therapeutic intervention.

Physiological anaemia

Physiological anaemia is the term often used to describe the fall in haemoglobin (Hb) concentration that occurs during normal pregnancy (Fig. 28.1). Blood plasma volume increases by approximately 1250 mL, or 45%, above normal by the end of gestation and although the red cell mass itself increases by some 25% this still leads to a fall in Hb concentration. Values below 10 g/dL are probably abnormal and require investigation.

Iron deficiency anaemia

Up to 600 mg iron is required for the increase in red cell mass and a further 300 mg for the fetus. Despite an increase in iron absorption, few women avoid depletion of iron reserves by the end of pregnancy.

In uncomplicated pregnancy, the mean corpuscular volume (MCV) typically rises by approximately 4 fL. A fall in red cell MCV is the earliest sign of iron deficiency. Later, the mean corpuscular haemoglobin

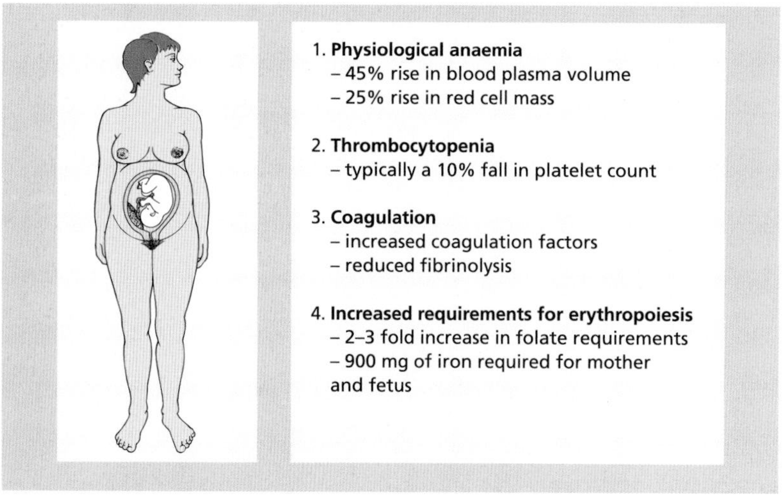

Fig. 28.1 Haematological changes during pregnancy.

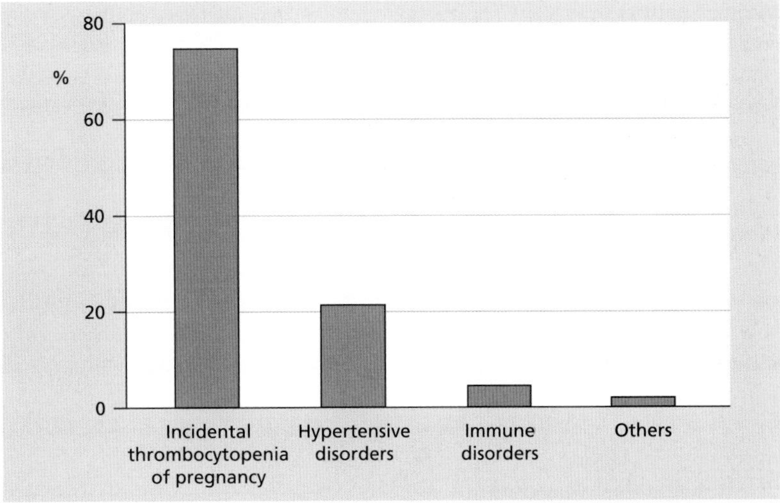

Fig. 28.2 Causes of thrombocytopenia during pregnancy.

(MCH) falls and finally anaemia results. Early iron deficiency is likely if the serum ferritin is below 15 μg/L together with serum iron <10 μmol/L and should be treated with oral iron supplements. The use of routine iron supplementation in pregnancy is debated but iron is probably better avoided until the Hb falls below 10 g/dL or MCV below 82 fL in the third trimester.

Folate deficiency

Folate requirements are increased approximately twofold in pregnancy and serum folate levels fall to approximately half the normal range with a less dramatic fall in red cell folate. In some parts of the world, megaloblastic anaemia during pregnancy is common because of a combination of poor diet and exaggerated folate requirements. Given the protective effect of folate against neural tube defects, folic acid 400 μg/day should be taken periconceptually and throughout pregnancy. Food fortification with folate is now being practised in many countries. Vitamin B_{12} deficiency is rare during pregnancy although serum vitamin B_{12} levels fall to below normal in 20–30% of pregnancies and low values are sometimes the cause of diagnostic confusion.

Thrombocytopenia

The platelet count typically falls by approximately 10% in an uncomplicated pregnancy. In approximately 7% of women this fall is more severe and can result in thrombocytopenia (platelet count $<140 \times 10^9$/L). In over 75% of cases this is mild and of unknown cause, a condition referred to as *incidental thrombocytopenia of pregnancy*. Approximately 21% of cases are secondary to a hypertensive disorder and 4% are associated with immune thrombocytopenic purpura (ITP; Fig. 28.2).

Incidental thrombocytopenia of pregnancy This is a diagnosis of exclusion and is usually detected at the time of delivery. The platelet count is always $>70 \times 10^9$/L and recovers within 6 weeks. No treatment is required and the infant is not affected.

Thrombocytopenia of hypertensive disorders This is variable in severity but the platelet count rarely falls to $<40 \times 10^9$/L. It is more severe when associated with pre-eclampsia and if severe the primary treatment is as rapid delivery as possible. The platelet count falls for a day or two after delivery and then recovers rapidly. The HELLP syndrome (haemolysis, elevated liver enzymes and low platelets) is a subtype of this category.

Idiopathic thrombocytopenic purpura (p. 281) In pregnancy, ITP represents a particular problem, both to the mother and to the fetus, as the antibody crosses the placenta and the fetus may become severely thrombocytopenic.

Like all adults, pregnant women with ITP and

platelet counts >50 × 10^9/L do not usually need treatment. Treatment is required for women with platelet counts <10 × 10^9/L and for those with platelet counts of 10–30 × 10^9/L who are in their second or third trimester or who are bleeding. Treatment is with steroids, intravenous immunoglobulin G (IgG) and splenectomy as appropriate.

At delivery, umbilical vein blood sampling or fetal scalp vein sampling to measure the fetal platelet count may be offered although their exact role is unclear. In general, caesarean section is not indicated when the maternal platelet count is >50 × 10^9/L unless the fetal platelet count is known to be <20 × 10^9/L. Platelet transfusion may be given to mothers in labour with very low platelet counts or who are actively bleeding.

Newborns of mothers with ITP should have a blood count measured for the first 4 days of life as the platelet count may progressively drop. A count greater than 50 × 10^9/L is reassuring. Cerebral ultrasounds may be performed to look for intracranial haemorrhage (ICH). In newborns without evidence of ICH, treatment with intravenous IgG is appropriate if the infant's platelet count is <20 × 10^9/L. Neonates with thrombocytopenia and ICH should be treated with steroids and intravenous IgG therapy.

Haemostasis and thrombosis

Pregnancy leads to a hypercoaguable state with consequent increased risks of thromboembolism and disseminated intravascular coagulation (DIC; p. 298). There is an increase in plasma factors VII, VIII, X and fibrinogen and fibrinolysis is suppressed. These changes last for up to 2 months into the puerperal period and the incidence of thrombosis during this period is increased. There is an association between thrombophilic conditions in the mother and with recurrent fetal loss. This is presumed to result from placental thrombosis and infarction.

Treatment of thrombosis

Warfarin has no role in management. It crosses the placenta and in addition is associated with embryopathy, especially between 6 and 12 weeks' gestation. Heparin does not cross the placenta but a significant side-effect of prolonged use is maternal osteoporosis. Low molecular weight heparin is now the treatment of choice because it can be given once daily and is less likely to cause osteoporosis.

Neonatal haematology

Normal blood count

The cord blood Hb varies between approximately 16.5 and 17 g/dL and is influenced by the timing of cord clamping (Fig. 28.3). The reticulocyte count is initially high (2–6%) but falls to below 0.5% at 1 week as erythropoiesis is suppressed in response to the marked increase in the oxygenation of tissues after birth. This is associated with a progressive fall in Hb to approximately 10–11 g/dL at 8 weeks from which point it recovers to 12.5 g/dL at around 6 months. In the blood film, nucleated red cells will be seen for the first 4 days and for up to 1 week in preterm infants. Numbers are increased in cases of hypoxia, haemorrhage or haemolytic disease of the newborn (HDN). MCV averages 119 fL but falls to adult levels by around 9 weeks. By 1 year, the MCV has fallen to around 70 fL and rises throughout childhood again to reach adult levels at puberty. Preterm infants have a more dramatic fall in Hb to 7–9 g/dL at 8 weeks and are more prone to iron and folate deficiency in the first few months of life. Neutrophils are initially high at birth and fall to plateau at 4 days—from this point on the lymphocyte count is higher than neutrophils throughout childhood.

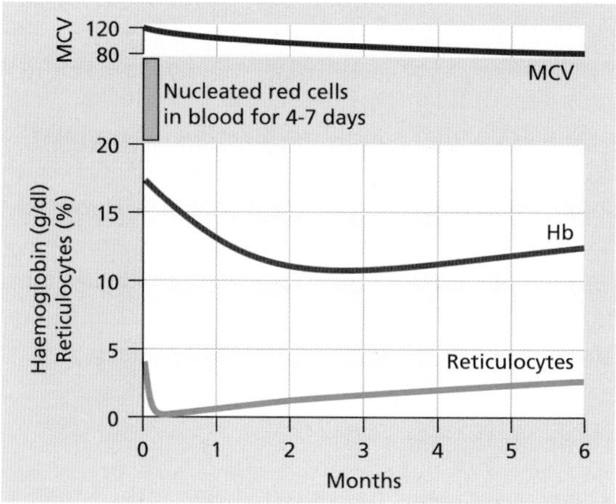

Fig. 28.3 Typical profile of the blood count in the neonatal period.

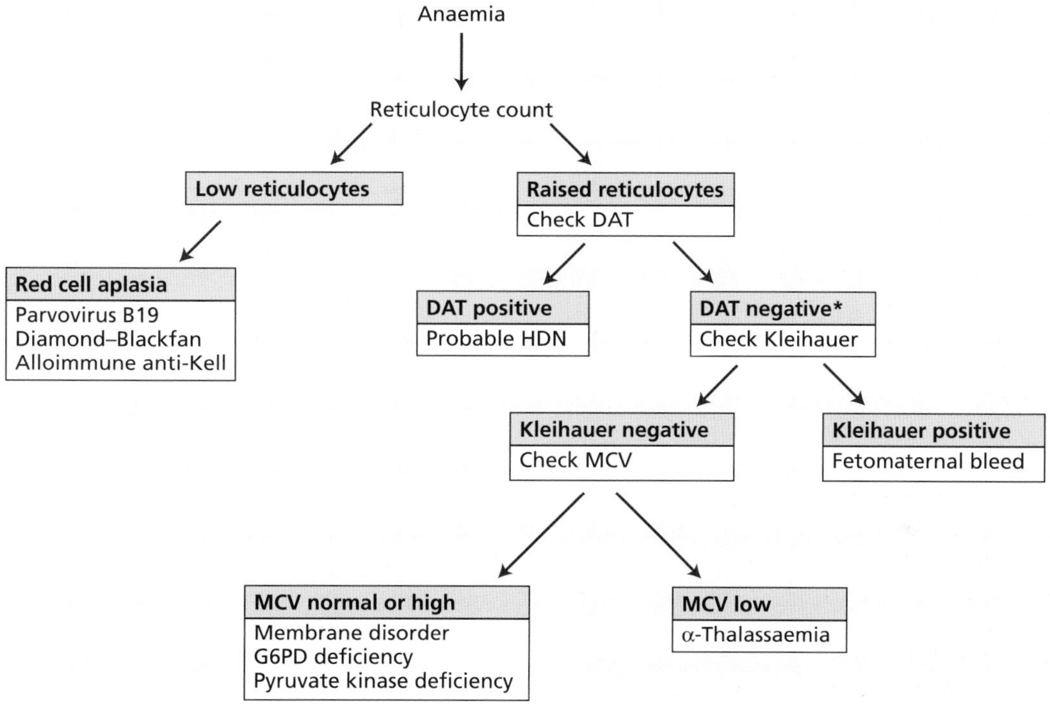

Fig. 28.4 The investigation of neonatal anaemia. * The DAT test may be negative in HDN, e.g. due to ABO incompatibility. DAT, direct antiglobulin test; HDN, haemolytic disease of the newborn; MCV, mean corpuscular volume.

Anaemia in the neonate

This should be considered for Hb <14 g/dL at birth. The clinical significance of anaemia is compounded by the high (70–80%) levels of HbF at birth, as this is less effective than HbA at releasing oxygen to the tissues (p. 17). Causes include the following (Fig. 28.4):

1 ***Haemorrhage*** Fetomaternal, twin–twin, cord, internal, placenta.

2 ***Increased destruction*** Haemolysis (immune or non-immune) or infection.

3 ***Decreased production*** Congenital red cell aplasia, infection (e.g. parvovirus). Anti-Kell causes alloimmune anaemia of the fetus and newborn with decreased erythropoiesis.

Generally, anaemia at birth is usually secondary to immune haemolysis or haemorrhage; non-immune causes of haemolysis appear within 24 h. Impaired red cell production is usually not apparent for at least 3 weeks. Haemolysis is often associated with severe jaundice and the causes include HDN, autoimmune haemolytic anaemia (AIHA) in the mother and congenital disorders of the red cell membrane or metabolism.

Red cell transfusion may be needed for symptomatic anaemia with Hb <10.5 g/dL or a higher threshold if there is severe cardiac or respiratory disease.

Anaemia of prematurity

Premature infants have a more marked fall in Hb after birth and this is termed ***physiological anaemia of prematurity***. Features include a slowly falling Hb, normal blood film and reticulocytopenia. It can be minimized by ensuring adequate iron and folate replacement and limiting phlebotomy. Erythropoietin is used in some centres.

Neonatal polycythaemia

This is defined as a venous haematocrit over 0.65 and can occur with twin–twin transfusion, intrauterine growth restriction and maternal hypertension or diabetes. If symptoms are present it should be treated with partial exchange transfusion using a crystalloid solution.

Fetomaternal alloimmune thrombocytopenia

Fetomaternal alloimmune thrombocytopenia (FMAIT) results from an immunological process similar to that which causes HDN. Fetal platelets that possess a paternally inherited antigen (HPA-1a in 80%; HPA-5b in 15%) that is not present on maternal platelets can sensitize the mother to make antibodies that cross the placenta, coat the platelets which are then destroyed by the reticuloendothelial system and lead to serious bleeding, including intracranial haemorrhage. Alloimmune thrombocytopenia differs from HDN in that 50% of cases occur in the first pregnancy. Its incidence is approximately 1 in 1000–5000 births.

Thrombocytopenia can lead to serious, sometimes fatal, bleeding *in utero* or after birth. Treatment is unsatisfactory. Severe postnatal cases may be treated with a platelet transfusion that is negative for the relevant antigen. Antenatal treatment may be either maternal intravenous immunoglobulin or fetal transfusion with HPA-compatible platelets.

Coagulation

Standard tests need to be interpreted with caution in the neonate. The activated partial thromboplastin time (APTT) and prothrombin time (PT) are prolonged because of reduced levels of the vitamin K-dependent factors II, VII, IX and X, and return to normal at around 6 months. The thrombin time (TT) is comparable with adult values. Neonates have an increased risk of thrombosis. This is a result of physiologically low levels of inhibitors of coagulation and the use of indwelling vascular catheters. Antithrombin (AT) and protein C levels are approximately 60% of normal for the first 3 months. Homozygous protein C deficiency is associated with fulminant purpura fulminans in early life. Therapeutic protein C concentrates are now available. Homozygous AT deficiency usually presents later in childhood but arterial and venous thrombosis may also occur in the neonate.

Haemorrhagic disease of the newborn is discussed on page 297.

Haemolytic disease of the newborn

HDN is the result of ***red cell alloimmunization*** in which IgG antibodies passage from the maternal circulation across the placenta into the circulation of the fetus where they react with fetal red cells and lead to their destruction. Anti-D antibody is responsible for most cases of severe HDN although anti-c, anti-E, anti-K and a wide range of other antibodies are found in occasional cases (see Table 27.2). Although antibodies against the ABO blood group system are most frequent cause of HDN this is usually mild. Within the UK, approximately 500 fetuses develop haemolytic disease each year and approximately 30 of these cases are fatal.

Rh HDN

When an Rh D-negative (p. 339) woman has a pregnancy with an Rh D-positive fetus, Rh D-positive fetal red cells cross into the maternal circulation (especially at parturition and during the third trimester) and sensitize the mother to form anti-D. The mother could also be sensitized by a previous miscarriage, amniocentesis or other trauma to the placenta or by blood transfusion. Anti-D crosses the placenta to the fetus during the next pregnancy with an Rh D-positive fetus, coats the fetal red cells and results in reticuloendothelial destruction of these cells, causing anaemia and jaundice. If the father is heterozygous for D antigen, there is a 50% probability that the fetus will be D-positive. The fetal Rh D genotype can be established by polymerase chain reaction (PCR) analysis for the presence of Rh D in a maternal blood sample.

The main aim of management is to *prevent* anti-D antibody formation in Rh D-negative mothers. This can be achieved by the administration of small amounts of anti-D antibody which 'mop up' and destroy Rh D-positive fetal red cells before they can sensitize the immune system of the mother to produce anti-D.

Prevention of Rh immunization

At the time of booking, all pregnant women should have their ABO and Rh group determined and serum screened for antibodies at least twice during the pregnancy. All non-sensitized Rh D-negative women should be given at least 500 units (100 μg) of anti-D at 28 and 34 weeks' gestation to reduce the risk of sensitization from fetomaternal haemorrhage. Fetal Rh D typing from DNA in maternal blood can be used before 28 weeks. If the fetus is Rh D-negative, no further anti-D prophylaxis is needed. In addition, at birth the babies of Rh D-negative women who do not have antibodies must have their cord blood grouped for ABO and Rh. If the baby's blood is Rh D-negative, the mother will require no further treatment. If the baby is Rh D-positive, prophylactic anti-D should be administered at a minimum dose of 500 units intramuscularly within 72 h of delivery. A ***Kleihauer test*** is performed. If the Kleihauer is positive many centres will perform flow cytometry for a more accurate estimate of the volume of feto-maternal haemorrhage (FMH). This uses differential staining to estimate the number of fetal cells in the maternal circulation (Fig. 28.5). The chance of developing antibodies is related to the number of fetal cells found. The dose of anti-D is increased if there is greater than 4 mL transplacental haemorrhage. Anti-D IgG (125 units) is given for each 1 mL of FMH greater than 4 mL.

Sensitizing episodes during pregnancy Anti-D IgG should be given to Rh D-negative women who have potentially sensitizing episodes during pregnancy: 250 units is given if the event occurs up to week 20 of gestation and 500 units thereafter, followed by a Kleihauer test. Potentially sensitizing events include therapeutic termination of pregnancy, spontaneous miscarriage after 12 weeks' gestation, ectopic pregnancy and invasive antenatal diagnostic procedures.

Treatment of established anti-D sensitization

If anti-D antibodies are detected during pregnancy they should be quantified at regular intervals. The strength of anti-D present in maternal serum is related to the clinical severity of HDN but this is also affected by such factors as the IgG subclass, rate of rise of antibody and past history. The development of haemolytic disease in the fetus can be assessed by velocimetry of the fetal middle cerebral artery by Doppler ultrasonography as increased velocities correlate with fetal anaemia (Fig. 28.6). If anaemia is detected, fetal blood sampling and intrauterine transfusion of irradiated Rh D-negative packed red cells may be indicated.

Clinical features of HDN

1 ***Severe disease*** Intrauterine death from hydrops fetalis (Fig. 28.7a).

2 ***Moderate disease*** The baby is born with anaemia and jaundice and may show pallor, tachycardia, oedema and hepatosplenomegaly. If the unconjugated bilirubin is not controlled and reaches levels exceeding 250 μmol/L, bile pigment deposition in the basal ganglia may lead to ***kernicterus***—central nervous system damage with generalized spasticity and possible subsequent mental deficiency, deafness and epilepsy. This problem becomes acute after birth as maternal clearance of fetal bilirubin ceases

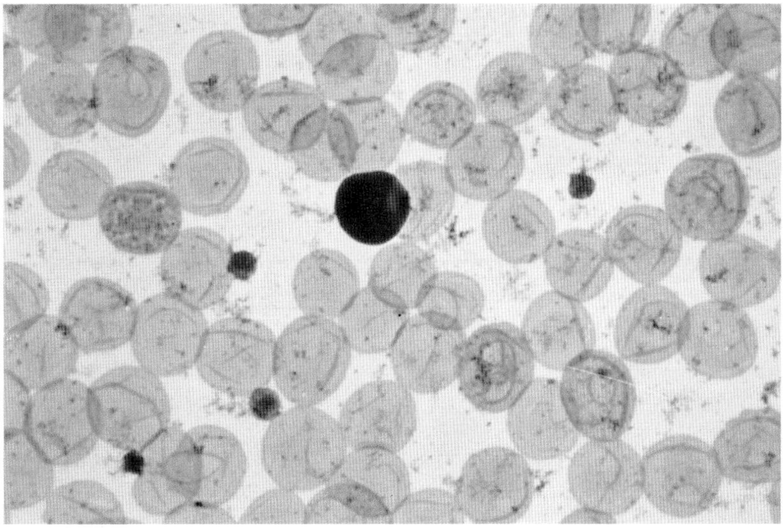

Fig. 28.5 Kleihauer test for fetal red cells; a deeply eosin-staining cell containing fetal haemoglobin is seen at the centre. Haemoglobin has been eluted from the other red cells by an incubation at acid pH and these appear as colourless ghosts.

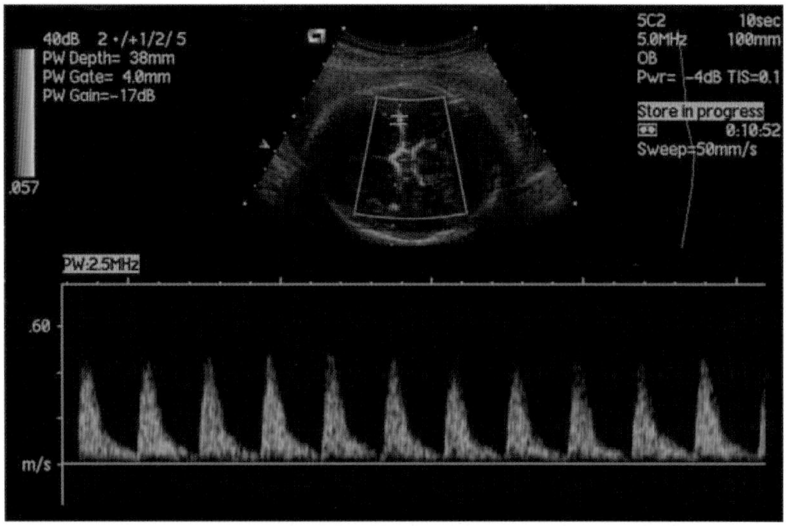

Fig. 28.6 Doppler ultrasonography of the circle of Willis in a fetus. The cursor is placed over the middle cerebral artery and an increased blood velocity correlates with anaemia. (From Kumar and Regan, 2005 with permission)

and conjugation of bilirubin by the neonatal liver has not yet reached full activity.

3 ***Mild disease*** Mild anaemia with or without jaundice.

Investigations will reveal variable anaemia with a high reticulocyte count; the baby is Rh D-positive, the direct antiglobulin test is positive and the serum bilirubin raised. In moderate and severe cases, many erythroblasts are seen in the blood film (Fig. 28.7b) and this is known as ***erythroblastosis fetalis***.

Treatment

Exchange transfusion may be necessary; the indications for this include severe anaemia (Hb <10 g/dL at birth) and severe or rapidly rising hyperbilirubinaemia. More than one exchange transfusion may be required and 500 mL is usually sufficient for each exchange. The donor blood should be less than 5 days old, CMV negative and irradiated. Rh D-negative and ABO compatible with the baby's and mother's serum. Phototherapy (exposure of the infant to bright light of appropriate wavelength) degrades bilirubin and reduces the likelihood of kernicterus.

ABO haemolytic disease of the newborn

In 20% of births, a mother is ABO incompatible with the fetus. Group A and group B mothers usually have only IgM ABO antibodies (p. 338). The majority of cases of ABO HDN are caused by 'immune' IgG antibodies in group O mothers. Although 15% of pregnancies in white people involve a group O mother with a group A or group B fetus, most mothers do not produce IgG anti-A or anti-B and very few babies have severe enough haemolytic disease to require treatment. Exchange transfusions are needed in only 1 in 3000 infants. The mild course of ABO HDN is partly explained by the A and B antigens not being fully developed at birth and by partial neutralization of maternal IgG antibodies by A and B antigens on other cells, in the plasma and tissue fluids.

In contrast to Rh HDN, ABO disease may be found in the first pregnancy and may or may not affect subsequent pregnancies. The direct antiglobulin test on the infant's cells may be negative or only weakly positive. Examination of the blood film shows autoagglutination and spherocytosis, polychromasia and erythroblastosis.

Bibliography

Finning K.M., Martin P.G., Soothill P.W., Avent N.D. (2002) Prediction of fetal D status from maternal plasma: introduction of a new non-invasive fetal RHD genotyping service. *Transfusion* **42**,1079–85.

Greer I.A. and Nelson-Piercy C. (2005) Low-molecular-weight heparins for thromboprophylaxis and treatment

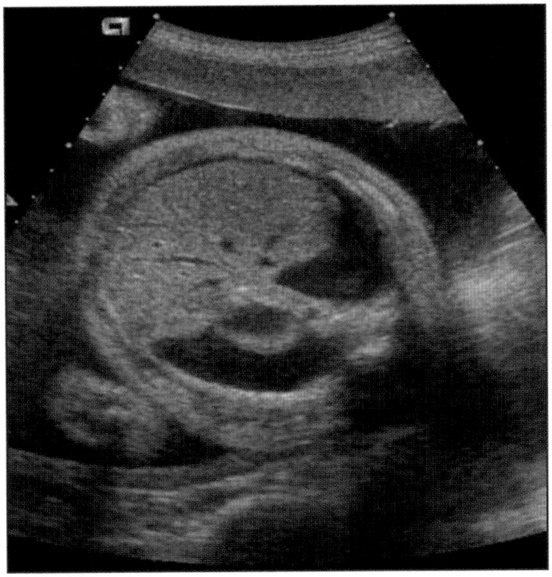

(a)

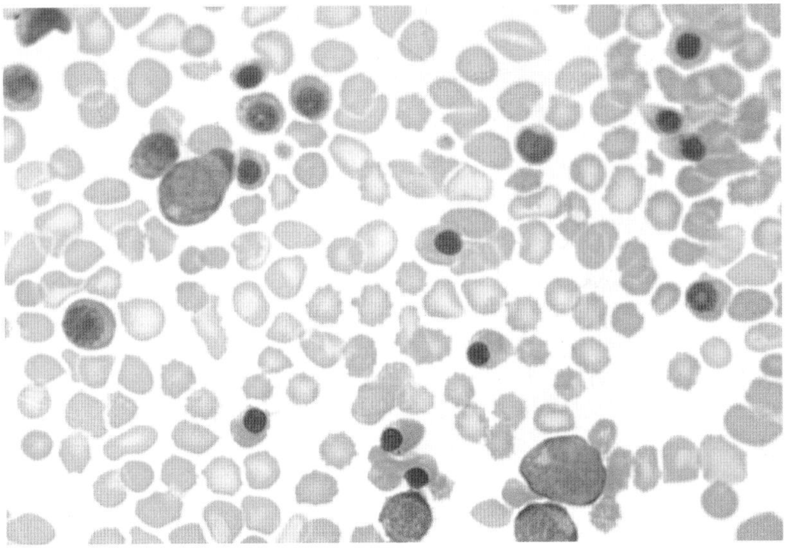

Fig. 28.7 **(a)** Ultrasound features of hydrops fetalis showing skin oedema, hepatomegaly and ascites. (From Kumar and Regan, 2005 with permission.) **(b)** Rh haemolytic disease of the newborn (erythroblastosis fetalis): peripheral blood film showing large numbers of erythroblasts, polychromasia and crenated cells. (b)

of venous thromboembolism in pregnancy: a systematic review of safety and efficacy. *Blood* **106**,401–7.

Kumar S. and Regan F. (2005) Management of pregnancies with Rh D alloimmunisation. *BMJ* **330**,1255–8.

Mari G., Deter R.L., Delle Chiaie L. *et al*. (2000) Noninvasive diagnosis by Doppler ultrasonography of fetal anemia due to maternal red-cell alloimmunization. Collaborative Group for Doppler Assessment of the Blood Velocity in Anemic Fetuses. *N Engl J Med* **342**,9–14.

Moise K.J. (2005) Red blood cell alloimmunization in pregnancy. *Semin Hematol* **42**,169–78.

Nathan D.G., Orkin S.H., Look A.T., Ginsberg D. (eds) (2003) *Hematology of Infancy and Childhood*. W.B. Saunders, Philadelphia.

Appendix 1

Principal features of known cluster differentiation (CD) molecules

Cluster	Main cellular distribution	Name/comments/function/diagnostic value
CD1a	Thymocytes, dendritic cells	Ligand for some $\gamma\delta$ T cells
CD1b	Thymocytes, dendritic cells	Ligand for some $\gamma\delta$ T cells
CD1c	Thymocytes, dendritic cells	Ligand for some $\gamma\delta$ T cells
CD2	Pan T cell, NK cells	SRCR, adhesion (LFA-2) binds LFA-3
CD3	Pan T cell	Signal transduction from the T-cell receptor
CD4	T-helper subset	Adhesion (binds class II MHC)
CD5	Pan T cell, B-cell subset	Expressed on B-CLL and mantle cell lymphoma
CD6	Subset of T cells	
CD7	Subset of T cells	
CD8	Cytotoxic T cell	Adhesion (binds class I MHC)
CD9	Pre-B cells, monocytes, platelets	
CD10	Precursor B and some mature B cells	Expressed in c-ALL (CALLA) and many cases of follicular lymphoma
CD11a	Leucocytes	Adhesion (combines with CD18 to form LFA-1 integrin)
CD11b	Granulocytes, monocytes, NK cells	Adhesion (combines with CD18 to form Mac-I integrin)
CD11c	Granulocytes, monocytes, NK cells	Adhesion (combines with CD18 to form p150,95 [$\alpha_X\beta_2$] integrin)
CD11d	Peripheral blood leucocytes	Adhesion (combines with CD18 to form $\alpha_D\beta_2$ integrin)
CD12	Monocytes, granulocytes	
CD13	Monocytes, granulocytes	An aminopeptidase
CD14	Monocytes, macrophages	Binds LPS
CD15	Granulocytes	Lewis X antigen (carbohydrate epitope)
CD16	NK cells, granulocytes, macrophages	FcγRIII
CD17	Granulocytes, monocytes, platelets	
CD18	Leucocytes	Adhesion (β chain of LFA-1 integrin family)
CD19	B cells	Modulates the threshold for signalling through B-cell receptor
CD20	B cells	
CD21	Mature B cells	CR2, C3dR, receptor for EBV. Complexes with CD19
CD22	B cells	Down-regulates B-cell activation
CD23	Activated B cells, macrophages, FDC	FcεRII. Positive on CLL
CD24	B cells, granulocytes	
CD25	Activated T cells, B cells, macrophages	α chain of IL-2 receptor. Expressed on hairy cell leukaemia. Marker of regulatory $CD4^+$ T cells

(Continued)

Cluster	Main cellular distribution	Name/comments/function/diagnostic value
CD26	Activated T cells, B cells, macrophages	
CD27	T cells, plasma cells	
CD28	T cells	Co-stimulation
CD29	Broad	Integrin β_1 subunit. Forms heterodimers with many integrin α subunits (e.g. CD49)
CD30	Activated T and B cells	Reed–Sternberg cells express; Ki detects
CD31	Monocytes, platelets, endothelium	Platelet endothelial cell adhesion molecule 1 (PECAM-1)
CDw32	Monocytes, platelets	FcγRII (receptor for aggregated IgG)
CD33	Monocytes, myeloid progenitors	
CD34	Precursors of haemopoietic cells	Marrow progenitors
CD35	Granulocytes, monocytes, B cells	C3b receptor, CR1
CD36	Monocytes, platelets	Platelet GPIIIb
CD37	Pan-13, some T cells, FDC	
CD38	Thymocytes, activated T cells, plasma cells	Plasma cell tumours
CD39	B cells	
CD40	B cells	Important co-stimulatory molecule for B cells
CD41	Platelets	Platelet GPIIb (forms complex with GPIIIa [CD61]), mutated in Glanzmann thrombasthenia
CD42a & b	Platelets	Form GPIb (platelet adhesion to von Willebrand factor)
CD43	Leucocytes	
CD44	Leucocytes, erythrocytes	
CD45	Leucocytes	Leucocyte common antigen. Low expression on malignant plasma cells
CD46	Leucocytes, epithelial cells, fibroblasts	Regulates complement activation
CD47	Broad	
CD48	Leucocytes	Binds CD2
CD49a–f	T cells, monocytes, platelets	α-integrin subunits. They can all form heterodimers with CD29 (to generate VLA1–6)
CD50	Leucocytes	ICAM-3
CD51	Platelets, megakaryocytes, activated T cells	Integrin α_V subunit. Can form heterodimers with β_1, β_3, β_5, β_6 or β_8
CD52	Lymphocytes and monocytes	Target for CAMPATH antibody (p. 192)
CD53	Leucocytes	
CD54	Leucocytes	Adhesion (ICAM-1 ligand for LFA-1)
CD55	Leucocytes and endothelium	Complement decay-accelerating factor (DAF)
CD56	Some T and B cells, neural and muscle tissue	NCAM. Expressed on malignant plasma cells
CD57	NK cells, subset of T cells	
CD58	Leucocytes, epithelial cells	Adhesion (LFA-3) ligand for CD2
CD59	Broad	Membrane inhibitor of reactive lysis (MIRL)
CDw60	T subset, platelets	
CD61	Platelets, megakaryocytes	Integrin β_3 subunit (associates with CD41 to form GPIIb/IIIa)
CD62 E, L and P	Endothelium (E), leucocytes (L), megakaryocytes and platelets (P)	Selectins. Recruit leucocytes to inflammation
CD63	Activated platelets, monocytes	
CD64	Monocytes, macrophages	FcγRI (high-affinity Fcγ receptor)
CD65	Granulocytes	
CD66a–e	Granulocytes (a–d)	Carcinoembryonic antigen (CEA) family. CEA is CD66e

(*Continued*)

Cluster	Main cellular distribution	Name/comments/function/diagnostic value
CD68	Monocytes, macrophages	
CD69	Activated B, T cells, macrophages, NK cells	
CDw70	Activated B, T cells	CD27Lm
CD71	Proliferating cells	Transferrin receptor
CD72	B cells	
CD73	B subset, T subset	Ecto 5′-nucleotidase
CD74	B cells, monocytes	MHC class II-associated invariant chain (Ii)
CDw75	Mature B cells	
CD76	Mature B cells	
CD77	Germinal centre B cells	
CD79a	B cells	Associated with B-cell antigen receptor complex (Igα)
CD79b	B cells	Associated with B-cell antigen receptor complex (Igβ). Negative on most cases of CLL
CD80	Monocytes/dendritic cells/B cells	B7-1. Involved in T-cell activation via CD28 and CD152
CD81	General expression	
CD82	General expression	
CD83	Dendritic cells/germinal centre B cells	
CD84	Macrophages and platelets	
CD85	Plasma cells/monocytes	Many lymphoid leukaemias
CD86	Dendritic cells and B cells	B7-2. Binds CD28 and CD152
CD87	Monocytes/granulocytes	Urokinase plasminogen activator receptor
CD88	Myeloid cells	Binds C5a
CD89	Phagocytic cells	IgA receptor, FcαR
CD90	Prothymocytes	Thy-1
CD91	Phagocytes	α_2-macroglobulin receptor
CD92	Myeloid	
CD93	Granulocytes, monocytes, endothelial cells	
CD94	NK cells, subset of T cells	Inhibitory receptor. Complexes with NKG2 and then binds HLA-E
CD95	Activated lymphocytes, monocytes, neutrophils	Fas. Triggers apoptosis
CD96	NK and T cells	
CD97	Granulocytes, macrophages	
CD98	Monocytes	
CD99	Leucocytes	
CD100	B, T and NK cells. Myeloid cells	
CD101	Monocytes, granulocytes and T cells	
CD102	Leucocytes and endothelium	ICAM-2. Ligand for CD11a/CD18 (LFA-1)
CD103	Intraepithelial lymphocytes	Useful in the diagnosis of hairy cell leukaemia. Integrin α_E subunit—with β_7 it binds to E-cadherin. Expressed on hairy cell leukaemia
CD104		Integrin β_4 subunit
CD105	Endothelial cells	Endoglin. Binds to TGF-β. Mutated in hereditary haemorrhagic telangiectasia
CD106	Endothelium	VCAM-1. Binds the integrins $\alpha_4\beta_1$ and $\alpha_4\beta_7$
CD107	Wide distribution	Lysosomal proteins
CD108	Lymphoid, myeloid, stroma	
CD109	Platelets	Can be target for alloantibodies

(Continued)

Cluster	Main cellular distribution	Name/comments/function/diagnostic value
CD114	Myeloid cells, endothelium, platelets	G-CSFR
CD115	Monocytes, macrophages	Macrophage colony-stimulating factor receptor (M-CSFR)
CD116	Monocytes, neutrophils, eosinophils, endothelial cells	α chain of GM-CSFR
CD117		*c*-kit, steel factor receptor
CD118	Broad	Interferon α/β receptor
CD119	Broad	α chain of IFN-γR
CD120	Broad	TNFRI, TNFRII
CD121	Broad	Components of the IL-1 receptor
CD122	B, T and NK cells	β chain of IL-2 receptor, IL-15R
CD123	Early and committed bone marrow progenitors	α chain of IL-3 receptor
CD124	Broad	α chain of IL-4R and component of IL-13R
CD125	Eosinophils and basophils	α chain of IL-5 receptor
CD126	Activated B cells, plasma cells and myeloma	α chain of IL-6 receptor
CD127	Lymphoid precursors and T cells	α chain of IL-7 receptor
CD128	Neutrophils	Component of IL-8 receptor
CD129	Erythroid and myeloid precursors, lymphocytes	α chain of IL-9 receptor
CD130	Broad	β chain of IL-6R, IL-11R
CD131		β chain of GM-CSFR, IL-3R and IL-5R
CD132		β chain of IL-7R, IL-9R, IL-15R
CD134	Activated T cells	OX40
CD135	Haemopoietic stem cells	FLT-3
CD136		Macrophage-stimulating protein receptor
CD137	Activated lymphocytes, monocytes	4-1BB
CD138	Pre-B cells and plasma cells	Syndecan-1. Detected by Mab BB4 and useful in the diagnosis of myeloma
CD139	Germinal centre B cells	
CD140	Broad	PDGF receptor
CD141	Endothelium	Thrombomodulin
CD142	Activated monocytes and endothelium	Tissue factor
CD143	Endothelium	Angiotensin-converting enzyme
CD144		VE-cadherin
CD145	Endothelium/stroma	
CD146	Endothelium/activated T cells	MUC-18
CD147	Broad	Extracellular matrix metalloproteinase inducer
CD148	Myeloid cells	
CD149	Broad	
CD150	Activated B and T cells	SLAM
CD151	Platelets, moncytes and endothelium	PETA-3
CD152	Activated T cells	CTLA-4. Binds CD80 and CD86
CD153	Activated T cells	CD30L
CD154	Activated T cells	CD40L. Mutations lead to hyper-IgM syndrome
CD155	Monocytes, macrophages, thymocytes	Poliovirus receptor
CD156	Monocytes, macrophages, granulocytes	ADAM-8
CD157	Monocytes, neutrophils, endothelium	BST-1

(*Continued*)

Cluster	Main cellular distribution	Name/comments/function/diagnostic value
CD158	NK cells and T-cell subsets	KIR
CD161	NK cells and some T cells	NKR-P1 family
CD162	Lymphocytes, neutrophils and monocytes	P-selectin glycoprotein ligand
CD163	Monocyte macrophage lineage	
CD164	Haemapoietic cells	MGC-24
CD165	Thymocytes, thymic epithelial cells	AD2/gp37
CD166	Thymic epithelial cells, activated T cells	CD6L
CD167	Epithelial cells	DDR1/receptor tyrosine kinase
CD168	Haemopoietic cells	RHAMM/hyaluronan-binding receptor
CD169	Macrophages	Sialoadhesin, siglec-1/cell–cell and cell–matrix interactions
CD171	Neurons, Epi (sub), lymphocyte (sub)	Homotypic and heterotypic cell adhesion
CD178	Activated T cells, neutrophils	FasL/cytokine
CD179a	Pro B and early pre B cells	VpreB/surrogate light chain
CD179b	Pro B and early pre B cells	λ5/surrogate light chain
CD184	Wide expression on haemopoietic cells	CXCR4/chemokine receptor/binds to SDF-1
CD233	Erythrocytes	Band 3/anion exchanger and attachment site for cytoskeleton
CD246	Few neural cells, subset of B-cell lymphoma	ALK/tyrosine kinase

ADAM, A disintegrin and metalloprotease; ALK, anaplastic lymphoma kinase; B-CLL, B-chronic lymphocytic leukaemia; c-ALL, common ($CD10^+$) acute lymphoblastic leukaemia; CD, cluster differentiation; C3dR, complement 3d receptor; EBV, Epstein–Barr virus; FcR, immunoglobulin Fc fragment receptor; FDC, follicular dendritic cell; G-CSFR, granulocyte colony-stimulating factor receptor; GM-CSFR, granulocyte–macrophage colony-stimulating factor; GP, glycoprotein; ICAM, intercellular adhesion molecule; IFN, interferon; Ig, immunoglobulin; IL, interleukin; Ki, antibody to CD30; KIR, killer inhibitory receptors; LFA, leucocyte function-associated antigen; LPS, lipopolysaccharide; Mac-I, integrin molecule; MHC, major histocompatibility complex; NK, natural killer; PDGF, platelet-derived growth factor; SRCR, sheep red cell receptor; TGF, transforming growth factor; TNFR, tumour necrosis factor receptor; VLA, very late antigens; w, workshop.

Appendix 2

Normal values

	Males	Females	Males and females
Haemoglobin	13.5–17.5 g/dL	11.5–15.5 g/dL	
Red cells (erythrocytes)	$4.5–6.5 \times 10^{12}$/L	$3.9–5.6 \times 10^{12}$/L	
PCV (haematocrit)	40–52%	36–48%	
MCV			80–95 fL
MCH			27–34 pg
MCHC			20–35 g/dL
White cells (leucocytes)			
total			$4.0–11.0 \times 10^9$/L
neutrophils			$2.5–7.5 \times 10^9$/L
lymphocytes			$1.5–3.5 \times 10^9$/L
monocytes			$0.2–0.8 \times 10^9$/L
eosinophils			$0.04–0.44 \times 10^9$/L
basophils			$0.01–0.1 \times 10^9$/L
Platelets			$150–400 \times 10^9$/L
Red cell mass	30 ± 5 mL/kg	27 ± 5 mL/kg	
Plasma volume	45 ± 5 mL/kg	45 ± 5 mL/kg	
Serum iron			10–30 μmol/L
Total iron-binding capacity			40–75 μmol/L (2.0–4.0 g/L as transferrin)
Serum ferritin*	40–340 μg/L	14–150 μg/L	
Serum vitamin B_{12}*			160–925 ng/L
Serum folate*			3.0–15.0 μg/L
Red cell folate*			160–640 μg/L

* Normal ranges differ with different commercial kits.
MCH, mean corpuscular haemoglobin; MCHC, mean corpuscular haemoglobin concentration; MCV, mean corpuscular volume; PCV, packed cell volume.

Appendix 3

Table 1 Proposed World Health Organization (WHO) classification of myeloid neoplasms.*

Myeloproliferative disease (MPD)
Chronic myelogenous leukaemia, Philadelphia chromosome (Ph1) [t(9;22)(qq34;q11), BCR/ABL] +
Chronic neutrophilic leukaemia
Chronic eosinophilic leukaemia/hypereosinophilic syndrome
Chronic idiopathic myelofibrosis
Polycythaemia vera
Essential thrombocythaemia
Myeloproliferative disease, unclassifiable

Myelodysplastic/myeloproliferative diseases
Chronic myelomonocytic leukaemia (CMML)
Atypical chronic myelogenous leukaemia (aCML)
Juvenile myelomonocytic leukaemia (JMML)

Myelodysplastic syndromes (MDS)
Refractory anaemia (RA)
  with ringed sideroblasts (RARS)
  without ringed sideroblasts
Refractory cytopenia (myelodysplastic syndrome) with multilineage dysplasia (RCMD)
Refractory anaemia (myelodysplastic syndrome) with excess blasts (RAEB)
5q-syndrome
Myelodysplastic syndrome, unclassifiable

Acute myeloid leukaemias (AML)*
Acute myeloid leukaemias with recurrent cytogenetic translocations
  AML with t(8;21)(q22;q22), AML1(CBFα)/ETO
  Acute promyelocytic leukaemia (AML with t(15;17)(q22;q11–12) and variants, PML/RAXα)
  AML with abnormal bone marrow eosinophils (inv(16)(p13q22) or t(16;16)(p13;q11), CBFβ/MYH11X)
  AML with 11q23 (MLL) abnormalities

Acute myeloid leukaemia with multilineage dysplasia
  with prior myelodysplastic syndrome
  without prior myelodysplastic syndrome

Acute myeloid leukaemia and myelodysplastic syndrome, therapy related
  Alkylating agent related
  Epipodophyllotoxin related (some may be lymphoid)
  Other types

(Continued)

Table 1 Proposed World Health Organization (WHO) classification of myeloid neoplasms (*Continued*).*

Acute myeloid leukaemia not otherwise categorized
- AML minimally differentiated
- AML without maturation
- AML with maturation
- Acute myelomonocytic leukaemia
- Acute monocytic leukaemia
- Acute erythroid leukaemia
- Acute megakaryocytic leukaemia
- Acute basophilic leukaemia
- Acute panmyelosis with myelofiborisis

Acute biphenotypic leukaemias

* Only major disease categories are listed.

Table 2 Proposed World Health Organization (WHO) classification of lymphoid neoplasms.*

B-CELL NEOPLASMS

Precursor B-cell neoplasm
- *Precursor B-lymphoblastic leukaemia / lymphoma (precursor B-cell acute lymphoblastic leukaemia)*

Mature (peripheral) B-cell neoplasms**
- *B-cell chronic lymphocytic leukaemia/small lymphocytic lymphoma*
- B-cell prolymphocytic leukaemia
- Lymphoplasmacytic lymphoma
- Splenic marginal zone B-cell lymphoma (+/– villous lymphocytes)
- Hairy cell leukaemia
- *Plasma cell myeloma* / plasmacytoma
- *Extranodal marginal zone B-cell lymphoma of MALT type*
- Nodal marginal zone B-cell lymphoma (+/– monocytoid B cells)
- *Follicular lymphoma*
- *Mantle cell lymphoma*
- *Diffuse large B-cell lymphoma*
- Mediastinal large B-cell lymphoma
- Primary effusion lymphoma
- *Burkitt's lymphoma / Burkitt's cell leukaemia*

T AND NK-CELL NEOPLASMS

Precursor T-cell neoplasm
- *Precursor T-lymphoblastic lymphoma / leukaemia (precursor T-cell acute lymphoblastic leukaemia)*

Mature (peripheral) T-cell neoplasms**
- T-cell prolymphocytic leukaemia
- T-cell granular lymphocytic leukaemia
- Aggressive NK-cell leukaemia
- Adult T-cell lymphoma / leukaemia (HTLV1+)
- Extranodal NK / T-cell lymphoma, nasal type
- Enteropathy-type T-cell lymphoma
- Hepatosplenic $\gamma\delta$ T-cell lymphoma
- Subcutaneous panniculitis-like T-cell lymphoma

(*Continued*)

Table 2 Proposed World Health Organization (WHO) classification of lymphoid neoplasms (*Continued*).*

Mycosis fungoides/Sézary syndrome
Anaplastic large-cell lymphoma, T/null cell, primary cutaneous type
Peripheral T-cell lymphoma, not otherwise characterized
Angioimmunoblastic T-cell lymphoma
Anaplastic large cell lymphoma, T/null cell, primary systemic type

HODGKIN'S LYMPHOMA (HODGKIN'S DISEASE)
Nodular lymphocyte predominance Hodgkin's lymphoma
Classic Hodgkin's lymphoma
Nodular sclerosis Hodgkin's lymphoma (Grades 1 and 2)
Lymphocyte-rich classical Hodgkin's lymphoma
Mixed cellularity Hodgkin's lymphoma
Lymphocyte depletion Hodgkin's lymphoma

* More common entities are in italics.
** B- and T/NK-cell neoplasms are grouped according to major clinical presentations (predominantly disseminated/leukaemic, primary extranodal, predominantly nodal).

Table 3 Mast cell diseases.

Cutaneous mastocytosis
Systematic mast cell disease (+/− skin involvement)
Systematic mast cell disease with associated haematological disorder (+/− skin involvement)
Mast cell leukaemia/sarcoma

Table 4 Histiocytic and dendritic-cell neoplasms.

Macrophage/histiocytic neoplasm
Histiocytic sarcoma

Dendritic-cell neoplasms
Langerhans cell histiocytosis
Langerhans cell sarcoma
Interdigitating dendritic cell sarcoma/tumour
Follicular dendritic cell sarcoma/tumour
Dendritic cell sarcoma, not otherwise specified (NOS)

Table 5 Plasma cell disorders: subtypes and variants.

Monoclonal gammopathy of undetermined significance (MGUS)
Plasma cell myeloma variants:
Indolent myeloma
Smoldering myeloma
Osteosclerotic myeloma (POEMS syndrome)
Plasma cell leukaemia
Non-secretory myeloma

Plasmacytoma variants:
Solitary plasmacytoma of bone
Extramedullary plasmacytoma

Table 6 Immunosecretory disorders (clinical manifestations of diverse lymphoid neoplasms).

Clinical syndrome	Underlying neoplasm
Waldenström's macroglobulinemia	Lymphoplasmacytic lymphoma
Heavy chain diseases (HCD):	
γ HCD	Lymphoplasmacytic lymphoma
α HCD	Extranodal marginal zone lymphoma (immunoproliferative small intestinal disorder)
μ HCD	B-cell chronic lymphocytic leukaemia
Immunoglobulin deposition diseases:	
Systemic light chain disease	Plasma cell myeloma, monoclonal gammopathy
Primary amyloidosis	Plasma cell myeloma, monoclonal gammopathy

Index

Note: Page numbers in *italic* refer to figures and tables

www.blackwellhematology.com

www.blackwellhematology.com